TEXTBOOK OF
COMPLETE DENTURE PROSTHODONTICS

TEXTBOOK OF
COMPLETE DENTURE
PROSTHODONTICS

Binu George BDS, MDS
Assistant Professor
Department of Prosthodontics
Sree Mookambika Institute of Dental Sciences
Kulasekharam, Tamil Nadu

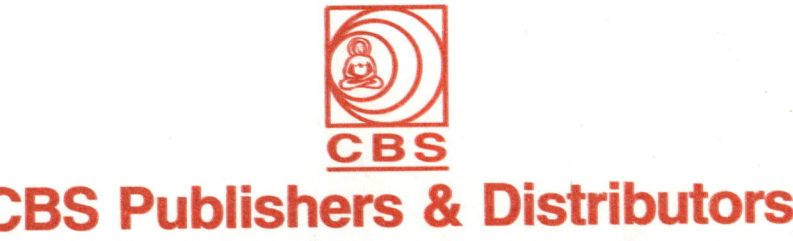

CBS Publishers & Distributors
New Delhi • Bangalore

Textbook of Complete Denture Prosthodontics

ISBN : 81-239-1333-8

First Edition : 2006
Reprint : 2008

Publishing Director : Vinod K. Jain

Published by :
Satish Kumar Jain for CBS Publishers & Distributors,
4819/X1, 24 Ansari Road, Darya Ganj, New Delhi - 110 002
E-mail : cbspubs@vsnl.com • Website : www.cbspd.com

Branch Office :
2975, 17th Cross, K.R. Road,
Bansankari 2nd Stage, Banglore - 560 070
Fax : 080-26771680 • E-mail : cbsbng@vsnl.net

Printed at : Swastik Packagings, Delhi - 110092

to
the everloving memory of
my mother, the late Mrs. Ponnamma George

List of Contributors

Dr. Saira Joseph BDS, MDS
Assistant Professor
Department of Prosthodontics
Sree Mookambika Institute of Dental Sciences
Kulasekharam, Tamil Nadu

Dr. Abdul Khader BDS, MDS
Senior Lecturer
Department of Prosthodontics
Royal Dental College
Trichur, Kerala

Dr. Anand KS BDS, MDS
Assistant Professor
Department of Prosthodontics
Sri Sidharatha Dental College,
Thumkur, Karnataka

Dr. Anoop M Azad
Former Assistant Professor
Department of Prosthodontics
B.P. Koirala Dental College
Nepal

Dr. J Srinivas Kumar BDS, MDS
Department of Prosthodontics
Government Dental College
Trivandrum, Kerala

Dr. Vinod Krishnan BDS, MDS
Assistant Professor
Department of Orthodontics
Sree Mookambika Institute of Dental Sciences
Kulasekharam, Tamil Nadu

Dr. Arun Sadasivan BDS, MDS
Assistant Professor
Department of Periodontics
Sree Mookambika Institute of Dental Sciences
Kulasekharam, Tamil Nadu

Dr. James Rex
Lecturer
Department of Prosthodontics
Sree Mookambika Institute of Dental Sciences
Kulasekharam, Tamil Nadu

Preface

Prosthodontics is a rapidly evolving branch of dentistry. Advancements have been made in every respect of prosthodontics. In preparing the first edition of this textbook, I have attempted to encompass all the various aspects of complete denture prosthodontics. Accordingly, I have arranged the chapters in such a manner that there is a certain continuity throughout the text. Chapter 1 deals with the branches of prosthodontics and also includes important historical aspects of prosthodontics. Chapter 2 covers all relevant details related to the evaluation of the patient and treatment planning. Chapter 6 entitled 'objectives of impression making' discusses retention, stability, support and esthetics in detail. Chapter 7 on 'complete denture impressions' includes routine impression procedures as well as impression procedures for medically compromised patients. Chapter 9 on 'posterior palatal seal' covers the anatomy, physiology, functions and also includes techniques for recording the same. Chapters 11, 12 and 13 deal with the various aspects of jaw relation. Chapter 17 includes a brief history and all relevant classifications of the 'articulators'. Chapter 25 on 'masticatory ability' describes in detail the factors important in mastication and the methods for evaluating masticatory efficiency. Chapter 30 entitled 'geriatric considerations in prosthetic dentistry' comprehensively covers the theories of aging, hard and soft tissue changes associated with aging, and the treatment methodology for senile patients. Chapter 32 entitled 'dental implants for the edentulous patient' includes a brief history, a note about biomaterials used, the type of restorations and advancements in dental implantology. In addition to these chapters, I have included chapters on gag reflex, dentogenic concept, pharmacotherapeutics, and failures and complications in complete dentures—the topics that are important to both the prosthodontist and the general dentist.

As this is the first edition of the book and my first venture, shortcomings may be present. I would be grateful if the readers send me their suggestions and comments at my e-mail address: binugeorge@hotmail.com

Dr. Binu George

Acknowledgements

I would like to thank all my teachers who guided me through my teething days in dentistry, especially Dr. Sudhakar Bhat and Dr. Prathyheek Shetty, Professors in Prosthodontics at CODS, KMC, Mangalore, and Dr. Mohan Baliga, Professor of Oral and Maxillofacial Surgery at CODS, KMC, Mangalore. I would also like to thank my wife Dr. Saira Joseph for all the help and support she gave me. Credit is also due to my brother, Mr. Anil George, who helped in correcting the manuscript and in designing the format. Last, but not the least, I would like to thank the publishers, CBS Publishers & Distributors, for their willingness and cooperation in bringing out this book.

Dr. Binu George

Contents

TEXTBOOK OF
COMPLETE DENTURE
PROSTHODONTICS

1

INTRODUCTION TO PROSTHODONTICS

Objectives of Prosthodontic Treatment

- Preservation of remaining oral structures
- Promotion of health
- Restoration of function and esthetics.

INTRODUCTION

The term **prosthodontics** has been derived from Latin (*pros*—replacement, *dons*—teeth, *ics* science). It is essentially the branch of dentistry dealing with the replacement of missing teeth and other oral structures with artificial substitutes. The **Glossary of Prosthodontic Terms (GPT-7)** has defined prosthodontics as the art and science that deals with the replacement of missing hard and soft tissue with artificial substitutes that may or may not be removed by the patient. **Boucher's clinical dental terminology** has defined prosthodontics as that branch of dentistry pertaining to the restoration and maintenance of oral function, comfort, appearance and health of the patient by the replacement of missing teeth, and contiguous oral and maxillofacial tissues with artificial substitutes.

Prosthetics. The art and science of replacing lost and damaged parts of the human body with artificial substitutes.

BRANCHES OF PROSTHODONTICS

Prosthodontics is broadly categorised as given

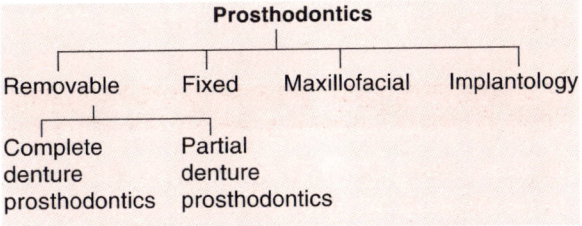

Removable Prosthodontics. It is the branch of prosthodontics dealing with the replacement of missing teeth by artificial substitutes that may be removed by the patient

Complete Denture Prosthodontics. That body of knowledge and skills pertaining to the restoration of the edentulous arch with a removable prosthesis.

Removable Partial Denture. Any prosthesis that replaces some teeth in a partially dentate arch. It can be removed from the mouth and replaced at will.

Fixed Prosthodontics. The branch of prosthodontics concerned with the replacement and/or restoration of teeth by artificial substitutes that are not readily removed from the mouth.

Maxillofacial Prosthetics. That branch of prosthodontics concerned with the restoration and/or replacement of the stomatognathic system and craniofacial structures with prosthesis that may or may not be removed on a regular or elective basis.

Implant Prosthodontics. The phase of prosthodontics concerning the replacement of missing teeth and/or associated structures by restorations that are attached to dental implants.

Prosthodontist. A dentist who has successfully completed an advanced education program in prosthodontics that is accredited by the appropriate accrediting body.

A **prosthesis** is defined as the replacement of an absent part of the human body by some artificial part, e.g. an eye prosthesis.

HISTORICAL REVIEW

The first attempts to replace teeth were by wax, skin of flax (Fig. 1.1) or suitably shaped bone. The earliest prosthesis to replace teeth dated to the third millennium before Christ (Fig. 1.2). This consisted of natural teeth attached to gold wires.

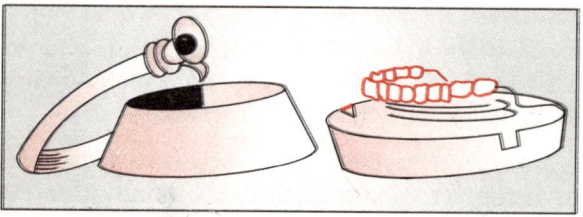

Fig. 1.1. Denture flasks.

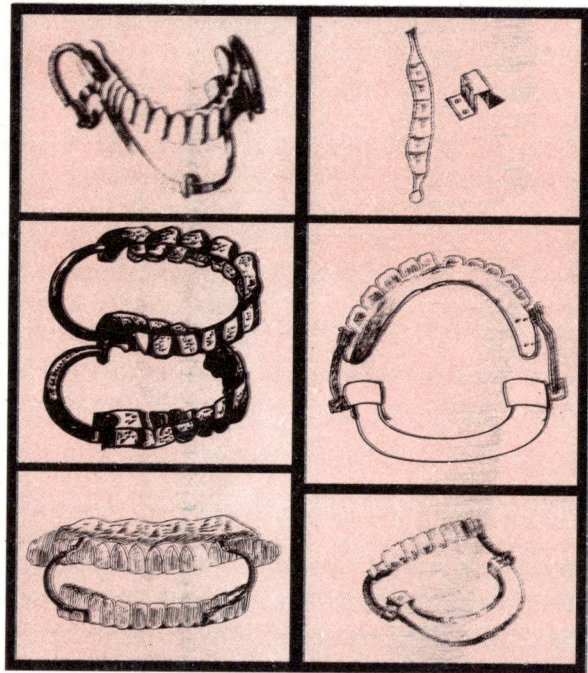

Fig. 1.2. Some of the earlier prosthesis.

References to this prosthesis were included in the work by Hippocrates and soon became a component part of Greek and Roman literature. In the early days prosthesis carved from bone were used by many including the Arabs.

Ambroise Pare, the famous French surgeon of the sixteenth century, described various. Prosthesis for closing defects of the hard palate. These included the button obturator. **Pierre Fouchard (1678-1761)** who is generally referred to as the father of modern dentistry described advanced prosthesis in his 18th century **Le Chirurgien Dentiste.** He described a prosthesis for replacing maxillary teeth and which was retained by spiral springs attached to a lower double bar which rested on natural posterior teeth.

In 1746, Mouton of Paris described the first gold crown. Philip Phaff of Berlin was the first with a maxillary impression from the jaw and a plaster casting made from it for prosthetic purposes. Bourdet of Paris was the first to try a gold base.

In 1757 **Bourdet** suggested the use of silk ligatures attached to natural teeth to retain extracted teeth. Philip Phaff advocated the use of plaster of Paris for making impressions.

The materials for making teeth included bones, ivory tusks from hippopotamus and walruses, human teeth from corpses and gold. Human teeth were found to be costly. Animal teeth were unstable towards corrosive agents in saliva and elephant ivory and bone contained pores that were easily stained. Mineral teeth or porcelain teeth greatly accelerated the end to the practice of transplanting freshly extracted human teeth.

After decades of effort, the Europeans mastered the production of fine translucent porcelains comparable to porcelains of the Chinese (by the 1720's). The use of feldspar to replace lime as a flux and high firing temperatures were both critical developments in fine European porcelain. In approximately 1774, a Parisian apothecary **Alexis Duchateau** with the assistance of a Parisian dentist Nicholas Dubois Dechemant (Fig. 1.3) made the first successful porcelain dentures at the Guerhard porcelain factory replacing the stained and malodorous ivory prosthesis of Duchateau. Dubosis Dechemant continually improved his porcelain formulations and received French and British patents. Nicholas Chemant characterized the dentures as *incorruptibles et sans odeur* (imperishable and odorless) later the descriptive toward incorruptibles became the term for the porcelain denture. **Jacques Gardette (1778)** developed the first adhering upper prosthesis by accident (Fig. 1.4). He had placed an upper prosthesis from the enamel of hippopotamus teeth into the maxilla of a female patient without springs. He found out later that the prosthesis was well retained without springs.

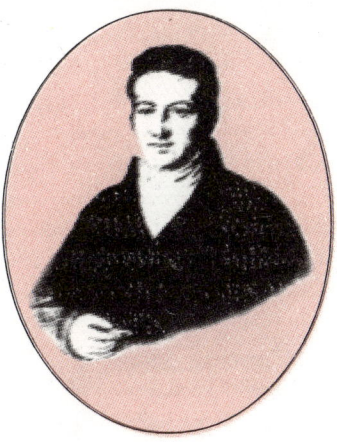

Fig. 1.4. Jaques Gardette.

In 1789 John Greenwood (Fig. 1.5), George Washington's dentist, carved a denture from hippopotamus bone and fitted it with 8 human teeth. Samuel Stockton White, in the later part of the nineteenth century introduced the SS White company. This company developed many tooth forms. (Stockton also introduced Dental Cosmos, a dental Journal).

In 1808 individually formed porcelain teeth that contained embedded platinum hooks were introduced in Paris by **Giuseppangelo Fonzi** (Fig. 1.6). These were called dents terro metalliques. The firing of porcelain teeth crossed the oceans into North America in 1817 through Antoine Plantou (who emigrated from Paris).

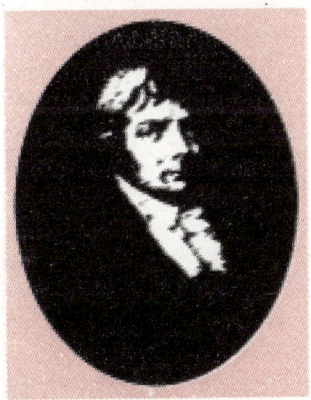

Fig. 1.3. Dubois Dechemant.

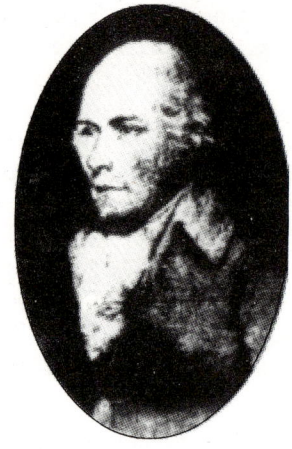

Fig. 1.5. John Greenwood.

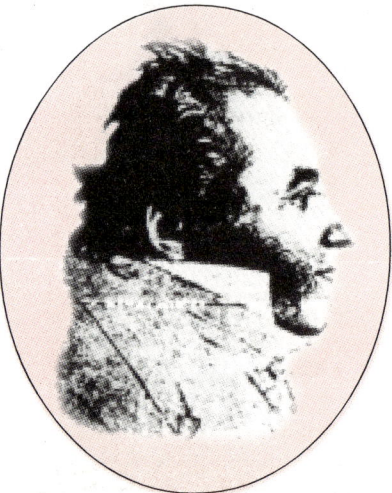

Fig. 1.6. Giuseppangelo Fonzi.

and production of mineral teeth was more accelerated in the United States of America than in Europe as the Americans were not influenced by traditions and theories as the Europeans, and were not under guild restrictions).

In 1820 Edward Hudson in Philadelphia was the first to cast the base of a prosthesis from tin, because of its weight it was suitable for only lower dentures. Even then the enamel from hippopotamus tusks remained the preferred material for bases.

Claudius Ash, who industrialized the dental kilns operated in London by other French immigrants was initially a goldsmith (Fig. 1.7). He was the founder of Ash Sons and Co which produced high quality teeth in 1837. In 1840, the same company introduced tube teeth, a type with central canal which was rivetted to a metal base with a post. This company had a monopoly for the rest of the nineteenth century.

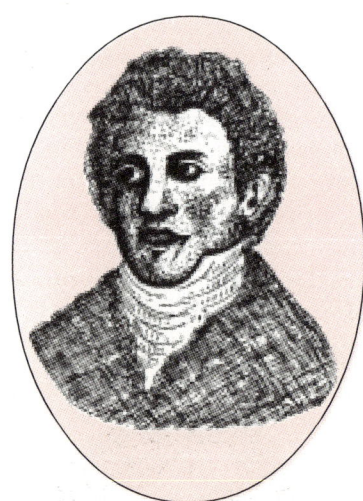

Fig. 1.7. Claudius Ash.

Delabarre in 1820 wrote a two-volume work on mechanical dentistry. He introduced a new concept for retaining obturators (using metal bands.) He reflected on times when war yielded their harvests, and the most beautiful teeth were to be had, healthy and beautiful for those lost by so many persons. In peace time supernumerary teeth or teeth from graves or cemeteries were used. In wars, like the Crimean war (1853-1856) teeth were harvested by the "hyenas of the battlefield". (The development

In 1840 Daniel T. Evan's articulator (Fig. 1.8) was patented and provided for lateral and forward movements.

In 1840 James Cameron, a dentist in Philadelphia patented a new and improved instrument for adjusting artificial teeth with

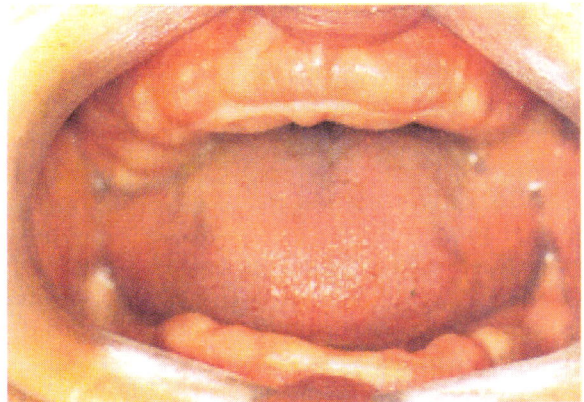

A. Maxillary and mandibular ridges

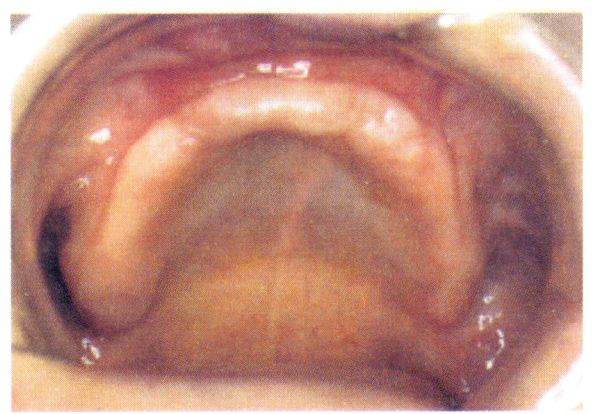

B. Flabby anterior ridge

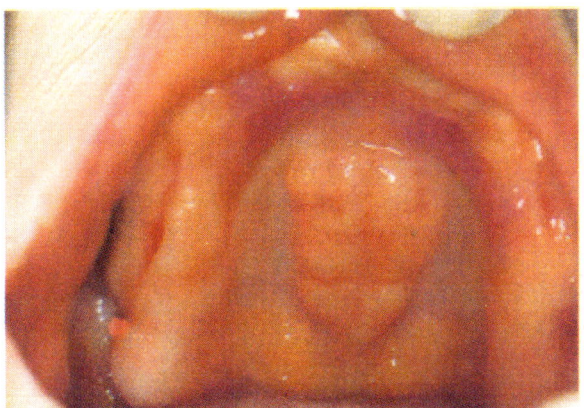

C. Torus palatinus

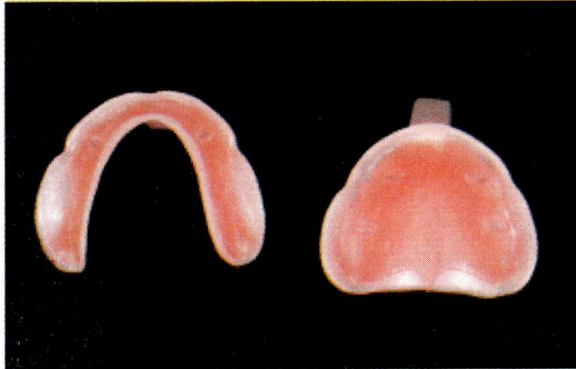

D. Acrylic special trays with wax spacer

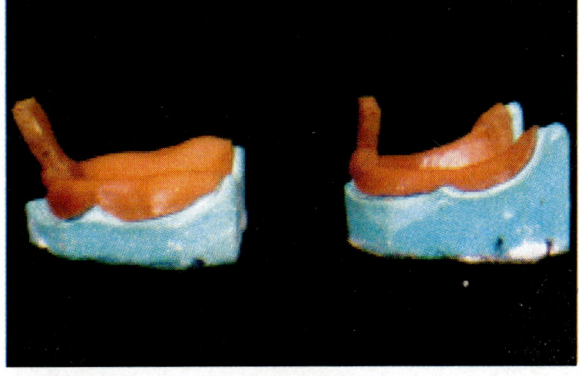

E. Special trays in shellac (Note the angulation of the handle for upper and lower trays)

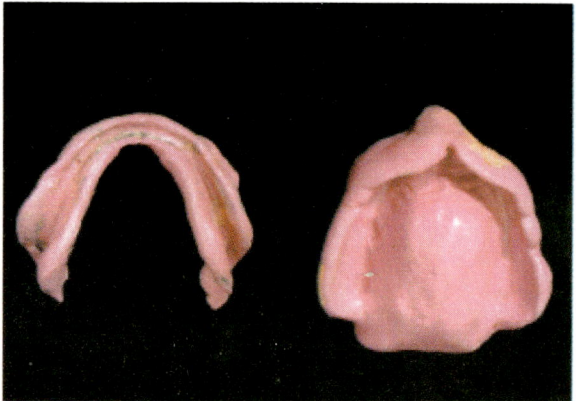

A. Secondary impression in addition silicone

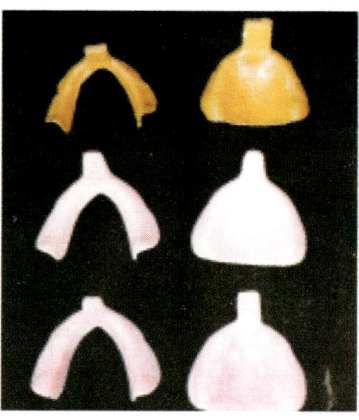

B. Special trays (in shellac, cold cure acrylic and heat cure acrylic)

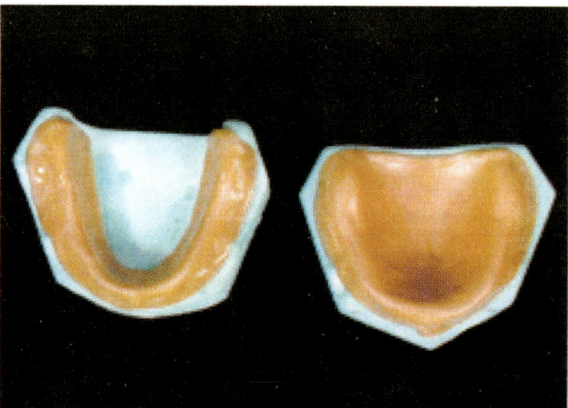

C. Temporary record base in shellac base plate

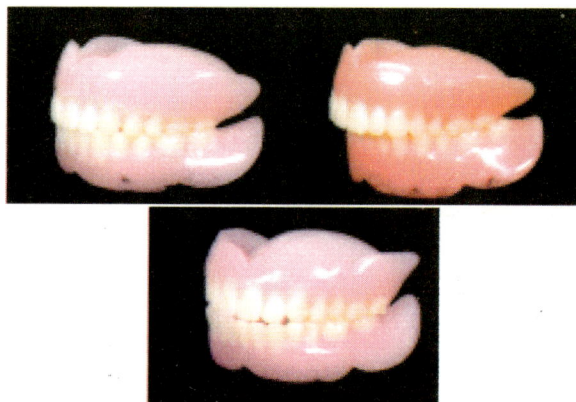

D. Class I, Class II and Class III dentures

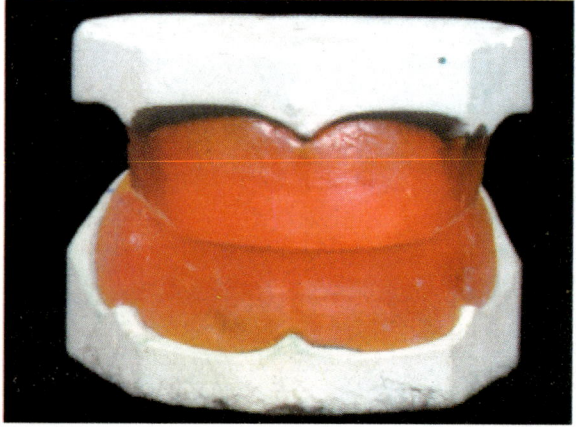

E & F. Maxillary and mandibular occlusal rim (frontal and profile view)

CASE 1

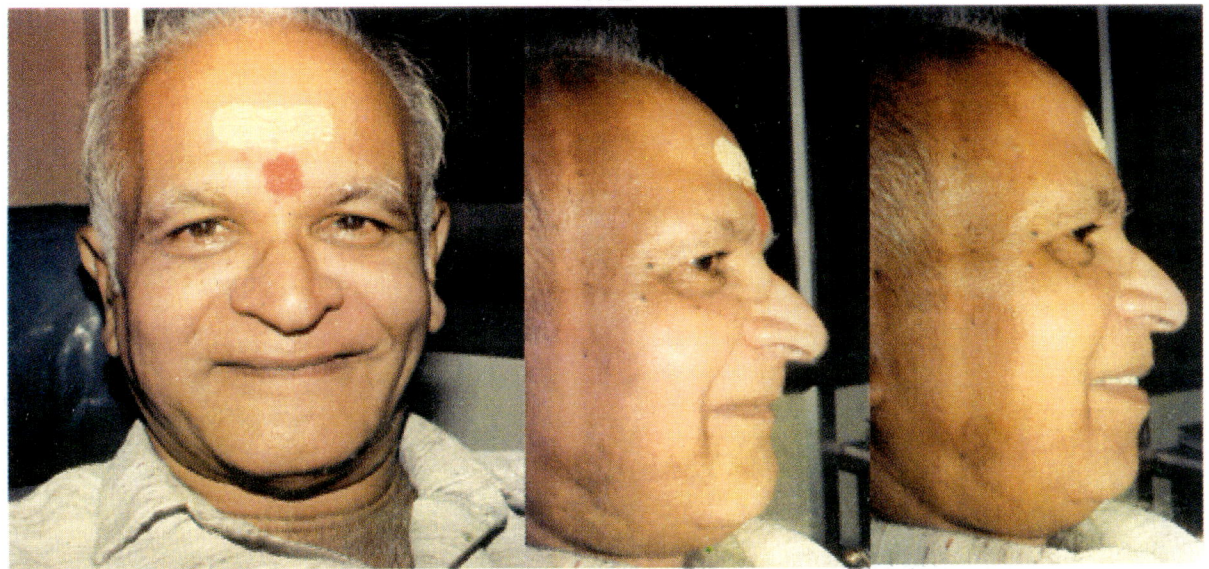

A. Preoperative view

B & C. Profile view: Without dentures, With dentures

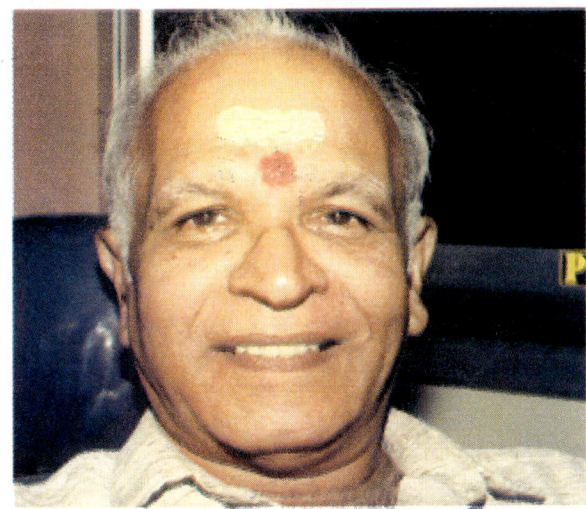

D. Post-insertion view

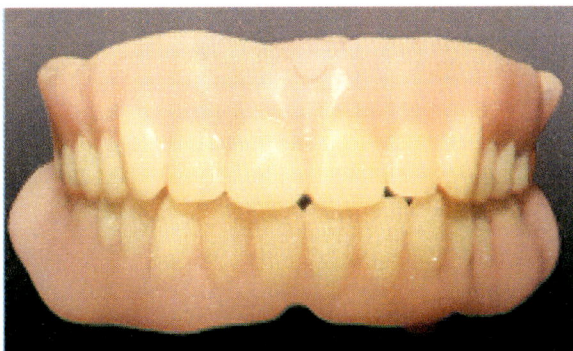

E. The prosthesis

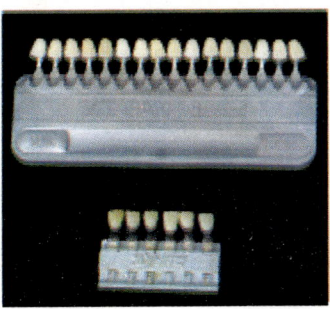

F. Porcelain and
acrylic shade
guides

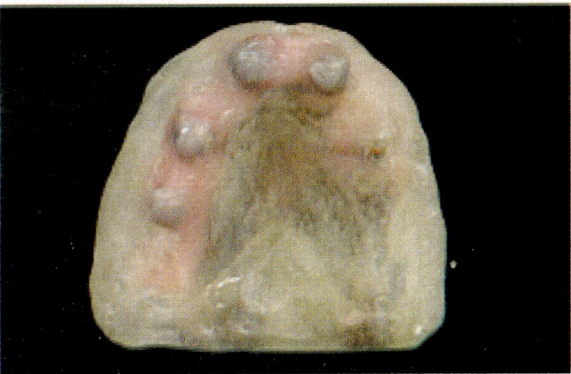

G. Template with ball bearings (to detect the magnification of the radiograph)

CASE 2

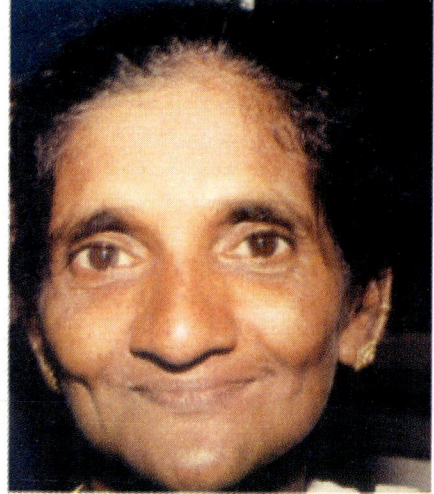

A. Preoperative view

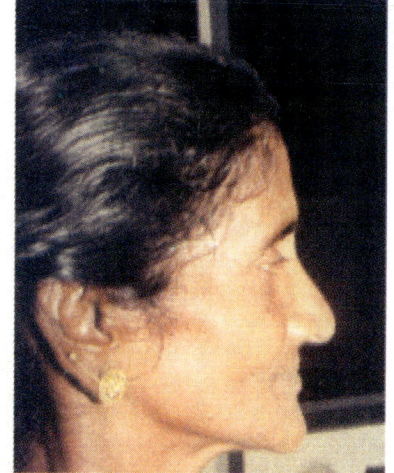

B. Profile view: Without dentures.

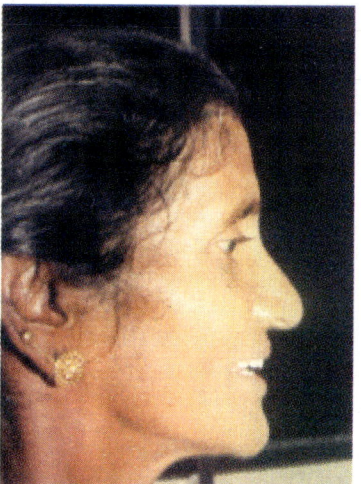

C. Profile view: With dentures

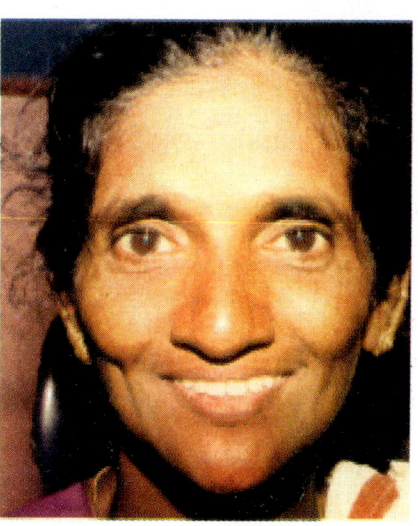

D. Post-insertion view

CASE 3

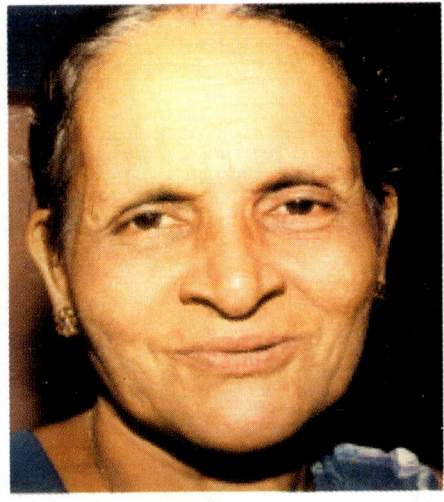

A. Preoperative view

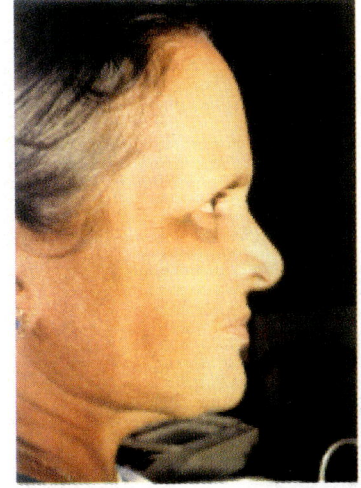

B. Profile view: without dentures

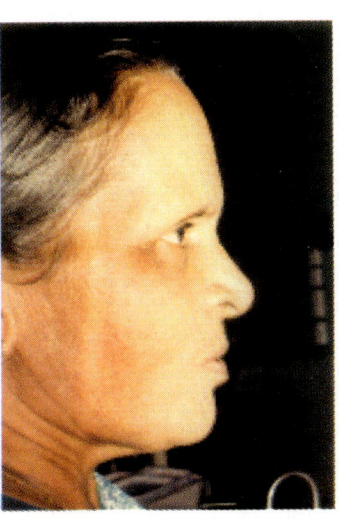

C. Profile view: with dentures

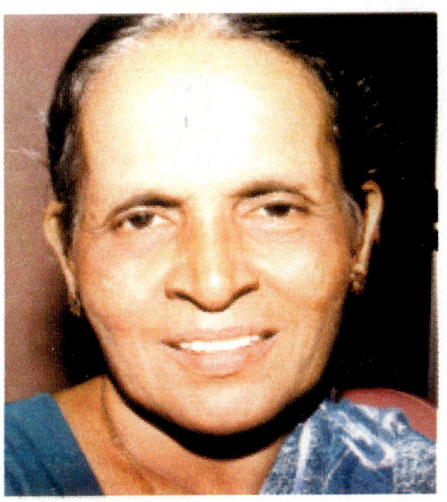

D. Post-insertion (frontal view)

CASE 4

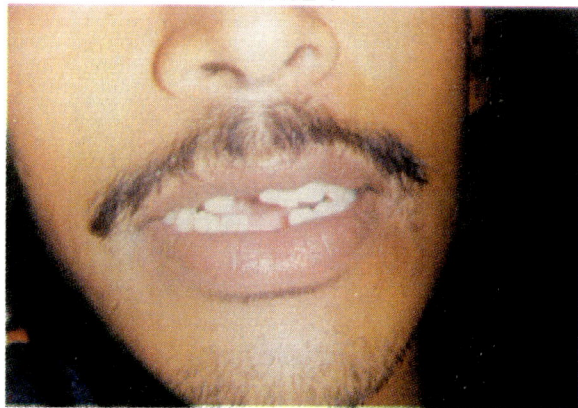

A. Preoperative view

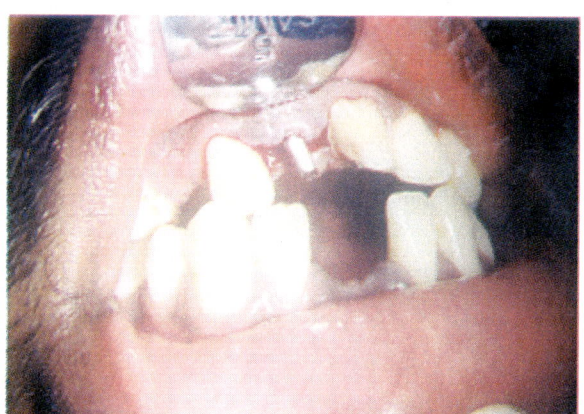

B. Preoperative view

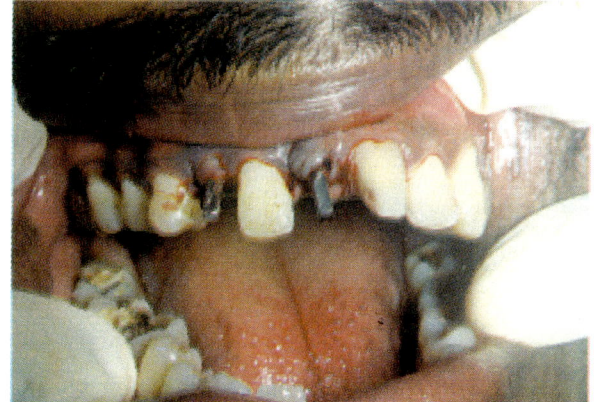

C. Preoperative view

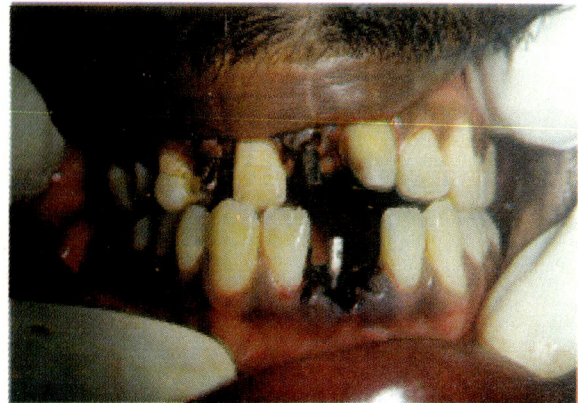

D. Implants placed in $\frac{31|}{|1}$ region

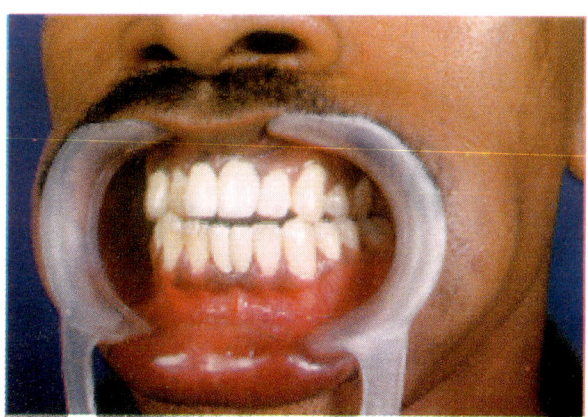

E. Postoperative view

CASE 5

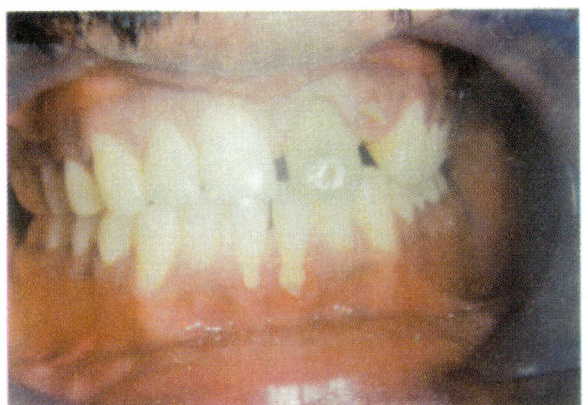

A. Preoperative view (with $\frac{|1}{}$ root stamp in $\frac{|2}{}$ region and periapically involved

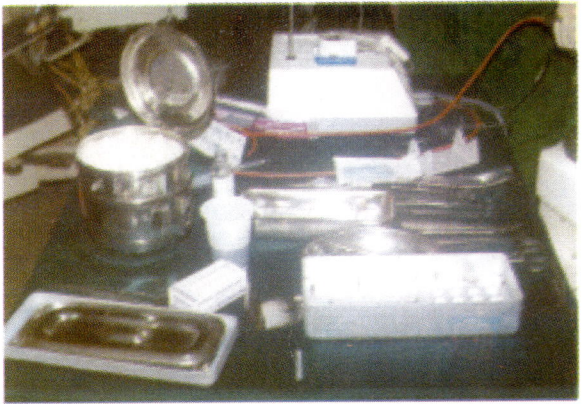

B. Armamentarium (including physiodispenser)

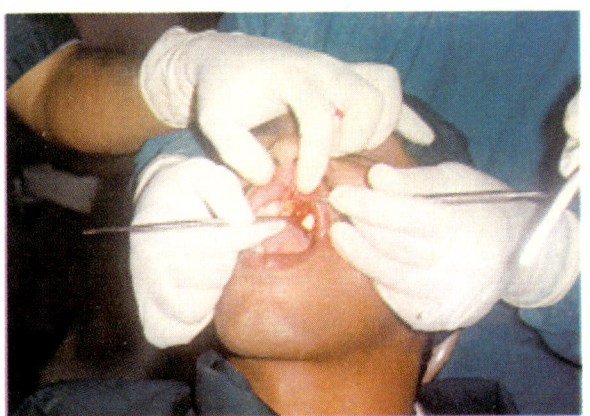

C. Elevation of mucoperiosteal flap

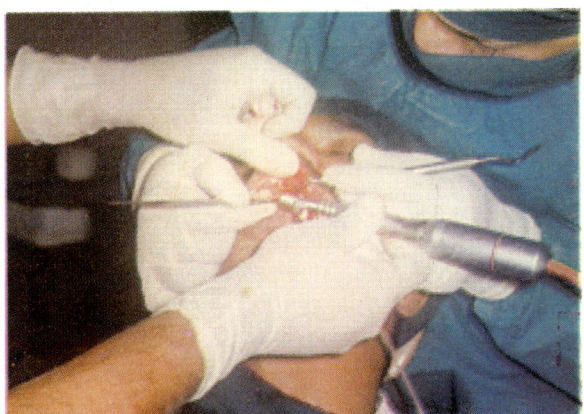

D. Use of round bur for initial entry into bone

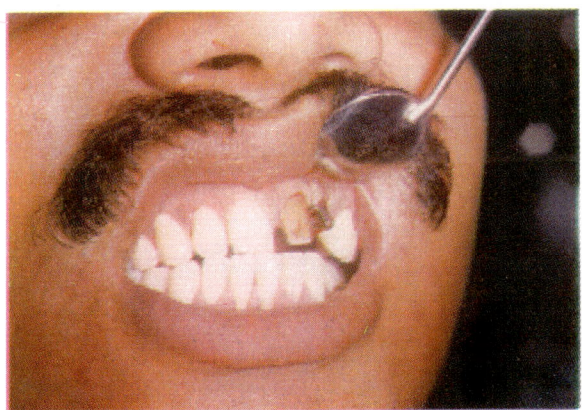

E. Implant placed in $\frac{|2}{}$ region

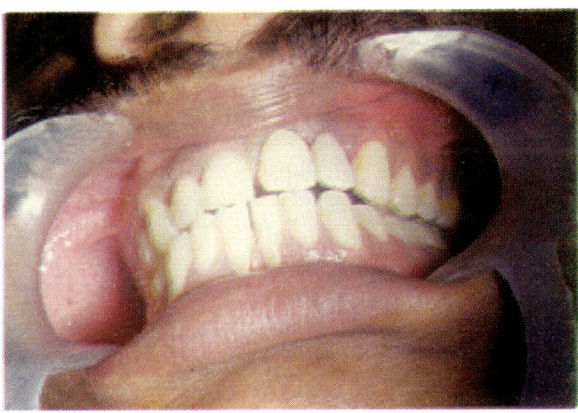

F. Postoperative view

CASE 6

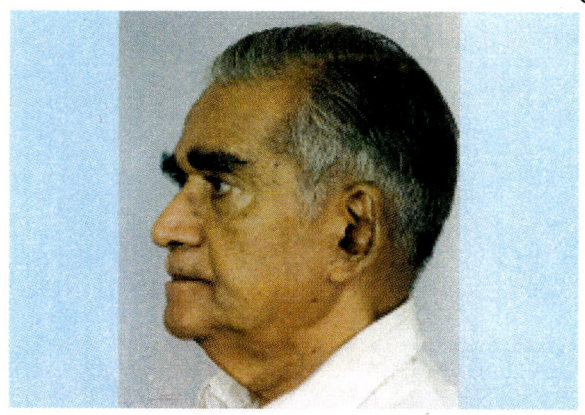

A. Preoperative view

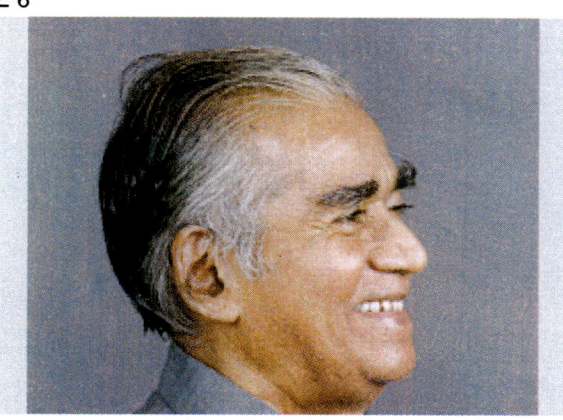

B. Postoperative view

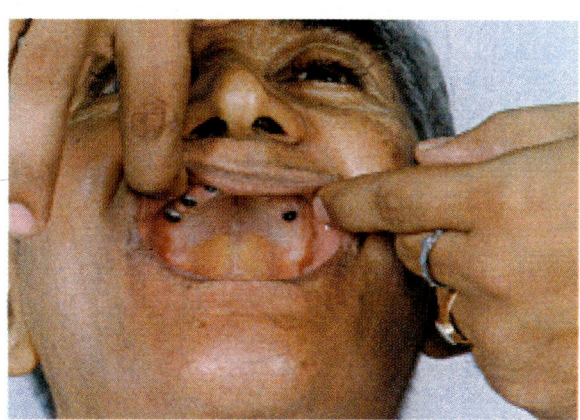

C. Cover screw has been exposed

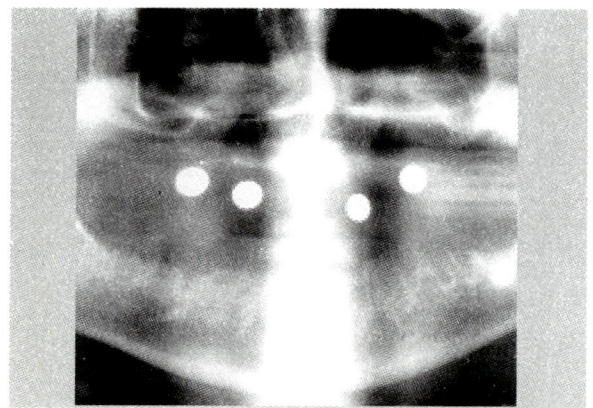

D. Radiograph taken after placing template with ball bearings (to determine amount of distortion)

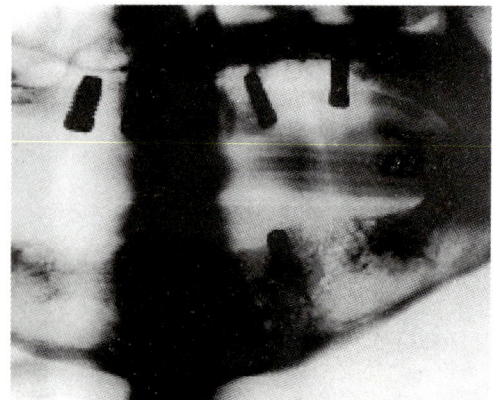

E. Radiograph taken after implant placement

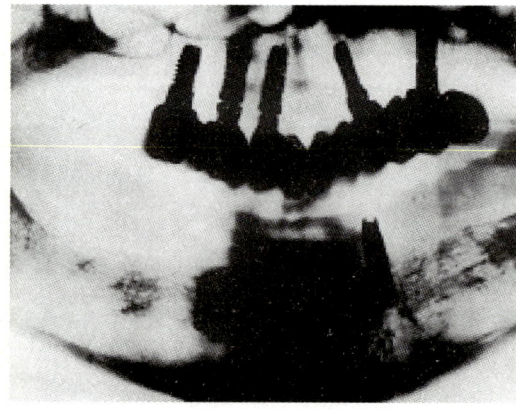

F. Radiograph of final prosthesis

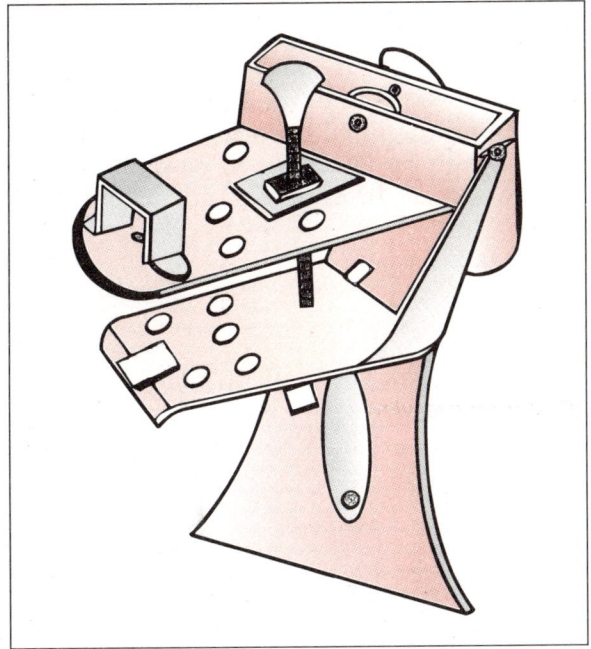

Fig. 1.8. Evan's articulator.

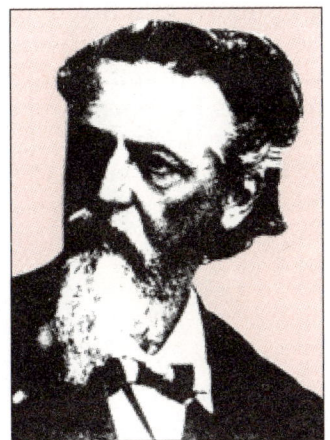

Fig. 1.9. William Bonwill.

which models were fastened in place on a support.

In 1848 Antoine Delabarre, the son of the reputed Parisian dentist recommended the use of gutta-percha for the bases of prosthesis.

In 1851 the American, Charles Goodyear succeeded in hardening resin from the rubber tree. This was first used in dentures by Thomas W Evans. The first articulator founded on geometrical, mathematical and mechanical laws was presented in 1864 by W G Bonwill (Fig. 1.9).

In 1866, Balkwall, a British dentist published his findings on articulation.

In 1886 Land introduced the first fused felds pathic porcelain inlays and crowns.

In 1889, Charles Elmer Luce in Boston investigated the physiology of the temporo-mandibular joint (TMJ) with the help of photography.

In 1890, the curve of occlusion or compensation was introduced by Graf Von Spee

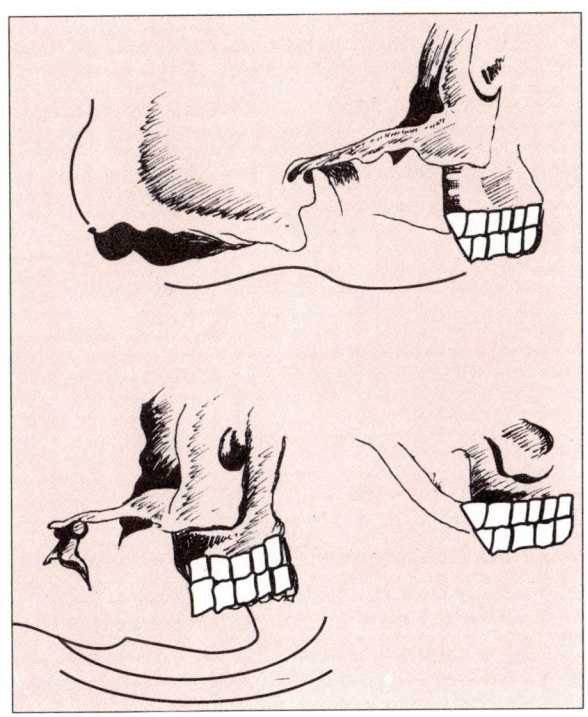

Fig. 1.10. The curve of spee.

and became an important part in artificial tooth se up (Fig. 1.10).

In 1908, Sir Norman G Bennett introduced the concept of Bennett movement. In 1924, the Vienna physician, Alphonse Poller introduced an impression material that remained plastic even after setting. It was agar-agar. The first methacrylate dental preparation in England appeared in 1935 as Kallodent and in 1936, the Kulzer Company in Frankfurt and Main brought out its own patented thermoplastic paladon, which could be polymerized by liquid monomer and powder polymers in offices.

In 1940, methylmethacrylate (MMA) was introduced and it soon replaced vulcanite as the principal denture base material because of its improved esthetic qualities and ease of manipulation. Elastic impression materials were developed from synthetic rubber by S L Pearson of the University of Liverpool in 1955.

MULTIPLE CHOICE QUESTIONS

1. **"Dents terro metalliques" refers to**
   a. Porcelain dentures
   b. Porcelain teeth with platinum hooks
   c. Natural teeth attached with silk ligatures
   d. None of the above

2. **The first successful porcelain dentures were made by**
   a. Ambroise Pare
   b. Guiseppangelo Fonzi and Delabarre
   c. Duchateau and D Chemant
   d. John Greenwood

3. **In 1808 _____ published a method for the manufacture of individual teeth with platinum hooks fired into them**
   a. J.C.F. Maury
   b. Fonzi
   c. J. Gardette
   d. None of the above

4. **S.S white is credited with**
   a. Developing tube teeth
   b. Introducing the Dental news letter that gave rise to Dental Cosmos
   c. Being George Washington's dentist
   d. Introducing gold clasps

5. **The "tube teeth" were introduced by**
   a. S.S. White
   b. Claudius Ash
   c. Gardette
   d. Gysi

6. **In _____, F.A. Wienand founded the first continental dental manufactory capable of offering commercial products**
   a. 1893   b. 1911
   c. 1908   d. 1907

7. **The typal form theory was introduced by**
   a. Gysi   b. Leon Williams
   c. Ash   d. T.W. Evans

8. **_____ investigated physiology of the TMJ with the help of photography**
   a. Spee   b. Luce   c. Balkwill   d. Bonwill

FAQs

1. **Define prosthodontics. What are its objectives ?**
2. **Branches of prosthodontics. Define.**
3. **Difference between a prosthesis and appliance.**

PATIENT EVALUATION AND TREATMENT PLANNING

There are a number of questionnaires available like the Cornell medical index (CMI), and the Minnesota multiphasic personality inventory. In prosthodontics the questionnaire used should help in building a healthy patient-physician relationship.

INTRODUCTION

For any disease or condition to be treated, it is very important to know the background and forms of the disease itself, so that it can be identified in the various patterns that it presents, and the necessary treatment be instituted. So, an accurate diagnosis is important.

In the complete denture patient, although the nature of the disease, the edentulism is the same, diagnosis is an entirely different process. It involves an evaluation of all pathologic and non-pathologic conditions. Many pertinent findings may remain elusive until the treatment nears completion. So, the treatment must be modified accordingly. Treatment planning is a consideration of all the diagnostic findings, (systemic and local) which may have an influence on the various phases of complete denture therapy.

CASE HISTORY CHART

1. Patient Data

Name   :
Age   :
Sex   :
Occupation   :

Chief Complaint :
History of
  Present Illness :

Medical History :
Systemic
  Examination   :
Personal History :
Cosmetic Index : Class I Class II Class III
Personality:

a. According to House
b. According to Blum

Medical History

General health   :

Pathology   :

Denture History :
Expectations
Years Edentulous   Maxillary
                          Mandibular

Previous Dentures
                          Maxillary
                          Mandibular

Existing or Current Dentures

Denture success
Pre-extraction Records

2. Physical Characteristics

Neuromuscular skills as evidenced by
a. Speech   Good   Fair   Poor
b. Coordination   Good   Fair   Poor

c. Posture and Walking pattern
d. Built and Nourishment

3. Clinical Evaluation

a. Facial Form (Williams)
b. Facial profile   Class I Class II Class III
c. Facial expression
d. Complexion
e. Hair
f. Eyes
g. Skin texture
   Others

h. Wrinkles   Due to age
                 Loss of vertical dimension
i. Vermillion Border

j. Lip
   Contour   -
   Mobility   Class I   Class II   Class III
   Length

k. Muscle Tone   Class I Class II Class III
l. Muscle
   Development   Class I Class II Class III
m.   Muscles of
   mastication   Class I Class II Class III

n. Temporomandibular Joint:
   Crepitus   Locking
   Clicking   Deviation
   Pain

o. Salivary Glands
p. Mandibular Movement
   a. Protrusive
   b. Right lateral
   c. Left lateral

Intraoral Examination

a. Arch size   Class I Class II Class III
b. Arch form
c. Ridge form
   Maxillary   Class I Class II Class III
   Mandibular   Class I Class II Class III

d. Height of residual ridge
   Maxillary   Class I Class II Class III
   Mandibular   Class I Class II Class III

e. Bony undercuts Class I Class II Class III
f. Tori   Class I Class II Class III
g. Interarch space Class I Class II Class III
h. Ridge
   Parallelism   Class I Class II Class III
i. Ridge Relation   Class I Class II Class III

j. Bone Quantity   Class A Class B Class C
   (See Fig. 2.17) Class D Class E
k. Bone Quality   Class I Class II
   (See Fig. 2.18) Class II Class IV

l. Lateral Throat
Form   Class I Class II Class III

m. Palatal Throat
Form   Class I Class II Class III

n. Palatal
Sensitivity   Class I Class II Class III

o. Shape of the
Hard Palate   Class I Class II Class III

p. Mucosa
Thickness   Class I Class II Class III

q. Mucosa
condition   Class I Class II Class III

r. Border
Attachments   Class I Class II Class III

s. Frenal
Attachment   Class I Class II Class III

t. Saliva   Class I Class II Class III

u. Tongue
    a. Size   Class I Class II Class III
    b. Position   Class I Class II Class III
    c. Shape

Existing Dentures

- Anterior Tooth Shade, Mold, Material
- Posterior Tooth Shade, Mold, Material
- Esthetics, phonetics, retention, stability, extensions, contours
- Centric relation and vertical dimension of occlusion
- Occlusal plane orientation
- Palate
- Post-dam
- Base adaptation
- Midline
- Buccal vestibule
- Cross bite
- Characterization
- Comfort
- Hygiene
- Wear

Radiographic Evaluation

Treatment Planning

CASE HISTORY

Patient Data

1. Name. Helps in the identification of the patient. It also aids in the development of a rapport between the dentist and patient. For example, Hello Mrs. Elizabeth is better than Hello madam.

2. Age. Age of the patient is very important while recording the history. As age advances, problems can be anticipated with: (i) adaptation to dentures, (ii) coordination, (iii) bone resorption, (iv) tissue sensitivity, (v) healing, and (vi) balanced nutrition.

3. Sex. In general, women are more difficult to please with the appearance of their dentures than men. Women during menopause can be difficult to treat due to psychologic problems, dry mouth, burning sensation in the mouth, and general vague pain.

4. Occupation and Social Position. The patient's occupation can give the dentist an indication of what he expects from his dentures. For example, tooth position is very important for a musician who plays a wind instrument.

5. Chief Complaint. The chief complaint should be written in the patient's own words. According to DeVan, the dentist should meet the mind of the patient before he meets the mouth of the patient. The patient should be questioned regarding his chief complaint. The patient's response will also allow the practitioner to assess whether the patient's expectations are realistic and attainable. The patient's psychological classification can also be determined.

6. Class I Cosmetic Index. High cosmetic index. The patients are often well dressed and are appreciative and cooperative.

Class III Low cosmetic index. Patients are often indifferent, uncooperative and place little value in the effort's of the prosthodontist.

House Classification (Sharry)

This classification was introduced by House in 1937.[1]

Philosophical Mind

- Those of a well-balanced mental type who have come previous to extraction. They have had no experience wearing artificial dentures and are dependent on the dentist for proper diagnosis, prognosis and education.
- Those who have worn satisfactory dentures, are in good health and are of the well-balanced type who may be in need of future service.

Exacting Type

- Those patients while suffering ill health and are seriously concerned about the appearance and efficiency of artificial dentures. They are willing to accept the advice of their physician and dentist, and are unwilling to submit to removal of their natural teeth.
- Those patients wearing artificial dentures, unsatisfactory in appearance and usefulness, and who doubt the ability of the dentist to render a service that will be satisfactory. They often insist on a written guarantee or expect the dentist to make repeated attempts at additional fee.

Hysterical Mind

- Those in bad health with long neglected pathological mouth conditions who dread dental service and submit to removal of teeth as a last resort. They are positive in their own minds that they can never wear artificial dentures.
- Those who have attempted to wear artificial dentures, have failed and are thoroughly discouraged, are of a highly nervous temperament, very exacting and will demand from artificial dentures efficiency and appearance equal to that of the most perfect natural dentures.

Indifferent Mind

Those who are unconcerned about the appearance and feel very little or no necessity for mastication. They are therefore non-persevering and will inconvenience themselves very little to become accustomed to the use of dentures.

Blum (1960) suggested a scheme for classifying patients:
- Reasonable or unreasonable
- Realistic or unrealistic.

Unreasonable Patients Have

1. Unreasonable expectations towards the doctor and towards medical science with regard to quickness and certainty of diagnosis and treatment and with regard to the power and selfless benevolence of the physician.
2. Unreasonable expectations about the fee and a basic unwillingness to pay unless completely satisfactory results are obtained.
3. Unreasonable beliefs about general incompetence or of physicians. These patients tend to have problems like nervous tension, superstition, oversensitivity, fearfulness, over critical natures, etc. They tend to be less educated and are more frequently labourers, semiskilled worker's etc. and have low incomes. (they often come from the lower middle classes.)

Definitions
Diagnosis. The determination of the nature of a disease.
Treatment plan. The sequence of procedures planned for the treatment of a patient after diagnosis.

GENERAL PHYSICAL STATE

It is important to know whether the patient suffers from any systemic illness. Diseases like diabetes, hypervitaminosis, or blood dyscrasciasis can affect the mucosal response to dentures. Prosthodontic treatment should be postponed until these diseases are controlled. Systemic diseases can be

1. Debilitating diseases
2. Diseases of the joints
3. Cardiovascular diseases
4. Diseases of the skin
5. Neurologic diseases
6. Oral malignancies
7. Climacteric.

Debilitating Diseases

Patients with diseases debilitating in nature should be kept under medical control. Diabetes, tuberculosis and blood dyscrasiasis are examples. These patients require extra instructions in oral hygiene, eating habits, and tissue rest. The physician should be consulted before treatment is instituted, frequent recalls should be done.

Hormonal Disturbances

1. Acromegaly—patient may require frequent adjustments and new dentures.
2. Hyperthyroidism—may be associated with reduced salivary flow and mucosal inflammation.
3. Hyperparathyroidism—may be associated with increased ridge resorption
4. Diabetes—can cause decrease in salivary flow, increased alveolar resorption, and impaired healing of mucosal ulcers.

Nutritional Disturbances

1. Avitaminosis—lowers the defence mechanism of the body.
2. Vitamin A deficiency—can cause hyperkeratosis.
3. Vitamin B deficiency—can cause angular cheilosis.
4. Vitamin D deficiency—can cause marked alveolar atrophy.

Infectious Diseases. Abnormal appearance of the mucosa may be due to tuberculosis, syphilis, scarlet fever, diphtheria, measles.

Anemias. These are the most common blood disturbances seen.

The appearance of changes in the oral mucosa in a patient should be suggestive of systemic conditions. The aid of a competent physician should be sought to establish the presence of a systemic condition.

Diseases of the Joint

Diseases involving the joints present a difficult problem. The weight-bearing joints are involved in osteoarthritis. Frequently the terminal joints of the fingers and the joints at the base of the thumb and big toe are affected.

Heberdens nodes are bony enlargements of the terminal joints of fingers. This will make it difficult for the patient to clean and insert dentures.

Osteoarthritis of the temporomandibular joint (TMJ) makes mandibular movements difficult. In some of these patients surgery may be indicated. Mouth opening may be limited, jaw relation records are difficult to obtain, and frequent occlusal correction may be needed.

Cardiovascular Diseases

Consultation with the patient's physician should be done. Short appointments with premedication may be required.

Diseases of the Skin

Dermatologic conditions like pemphigus may have oral manifestations. In these patients, constant use of dentures is contraindicated, and their use is primarily for mental comfort.

Neurologic Conditions

Bell's palsy and parkinsonism are commonly seen. In such patients, denture retention and maxillomandibular record taking are problems.

Oral Malignancies

Most oral malignancies are detected by the dentist. These should be confirmed by biopsy and treated. Prosthodontic treatment can be carried out later. The time that should elapse after radiation therapy (before prosthodontic treatment can be initiated) depends upon the prognosis of the tumor, the amount of radiation received and the condition of oral tissues. The radiation therapist should be consulted and treatment should be decided with his approval.

Climacteric

Climacteric is one of the periods in life of both the male and female when an important change in bodily function occurs. In females this period is referred to as menopause. There are changes in glandular functions. In some patients mental disturbance may be seen. Some of the other symptoms seen include burning tongue and palate, tendency to gag, inability to adjust, etc.

EXTRAORAL EXAMINATION

Tone of Facial Tissues

A close inspection of the skin of the face will reveal the tone of the facial tissues. This is important because two factors affect the tissue tone. First the age and health of the patient will influence the intrinsic structures of the facial tissues.

The tone of the facial tissues may indicate the limitations in what might be done to improve the patient's facial contours. A face that has poor tissue tone with loose or wrinkled tissues throughout cannot be made to appear youthful by new dentures.

Secondly, poor tissue tone can be due to poor support by the intraoral structures. This can be improved by proper support to tissues by the denture base and teeth.

Temporomandibular Joint Examination

Temporomandibular joint should be thoroughly examined. Any pain on palpation or mandibular movement must be noted. Muscles of mastication must be examined for any tenderness. The range of mouth opening and deviation must be noted. Joint sounds if present like crepitus, clicking or popping sounds must be investigated. Presence of these symptoms with or without any disease affects the treatment planning. Any pre-existing disease must be appropriately treated. Alteration of the existing prosthesis may also be required (like vertical dimension). Occlusal scheme selected must be on the basis of the health of the temporomandibular joint.

Salivary Gland

The various structures of the face are best examined with bimanual palpation.

Any lesions of the parotid gland must be noted. The parotid duct is usually identifiable intraorally and manipulation of the duct should elicit a flow of clear watery fluid. Submandibular gland is identified by intraoral and extraoral palpation. Patency of the duct can be noted by the salivary flow.

A quantitative and qualitative evaluation of the saliva is most important for prognosis. Saliva from the parotid duct is primarily serous, that from the sublingual and submandibular glands mucinous and serous. Palatine glands are purely mucinous.

Copious amount of serous saliva adversely affects the retention of complete dentures by disrupting the border seal. Excess saliva will complicate impression making and can be an annoyance to patients. It can also cause problems to patients who are wearing new dentures. (which itself will stimulate salivary secretion). **Xerostomia** also presents serious problems and there is reduced retention in these patients. Lack of saliva also causes sticking of the denture to the mucosal tissues. Ideally there should be moderate flow of saliva which is of the serous type.

Facial Form (Classification According to Leon Williams)

Leon Williams classified the form of the human face in to 3 types: square, tapering, and ovoid, each type merging with the other without any line of demarcation.

In order to determine what type a patient belongs to, the operator imagines two lines—one on either side of the face, running about 2.5 cm in front of the tragus of the ear and through the angle of the jaw.

If these lines are almost parallel, the type is square, if they converge towards the chin it is tapering, and if it is diverging it is ovoid.

The facial form can also be determined using a Trubyte tooth indicator.

Facial Profile

Class I–normal
Class II–retrognathic
Class III–prognathic

Facial profile is determined by considering the glabella, point A and the pogonion (Fig. 2.1).

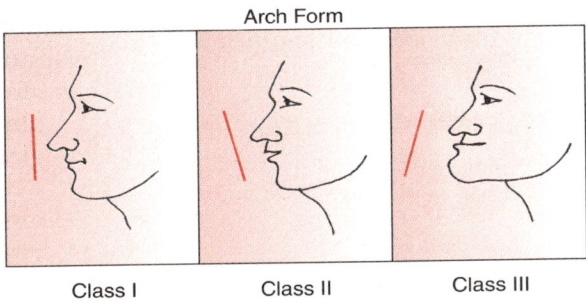

Arch Form

Class I   Class II   Class III

Fig. 2.1. Face profile.

Facial Expression

An absence of facial expression may indicate a loss of muscle tonus. A mask-like expression may be due to numerous surgical procedures. It can also occur in patients with central nervous system (CNS) disorders like paralysis agitans, or endocrine disorders like hypothyroidism.

Complexion

Pallor may be indicative of nausea, hypothyroidism or nephrosis. It also occurs in patients with systemic debilitating diseases. Ruddy complexion may be seen in polycythemia, chronic alcoholics or neoplasms.

Bronzed skin may be seen in Addison's disease and may be seen in patients who have received radiation therapy. Lemon-yellow complexion occurs in patients with jaundice due to gall bladder, bile duct or hepatic disorders.

Hair

Hair may be black, blonde, brown, brunnette, white or black.

Eyes

Eyes may be black, blue, brown, gray hazel. The shade of hair and eyes in selection of teeth is irrelevant.

Lip

Lip can be: (i) supported, and (ii) unsupported

Lip Support. If the tissues around the mouth have wrinkles and the rest of the face does not, then significant improvement is possible. The wrinkles can be avoided by adequate support provided by the placement of anterior teeth in the correct anteroposterior position. If the wrinkles are long standing (for e.g. vertical lines in the lower half of the lip), then significant improvement may not occur. In an attempt to provide support, if the upper anteriors are placed too far labially, unfavourable leverages may be exerted on the denture.

Lip Mobility
Class I–normal
Cass II–reduced
Class III–paralysis.

Lip Thickness. In patients with thin lips, any slight change in the labiolingual position of teeth makes an immediate change in the lip contour. Thick lips give a little more room for alteration in the tooth position before obvious changes occur in lip contour.

Lip Length. Patients with short upper lip will expose all the upper anterior teeth and denture base.

Posture and Walking Pattern

- Stooped shoulders may indicate changes in the spine.
- Tremor of the head occurs in parkinsonism.
- Tremor of the head is seen in patients on tranquilizers.
- Involuntary hurried walking occurs in patients with CNS disorders especially parkinsonism.
- Slapping of the sole of the foot may occur in tabes dorsalis or may follow injury to the spine.
- Drooping of the toe may occur as a result of poliomyelitis.
- Staggering may occur due to excessive alcohol, excessive medication with muscle relaxant drugs, hyperventilation or from damage to the spinal cord.

Expectations. The reason the patient seeks prosthetic treatment is of critical importance. The patient's expectations should be determined and evaluated to see if they are realistic and attainable.

Years of edentulousness of maxilla/mandible—gives information about bone resorption patterns, progression, and cause and timing of tooth loss.

Previous Dentures. The patient should be questioned regarding the number and type of previous dentures. The reason for replacement of earlier dentures should be found out.

Existing or Current Dentures

The time the patient has worn the current dentures should be recorded. Responses obtained should be compared with clinical observations. Denture experience, denture care, dental knowledge, parafunctional habits should be understood.

Denture Success. The esthetics and function of existing dentures should be evaluated. Denture success for each arch can be favourable or unfavourable.

Breathing Pattern

Wheezing is seen in bronchial asthma, emphysema, bronchial infection and heart failure. Erratic breathing, continuous hyperventilation, and periodic variations in breathing may be due to serious pulmonary, renal or cardiac problems.

Muscle Tone

Class I. The patient exhibits normal tension, tone and placement of the muscles of mastication and facial expression. No degenerative changes are present.[1]

Class II. The patient displays approximately normal function but slightly impaired muscle tone.

Class III. The patient exhibits greatly impaired muscle tone and function coupled with poor health and inefficient dentures.

Muscle Development

Class I–heavy
Class II–medium
Class III–light

Muscles of Mastication

Class I. Muscles of mastication are normal in tone and function.[1]

Class II. Muscles of mastication are near normal.

Class III. Muscles of mastication are subnormal in function and tone.

Mandibular movement—can be normal, excessive or limited.

INTRAORAL EXAMINATION

Color of the Mucosa. The color of the mucosa will reveal much about its health. The differences in appearance between a healthy pink mucosa and red inflamed tissue are apparent.

Some tissues will recover by rest, others require tissue conditioning material or surgery. Regardless of the method used, prior to obtaining impressions the tissues should be healthy. If the dentures are made over inflammatory tissue, the dentures may not fit.

Arch Size

Class I (large). The alveolar ridge is of adequate height to give support and to resist lateral movement of the denture base.

Class II (medium). Alveolar ridge has undergone some resorption. Bone is adequate to resist lateral movement.

Class III (small). The alveolar ridge is almost or completely resorbed. There is no resistance to lateral movement of the denture.

Shape of the Residual Ridge

Vertical forces that are placed on the denture are resisted in part by the residual ridge[2] (Fig. 2.2).

Class I. The ridge is U-shaped in its cross-section. The broad, flat ridge crest offers excellent vertical support.

Class II. The ridge is more "V"-shaped in cross-section.

Class III. (Knife-edged ridge). The remaining ridge has a narrow, sharp ridge crest that offers little or no vertical support.

Arch Form

Arch form is generally classified as square, tapering or ovoid. It is important in offsetting

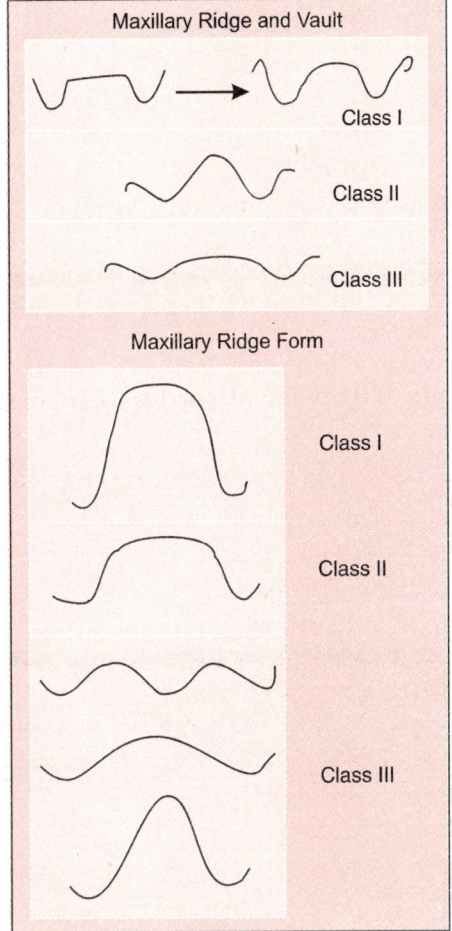

Fig. 2.2. Ridge from.

rotational movement of the denture base (Fig. 2.3).

Class I. The square arch is the best form to prevent rotational movement.

Class II. The tapering form offers some resistance to movement but to a lesser degree than the square arch.

Class III. The ovoid form because of its rounded shape offers little or no resistance to rotational movements.

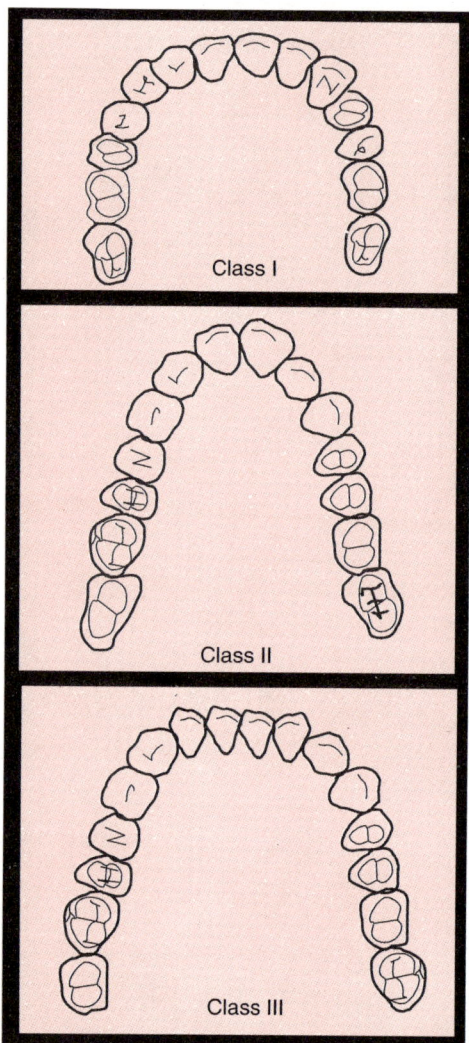

Fig. 2.3. Arch form.

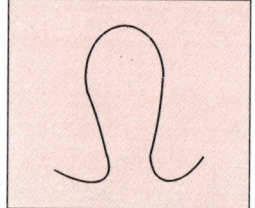

Fig. 2.4. Undercut.

Bony Undercuts

A residual ridge with bony undercuts is most unfavourable to a stable denture and surgical reduction may be required (Fig. 2.4).

Class I. Bony undercuts are absent.

Class II. There are small undercuts over which the denture can be placed altering the path of insertion.

Class III. Prominent bilateral undercuts are present that must be corrected by surgery.

Tori

Class I. Tori are so small that they do not interfere with the fabrication of complete dentures.

Class II. Tori that offer mild difficulties for the adaptation of dentures. Surgical intervention is optional.

Class III. Tori are excessively large, with undercuts or extend to the posterior palatal seal. Surgical intervention is needed (Colour Plate 1).

Interarch Space

Class I: The patient has enough interarch distance to accommodate the denture (Fig. 2.5).

Class II. There is excessive space. The denture is usually less stable because there is too much distance between the denture and the ridge.

Class III. Interarch space is limited, placement of artificial teeth can be difficult.

Ridge Parallelism

When teeth are gradually lost, the residual ridges will diverge from each other. If the ridges are not parallel to the occlusal plane, dentures will slide over the basilar tissues when occlusal forces are applied to them (Fig. 2.6).

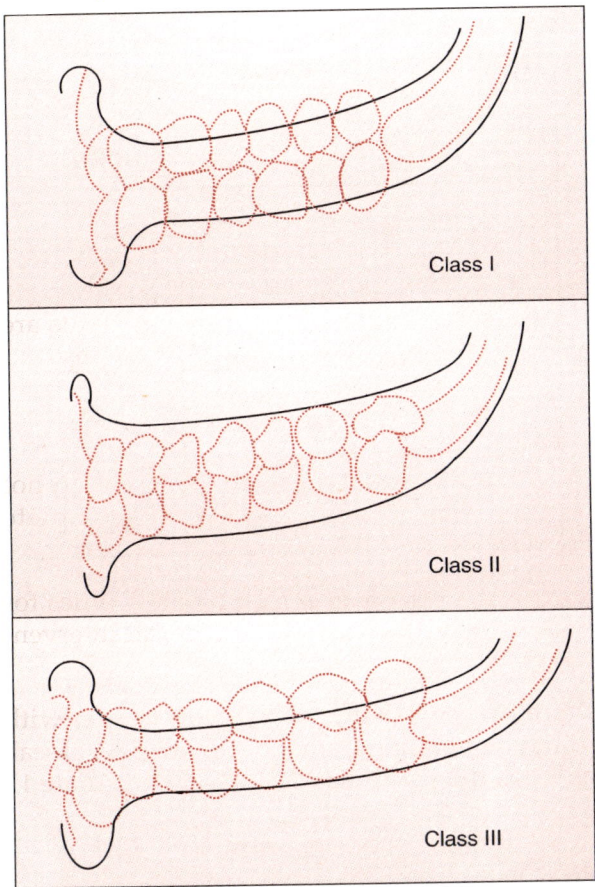

Fig. 2.5. Interach space.

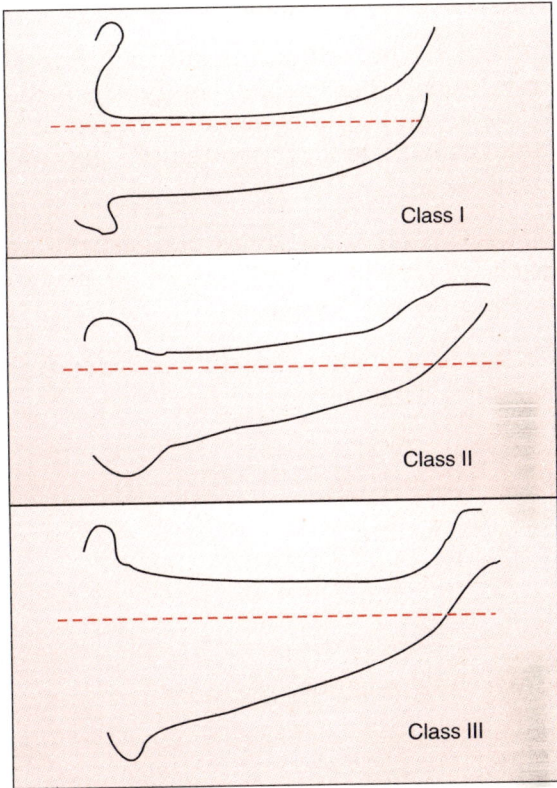

Fig. 2.6. Ridge parallelism.

Class I. Both ridges are parallel to the occlusal plane.

Class II. Either the mandibular ridge or the maxillary ridge is divergent anteriorly.

Class III. Both ridges diverge anteriorly. Both dentures will tend to slide forward.

Shape of the Hard Palate

Vertical support and retention for the maxillary denture are determined by the shape of the hard palate. The palate may be flat, V/U-shaped (Fig. 2.7).

Class I. Broad flat palate offers the best vertical support and retention.

Class II. V-shaped palate form gives more adequate denture support and retention.

Class III. U-shaped palate offers little vertical support.

Palatal Sensitivity

Class I–normal
Class II–subnormal
Class III–supernormal
Palatal sensitivity can be evaluated by running a dry gauze across the palate. A Class-III patient will immediately gag.

Slope of the Soft Palate

Class I: The soft palate slopes gradually down from the hard palate. This type generally allows several millimeters of soft, relatively immovable tissue for formation of a good seal (Fig. 2.8).

Class II. Soft palate slopes more sharply than the class I type thus limiting the seal area and posterior denture length.

Class III. The soft palate drops sharply down from the hard palate.

Mucosa Condition

Class I–healthy
Class II–irritated
Class III–pathologic

Border Attachments

These are subject to change in the edentulous mouth.

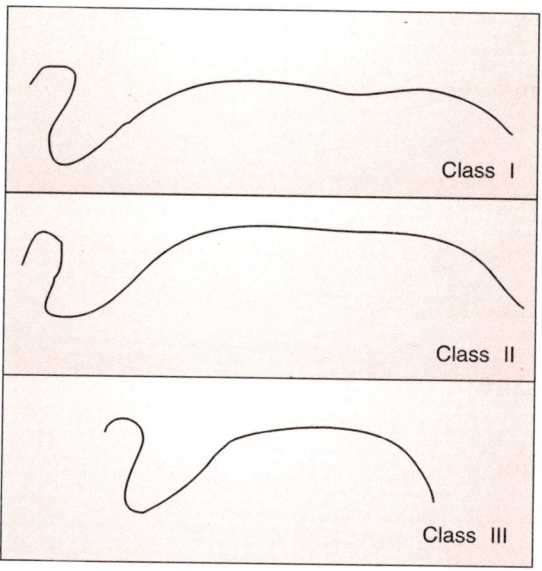

Fig. 2.8. Palatal throat form.

Class I. Conditions are most favorable when there are approximately 12 mm of attached gingiva extending from the crest of the residual ridge to the vestibule.

Class II. There are from 8 to 12 mm of attached gingiva.

Class III. Limited success can be expected with dentures when the attached gingiva is less than 8 mm.

House has classified border attachments into:

Class I. Attachments are high in maxilla or low in the mandible in relation to the ridge crest (0.5 inches or more between the level of attachment and the crest of the ridge).

Class II. Attachment height in relation to the crest of the ridge is between 0.25 and 0.5 inches.

Class III. Attachment height is less than 0.25 inches from the ridge crest.

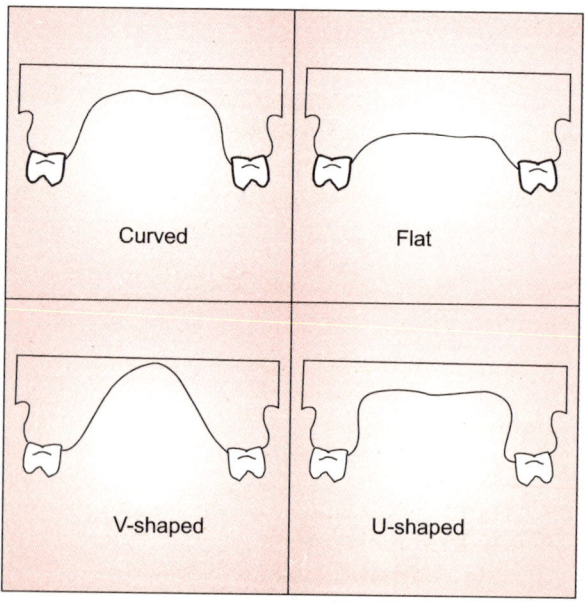

Fig. 2.7. Different types of palate forms.

Frenum Attachment

Class I. High in the maxilla or low in the mandible with respect to crest of the ridge.

Class II. Medium.

Class III. Frenum encroaches on the crest of the ridge and interferes with border seal. Surgical correction may be needed.

Saliva

Class I. Normal quantity and quality of saliva.

Class II. Excessive saliva contains much mucus (Ptyalism).

Class III. Xerostomia.

Tongue

Size

Class I. Tongue is of adequate size to fill but not over fill the floor of the mouth.

Class II. Tongue slightly overfills the floor of the mouth and covers the alveolar ridge.

Tongue Position

Class I. Tongue is in the correct position. The tip is relaxed and it rests in the area of the lingual surface of the lower anterior teeth. The lateral borders of tongue contact the lingual surfaces of the premolars.

Class II. Lateral borders of tongue are in correct position but the tip turns up or down.

Class III. Tongue is in a retracted position. Tip does not touch the lower denture or ridge.

Tongue Shape

- Broad flat, thick
- Long, tapered, narrow.

Ridge Form

A systematic examination of the edentulous oral cavity begins with the residual alveolar ridges. It is characterized by its cross-sectional contour and is classified traditionally as being U-shaped, V-shaped, and flat. Although the amount of ridge available is important, its relationship to the contours of the hard palate are even more critical. The U-shaped ridge in either arch is generally favourable for supporting a denture. This is because it has a broad base for the resistance to occlusal stresses and parallel sides that enhance adhesion and resistance to displacement as well as encourage border seal (Colour Plate 1).

A V-shaped ridge[4] has a narrow crest not conducive to receiving stresses without irritation and discomfort. As the surface decreases, retention is more difficult to achieve. Mandibular V-shaped ridges which are thin and sharp provide the most formidable challenge. If surgical reduction is considered, then the opportunity for lateral stability and resistance to horizontal displacement are sacrificed. However without protection by redistribution of stresses or the use of resilient base materials and acrylic resin teeth, the thin ridge is usually a constant source of pain and discomfort for the patient.

A flat residual ridge most frequently confronts the clinician and is difficult to restore. Bulbous ridges are usually thinner at the base than at the crest and is usually considered undercut. Thin type of ridge is unfavourable for border seal since base relief is a must for proper sealing of the prosthesis. Variations in the ridge contour can also occur. Exostoses, irregular bone resorption, retained roots causing sharp spicules or prominence on the ridge crest are common causes of such variations (Figs 2.9 and 2.10).

Palate

Bone of the palate has a periosteal attachment and mucosal covering with underlying connective and glandular tissue elements. Palpation normally reveals the characteristic features of these structures. The anterior

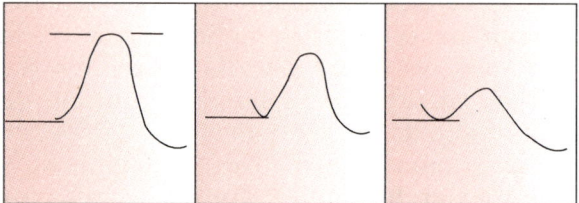

Fig. 2.9. Different types of V shaped ridges (high to low ridges).

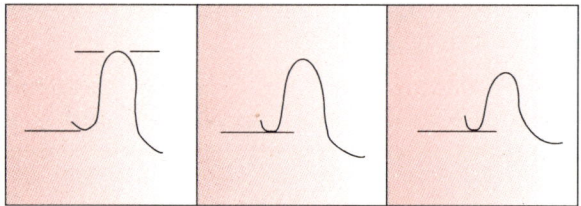

Fig. 2.10. Different types of knife-edged ridges.

palatine foramina marked by the incisive papilla lies on the anterior part of the median palatine suture. Traumatic forces should not be applied to this area. In its anteroposterior extent, the median palatine suture can vary from a midline depression to an extensive undercut torus palatinus. The suture is covered by relatively thin mucoperiosteum. Classifying palatal throat form is very important because of the wide range of three-dimensional movements occurring during speech and deglutition. Movement of the soft palate at the vibrating line in the midline involves a thin, tendon-like band, the palatine aponeurosis, which supports the palatal muscles, strengthens the palate and attaches anteriorly to the posterior border of hard palate. In 1958 House classified palatal throat form into:

Class I. The palate has a gradual inferior slope with less active movements at the junction of the hard and soft palates and can therefore be covered beyond the junction to enhance extension and seal. It is the most favourable condition.

Class II. has a more acute slope and is more active than a class I palate but generally

demonstrates less movements than Class III. The soft palate turns downward approximately at an angle of 45°.

Class III. slopes down sharply at an angle of about 70°. Denture base impingement can lead to soreness, loss of border seal and gagging. The space available for the posterior palatal seal is minimum.

Lateral Throat Form

In 1932, Neil described the lateral throat form as the contour of the hard lingual surface of the mandibular ridge in the molar area and the velum- like tissue distal to the mylohyoid ridge in the retromylohyoid fossa as it functions under the influence of the tongue.

Lateral throat form is classified according to the extent of the anterior movement of the retromylohyoid curtain as the tongue is extended anteriorly beyond the vermilion border of the lower lip. (With the index finger passively contacting the curved wall of the mucosa in the retromolar fossa with the tongue at rest, the patient is asked to protrude the tongue).

Class I. Minimal or no pressure is exerted on the finger (Fig. 2.11).

Class II. Any position of the tissues between the extremes (Fig. 2.12).

Class III. Heavy pressure is placed on the finger. This is important for ascertaining the border extension in this area. Overextension in the retromylohyoid area results in loss of border seal, displacement of the denture or soreness that readily radiates to the floor of the mouth, throat and neck (Fig. 2.13).

Jaw Relationship

Smith (1951) described jaw relationship as the anteroposterior position of the mandibular residual alveolar ridge relative to the maxillary residual ridge when the jaws are in centric relation (Fig. 2.14).

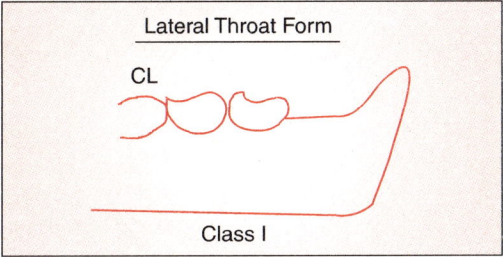

Fig. 2.11. Lateral throat form.

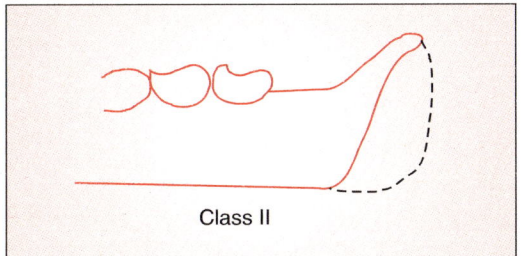

Fig. 2.12. Lateral throat form.

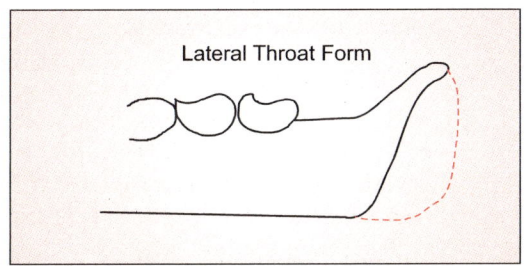

Fig. 2.13. Lateral throat form.

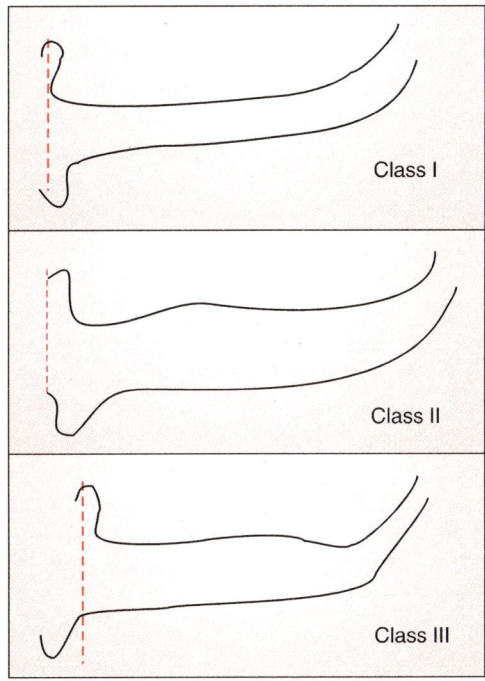

Fig. 2.14. Ridge relationship.

Jaw relationships can be:

Normal (Angle class I). Anterior segment of the mandibular ridge is directly below or slightly posterior to the maxillary anterior ridge segment.

Orthognathic (Angle class II). Anterior segment of the mandibular ridge is retruded beyond the normal position as it relates to the maxillary anterior ridge segment.

Prognathic (Angle class III). Anterior segment of the mandibular ridge is protruded beyond the normal position as it relates to the maxillary anterior ridge segment.

Cross bite A. Anterior ridge relation is prognathic but posterior ridge relation is normal.

A critical evaluation of the arch alignment and the interarch ridge relationship is necessary for formulating an approach to the treatment. Tray selection, impression technique, tooth form and position, division of interarch space, occlusal scheme and base materials are some inter-related aspects of this observation. Colour Plate 2 shows dentures fabricated accordingly.

Tongue

The success of complete denture service is directly related to a thorough understanding of the morphology and physiology of the tongue. Smith described two anatomic tongue types: (i) long, narrow and tapered, and (ii) short, broad and thick.

Thick broad tongue fills more space in the floor of the mouth so as to provide a positive contacting surface for the lingual denture flange and hence a better border seal. However its morphologic features complicates impression procedures and renders it more susceptible to irritation and occlusal trauma from the teeth. Wright and coworkers studied tongue positions and their effect on the stability of the mandibular denture. They found that 75% of all the patients observed had normal tongue position, in which the tongue completely filled the floor of the mouth, had a dorsal surface that was round, smooth and free of muscular contractions, and had lateral borders which rested on the incisal edges of the lower anterior teeth or anterior edentulous ridge crest.

Retracted tongue positions were found in 25% of the patients.

Normal tongue position contributes to enhanced retention of both the maxillary and mandibular dentures. Habitual tongue thrust is detrimental to the stability and encourages mandibular protrusion to the extent that balanced occlusal relationships are difficult to maintain. Posture of the tongue is also related to the maxillomandibular relationship. The patient with a retrognathic mandible carries the lower jaw in an anterior position to facilitate mastication, speech and closure of the lips. The tongue of a prognathic patient will fill the floor of the mouth. Poor tongue habits and undue pre-occupation with position usually results in an unsuccessful denture experience.

Mucosa Masticatory mucosal displaceability is classified by House as:

Type I. Tissue can be displaced approximately 2 mm, cushion like yet will not permit gross positional displacement (Fig. 2.15).

Type II a. Tissue thinner than 2 mm, usually unyielding, often atrophic with smooth surface.

Type II b. Tissue thicker than 2 mm, easily displaced, poor stress bearing usually occurs

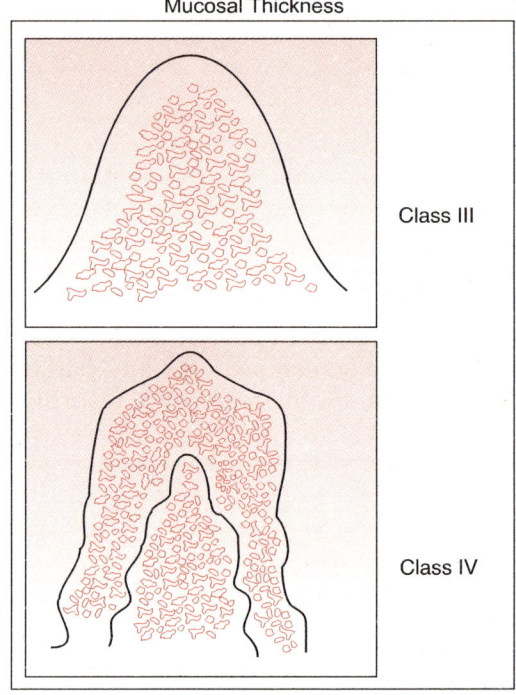

Mucosal Thickness

Class III

Class IV

Fig. 2.15. Mucosal thickness.

as flabby redundancy in regions of excessive bone resorption, under ill-fitting or mal-occluded prosthesis. It may also occur where severe bone resorption has occurred laterally.

Type III. Excessively flabby to the degree that surgical excision is indicated.

Floor of the Mouth. It presents a wide variety in anatomy and functional relation to the ridge crest. If the floor of the mouth is near the ridge crest at rest or the magnitude of the movement is great, retention and stability of the denture will be poor. Floor of the mouth in the sublingual and mylohyoid area may be very high and close to the ridge crest. At times it may be above the level of ridge crest and may eliminate the alveolo-lingual sulcus totally. If these tissues cannot be selectively placed by the denture flange, the prognosis of the mandibular complete denture will be poor.

ROENTGENOGRAPHIC EXAMINATION

Roentgenographic examination is an essential part of diagnosis and treatment planning in complete denture service. Periapical surveys of edentulous jaws may be used but panoramic radiographs are faster, reduce the exposure to radiation, and an entire image of maxilla or mandible can be obtained in a single film. It can be used to screen jaws for any pathology or for determining the amount of resorption.

The interpretation of the panoramic radiograph should follow a five-step analysis as outlined by Chomenko:

1. Screen jaws for defects in the structure and for reactive new bone formation, bone enlargements and displacement of jaw parts.
2. Describe the appearance of the lesion as well as bony changes with its radiographic pattern.
3. Correlate it with clinical, histological and laboratory findings.
4. Perform a differential diagnosis.
5. Estimate the growth of the lesion.

Any lesion which requires definitive management must be referred to the oral pathologist and oral surgeon.

A panoramic radiograph is useful in assessing the amount of ridge resorption. ***Wical and Swoope***[4] found that the mental foramen divided the mandible into thirds in normal dentulous panoramic radiographs. If the distance from the inferior border of the mandible to the lower border of the mental foramen was measured and multiplied by 3, it gave the actual height of the alveolar ridge crest (Fig. 2.16).

Class I (mild resorption) loss of up to 1/3rd of the vertical height.

Class II (moderate) loss of 1/3rd to 2/3rd of the original vertical height.

Class III (severe) loss of more than 2/3rd of the original vertical height.

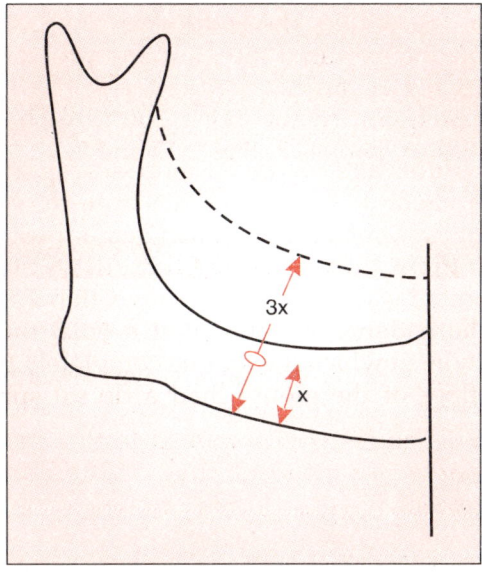

Fig. 2.16. Wical and Swoope's method for determining the original alveolar crest height.

Evaluation of the Old Denture

The patient's experience with previous dentures must be charted out. It can give an insight into whether the patient's expectations are realistic and also if the present denture service can satisfy the patient. The following should be evaluated.

1. Occlusion should be evaluated by light closure of the jaws as the dentist guides the mandible into centric relation. There should be bilateral simultaneous contact. Any slide is unacceptable.
2. Occlusal vertical dimension must be evaluated in profile view at occlusion.
3. The denture should be evaluated for proper basal seat coverage.
4. Retention and stability should be evaluated and correlated with the existing residual alveolar ridges.
5. Esthetics can be evaluated by the effect of dentures on the appearance.
6. Phonetics must be evaluated by the efficiency of the patient to converse normally.

7. On the whole, the comfort of the patient must be enquired into and any problem in this regard noted.

Bone quantity and bone quantity characteristics are shown in Figs 2.17 and 2.18.

TREATMENT PLAN

Considerations in Treatment Planning

Evaluation of the patient involves assessment of mental as well as physical conditions. Knowledge and skills applied to this process will determine the quality of the clinical judgement.

Personal Factors

The key to planning successful treatment is the mutual understanding between the dentist and the patient regarding what is to be done. Regarding the patient includes:
1. Desire for or dissatisfaction with the prosthesis.
2. Health and living patterns
3. Condition of oral and perioral tissues and structures
4. Adequacy of the prosthesis being worn.

Patient's chronologic age is less important than the physiologic age in any treatment planning. Patient's profession and social status may be very critical factors in deciding both the treatment planning and acceptability of the prostheses. Patients under abnormal stress readily express their anxiety and commonly attempt to transfer them to the dentist.

Physical Factors

The contents of the oral cavity cannot be dissociated from the body, as a whole in treatment planning. Many metabolic processes affect oral health.

Bone. Clinical factors related to the resorption of bone are numerous and varied.

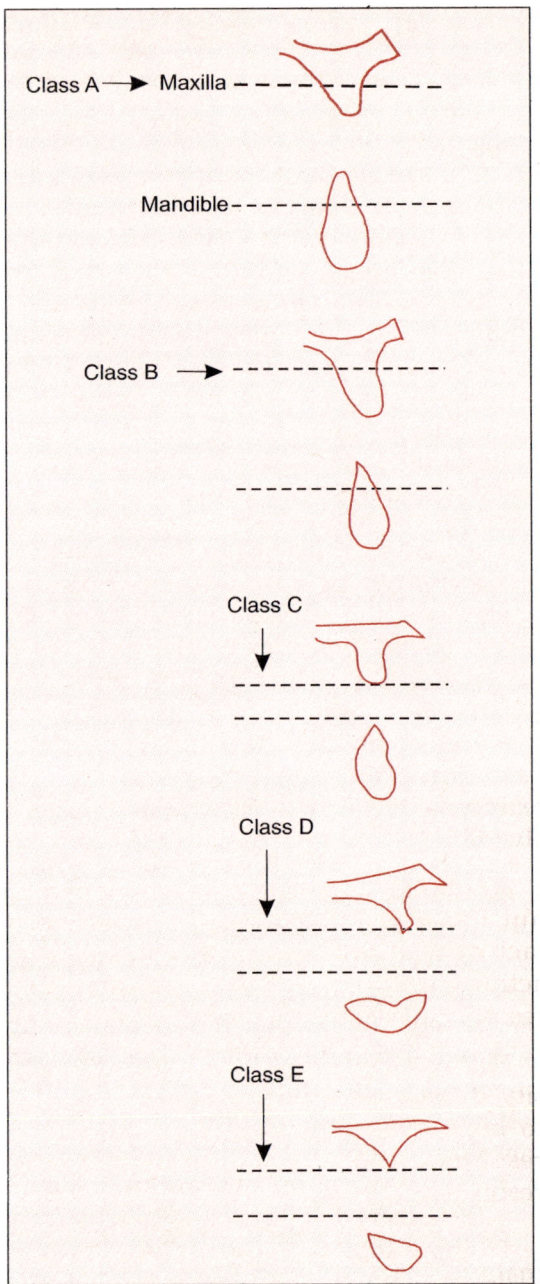

Fig. 2.17. Bone quality.

Anatomic Factors. The size, shape and density of the ridges, the thickness and characteristic of mucosal covering, ridge

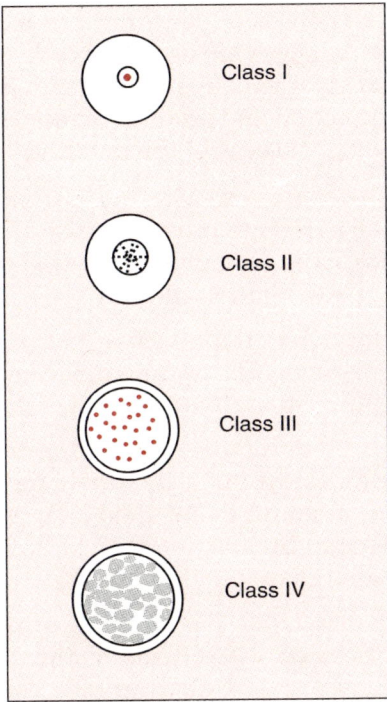

Fig. 2.18. Bone quality.

relationships and the number and depth of the alveoli.

Metabolic Factors. All of the multiple nutritional hormonal and other metabolic factors that influence the relative cellular activity of the bone forming cells and bone resorbing cells should be considered.

Functional Factors. The frequency, intensity, duration and direction of force application to bone are translated into cellular activity resulting in either bone formation or bone resorption.

Prosthetic Factors. The techniques, materials, principles, concepts and practices that are incorporated into the prostheses are important.

Control Factors. There are numerous control factors at genetic, systemic and local level for control of modelling and remodelling behavior.

Various local control mechanisms include biomechanical factors, neurotrophic factors, pH, bioelectric potential, temperature, nerve and neuromuscular reflex. However present knowledge on the effect of the above factors on complete denture prosthodontics still remain elusive.

Biomechanical Considerations

A number of factors influence the choice of methods to be used and the difficulties that will be encountered in providing complete denture service. These factors cannot be eliminated. The procedures may have to be altered for these factors.

Arch Size. The size of the mandible and maxilla determine the ultimate support available for the complete dentures. Large jaws produce more support than small jaws and the difference is directly proportional to their sizes.

If the jaws are small, the impressions must be as accurate as possible because a small error would be relatively larger than the same error in the impression of a patient with a large mouth.

Disharmony in Jaw Sizes. Some patients may have large maxillary and small mandibular jaws or vice versa. These conditions arise from genetic factors and from improper growth and development.

Maxillary protrusion is the least favorable condition because the area of coverage of the mandible is less than normal. The occlusal contact area in the premolar and molar regions is decreased.

In patients with Class II or Class III malocclusions the artificial teeth should be placed in the same basic position as the natural teeth and occlusion will have to be developed in harmony.

Ridge Form. In situations where the mandibular ridge is sharp with sharp bony spicules, a selective pressure technique should be used so that more occlusal force is placed on the buccal shelf.

Vault Form. Affects the retention of the maxillary denture. A U-shaped vault produces the most favourable prognosis. A V-shaped vault resists vertical displacement but provides no resistance to lateral shift.

A high arched vault resists lateral shifts, but vertical displacement tends to break the seal in all areas at once.

Ridge Relation. Ridge relation changes as the shrinkage occurs.

Muscle Control. Good muscular control and coordination are essential for effective wearing of the complete denture. For example, if the tongue movements are used for manipulating the lingual flanges in border molding, the timing, direction, and amount of movement are critical for the success of the molding.

If tongue movements are too slow, too fast or in a wrong direction, more time and effort will be needed to complete the procedure successfully.

Muscle Tonus. The tone of the facial tissue is critical to several steps of denture fabrication. If the muscles are too tense, the cheek and lip manipulations will be difficult, but if too slack, the lips and cheeks may be easily displaced by the denture.

Muscular Control. Good muscular control and coordination are essential to the effective wearing of complete dentures. For example if tongue movements are used for border molding the lingual flanges of a mandibular denture, the timing, direction and amount of movement are critical to the success of the molding.

Jaw Movements. The ability or lack of ability of a patient to move the mandible to the right place at the right time will reveal problems in making jaw relation records.

Gagging. A patients active gag reflex can compromise a dental treatment. It can frustrate both the dentist and patient.

Temporomandibular Joint Problems. The temporomandibular joint must be healthy before new dentures are made. A unhealthy temporomandibular joint will complicate the registration of jaw relation records.

Cheek and Lips. The muscles of the cheek and lip have a critical function in the successful use of dentures. The denture flanges must be properly shaped so that they aid in maintaining the dentures in place without conscious effort on the part of the patient. Correct arch form, tooth position, and shape of the polished surface is necessary for this.

Arch Shape. It helps in determining the: (i) form of the teeth to be used, and (ii) relative development of the lower third of the face. This may help in arrangement of teeth.

Further Reading

1. House MM. The relationship of oral examination to dental diagnosis. J Prosth Dent. 1958; 8(2):208-19.
2. Rayson J.H. et al. Diagnosis and treatment planning.
3. Kelly K. Changes caused by a mandibular removable partial denture opposing a maxillary complete denture. J Prosth Dent. 1972; 2:140-50.
4. Wical Swoope. Studies of residual ridge resorption. J Prosth Dent. 1974; 1 32: 07-12.

MULTIPLE CHOICE QUESTIONS

1. **A patient with hyperparathyroidism may suffer from**
   a. Reduced salivary flow
   b. Increased ridge resorption
   c. Angular cheilosis
   d. Hyperkeratosis

2. **A ruddy complexion of the skin may be indicative of**
   a. Hypothyroidism
   b. Polycythemia
   c. Addison's disease
   d. Jaundice

3. _____ **type of arch form is considered ideal to resist rotational movement**
   a. Square   b. Tapering
   c. Ovoid   d. None of the above

4. **Excessive interarch space is seen in**
   a. Class I   b. Class II
   c. Class III   d. None of the above

5. _____ **vault form provides the most favourable prognosis**
   a. Class I   b. Class II
   c. Class III   d. None of the above

6. **According to house personality classification, the patients who are considered ideal are**
   a. Philosophical   b. Hysterical
   c. Skeptical   d. Indifferent

7. **Diagnosis is**
   a. The determination of the cause of the disease
   b. The determination of the prevalence of a disease
   c. The determination of the nature of a disease
   d. None of the above

8. **In diabetic patients, the features seen are**
   a. Increase in salivary flow
   b. Increased ridge resorption
   c. Impaired healing
   d. b and c

9. **Xerostomia may cause**
   a. Increase in retention of the denture
   b. Decrease in retention of the denture
   c. Decrease in support of the denture
   d. Decrease in stability

10. **A class II interarch space is associated with**
    a. Decreased interarch space
    b. Increased interarch space
    c. Denture will not have adequate stability

FAQs

1. **House personality classification**
2. **Systemic conditions influencing treatment planning**
3. **Biomechanical consideration in treatment planning**

3

PREPROSTHETIC SURGERY

INTRODUCTION

The basal seat area serves as the foundation for the denture. Dentures are rigid pieces of acrylic resin which are shaped to fit the basal seat area. No denture regardless of how well it is constructed can be better than the foundation on which it is placed.

The goal of preprosthetic surgery is to modify the oral environment to render it free of disease and to make its form more compatible with the requirements of complete denture wearing. Goodsell has elaborated some of these requirements. They are:

1. Ridges that are broad and flat with vertical height (minimum of 5 mm) provided by nearly parallel non-undercut bony walls.
2. A firm, resilient mucosal covering with nicely shaped buccal and lingual sulcus that are uninterrupted by flange, scars or redundant tissue folds.

3. An interarch distance (minimum 16 to 18 mm) and relationship that allows room for the denture and its components.

Prior to preprosthetic surgery the patient's attitude towards treatment should be evaluated. A complete understanding and acceptance of limitations of denture performance must be accomplished before treatment is begun.

Preprosthetic Surgery. Surgical procedures designed to facilitate fabrication or to improve the prognosis of prosthodontic care.

Allograft (Homograft). A graft of tissue between genetically dissimilar members of the same species.

Alloplast. A material originating from a non-living source that surgically replaces missing tissue or augments that which remains.

Autogenous Graft. A graft taken from the patient's own body.

Autograft (Autochthoxnousgraft). A graft of tissue derived from another site in or on the body of the organism receiving it.

Initial Preoperative Examination Procedures. This include radiographic evaluation. Pantographic and periapical radiographs supplemented with lateral jaw and overall

28

radiography is required if pathology is suspected. Cephalogram is necessary if orthognathic surgery is needed.

Secondary Preoperative Examination Procedures. This includes treatment and care for abused and distorted tissues caused by the use of existing malfitting dentures. Such procedures either eliminate the need for surgery totally or reduce the complexity and extent of planned surgery, or make the outcome of surgery more predictable.

The simplest procedure is to remove the existing denture from the oral cavity for a period of time accompanied by soft tissue stimulation with a soft toothbrush or a damp wash cloth. This is often augmented by the use of a tissue conditioning material.

INITIAL HARD TISSUE PROCEDURES

Definition: These surgical procedures involve teeth and bone and are most often done in the private office by the general practitioner. These include:

1. The Extraction of Teeth. It should preserve as much bone and soft tissue as needed and the bony alveolar margins should be palpated through their soft tissue covering to discover sharp bony projections that act as potential fulcrum points for denture movement and soreness.

2. Root Tips. Those showing radiographic evidence of pathologic change should be removed and that covered by sound bone with no evidence of pathologic change can be left undisturbed. If left in place, the patient should be advised of its presence, its location and asked for periodic recall and observation. Removal of root tip should provide for the preservation of bone and soft tissue.

3. Unerupted Teeth. This should be evaluated for evidence of pathologic activity, location, age of the patient, history of symptomatology, and past prosthodontic history. Majority of unerupted teeth have to be removed because of risk of development of dentigerous cyst or ameloblastomas. Those unerupted tooth showing evidence of pathologic activity must be sent for microscopic examination.

An asymptomatic impacted tooth covered with sound bone can be left in place to preserve arch morphology.

4. Non-pathologic Bony Conditions. Alveoloplasty is the surgical reshaping of alveolar ridge. It is indicated where uneven interseptal spines or bilateral bony undercuts exist.

In patients with advanced periodontal disease, surgery is limited to tooth removal, rounding of uneven or sharp bony areas and removal of excess or inflamed soft tissue.

5. Intercortical Alveoloplasty. It is done when alveolar process is prominent but regular. It is performed by removing the interseptal bone and collapsing the labial or buccal cortical plates so that they meet the lingual/palatal cortical plates. It is an ideal procedure for immediate denture cases. The septa are removed to the base of the socket with a rongeur and cortical plate fractured in by finger pressure.

6. Mylohyoid Ridge Reduction. It is done to lessen the amount of undercut present or to relieve the irritation of the mucosa over that shelf like bony projection. Bone is removed with a bur or osteotome and smoothened with a bone file. Care is taken not to displace bony fragments into the submandibular space.

7. Knife-edged Ridge. In atrophic mandible the alveolar process because of lateral resorption forms knife-edged ridge. The overlying soft tissue is often rolled with a movable fibrous base. Surgical correction will leave the patient with a less vertical tissue height and continued bone resorption. Even ridge augmentation with synthetic implant materials have produced migration and obliteration of the vestibule in the area of augmentation.

8. Alveolar Tubercle. They often present bilateral buccal undercuts that become a problem during impression making and insertion/removal of the denture. Grinding from the tissue surface leads to problems of retention and food accumulation. If no undercut is present in the anterior section of the arch, it is not necessary to remove the undercuts from both tubercles. Adequate room should exist in a horizontal direction to allow free passage of the coronoid process.

Another condition occasionally seen is when the alveolar tubercle approximates the retro-molar papilla and the pad area to the extent that adequate denture base coverage and correct placement of occlusal plane is not possible. Both bone and soft tissue removal is required with care taken not to damage the greater palatine artery or the maxillary sinus.

9. Preirradiation Alveolectomy. Patients with oral cancer who require multiple extraction of teeth before radiation should have immediate closure of gingival tissue over the sockets. This will require radical removal of bone and is called alveolectomy.

The surgical technique of alveoloplasty requires an adequate mucoperiosteal flap to allow removal of bone with a minimum of soft tissue trauma. The alveolar process should be smoothed and the wound cleaned of debris. The flap should be reapproximated and carefully sutured. A surgical splint can be constructed that will protect the area from trauma until it is healed. Such a splint should not be opposed by a functional denture and should avoid placing undue pressure on the surgical site to avoid possible impingement on the vascular supply of the newly repositioned flap.

10. Exostoses. These are bony nodules situated on the alveolar process of the mandible or the maxilla. They are covered with a thin, friable mucosa that is easily injured and does not tolerate pressure from a denture. The buccal aspect in the molar region of the mandible and the buccal aspect from the premolar, posteriorly to the alveolar tubercle in the maxilla are the most frequent locations. These exostoses present undercuts to the path of insertion and removal and should be removed by alveoloplasty.

11. Tori. These are bony hyperostoses common to both maxilla and mandible. In maxilla, small tori that do not act as fulcrum points under a denture may not require removal. The torus even small in size may act as a fulcrum. In such instances, the denture base over the area must be relieved or the torus should be surgically removed.

Large torus with gross undercuts or located posteriorly where the posterior palatal seal has to be placed should be surgically removed. Careful radiographic examination is required to rule out the possibility of pneumatization.

Torus mandibularis: It is found on the lingual cortical surface of the mandible, is usually bilateral and is located in the premolar area. Most mandibular tori must be removed before denture construction because relief in the denture base rarely provides comfort. Mucoperiosteal flap of adequate size is reflected to avoid the use of vertical releasing incisions. Torus is removed with a bur or an osteotome and smoothened with a bone file. The bony reduction should be limited to a level above the attachment of the mylohyoid muscle. A surgical splint is not necessary because the mucoperiosteal covering can be readapted, it is vascular and heals rapidly.

12. Genial Tubercles. These are prominent following advanced alveolar ridge resorption in the anterior area of the mandible. They are covered with thin mucosa that cannot tolerate the pressure of a denture flange located in this area. The superior portion of these prominences are removed and that portion of the genio-glossus muscle that is attached in the area is usually left free. If necessary, it may be reattached by suturing it to the muscle layer located below. Complete removal of the genial tubercles should be avoided because lack of attachment of the genioglossus and geniohyoid could lead to impaired tongue function.

Pathologic Bony Conditions

Small cystic lesions are removed by enucleation and large cystic lesions are marsupialized to allow shrinkage and bone fill in and to prevent surgical fracture or damage to adjacent structures. In several months as shrinkage occurs enucleation should be performed.

Tumors

In all instances histologic diagnosis and radiographic findings are necessary. Surgical care for a tumor is dictated by the nature and extent of the tumor. Attempts should be made to preserve as much residual ridge as possible for best denture support.

INITIAL SOFT TISSUE PROCEDURES

Initial soft tissue procedures are defined as those surgical procedures that are usually performed by a general practitioner in a private office.

Alveolar Tubercle. Alveolar tubercle frequently approximates the retromolar pad and papilla, is pendulous and consists mainly of fibrous connective tissue. These are removed by a series of wedge-shaped incisions.

The goal of this procedure is a firm, well-defined tubercle that will provide support and stability to the maxillary denture.

Frenae. The maxillary and mandibular labial and buccal frenae as a result of resorption become attached to or near the crest of residual alveolar ridge. The labial frenum sometimes becomes hyperplastic and interferes with the border extension and exerts a dislodging influence on the denture.

A frenectomy accomplishes two important things (i) it allows increased border extension, and (ii) it releases a mobile band of tissue that is in contact with the denture.

Various surgical procedures have been suggested varying from simple incisions for narrow attachments to incisions with mucosal undermining for larger attachments to more complicated Z or V-Y plasties for broad based attachments. The last two procedures will both remove the frenal attachment and lengthen the vestibule.

Lingual Frenum. If the attachment results in a partial ankyloglossia, a simple release is sufficient. A wide attachment that is strong and resistant to displacement when the tongue is elevated will necessitate an alveolar detachment as an additional dissection.

Individual Isolated Muscle Origins. These are handled with single transverse excisions and sutured through the firm attachment tissue at the base of the incision to ensure firm immobilization.

Scar Contractures. These present in the vestibule are handled much like frenal attachments, but they tend to recur unless a surgical splint is provided immediately after surgery for a period of 10 to 14 days.

Benign Soft Tissue Lesions

Lips. All pathologic conditions of lips including ulcers, fistulas and masses must be removed before beginning denture construction. Unhealed ulcers must be biopsied.

Palate. Epulis fissuratum results from chronic denture irritation. It is frequently seen in the anterior vestibule when the patient has natural mandibular anterior teeth that occlude against an opposing maxillary complete denture.

Inflammatory hyperplasia of palate. It is seen under old, ill-fitting maxillary dentures.

Treatment consists of (i) removal of the irritant and placement of soft lining materials in the denture to reduce inflammation and bleeding during surgery, and (ii) surgical removal of the tissue by excision or cautery with care taken to preserve the periosteum and underlying structures.

Hyperkeratosis and Dyskeratosis. These must be differentiated by surgical biopsy and histologic examination. Hyperkeratosis is removed by stripping with low intensity electrocautery.

Lichen Planus. Lichen planus occurs most frequently on the buccal mucosa and must be differentiated from dyskeratotic lesions by biopsy. Dentures are not contraindicated but patients with erosive type of lichen planus may have continuous soreness of erosive lesions and have difficulty with dentures.

Mucoceles and Retention Cyst. These are the result of mucus pooled in the connective tissue stroma due to trauma from lip or cheek biting. These are treated by surgical excision.

Ranula are large and seen in the floor of mouth are treated by marsupialization

Dermoid Cyst. Seen as a midline swelling in the floor of the mouth. It must be differentiated from a ranula. These are treated by surgical enucleation or excision.

Papillomas and Fibromas. Benign neoplasms of the oral mucosa are treated by excision before denture construction.

Hypermobile Tissue. Hypermobile tissue on the crest of the ridge is formed because of excessive submucosa that developed during extended period of periodontitis and accompanying bone resorption. After the loss of teeth, this tissue undergoes fibrosis producing a pendulous mobile structure. This problem can also occur after extraction (from alveolar bone resorption) under an ill-fitting denture or from excessive force placed on the alveolar process when natural teeth in one arch occlude against a denture in the other. Treatment for pendulous tissue consists of simple excision or

excision combined with alveoloplasty or vestibuloplasty (Fig. 3.1).

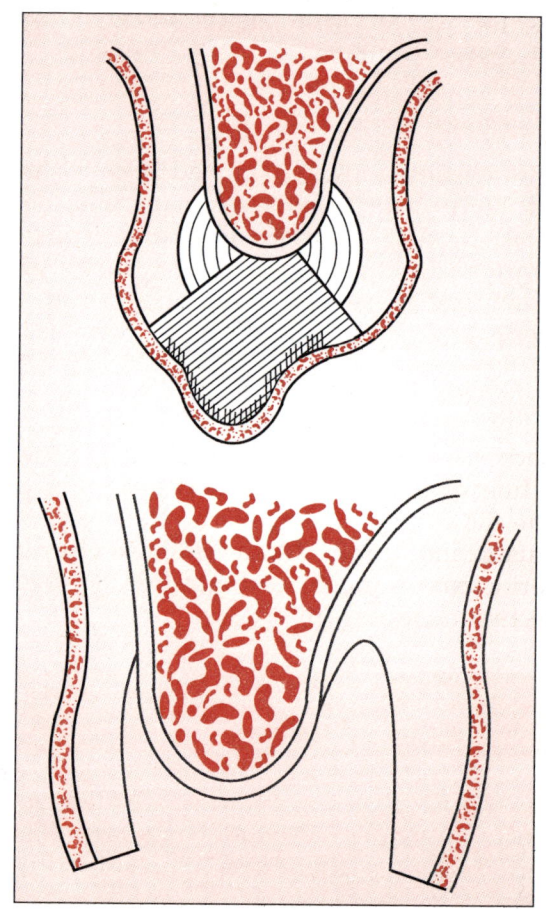

Fig. 3.1. Removal of excessive tissue in the alveolar tubercular area.

- If the buccal and lingual sulcus is adequate for denture construction and the ridge is not too sharp, it can be treated by simple excision of the pendulous tissue.
- If the ridge is already atrophic and the underlying bone is thin and sharp, excision may lead to a greater deficiency of the denture base, inadequate soft tissue coverage, pain and discomfort. To avoid this, the soft tissue procedure can be combined with minor alveoloplasty if the alveolar

height is adequate or with alveoloplasty and subsequent vestibuloplasty if it is not. Another alternative is the use of a sclerosing solution. This is done primarily if the hypermobile tissue has good contour.

Sclerosing Procedure

Indication. Excessively mobile ridge tissue in both maxillary and mandibular arches that have acceptable contours, are ideal for this procedure.

The technique consists of injecting, 5 % solution of sodium morrhuate using a Luer-Lok syringe, (supraperiosteally and infiltrating with in the tissue).

Impressions for denture construction are made 4 to 6 weeks later.

Injection of sclerosing solution produces fibrosis in the soft hyperplastic tissue and causes binding of the alveolar soft tissue to the periosteum thereby increasing firmness and decreasing mobility.

SECONDARY HARD TISSUE PROCEDURES

Maxillary Ridge Augmentation Procedures

- One procedure takes advantage of the osteogenic potential of hematopoetic bone marrow through the use of participate bone marrow and cancellous bone chips, contained within a metal crib (mesh). The mesh is left in place over the graft and acts to protect and contain the bone graft for a period of 10-14 weeks. Soft tissue procedures are instituted thereafter to reconstruct the vestibules to supply adequate soft tissue (to cover the graft).

    Complications include high rate of dehiscences over the metal crib and a high resorption rate of the graft under the prosthesis.

- Another procedure for maxillary ridge augmentation is a combination of the classic Le-Fort I maxillary osteotomy with down fracture of the maxilla and the total alveolar maxillary osteotomy which leaves the palate in place but allows downward movement of the alveolar ridge segments.

Interpositional or Inlay Bone Grafting with iliac crest bone (used as blocks) along with particulate and marrow, are used in both these procedures to fill voids. These two techniques might be called composite or combination procedures because they combine the separate techniques of osteotomy and bone grafting.

Vestibuloplasties are often required following these procedures. A maxillary splint constructed on the mounted diagnostic cast after surgery is used (i) to keep the soft tissue and graft adapted during healing, (ii) to prevent hematoma formation, and (iii) for fixation of the maxilla during the healing period.

Mandibular Ridge Augmentation Procedures

These procedures in addition to restoring the ridge shape also strengthen the severely atrophic mandible that is in danger of spontaneous pathologic fracture. Patient selection must be based on patient motivation and mental and physical health of the patient.

Autogenous graft material used for onlay or inlay grafting for mandibular augmentation include iliac crest, cancellous bone and marrow, or a combination of these.

- Use of rib graft for mandibular augmentation showed a high resorption rate of 50 % in the first 2 years In this procedure, two ribs or one rib and bone particles from the iliac crest are used. The rib is placed on the ridge and the spaces remaining are filled with bone particles from the second rib or the iliac crest. Graft material will mature in 4 months' time following with which vestibuloplasties are done. A long healing period is allowed because the functional shape of the alveolar ridge must remodel before dentures can be constructed (Fig. 3.2).

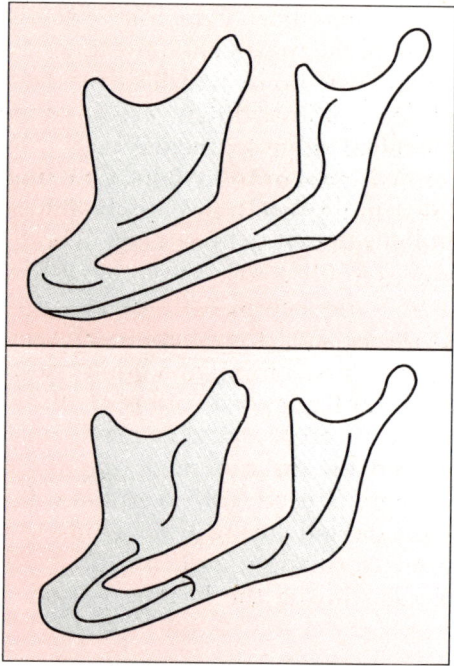

Fig. 3.2. Superior border onlay rib graft.

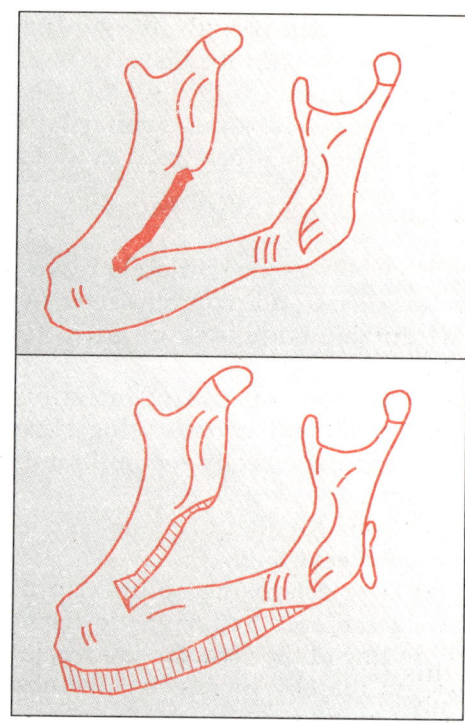

Fig. 3.3. The inferior border onlay rib graft.

Inferior Border Rib Grafting (by Sanders and Cox)

The advantages of this procedure are that the graft does not have to bear the weight of the denture, the vestibules are preserved, no splint is required, and the healing period is reduced (Fig. 3.3).

Disadvantages include sensory or motor nerve deficiency (that can lead to lip biting) and changes in facial appearance.

• MacIntosh et al suggested the use of iliac crest for onlay or inlay grafting through an extraoral or intraoral approach. This procedure was supplemented by osteotomy techniques with interpositional grafting. Donor blocks of iliac crest provide the cortical bone framework and cancellous marrow is used to fill the space between segments of cut cortical bone. The pieces are wired into place. The resulting ridge will be both wider and higher than that before

surgery. Vestibuloplasties are performed 4-6 months after the healing is complete.

The procedure of choice for mandibular ridge augmentation includes the combination of osteotomy techniques (horizontal or vertical) with interpositional bone grafting.

These procedures involve the movement of a pedicle of bone along with its blood supply. The viability of the bone will be greater and the resorption decreased because the blood supply to the bone is maintained.

Horizontal Osteotomy Techniques

For these techniques, an adequate vertical height of the mandible must exist so that the mandible can be cut horizontally. This cut is placed below the level of the mandibular canal and mental foramen to avoid injury to the mandibular nerve. The superior part of the ridge is elevated and the iliac bone blocks, particulate bone and marrow are sandwiched in between. Transosteal wires hold the components in place. Model surgery is necessary before carrying out the procedure.

Advantages
- Increased ridge height which is stable
- Shortened postoperative period (3 months).

Disadvantages
- Nerve trauma
- Paresthesia
- Mandibular fracture
- Flap dehiscence

Vertical or Visor Osteotomy. It was introduced by Harle and modified by Peterson and Slade. This is used in situations where insufficient vertical mandibular bone height is present (for the horizontal osteotomy) but adequate bone width (approx 10 mm) is present.

In this technique, the mandible is split vertically and the lingual section is elevated to increase the mandibular height. Cancellous bone or particulate bone and marrow is placed to correct the contours and to fill in the gaps on the facial side of the elevated segments.

Transosteal wires hold the segments in place for a period of 3-4 months before vestibuloplasties are performed.

Disadvantages
- Greater chance for nerve trauma and paraesthesia.
- All osteotomy techniques must be performed with extreme care because procedures will alter the spatial relationships of the arches.

The graft material may bond with bone as a result of deposition of new bone mineral on the supporting matrix of hydroxyapatite.

Hydroxyapatite is mixed with various materials such as freeze dried bone, bone morphogenic protein or purified fibrillar collagen. These materials are placed by tunneling beneath the mucosa and periosteum. The graft is placed directly on the bone surface to be augmented, with the help of a syringe.

Use of a splint has proven to be troublesome. This is because the actual area of material deposition as influenced by the anatomic and surgical limitations differs from the ideal area as determined on the presurgical casts. A splint fabricated using a predicted location displaces the material into the tissue, where it acts as an irritant beneath the denture (Fig. 3.4).

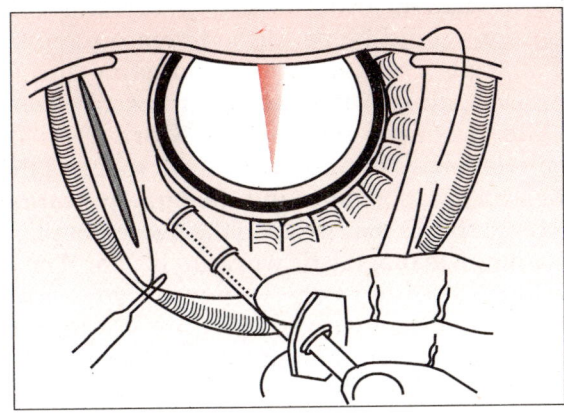

Fig. 3.4. Augmentation of mandibular ridge using hydroxyapatite placed with a syringe.

Vestibuloplasties are done 10 weeks after graft placement.

Another technique creates a defined subperiosteal tunnel through the use of silicone tissue-expanding implants which become encapsulated with fibrous tissue and are later removed. The hydroxyapatite is injected into the defined space later.

Other techniques involve the use of resorbable material (plaster or collagen cylinders) to confine the hydroxyapatite to minimize the problem of displacement.

RIDGE RELATIONSHIP PROCEDURES

Ridge relationship procedures involve the correction of discrepancies of both arch size and arch relationship to each other in space.

Improper relationships of this nature create both functional and esthetic problems for the patient. Disharmonies of tooth relationships and occlusal contacts that result from skeletal disharmonies in the natural dentition are an index to the problems in tooth arrangement that will be present when the patient receives complete dentures.

Malrelated jaws should be analyzed early in the diagnostic procedure and surgical corrections should be performed before removal of all teeth. The teeth act as landmarks during the orientation of jaws and also act as stabilizers while the jaws are healing. Correction of malrelation in the absence of teeth requires the construction of splints and the immobilization of these splints may prolong the treatment plan.

Complete diagnostic work-up is vital. These include radiographs, photographs and mounted diagnostic casts. Cast surgery is critical to evaluate the success of the procedure. Psychologic evaluation of the patient is necessary to evaluate the patient's ability to adopt to stress and change. Relationship of the ridges in all three planes of space must be considered.

The gunning type of splint made on these preoperatively altered casts will accurately reposition the segments and provide for proper fixation.

Relapse tendencies in both the vertical and horizontal directions due to muscle pull can be decreased with the use of skeletal fixation.

Maxillary Advancement Procedures

Maxillary advancement procedures are used to correct problems of maxillary retention. This may involve a combination of true skeletal maxillary retrusion and pseudoretrusion due to resorption of the small maxilla. Lateral, anteroposterior and vertical relationship of the arches must be considered.

The procedure of choice is Le-Fort I osteotomy with or without interpositional grafting.

Mandibular Advancement Procedures

Mandibular advancement procedures are less commonly performed; because in the retrognathic mandible there is less bone and soft tissue for the surgeon to work with.

The procedure of choice is sagittal osteotomy or several of its variants performed from an intraoral approach.

Contraindications. A thin ramus or severe mandibular atrophy in the posterior region of the mandible. If an advancement of more then 8 mm is required, use of bone grafts is necessary. Prosthodontic procedures are performed after skeletal fixation for a period of 6-8 weeks.

Mandibular Retrusion Procedures

Mandibular prognathisms can either be true or acquired. The currently accepted procedure involves an osteotomy procedure in the subcondylar region or an osteotomy in the ramus.

The Subcondylar (oblique) Osteotomy. Intraoral approach is used when less than 10 mm movement is required. Extraoral approach that allows good access for muscle and bone surgery is used when movement of 10-12 mm is required.

Ramus Osteotomy (or) Sagittal Osteotomy. This procedure is indicated where extreme movement (> 10 mm) is required and when symmetry of the segments to be moved is present.

An additional procedure may be performed in the body of the mandible when symmetry is lacking or a greater amount of movement is required (of one segment). Intermaxillary fixation is required for 4-6 weeks and surgical splints should be worn until definitive complete dentures are inserted.

SECONDARY SOFT TISSUE PROCEDURES

Ridge extension procedures are needed when years of denture wearing and neglect injure and modify the basal seat area and make successful denture wearing difficult. These procedure are preferred over hard tissue procedures when adequate bone exists beneath the soft tissue and muscle covering. This bone must be uncovered by modifying the relationships of hard and soft tissues. Thus the existing bone is made available for use in the support and retention of the denture.

Thorough presurgical evaluation and diagnostic work-up is necessary. It is valuable to observe structures that could limit the success of extension procedures. In the maxilla these include the malar buttresses and anterior nasal spine.

In the mandible they are the mental foramen, genial tubercles and the inferior border of the mandible.

Maxillary Ridge Extension Procedures (Vestibuloplasty/sulcoplasty/ridge extension/sulcus extension)

There are various techniques for vestibuloplasty like:
1. Secondary epithelialization vestibuloplasty.
2. Soft tissue graft vestibuloplasty with skin or oral mucosal tissue.

Submucosal Vestibuloplasty

Submucosal vestibuloplasty was described by Obwegeser in 1959 as a closed procedure for both the maxilla and mandible. It is indicated in areas where enough bone and healthy mucosa exist, but where muscle attachments are close to the crest of the alveolar ridge. This procedure has remained mainly as a maxillary procedure because of relapse that occurs in the mandible.

Assessment of whether enough mucosa exists or not is done by placing a mouth mirror into the sulcus and depressing the tissue. If the vermilion of the lip is not displaced or distorted, then it is presumed that an adequate mucosa exists. Likewise the mirror test can be done in the posterior region and the pull on the buccal

tissues should be observed. If there is insufficient mucosa, a secondary epithelialization or graft procedure is preferable.

Procedure. A vertical incision is placed in the area of the maxillary labial frenum. A submucosal tunnel is created in the unattached mucosa with a scissors along the alveolar process and extending into the lip and cheeks on both sides of the incision. If there is inadequate access, a vertical incision can be made in the canine or first premolar region. Next the submucous layer (muscle and connective tissue) is dissected free of the overlying mucosa and underlying periosteum by a blunt and sharp dissection. The middle layer of the submucosa is resected.

A surgical splint is placed for 10 days and is held with perialveolar wires, staples or a midpalatal screw.

Disadvantages
- It is a blind procedure.
- Fifty percent relapse rate is found in the first 3 years.

Submucosa Resection

- Submucous resection Wallenius (1963) suggested a submucosa resection via an open technique.

Procedure. A facial incision is made at the mucogingival junction. This incision is carried to the periosteum if the mucogingival junction is lateral to the alveolar crest or to a depth equal to half the thickness of soft tissue if the mucogingival junction is occlusal to the alveolar crest. The hypermobile soft tissue is directed supraperiosteally and bisected supracrestally stopping 2-2.5 mm short of the soft tissue crest. The superfluous spongy connective tissue is removed from the inner side of the flap and from the palatal aspect of the ridge, and care is taken to ensure that a uniform 2-2.5 mm of mucosa remains.

The mobilized thin, keratinised mucosa is held firmly against the alveolar crest and an incision is made at its border into the alveolar mucosa. This mucosa is then sharply dissected from the alveolar ridge periosteum in a coronal direction. The mobilized mucosa is then sutured to the periosteum with interrupted mattress sutures. A soft lined splint is placed for 7-10 days. Prosthetic treatment is started after 4-6 weeks.

Secondary Epithelialization

Kazanjian in 1935 described a method for deepening the vestibule in which a labial flap pedicled off the alveolar process was used to cover the newly exposed bone while the lip surface was permitted to re-epithelialize.

The major disadvantage of all these techniques was scar contracture on the labial aspect that resulted in a loss of vestibular depth.

To overcome this disadvantage, Clark recommended a vestibuloplasty procedure in which the flap was pedicled off the lip rather than the alveolar process. Since the raw surface is on the bone rather than on the lip, less contracture occurs as the wound granulates and re-epithelializes (Figs 3.5 and 3.6).

Soft tissue Graft Vestibuloplasty

Soft tissue graft vestibuloplasty includes the use of: (i) free mucosal graft, and (ii) split-thickness skin graft.

Indications
- Expected presence of adequate bone for denture success after the procedure is

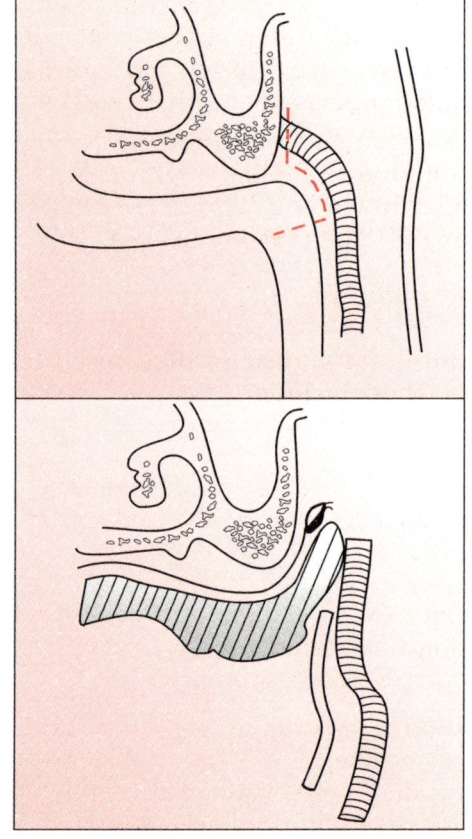

Fig. 3.6. The secondary epithelialization procedure in the posterior region.

performed and after the expected 20-30% relapse has occurred
- Presence of poor mucosal covering that would be best removed and replaced.

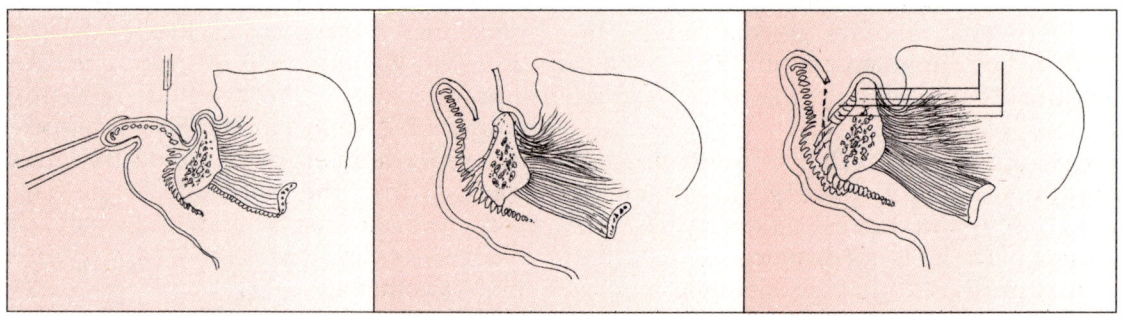

Fig. 3.5. The secondary epithelialization or the reverse anterior sulcus slide procedure.

- Planned use of bone graft material for ridge augmentation.

Use of skin graft is controversial. Some are of the opinion that it is not wetted well by oral fluids and thus will not provide the required retention for the maxillary denture.

Availability of large amount of skin and the rapidity of healing favours its use.

Mandibular Ridge Extension Procedures

Procedures are similar to those used for the maxilla. These include
- Sub mucous resection vestibuloplasty.
- Secondary epithelialization vestibuloplasty.
- Transpositional flap vestibuloplasty (lip switch).
- Soft tissue graft vestibuloplasty.

A minimum of 15 mm of bone must be available for the success of mandibular ridge extension.

Secondary Epithelialization Vestibuloplasty

Sulcus Slide. A supraperiosteal flap is raised from an incision on the ridge side or labial side of the sulcus. The flap is repositioned and sutured at the depth of the new sulcus.

Reverse Anterior Sulcus Slide. The initial incision is placed on the lip side of the suture.

Use of splint is controversial and relapse is a severe problem.

Transpositional Flap Vestibuloplasty

(Lip-switch). This technique was originally developed by Kethley and Gamble (Fig. 3.7).

Indication. Patients who require mandibular ridge extension procedures but are medically unable to tolerate more extensive procedures.

Technique. A split-thickness mucosal flap is dissected from a periosteal flap. The periosteal flap is used to cover the raw soft tissue surface and the mucosal flap is used to cover the raw bony surface.

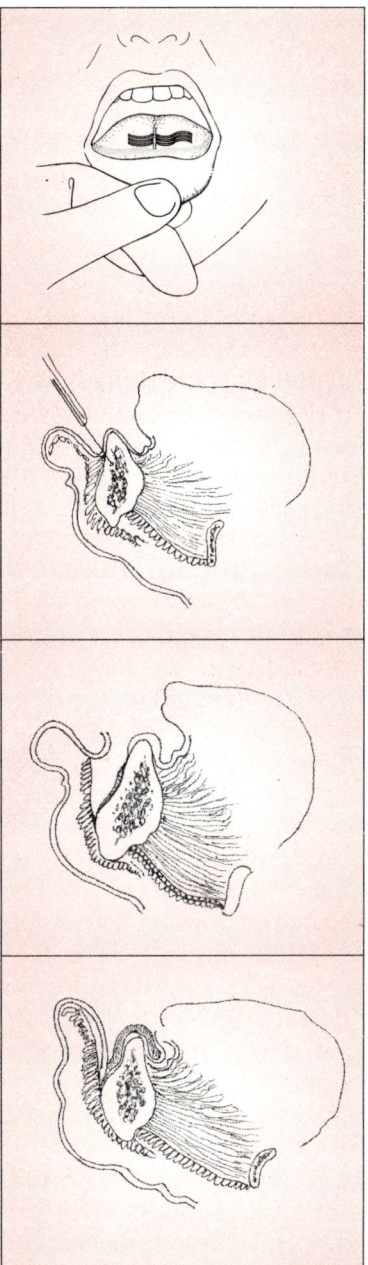

Fig. 3.7.

Advantages
- Applicable in most patients
- Presence of a raw surface that needs a lengthy healing period is eliminated

- Bony recontouring/ridge augmentation can be done at the same time as the lip switch
- Very little regression.

Disadvantages. Lip distortion may occur as healing progresses.

Soft Tissue Graft Vestibuloplasty

Soft tissue graft vestibuloplasty can be done using: (i) mucosal graft, and (ii) split-thickness skin.

Technique. The surgical procedure is essentially the same as that performed for the secondary epithelialization procedure. The soft tissue graft is placed over the de-epithelialized site. The graft is secured in place (with the bleeding surface upward) with a newly relined splint, with tincture of benzoin or dermatome glue. Excess graft material is trimmed off and splint is placed over the ridge and wired to place. The wires are removed in 7 to 10 days. The redundant graft material is excised and the splint is relined with the soft liner material. The graft material is allowed to mature for 3 to 5 weeks after which the prosthesis is made.

A second splint is used to cover the intraoral donor site, for 7 to 10 day's to cover and protect the donor side and improve the patient comfort. Removal of this splint will reveal a white surface covering a granular bleeding surface which will heal in 3 weeks. Antibiotic coverage and use of drugs like dexamethasone are recommended.

Complications include mental nerve involvement, painful swallowing, swelling causing difficulty in breathing. Hospitalization is desired and oral feeding is discontinued until swallowing can be accomplished comfortably.

Free Mucosal Graft

The free mucosal graft may be taken from any area of the oral cavity but cheek and palate are the frequent choices. The amount of donor tissue is limited by these sites, but the donor graft may be enlarged by fenestration or meshing.

Some prefer the use of well-keratinized palatal mucosa to produce a superior denture bearing area which is capable of providing better support and retention. Air-driven dermatomes make graft harvesting quicker, easier and controlled.

If a large amount of donor graft tissue is required, skin graft is a better choice than mucosa.

The mucosal graft may either be secured to the graft receptor site or it may be sutured to the site after fenestrating the graft to allow for the escape of blood and fluids.

Some surgeons prefer to use a soft lined surgical splint. Others feel that careful suturing followed by controlled pressure to prevent hematoma formation without the use of the splint avoids the problems of pressure necrosis and the time-consuming complications of splint fabrication and adjustment.

If no splint is used following surgery, one is usually placed in 7 to 10 days. This splint is soft-lined and used until a new denture is inserted.

Great care must be exerted not to overextend this splint. It should terminate just at or slightly short of the vestibular reflection to avoid pressure on the suture line.

Disadvantages

- About 20-30% shrinkage and relapse may be expected from the procedure during healing. This amount may be compensated for during surgical planning.
- Donor site problems like hemorrhage, scaring.
- Sharp nature of the vestibule
- Loss of the graft
- Production of tunnels that are due to local complications at the graft site.

Advantages

- Procedure is performed on an outpatient basis.
- Absence of extraoral scar and skin graft donor site problems.

Skin Graft Vestibuloplasty

Skin graft vestibuloplasty uses hairless donor skin from the buttocks, inner thigh or abdomen. A thin graft of uniform thickness of 0.0125–0.015 inches is obtained with an electric dermatome.

Thicker grafts may be preferred because they tend to ulcerate and contract less during healing, but the presence of hair follicles and other adnexal structures in thicker skin sections is a long-term problem for the patient and prosthodontist.

The donor site should be covered carefully for patient comfort postoperatively. The site should be left undisturbed for a period of 10-14 days. Healing will be essentially complete in 2-3 weeks. A softlined splint is often required to protect the graft and prevent hematoma formation.

One problem with skin graft vestibuloplasty is the color and consistency of the ridge tissue. This tissue being different from mucosa is hard to "read" when the dentist examines for pressure spots and denture abrasion.

Maxillary Oral Implants

Maxillary implants are indicated for those patients who cannot adapt to a properly made maxillary complete denture. This may be due to physical, anatomic or psychologic reasons. The bone of the maxilla, being more spongy in nature, and the presence of anatomic limitations, such as the maxillary sinus, make maxillary implantation risky and less predictable.

Maxillary subperiosteal implants of various designs were described in the early 1950s. Many of the surgical and prosthodontic techniques that were developed with minor modifications remains unchanged. The success rate of maxillary subperiosteal implants has never approached that of those placed in the mandible.

Maxillary Endosseous Implants

The use of these implants requires careful diagnosis and evaluation. Casts and radio-graphs must be carefully examined and three dimensional pictures of available bone must be developed. Size and location of the maxillary sinus and floor of the nose place definite limitations.

Mandibular Oral Implants

Indication
- Severe mandibular atrophy with dehiscence of the mental nerve. Intolerance to conventional lower denture resulting from the lack of adequate bony support.

Contraindications
- Impacted tooth
- Bony pathology
- Recent extraction
- Sharp alveolar ridges requiring alveoloplasty

Attachment Systems

Different types of attachment systems allow the dentist great design flexibility when individual attachments are used.

One form of attachment is the closed field magnet system which uses a ferromagnetic stainless steel keeper and a permanent rare earth magnet.

Advantages
- They have 20-50 times the attractive force of earlier magnets.
- Maintenance requirements are absent
- Magnet technique is simple.
- Parallelism of implants or ridges is not a requirement.
- Magnets are self-seating and have no moving parts to wear or break during function.
- They allow for a stress breaking design which places good vertical but little lateral loading.

A rounded magnet and keeper are usually chosen to avoid clicking.

Problems with Magnets
- They include iron parts which are prone to corrosion
- Metallic magnets are soft and will wear in function.

• Increasing the space between the magnets decreases the magnetic retention.

Distraction Osteogenesis and its Application in Prosthodontics

Distraction osteogenesis or the Ilizarov technique is a surgical procedure for the reconstruction of skeletal deformation. It involves the gradual controlled displacement of surgically created fractures which results in simultaneous expansion of soft tissue and bone volume.

Indications. Primary indications are for combined deficiencies in bone and soft tissue.

Secondary indications include expansion of the alveolar housing to create a site for dental implants, to improve ridge esthetics for placement of a pontic and to improve the periodontal environment adjacent to teeth. The limitations include the requirement of a minimum amount of bone.

Distraction osteogenesis is a surgical procedure involving new bone formation between vascularised bone surfaces following osteotomy or corticotomy as a result of regular distraction achieved by means of functionally stable devices.

MULTIPLE CHOICE QUESTIONS

1. **An allograft is**
   a. A material originating from non living source
   b. A graft of tissue between genetically dissimilar members of the same species
   c. A graft derived from another site on the body of the organism receiving it
   d. None of the above

2. **Statement that is true regarding an exostosis**
   a. These are bony nodules situated on the alveolar process of maxilla and mandible
   b. Are frequently removed by alveoloplasty
   c. Are seen frequently in the buccal aspect of the molar in the mandible
   d. All of the above

3. **V or Z plasties are surgical procedures for**
   a. A knife edge ridge
   b. Bulbous tuberosity
   c. Broad based frenum attachments
   d. High genial tubercules

4. **Statement that is true regarding visor osteotomy**
   a. It is used in situations where insufficient vertical mandibular bone height is present but adequate width is present

   b. Is used in situations where insufficient mandibular width is present
   c. Involves splitting of the mandible vertically
   d. a and c are true

5. **Interpositional or inlay bone grafting is used to**
   a. Correct ridge relation problems
   b. For maxillary ridge augmentation procedures
   c. For mandibular ridge augmentation
   d. None of the above

6. **The procedure of choice for maxillary advancement is**
   a. Sagittal osteotomy
   b. Lefort I osteotomy
   c. Subcondylar osteotomy
   d. None of the above

7. **In Kazanjian's secondary epithelialization technique**
   a. A labial flap predicled off the lip is used to cover newly exposed bone
   b. A labial flap predicled off the alveolar process is used to cover the exposed bone, lip is allowed to reepithelialize
   c. It is a vertibuloplasty technique
   d. b and c are true

8. **The lip-switch vestibuloplasty technique was introduced by**
   a. Kazanjian
   b. Clark
   c. Kethley and Gamble
   d. Obwegeser

9. **_____ is a graft taken from a non - living source**
   a. Autograft
   b. Alloplast
   c. Homograft
   d. Allograft

10. **Of the following the most commonly used sclerosing solution is**
    a. 5% NaCl
    b. 5% of Sodium bromide
    c. 5% of Sodium morrhuate
    d. 5% Potassium murrhuate

4

RESIDUAL RIDGE RESORPTION

INTRODUCTION

After the extraction of teeth, the empty dental alveoli fill up with blood, which sequentially clot, and is subsequently replaced with new bone. The mucoperiosteum covers over the remaining alveolar bone and healing alveoli.

The residual ridges to which the prosthesis are meticulously fitted change shape and are reduced in size at varying rates in different individuals and in the same individual.

Residual ridge resorption is a chronic, progressive irreversible and disabling disease probably, of a multifactorial origin.

PATHOLOGY OF RESIDUAL RIDGE RESORPTION

The basic structural change in residual ridge resorption (RRR) is loss of bone.[1] In certain situations, the loss of bone may leave the overlying mucoperiosteum excessive and reduntant, and in other cases there are no reduntant soft tissue overlying the bone.

A simplified method for categorizing the most common residual ridges configurations, follows:

Order I—Preextraction
Order II—Postextraction
Order III—High well rounded
Order IV—Knife edge
Order V—Low well rounded
Order VI—Depressed

A gross finding, on dry specimens is that the external surface of the maxilla and mandible are uniformly smooth, but the crestal areas of the residual ridges have a different appearance and shows many more porosities and imperfections irrespective of the stage of residual ridge configuration. Bones with the most severe RRR may display the gross porosity of medullary bone on the crest of the ridge and eventually may even display the uncovering of the inferior alveolar canal on the mandible.

In the maxilla, cases have been reported where there are virtually no maxillary alveolar processes. But in the mandible, although complete resorption of the body of the mandible has not been recorded, cases have been reported with only a thin cortical plate on the inferior border.

44

To determine the amount of bone loss there are several methods:

- Examination by visualization. The problem with this technique is that a knife-edged ridge may be mistaken for redundant or inflamed soft tissue.
- One can more accurately determine the amount of bone loss by palpation in the mouth.
- To determine the rate of bone resorption over a long period of time, the best method is to take a lateral cephalometric radiograph.
- According to Wical et al, the orthopanoramic radiograph (OPG) is the simplest and useful method.

Microscopic Pathology

The microscopic studies have revealed the evidence of osteoclastic activity on the external surface of the crest of residual ridges as a mechanism by which gross bone loss occurs. However there are no reports of new bone formation or reversal lines on the external surface of the residual ridge.

A microradiographic study of 21 mandibles showed wide variation in the configuration, density and porosity of not only the residual ridges, but also the entire cross-section of the anterior mandible. This study pointed out the presence of smooth lamellar bone on the labial, lingual and inferior surfaces of the mandible and the total absence of such lamellations on the crest of the residual ridges of all 21 specimens.

PATHOPHYSIOLOGY

The pathophysiology[1] deals with the mechanism of disordered function. In the normal function of the bone, there will be constant remodeling throughout life through the process of bone resorption and formation. This bone resorption and bone formation will always maintain the equilibrium except during growth where bone formation exceeds bone resorption.

In the case of osteoporosis and periodontal disease, there will be either localized or generalized destruction of bone around the teeth due to certain pathologic processes. In both these cases, i.e. osteoporosis and periodontal disease, once the bone matrix is lost, it does not ordinarily return.

Similarly residual ridge resorption is a localized pathologic loss of bone, i.e. it is not built back by simply removing the causative factors. To date the process of RRR has not been reversed such that the residual ridge has increased in size.

According to Enlow's principle[2], the reduction of the metaphysis of a long bone can be illustrated diagrammatically by the principle of 'V' with the minus symbols representing the periosteal resorption and plus symbols representing endosteal deposition. Similarly in the mandible, the RRR can be explained based on the same principle.

PATHOGENESIS

The life history of RRR can be illustrated diagrammatically and radiographically.[3]

Immediately following the extraction any sharp edges remaining are rounded off by external osteoclastic resorption, leaving a high well-rounded residual ridge. As resorption continues from the lingual and labial aspect, the crest of the ridge becomes increasingly narrow and ultimately becoming knife edge. As the process continues, the knife edge becomes shorter and eventually disappears, leaving a low well rounded or flat ridge (order V). Eventually this too resorbs leaving a depressed ridge (order VI).

Usually RRR proceeds slowly over a long period of time. The most standardized data with significant number of patients can be found in the postextraction study of mandibular bone loss by Carlsson. Carlsson et al in their study over a period of 5 years of postextraction mandibular bone loss found that there is a 7.25 folds of difference in the resorption between the patient with least RRR and the patient with most RRR. His study shows a remarkable difference in the mean rate for different time periods in the first five years following extraction.

In this the most interesting feature is the difference between the two patients who represent the minimum and maximum rates in his group. The patient with the most RRR in the early post extraction period continued to have the highest rate of RRR in the later stages of study. Over the five-year period, there was 7.25 fold difference in RRR between the two extremes.

EPIDEMIOLOGY OF RESIDUAL RIDGE RESORPTION

The epidemiology is the study of the distribution and determinants of disease in man. Epidemiology contributes to the understanding of the etiology of the specific disease.

How Prevalent is Residual Ridge Resorption?

Cephalometric studies have shown that the presence of RRR is worldwide, occurs in males and females, young and old, with or without dentures and is unrelated to the primary reason for the extraction of the teeth (caries, or periodontal disease). It is more common in Great Britain, Sweden, USA Australia and Japan.

ETIOLOGY OF RESIDUAL RIDGE RESORPTION

The residual ridge resorption is a multifactorial disease and the rate of RRR depends on the concurrence of two or more factors which may be called the cofactors. For convenience these

Table 4.1. Etiologic factors and residual ridge resorption (RRR)[6]

Etiologic factor	Correlation with RRR
Anatomic Factor	4 × more RRR
Mandible	than normal
Large-alveolar process	Increased RRR
Labial alveoloplasty	Increased RRR
Density of given bone	No correlation
Prosthodontic factor	
Immediate denture	Decreased RRR
Zero degree teeth	Increased RRR
Metabolic and Systemic factor	
Age and Sex	No correlation
Osteoporosis	Decreased RRR
Ca and Vitamin D Supplement	
Functional Factor	
Intensive denture wearing	Increased RRR
Regular denture wearing	No correlation
Other factors	
Bielectric potential	Decreased RRR

cofactors can be divided into four categories.
- Anatomic,
- Metabolic,
- Functional,
- Prosthetic.

For further convenience, since the functional factors must function through the prosthetic factors, they may be grouped together as mechanical factors. This gives three groups of cofactors anatomic, biologic, and mechanical.

Anatomic Factors

The anatomic factors include:
- The size and shape of ridge
- The type of the bone
- The type of mucoperiosteum.

The residual ridge resorption varies with the quantity and quality of the residual ridge. If a ridge has existed as a high and well rounded one for several years, it will continue to do so. If the residual ridge has gone from an Order I to and Order IV in a span of 2 years, it will probably continue to resorb rapidly. If a low depressed ridge has existed, for many years, future RRR will be at a lower rate.

Another way to evaluate the anatomic factors is to consider the mechanical factors that would be favorable to stability and retention of the denture. Thus, well rounded ridges and broad palates would seem to be favorable anatomic factors.

Tallgren has correlated the shape of the mandible with that of the anterior mandibular bone loss. He indicated a pronounced resorption in subjects with a marked mandibular base and a less marked resorption in subjects with a flattened mandibular base.

Metabolic Factors

Metabolic factors include age, vitamins, diet, and osteoporosis.

Age. It is well known that an older person is likely to have a great deal of more alveolar ridge resorption than a younger person. According to Jowson in 1916, preliminary studies have shown that in growing persons, bone formation outweighs the resorption. But in aged the resorption may not be compensated by formation of bone resulting in senile osteoporosis.[5]

Residual ridge resorption varies directly with certain systemic or localised bone resorptive factors and inversely with certain bone formation factors.

$$RRR = \frac{Bone\ resorption\ factors}{Bone\ formation\ factors}$$

In residual ridge resorption certain local bone resorbing factors could be very important. This include endotoxins from dental plaque, osteoclast activating factor, prostaglandins, human gingival bone resorptive stimulating factors and others. Plaque can occur in edentulous mouths especially in patients who do not properly clean their dentures.

Systemic factors also influence the balance between normal bone formation and resorption, for, e.g., systemic diseases such as diabetes and tuberculosis can influence alveolar resorption.

Hormones

It is well known that hormones and vitamins influence the bone resorption. Parathyroid hormone (PTH) is the most important of the hormones so far as alveolar ridge resorption is concerned.

Parathyroid hormone is responsible for the maintenance of normal blood calcium levels of 10-12 mg%. It is generally assumed that the blood concentration of ionic calcium regulates PTH activity.

When the circulating level of PTH is abnormally high, a general picture of osteoporosis ensues. The level of blood calcium will be elevated and that of blood phosphorus decreased.

A decrease of PTH results in an increased formation of bone and possibly in a deposition of calcium salts in other organs. Here the blood calcium concentration falls and that of phosphates increases. These conditions may lead to generalized osteosclerosis.

Wical in 1961 in his investigation regarding the relationship of dietary, calcium, phosphorus and alveolar bone resorption in edentulous patients found positive correlation among low calcium intake, calcium phosphorus imbalance and severe ridge resorption.

Vitamins

The vitamins play an important role in bone physiology and it may be well for practitioners to look to the dietary intake of their patients. Although it cannot be said that alveolar resorption is attributable to deficiency, clinical or subclinical, it is wise to maintain the overall health of the patient so that any possible factor which contributes to alveolar resorption may be eliminated.

Vitamin D. by regulating the absorption of calcium from the intestine can aid in maintaining normal blood calcium levels. Furthermore, it has been shown that Vitamin D actually inhibits the action of PTH, rather than supporting it.

Vitamin A. This vitamin does not play so important a role in bone physiology as vitamin D, but certain influences on bone appear to be attributable to both hyper- and hypovitaminosis. A. It is believed that hypovitaminosis-A, results in overall bone growth being retarded and in the later stages of the disease, endochondrial bone growth may cease entirely.

Vitamin C. Vitamin C deficiency is characterized by a decreased activity of fibroblasts, osteoblasts and odontoblasts, which ultimately affects collagen production.

Mechanical Factors

Mechanical factors includes both functional and prosthetic factors. The functional factors depend on the frequency, direction and amount of force applied to the ridge. Prosthetic factors depend on the form and type of teeth and interocclusal distance.

Some postulate that RRR is an "abused" bone resorption due to excessive forces transmitted through dentures, whereas others postulate that RRR is inevitable disuse atrophy.

In considering forces one must be concerned not only with the amount of forces, but also the frequency of forces, duration of force, direction of force, area over which force is distributed and the damping effects of underlying tissue.

Amount of force applied to the bone may be affected inversely by the "damping" effect or energy absorption. Damping effect may take place in the mucoperiosteum which may be considered as a viscoelastic material. In addition the damping effect of bone itself should be considered.

MANAGEMENT

Ridge Augmentation

Preprosthetic surgery is an important aspect of the surgical rehabilitation of the edentulous and partially edentulous patient presenting with severe alveolar atrophy and of the postresection patient presenting with total or partial resection of mandible or maxilla.

As life expectancies increase, the severely resorbed ridge is becoming more common. With the refinement of older techniques for ridge augmentation and the development of newer ones, a better treatment can be given for these patients.

The goal of these procedures[7] is to recreate an edentulous ridge with characteristics that are compatible with the requirements of denture wearing. Many variables affect the success of these procedures. These include the materials used, the augmentation site, surgical design, prosthodontic design, patient interest, prosthodontic follow-up and skill of the surgeon and prosthodontist.

Definitions

Augmentation (To Increase in Size Beyond the Existing size)—in alveolar ridge augmentation, bone grafts or alloplastic grafts are used to increase the size of an atrophic alveolar ridge.

Autogenous—originating or derived from within the same individual (self-produced, self-generated, autologous).

Autograft—a graft of tissue derived from another site in or on the body of the organism receiving it—also called autochthonous graft, autogenous graft, and autoplast.

Autogenous graft—a graft taken from the patient's own body (autograft).

Osteogenesis (GPT-7)—development or formation of bone (Misch) osteogenesis is the capability of a material to form bone even in the absence of undifferentiated mesenchymal cells.

Osteoinduction—the capability of chemical procedures, etc. to induce bone formation through the differentiation of osteoblasts (Misch) an osteoinductive material is one capable of inducing the transformation of undifferentiated cells into osteoblasts or chondroblasts in an area where it is not common.

Osteoconduction—characteristic bone formation, apposition from and on existing bone.

History of Atrophic Ridge Management

Methods to increase alveolar ridge height in the past have included onlay bone grafting, interpositional bone grafting, and use of metallic dental implants. Materials like acrylic, silicone rubber, proplast have not performed well because of extrusion, infection, poor physical properties and technical problems.

Materials Used for Ridge Augmentation. These materials can be classified: (i) metallic, and (ii) Non-metallic materials.

Non-metallic Elements

1. Autogenous grafts—obtained from the same individual, e.g. iliac crest grafts or rib grafts.
2. Allografts—obtained from same species but a different genotype, e.g. demineralized freeze-dried bones (DFDBs), freeze dried bone, frozen bone.
3. Xenografts—obtained from a bovine source.
4. Alloplasts—e.g. ceramics, polymers, composite.
   Ceramics can be (i) Bioactive, e.g. HA, TCP, durapatite, and (ii) bioinert, e.g. Al_2O_3, TiO_2.

Metallic Elements

1. Ni-Cr alloys in mesh form
2. Pure titanium in mesh form
3. Dental implants
   Materials can be classified based on the effect they have on bone.

1. Osteoconductive materials—forms bone by apposition, e.g. ceramics, frozen bone.
2. Osteoinductive materials—e.g., frozen bone, DFDBs, freeze dried bone.

It is capable of inducing the transformation of undifferentiated cells into osteoblasts or chondroblasts in an area where this is not an expected behavior.

Osteogenesis—refers to a material capable of forming bone, even in the absence of local undifferentiated mesenchymal cells, e.g. autogenous bone.

Calcium Phosphate Ceramics

Plaster of Paris was used by Dreesman to fill bone defects in 1894. The first study on clinical use of calcium phosphate powder dates to 1920 when Albee found a positive influence of triple calcium phosphate on healing of bone fractures. Hydroxyapatite and Beta-whitlockite are used commonly.

Initially powders were available for clinical use but in 1971, two techniques were developed to produce blocks.

* By sintering of calcium phosphate powders
* By adding controlled amount of calcium oxide and phosphorus pentaoxide (P_2O_5) to silicate glasses and obtain a interface layer of calcium phosphate (bioglass, glass ceramics) These materials form a high bond with bony tissues. Other ceramics, like Al_2O_3 do not have this property and are called bioinert ceramics.

Composition

* Brushite ($CaHPO_4$) is stable as aqueous solution at a temperature 25°C at pH 4-5.
* Apatite is stable at pH 7.4-5 .
* Beta-whitlockite is not stable as aqueous solution at 25°C.
* Magnesium containing Beta-whitlockite is stable in aqueous solution at 25°C.

Microstructure. As described by Peelen, an important microstructural property of calcium phosphate ceramics is their porosity.

Two types of pores are seen:
- Macropores relate to pores with a diameter of 100 microns.
- Micropores relate to spaces between powder particles that are not sintered together.

Dense ceramics have macropore volume (V macro = 0) and micropores less than 5%

Macropores enhance tissue ingrowth and enhance available surface for cellular integration.

Degradation of Calcium Phosphate Ceramics.

It occurs in two steps: (i) physiochemical processes in which individual powder particles are loosened from implanted ceramic, and (ii) ingestion and intracellular dissolution of these particles occur.

The rate of loosening of individual powder particles from the ceramic surface depends on available surface. As V macro increases the number of particles released per unit of time will increase. Rate of loosening also depends on the diameter of the necks and on solubility rate of the material.

Ceramics cannot be used in large defects because tensile loading can lead to fatigue failure.

In dentistry ceramics are used : (i) as granules to repair periodontal defects, (ii) as tooth roots to prevent resorption of jaws, and (iii) as granulate blocks to augment the ridge.

When particles are used they have a diameter of 0.1 to 0.5 mm (so called granulate).

Dense Hydroxyapatite (HA).

A popular bone substitute, is non-resorbable and osteophilic when in a tightly dense crystalline structure. It is an inorganic material and cannot grow or fixate itself to the implant. It is very hard and is difficult to cut with a knife or bur. This material is used for ridge augmentation and is commonly used to recontour the facial plate.

Porous Hydroxyapatite.

These are resorbable when placed into bone or soft tissue. Their primary indication is when bone can grow next to the material and then replace it.

All calcium phosphate compounds resorb at low pH.

Advantages of Dense Non-resorbable HA

- These are inert, biocompatible,
- Do not induce inflammatory or foreign body reaction when implanted into tissues.
- No immune reaction, no local or systemic toxicity.
- Bone can grow to surface of HA without any interposing connective tissue and an ionic bond may form between bone and implanted material.

Bone Physiology

The cells responsible for formation of bone are the osteoblasts. The cells responsible for resorption are osteoclasts. Both osteoblasts and osteoclasts are derived from undifferentiated mesenchymal cells. The materials used for ridge augmentation (except materials that act by osteogenesis) influence one of these processes. Osteoinductive materials act on undifferentiated mesenchymal cells whereas osteoconductive materials act on osteoblasts. Osteogenesis takes place independent of the presence of these cells.

Preprosthetic Surgery Involving Bone Grafting

Classic methods of preprosthetic rehabilitation have involved bone grafting with particulate and other forms of autogenous osseous material, followed by vestibuloplasty to provide vestibular depth for later construction of a conventional prosthesis. In the fully resected and hemiresected mandible, titanium mesh implants have been used to control bone regeneration and to contain the bone graft material.

Use of Bone Grafts to Restore Ridges.

In the past, patients presenting with excessively resorbed alveolar ridges underwent grafting procedures with autogenous bone using rib grafts or iliac crest grafts.

Disadvantage. They maintain the ridge for 1-3 years but get resorbed over a period of time.

Use of Particulate Ceramic Implants in Restoring Alveolar Ridges.
Hydroxyapatite particles were used for augmenting ridge.

Disadvantages

- Hydroxyapatite alone does not produce bone regeneration; it requires osteoblasts for bone formation.
- Soft tissue covers the hydroxyapatite particles and this mass can lead to micro and macro movements. This is inconsistent with good prosthodontic base support and can lead to paresthesia and discomfort.

Use of Particulate Ceramic Implants Together with Autogenous Cancellous Bone.
Hydroxyapatite particles were utilized along with autogenous bone grafts. It was done in order to produce a lamellated structure of alveolar bone to slow the resorptive process.

Xenografts to Restore Alveolar Ridges.
A porous xenograft obtained from bovine sources has been used to restore alveolar ridges. This graft is subjected to a series of procedures that results in elimination of the organic material. The inorganic portion is left behind (contains HA and other materials like carbonate and tricalcium phosphate). Due to this, there will be some osteoclastic resorption of the material. This, along with favorable remodeling of bone helps to maintain the ridge for some time.

Use of Endosteal Implants in Maintaining Alveolar Bone.
A recent development in preprosthetic surgery has evolved with the use of endosteal implants in minor types of bone reconstruction.

Precautions to take during extraction to reduce ridge resorption.
The labial plate of bone is thinner than the palatal plate and so is remodeled or lost after extraction, periodontal disease or trauma to a greater extent. When a tooth is being-removed the labial plate should be preserved. The labial periosteal covering should remain intact as its inner layer is responsible for bone remodeling. The cortical bone receives 80% of its arterial supply and 100% of its venous return from the periosteum. So, careful extraction is indicated to reduce bone loss. If bone has to be removed it should be at the expense of the palatal plate. Also, pathologic tissue remaining should be removed after extraction.

Bone Augmentation Processes

Osteoconduction. Characterizes bone growth by apposition, from and on existing bone. This process occurs in the presence of bone or differentiated mesenchymal cells.

The healing of bone around an osseo-integrated implant is an osteoconductive process and follows typical remodeling at the bone-implant interface.

The most commonly used osteoconductive materials are alloplastic products. These are synthetic and come in a variety of textures, particle sizes, and shapes. These are: (i) ceramics, (ii) polymers, and (iii) composites.

Ceramics are most commonly used and can be (i) bioactive, e.g. calcium phosphatic materials, and (ii) bioinert, e.g. Al_2O_3, TiO_2.

These do not have any direct bonding with host bone and are mechanically held in contact with bone.

Bioactive materials form a chemical bond with the bone, e.g. HA, beta tricalcium phosphate.

Allografts have also been used, e.g. frozen bone.

Disadvantages

- Contamination or allergic reaction can occur.
- Disease transmission can occur.
- Additional surgical site may be needed.

Osteoinduction. It is capable of inducing the transformation of undifferentiated cells into osteoblasts or chondroblasts in an area where this is not an expected behavior. The most common osteoinductive cells are allografts.

Advantages

- Elimination of donor site in the patient.
- Availability.

It is obtained from cadavers, is processed and stored in various sizes and shapes in bone banks for future use. These are of three types:

- *Frozen bone* is removed from cadavers, directly frozen, and irradiated to reduce the immense reaction in the patient.
- *Freeze dried bone* includes an additional desiccating step. It works mainly through an osteoconductive process.
- *Demineralized freeze-dried bone (DFDBs)* are also obtained from a disease-free person. The bone is washed in distilled water and ground to a particle size of 25-150 mm. The powder is demineralized in 0.6 N HCI or nitric acid for 6-16 hours.

After dehydration, it is sterilized in ethylene oxide and freeze dried to further decrease antigenicity. Several tests are done to evaluate the safety of this process, and acid demineralization process destroys any viruses and pathogens. The calcium and phosphate salts are removed form bone in the reducing process.

The bone remaining from this treatment possesses organic osteogenic growth factors in the matrix necessary for bone formation like BMP, platelet-derived growth factor and transforming growth factor. Cortical bone contains most of the BMP in bone.

Osteogenesis. Refers to a material capable of forming bone even in the absence of local undifferentiated mesenchymal cells. Osteogenic graft materials are composed of living bone cells which produce large amounts of growth factors for bone, e.g. autogenous bone.

Autogenous iliac bone grafts or local bone grafts from maxillary tuberosity, ascending ramus or mental symphysis are common donor sites. Medullary or trabecular bone contains bone cells in largest concentration. Cells should be stored in sterile saline, Ringer's lactate solution, or sterile 5% dextrose and water to maintain cell vitality. Distilled water is contraindicated for this purpose.

Autogenous bone has an inorganic matrix containing osteoblasts, osteocytes, osteoclasts, and osteogenic proteins.

Membranous bone harvested from the mandibular symphysis represents an excellent source of autogenous bone. It has characteristics like early revascularization, high BMP potential, and number of living cells.

Applications

- Five-wall defect.
- Healthy tooth extraction
- Cyst on lateral aspect of bone.
- Four-wall defect, e.g. loss of labial wall on extraction site. Use DFDB's on bone.
- Two-wall to three-wall defect, e.g. periodontal infected tooth extraction autogenous bone chips on bone.
- One-wall defect, e.g. onlay graft, autogenous bone block on bone, and DFDB on autogenous graft.

Procedures for Ridge Augmentation

Procedures can be divided into two parts: (i) techniques to correct the condition, and (ii) techniques to compensate for the problem.

The ultimate selection of the technique depends upon health of patient, anatomic conditions and experience of the operator. Those techniques that retain original bone composition in denture-bearing area give the best result.

Techniques to Correct Alveolar Atrophy

- Direct augmentation of superior border of mandible
- Direct augmentation of atrophic maxilla
- Augmentation of inferior border of mandible
- Augmentation of inferior border of mandible with pedicle and interpositional bone grafts.
- Combined vertical and horizontal osteotomies for mandibular augmentation.
- Augmentation of atrophic maxillary ridge with pedicle and interpositional bone grafts.

- Augmentation with synthetic graft materials.
- Labial augmentation of undercut anterior mandibular ridge.
- Lingual rest technique.
- Visor osteotomy.

Techniques to Compensate for Alveolar Atrophy

- Vestibuloplasty (submucosal vestibuloplasty)
- Lowering of the floor of the mouth (lingual vestibuloplasty)
- Prong dentures
- Implants
- Zygomaticoplasty, tuberoplasty
- Lowering the mental foramen.

Direct Augmentation of the Superior Border of Mandible

Procedure

- The mucosa is infiltrated with LA containing epinephrine.
- An incision is made down to the bone from one end of the retromolar pad to the other, splitting the crestal tissue.
- The buccolabial mucoperiosteal flap is reflected.
- Mental nerves are identified and freed to prevent them from being stretched.
- The lingual flap is reflected to the level of the mylohyoid muscle (additionally loosened by submucous dissection).
- If autogenous graft is to be used for this procedure, two segments about 15 cm long are obtained from fifth to ninth ribs.
- One rib is contoured by vertical scoring on the inner surface or by bending with a curved forceps.
- The second rib is cut into pieces of 4-6 mm and is used to be packed against the first rib.
- Before placement, the level of remaining ridge is evaluated and if needed, grooves are cut to reduce the height.
- The posterior aspect of rib should be placed towards the mylohyoid shelf.
  The rib is fixed by three intraosseous ligature wires: one placed through each mylohyoid shelf, and one placed anteriorly in the midline.
- Closure of the flaps is done with a continuous polyglycolic acid horizontal mattress suture starting in retromolar pad region. After the first two sutures are placed, bone chips are placed in the region between the flap and first rib to increase the width of the ridge.
- After the flaps are completely adapted with horizontal mattress sutures, a spiral suture is used to provide a tighter closure.

A vestibuloplasty is then done after 3-6 months to appose the denture-bearing area that has been newly added. When iliac bone is to be used for mandibular augmentation, cortico-cancellous bone and marrow is obtained. (Guersey, 1979). Grafts are fixed to the mandible with circum mandibular wires passing through holes in the grafts. Cancellous bone and marrow are packed into any spaces between graft and flap.

Direct Augmentation of Atrophic Maxilla (Baker and Connole)

- A contoured rib was used for augmentation of maxilla. A crestal incision is made starting at the tuberosity and continuing forward till mobile tissue is encountered.
- The palatal and buccolabial flaps are elevated maximally. The ribs are contoured and placed so that it is lateral to the crest of ridge in the posterior areas and in front of the ridge anteriorly. It is secured with four inter-osseous wires and cancellous chips and marrow are packed lateral and medial to the rib and in any gaps between the rib and maxilla.

Augmentation of Inferior Border of Mandible. (Reported in use by Sanders and Cox).

Advantages

- Does not obliterate the vestibule thereby permitting an interim denture to be worn immediately.
- Does not change vertical dimension.

- Makes secondary vestibuloplasty much easier.
- Does not subject graft to high masticatory forces.

Disadvantages

- An extraoral scar.
- Possibility of altering facial appearance.
- Failure to change the shape of the superior surface of the mandible.

Technique. (by Sanders) involves a continuous submandibular incision from angle to angle. Two ribs approximately 15-20 cm long are obtained and bent by scoring and removal of inner cortex. Three or four transosseous holes are drilled in the lower border of the mandible and 21 gauge wires are passed through them. One rib is then abutted against the lingual aspect of the lower border and the other against the buccal border. The space between the ribs is packed with cortical chips and the entire graft is fixed by tightening the wires around it in a circumferential manner. The wound is then closed in layers and a pressure dressing is placed. Vestibuloplasty can be performed in 3-6 months.

Further Reading

1. Atwood DA. Some clinical factors related to rate of resorption. J Prosth Dent. 1962; 12(3): 441-48.
2. Klemeth E. A review of residual ridge resorption and bone density. J Prosth Dent. 1996; 75: 512-4.
3. Ronald V Lams. Contour changes of the alveolar process following extractions. J Prosth Dent. 1960; 10(1):25-32.
4. Kelsey CC. Alveolar bone resorption under complete dentures. J Prosth Dent. 1971; 25(2): 152-61.
5. Sobolik C F. Alveolar bone resorption. J Prosth Dent. 1960; 10(4):612-19.
6. Jehangiri L et al. Current perspectives in residual ridge remodelling. J Prosth Dent.1998; 80:224-37.
7. McCord et al. Registration stage I. Br. Dental J. 2000; 188(10): 529-36.

MULTIPLE CHOICE QUESTIONS

1. **Residual ridge resorption may increase**
   a. After labial alveoloplasty
   b. Patient wearing immediate dentures
   c. Denture with zero degree teeth
   d. a and c

2. **_____ is the capability of a surgical procedure to induce bone formation through the differentiation of osteoblasts**
   a. Osteogenesis
   b. Osteoconduction
   c. Osteoinduction
   d. None of the above

3. **An example for an allograft is**
   a. Rib graft   b. Freeze dried bone
   c. Ceramics   d. Composite

4. **DFDB's show _____ phenomenon**
   a. Osteoinduction
   b. Osteoconduction
   c. Osteogenesis
   d. None of the above

5. **Frozen bone is**
   a. Removed from cadavers, frozen and irradiated
   b. Is obtained from a disease free person and washed in distilled water
   c. Are grafts obtained from intraoral sites. Ex : Maxillary tuberosity
   d. None of the above

6. **An order IV type of residual ridge is**
   a. Knife edged
   b. High well rounded
   c. Post extraction
   d. Severely resorbed

7. **Statement that is false is**
   a. Increase in PTH results in more resorption of bone
   b. Decrease in vitamin D results in less resorption of bone
   c. "The damping effect" of bone and mucoperiosteum can reduce resorption
   d. All are false

Short notes

1. **Factors influencing residual ridge resorption.**

5

ANATOMICAL CONSIDERATIONS IN IMPRESSION PROCEDURES

Introduction
Macroscopic anatomy, maxillary limiting, and supporting
    structures, Microscopic anatomy
Macroscopic anatomy, mandible, limiting and supporting
    structures, Microscopic anatomy

INTRODUCTION

For the dentures and their supporting tissues to coexist for a reasonable period of time, an understanding of the macroscopic and microscopic anatomy of the supporting and limiting structures involved is necessary. This will help to determine the form of the denture borders that will be harmonious with the normal function of the limiting structures around them and will help determine the selective placement of forces by the denture bases on the supporting tissues.

The foundation for dentures is made up of bone covered by mucous membrane

Each type of tissue found in the oral cavity has its own characteristic ability to resist external forces. This is important for the maintenance of health of the tissues of the basal seat and also for ensuring stability and support of the dentures. For example, nature has placed fibrous connective tissues in places where external forces are applied whereas glandular tissues are never found in such areas. The distribution of forces applied to the basal seat by dentures should be planned in relation to types of tissues seen in various parts of the basal seat.

Definitions

Retromylohyoid Area. That area in the alveolingual sulcus just lingual to the retromolar pad and that extends lingually down to the floor of the mouth and back to the retromylohyoid curtain. It is bounded anteriorly by the lingual tuberosity.

Sublingual Crescent. That crescent-shaped area on the anterior floor of the mouth formed by the lingual wall of the mandible and the adjacent sublingual fold.

Sublingual Fossa. A smooth depression on the lingual surface of the body of the mandible near the midline, above the mylohyoid line and below the alveolar crest.

Support for the Maxillary Dentures. The maxillary denture is supported by two pairs of bones, the maxillae and the palatine bones.

Maxilla. There are two maxillae, each consisting of a central body and four processes.

Areas of the body and two of the processes are involved in the support of the maxillary denture.

Maxillary Tuberosity. The posterior surface of the maxillary body ends inferiorly as a convexity termed the maxillary tuberosity.

This is important for the support of the denture. They provide resistance against the horizontal movements of the maxillary denture. The medial and lateral walls resist the horizontal and torquing forces that would move the denture base in a lateral or palatal direction. The posterior wall resists movement in an anterior direction.

Alveolar Processes. These arise from the body of each maxilla. The alveolar process consists of two parallel plates of cortical bone, buccolingual or labiolingual which unite behind the last molar tooth to form the maxillary tuberosity. They develop as the teeth form and are resorbed when teeth are lost.

The socket surrounding the root of each natural tooth is the alveolus, and the bony ridge that supports the teeth is the alveolar ridge. The bony process remaining after teeth has been lost is the residual alveolar ridge.

After the natural teeth are lost, shrinkage of the alveolar ridge occurs. This is rapid at first, but then continues at a reduced rate throughout life.

If a denture is made soon after the teeth are removed, the foundation may be large but may also be tender to pressure. This may be due to incomplete healing resulting in a lack of cortical bone over the crest of the residual alveolar ridge.

If on the other hand, the teeth have been out for many years the residual ridge may become quite small, and there may be large nutrient canals and sharp bony spicules near the crest of the ridge which may limit the pressure applied.

Palatine Processes. The palatine processes of the maxillary bones arise as broad, horizontal plates from the bodies of the maxillae. The two horizontal plates are united in the midline by the midpalatal suture. The horizontal palatine processes of the maxillae appear to resist resorption.

Due to the resorption of adjacent structures, this area may become prominent and may act as a fulcrum point around which the maxillary denture will rotate.

Incisive Fossa. It is located in the midline of the palate, posterior to the maxillary central incisors or in the edentulous mouth slightly to the palatal side of the anterior palatal alveolar plate. The nasopalatine nerve and vessels exit to the palate at right angles to the margins of this bony fossa.

The denture base should be relieved over this area. Failure to do so will result in pressure in the nerves and blood vessels with a decrease in blood supply to the anterior part of the palate, nerve irritation and burning symptoms.

Palatine Bones. The horizontal plates of the palatine bones[1] articulate with the posterior rough border of the horizontal palatal processes of the maxilla. The posterior border of the horizontal plates of the palatine bones unite in the midline to form the sharp posterior nasal spine (the posterior margins of the hard palate serve as the anterior attachment for the aponeurosis of the soft palate).

Greater Palatine Foramina. It is located medial to the third molar at the junction of the maxillae and the horizontal plate of the palatine bone. A groove extending anteriorly from the foramen contains anterior palatine nerve and vessels.

Bone of the Basal Seat. Factors that influence the form and size of the supporting bone of the basal seat include: (i) its original size and consistency, (ii) patient's general health and resistance, (iii) force developed by the musculature, (iv) severity and location of periodontal disease, (v) forces occurring from wearing of dental restorations, (vi) surgery at the time of removal of teeth, and (vii) relative length of time-different parts of the jaws have been edentulous.

Pterygoid Hamulus. It is a thin curved process at the terminal end of the medial pterygoid plate of the sphenoid bone. The hamular notch is located between the pterygoid hamulus and the alveolar tuberosity.[2]

MACROSCOPIC ANATOMY

Table 5.1 gives correlation of anatomic landmarks.

Table 5.1. Correlation of anatomic landmarks

Mandibular		
Labial frenum	→	Labial notch
Labial vestibule	→	Labial flange
Buccal frenum	→	Buccal notch
Buccal vestibule	→	Buccal flange
Residual alveolar ridge	→	Alveolar groove
Retromolar pad	→	Retromolar fossa
Maxilla		
Labial frenum	→	Labial notch
Buccal frenum	→	Buccal notch
Coronoid bulge	→	Coronoid contour
Residual alveolar ridge	→	Alveolar groove
Maxillary tuberosity	→	Maxillary tubercular fossa
Hamular notch	→	Pterygomaxillary seal
Posterior palatal seal region	→	Posterior palatal seal
Fovea palatinae	→	Fovea palatinae
Median palatine raphae	→	Median palatine groove
Incisive papilla	→	Incisive fossa
Rugae	→	Rugae

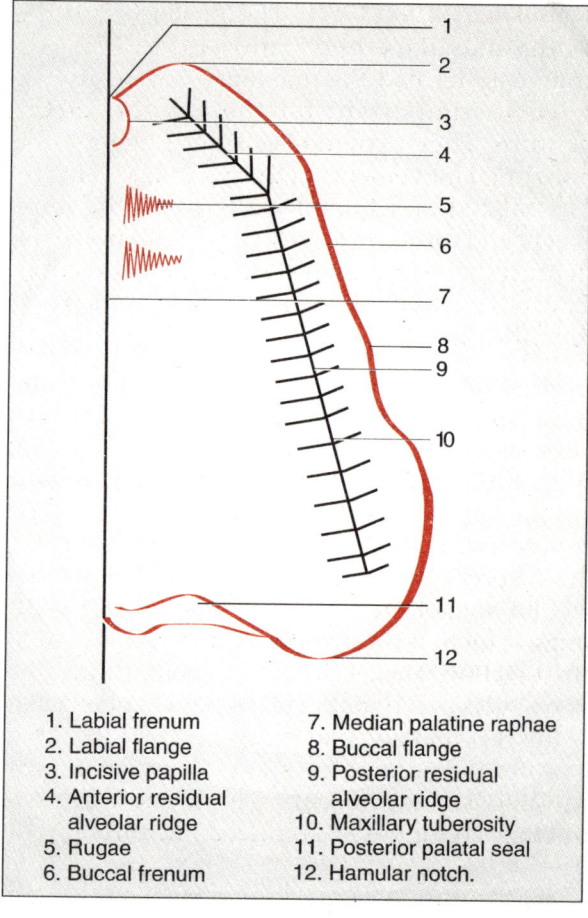

1. Labial frenum
2. Labial flange
3. Incisive papilla
4. Anterior residual alveolar ridge
5. Rugae
6. Buccal frenum
7. Median palatine raphae
8. Buccal flange
9. Posterior residual alveolar ridge
10. Maxillary tuberosity
11. Posterior palatal seal
12. Hamular notch.

Fig. 5.1. The maxillary denture base, anatomic and denture landmarks.

Maxillary Limiting Structures

The denture base should cover the maximum area possible within the limits of the health and function of the tissue it covers and contacts. This means that the denture should be made in such a manner that it covers all the available basal seat tissues without causing soreness at the denture border and without interfering with the action of the structures that contact or surround it (Fig. 5.1).

Labial Frenum

Labial frenum is a fold of mucous membrane located at the median line. It contains no muscle of significance and so can be surgically excised if it extends close to the ridge. This band of tissue starts superiorly in a fan shape from the mucous membrane of the lips and converges, to its terminal attachment on the labial side of the ridge. It can be single or double and it inserts in a vertical direction.

Significance. The labial notch in the labial flange of the denture should be wide and deep enough to allow the frenum to pass through it without manipulation of the lip.

Labial Vestibule

The area that extends on both sides from the labial frenum to the buccal frenum is the labial vestibule. The reflection of the mucous membrane superiorly determines the height.

Orbicularis Oris[4]

Orbicularis oris muscle rests on the labial flange and teeth of the denture. Its tone depends on the support it receives from the thickness of the labial flange and position of the arch of teeth.

The fibers of the orbicularis oris passes horizontally through the lips and anastomoses with fibers of the buccinator muscle. They have only an indirect effect on the extent of the impression and denture base.

Buccal Frenum

Buccal frenum is a fold of mucous membrane that extends from the buccal mucous membrane reflection area towards the slope or crest of the residual ridge.

It can be a single or double fold or broad and fan-shaped.

The caninus muscle attaches beneath and influences the position of the buccal frenum. In addition to this, the orbicularis oris pulls the frenum forward and the buccinator muscle pulls it backward.

Significance of this frenum is that the buccal notch in the denture should be broad enough to allow movement of the frenum. Inadequate relief can lead to dislodgement of the denture when the patient smiles.

Buccal Vestibule

Buccal vestibule is located opposite the tuberosity and extends from the buccal frenun to the hamular or pterygomaxillary notch. The size of the buccal vestibule is influenced by
- Contraction of the buccinator
- Position of the mandible
- Amount of bone lost from the maxilla
- Distal end is affected by the masseter
- Movement of the mandible.

The width of the buccal vestibule is reduced as the mandible moves forward or to the opposite side. The width and shape of the posterior part of the buccal vestibule are altered by lateral movements of the mandible.

The buccal vestibular space area is higher than any other part of the border.

Pterygomaxillary or Hamular Notch

Pterygomaxillary or hamular notch is located between the tuberosity of the maxilla and hamulus of the medial pterygoid plate. The posterior palatal seal should be placed through the center of the deep part of the hamular notch, because no muscle or ligament is present at a level necessary to prevent placement of extra pressure.

The thickness of the distal end of the buccal flange of the denture should be adjusted to accommodate the ramus, coronoid process and masseter as they function.

If the distal end of the flange is thick, the denture will be displaced during opening or lateral movements of the mandible.

Fovea palatinae[8] are indentations near the midline of the palate. It is formed by a coalescence of several mucous gland ducts. They are close to the vibrating line and always in soft tissue.

MICROSCOPIC ANATOMY

Maxillary Structures

The clinical procedures used in making impressions are directly related to the gross anatomic structures of the oral cavity and their function. The response of the individual cellular components that make up the basal seat determines the ultimate success of the dentures in terms of preservation of the residual ridges and comfort of the patient.[5]

An awareness of the microscopic anatomy of the mucous membrane and bone that form the residual ridge is essential in the development of a border in form and length and in the elective placement of pressures on the basal seat during impression making. The **mucosa** of the oral cavity is formed by stratified squamous epithelium and an adjacent layer of connective tissue called the lamina propria.

The **submucosa** is formed by connective tissue that varies in character from dense to loose areolar tissue. It may contain glandular, fat, or muscle cells and transmits the blood and nerve supply to the mucosa.

The submucosa is largely responsible for offering support to the denture because it forms the bulk of the mucous membrane.

When the mucosal layer is thin over the bone, the soft tissue will be non-resilient and will not aid in the retention of the denture. It may be loosely attached to the periosteum of the residual ridge or may be inflamed or edematous.

Oral Mucosa

Masticatory Mucosa. Covers: (i) the crest of the residual ridge including the residual attached gingiva firmly attached to underlying bone, and (ii) Hard palate—it is characterized by a well-defined keratinized layer on its outermost surface that is subject to changes depending on the stimulus.

Lining Mucosa. It is found on mucous membranes that are not firmly attached to the periosteum of the bone. It covers the lips and cheeks, vestibular spaces, alveololingual sulcus, soft palate, ventral surface of the tongue and unattached gingiva found on the slopes of the residual ridges.

It is devoid of a keratinized layer and is freely movable.

Residual Ridge

Mucous Membrane. This is firmly attached to the periosteum of the bone of the maxilla by the connective tissue of the submucosa. The stratified squamous epithelium is thickly keratinized.

Submucosa. It is devoid of glandular or fat cells. It has dense collagenous fibers that are contiguous with lamina propria.

It provides the resiliency for the primary support of the upper denture.

Bone. The outer surface of the bone in the region of the crest of the upper residual ridge may be compact in nature, being made up of haversian systems. The compact bone and the tightly attached mucous membrane make the crest of the residual ridge histologically best able to provide primary support for the upper denture.

As the mucous membrane extends from the crest along the slope of the upper residual ridge to the reflection, it loses its firm attachment to the underlying bone. This marks the end of the residual attached mucous membrane. This area has non-keratinized or slightly keratinized epithelium, and submucosa has glandular tissue and elastic fibers. Lesser stress will be placed in this region during the impression procedures because the impression material in this area is closer to escape ways.

Hard Palate. The epithelium is keratinized. The soft tissue varies in consistency and thickness in different locations.

Anterolaterally, the submucosa of the hard palate contains adipose tissue and postero-laterally it contains glandular tissue. These tissues should be recorded in the resting condition. If they are displaced in the final impression, they tend to return to normal form within the completed denture base, creating an unseating force on the denture or causing soreness in the patient's mouth.

In the median palatal suture area, submucosa is extremely thin. The mucosal layer is nearly in contact with the underlying bone. As a result of this, tissue in this area is non-resilient and no stress should be placed here during the impression procedure. If pressure is placed: (i) denture may rock over the centre of the palate when vertical forces are applied to the teeth, and (ii) Extra pressure can result in excruciating pain.

Incisive Papilla

In the submucosa nasopalatine vessels and nerves are present.

Limiting Structures

Vestibular Spaces. The epithelium is thin and non-keratinized. The submucosa is thick and contains large amounts of loose areolar tissue and elastic fibers. The nature of the submucosa makes this region easily movable.

Hamular Notch. The submucosa is thick and is made up of loose areolar tissue. Additional pressure can be placed on this tissue at the center of the notch to complete the posterior palatal seal. The histologic structure allows it to be displaced without any trauma.

MACROSCOPIC ANATOMY

Mandible

The mandible is the movable member of the stomatognathic system. The body of the mandible is horseshoe-shaped and carries the alveolar process (Fig. 5.2.).

The distal portion of each side continues upward and backward into the mandibular ramus.

The ramus divides into the coronoid and condylar process. The condyle is the articular surface of the condylar process. The condyle is connected with the ramus by the constricted mandibular neck.

Coronoid Process

Coronoid process is a triangular bony projection that varies in shape and size. The convex anterior border of the coronoid process continues into the anterior border of the ramus. When the mandible is protruded, the anterior border of the ramus extends toward the alveolar tuberosity which is located medial to the ramus and so if the distobuccal flange of the maxillary denture is too thick, the denture may be dislodged during lateral excursions.

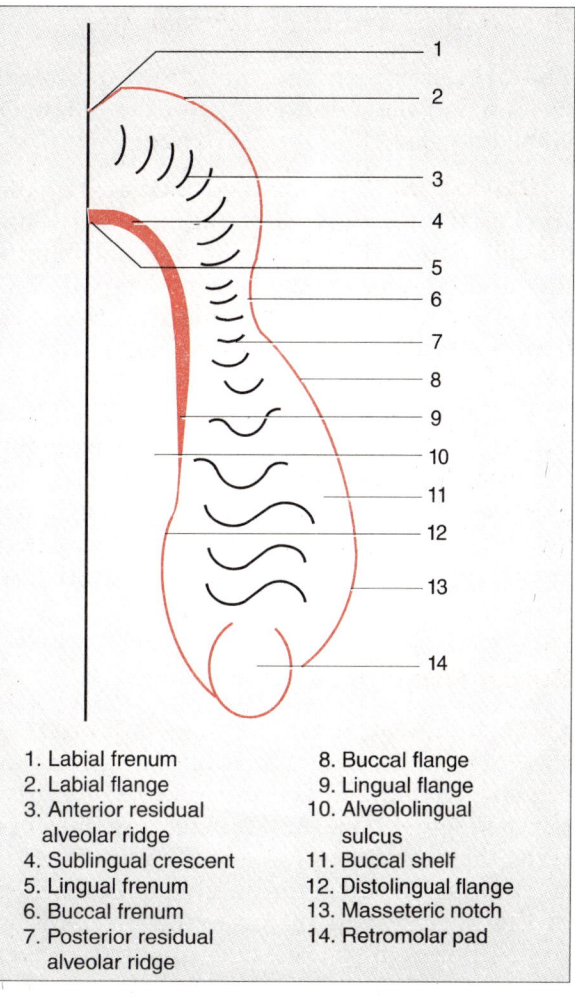

1. Labial frenum
2. Labial flange
3. Anterior residual alveolar ridge
4. Sublingual crescent
5. Lingual frenum
6. Buccal frenum
7. Posterior residual alveolar ridge
8. Buccal flange
9. Lingual flange
10. Alveololingual sulcus
11. Buccal shelf
12. Distolingual flange
13. Masseteric notch
14. Retromolar pad

Fig. 5.2. The mandibular denture base anatomic and denture landmarks.

Crest of the Residual Ridge

The crest of the alveolar ridge is covered by fibrous connective tissue that in most cases is firmly attached to the underlying periosteum. But the crest is not suitable for resisting external forces because in many cases the underlying bone is cancellous and without a good cortical plate covering it. It is considered as a secondary stress bearing area.

Buccal Shelf and Buccal Flange Area

The area between the mandibular buccal frenum and the anterior edge of the masseter is the buccal shelf or buccal flange.

Boundaries. It is bounded medially by the crest of the residual ridge, anteriorly by the buccal frenum, laterally by the external oblique line and distally by the retromolar pad. The buccal shelf is very wide and is at right angles to the vertical occlusal forces. So, it is a primary stress-bearing area.

The bone of the buccal shelf area is very dense because the trabeculation of bone is so arranged to resist the forces of the elevator muscles.

Its density, mucosal covering, relation to the vertical closure of the jaws are favorable to best resist the forces transmitted through the denture base.

Buccal Flange Area

The mandibular attachment of this muscle is close to the crest of the ridge in the molar regions. Here the fibers run anteroposteriorly, paralleling the bone, and the denture does not resist the contracting force of the muscle.

The inferior part of the buccinator is attached in the buccal shelf of the mandible, and so contraction of the muscle does not lift the lower denture.

Mylohyoid Ridge

The shape and inclination of the mylohyoid ridge varies greatly among edentulous patients. It is an irregular bony crest extending from the third molar region to the lower border of the mandible in the region of the chin. It is more prominent from the third molar to the second bicuspid area.

Relation of the mylohyoid and level of the muscle. Anteriorly, the muscle attaches close to the inferior border of the mandible and as the ridge goes posteriorly the muscle may be flush with the superior border of the residual ridge.

Anteriorly only the height of the lingual flange will be affected by the muscle, posteriorly the angle of the posterior lingual flange in the molar region is also affected.

The contour of the mylohyoid ridge also affects the lingual flange.

Lingual Tuberosity

The lingual tuberosity is an irregular bony prominence on the distal end of the mylohyoid. When this area is excessively prominent or rough, it may become an undercut area which may have to be removed surgically.

Mental spines are situated on the lingual aspect of the mandibular body in the midline slightly above the border. These may be divided into a superior and inferior section or right and left prominence.

Limiting Structures

Mandibular dentures should extend as far possible within the limits of health and function of the tissues and structures that surround and support them. This is more difficult to achieve in the mandible because the structures in the lingual side of the mandible are more complicated and difficult to control than those on the buccal and labial. This is because there is a greater range of movement and speed of action of these structures.

Labial Frenum

The labial frenum contains a band of fibrous connective tissue that helps to attach the orbicularis oris. The frenum is quite sensitive and active and must be carefully fitted to maintain seal without causing soreness.

Labial Flange

Labial flange is the part of the denture that extends between the labial frenum and the buccal frenum.

This flange is limited in extension because the fibers of the orbicularis oris and the incisivus labi inferioris are close to the ridge. It is limited inferiorly by the reflection of the mucous membrane, labially by the lip and internally by the residual ridge.

The labial flange can be extended in length and thickness to supply necessary support to the lip because there is no muscle extending from the residual ridge to the lip.

Buccal Frenum

Buccal frenum is a fold of membrane extending from the buccal mucous membrane reflection to or towards the slope of the crest of the residual ridge in the region just distal to the cuspid eminence. It may be single or double, broad U-shaped or narrow V-shaped. The reflection is in an anteroposterior direction. In the areas of the buccal frenum, there should be less extension of the denture because of the muscular and fibrous tissues present there.

Buccal Vestibule

Buccal vestibule extends from the buccal frenum posteriorly to the outside back corner of the retromolar pad and from the crest of the residual alveolar ridge to the cheek.

External Oblique Ridge and Buccal Flange

External oblique ridge is a ridge of dense bone extending from just above the mental foramen superiorly and distally becoming continuous with the anterior border of the ramus.

The buccal flange area that begins immediately posterior to the buccal frenum and extends to the anterior border of the masseter swings wide into the cheek at nearly right angles to the biting force, providing the lower denture with its greatest surface for resistance to vertical occlusal forces.

The external oblique ridge does not govern the extension of the buccal flange because resistance encountered in the region varies widely.

The buccal flange may extend to, onto or over the external oblique ridge depending on the location of the mucobuccal fold. The palpation of the external oblique ridge is valuable in helping to ascertain the relative amount of resistance of the border tissues in this region.

Masseter Muscle Region

The distobuccal borders of the mandibular denture must converge rapidly to avoid displacement because of contracting pressure of the masseter muscle whose anterior fibers pass outside the buccinator in this region.

When the masseter contracts it alters the shape and size of the distobuccal end of the lower buccal vestibule. It pushes inward against the buccinator muscle and suctorial pad of cheek.

The factors that influence the action of masseter muscle are: (i) shape of the mandible, and (ii) origin of the muscle.

Distal Extension of Mandibular Impression

The distal extent of the mandibular impression is limited by: (i) ramus of the mandible, (ii) by buccinator fibers that cross from the buccal to the lingual as they attach to the pterygo-mandibular raphe and superior constrictor, and (iii) sharpness of the lateral bony boundaries of the retromolar fossa.

The retromolar fossa is formed by the crossing of the internal and external oblique ridges ascending the ramus. If impression extends on to the ramus, the buccinator and adjacent tissues will be compressed between the hard denture border and sharp external oblique ridge.

This will cause soreness and will also limit the action of the buccinator. The desirable distal extension is slightly to the lingual of these bony prominences and includes the retromolar pad.

Retromolar Pad and Region

The retromolar pad forms the posterior limit of the lower denture. It is a triangular soft pad of tissue at the distal end of the lower ridge and should be covered by the denture to provide the seal in this region.

Structures, seen are:

1. Buccinator fibers that enter it from the buccal side
2. Superior pharyngeal constrictor fibers that enter it from the lingual side
3. Pterygomandibular raphe enters it from the superoposterior inside corner. These structures, limit the extent of the denture and prevent placement of excess pressure in this area.

Retromolar Papilla

Retromolar papilla is a small pear-shaped area anterior to retromolar pad. It has dense fibrous connective tissue.

Lingual Borders

The lingual tissues offer more direct resistance than the labial and buccal tissues and so will not tolerate overextension of the lingual flange. They are easily distorted during the impression procedure and overextension will cause soreness and dislodgement of the denture by tongue movement.

The lingual borders of the mandibular impression are easily carried down along the bony surface of the mandible into the undercut below the mylohyoid ridge but extension of the lingual flange under the mylohyoid ridge cannot be tolerated in function because it will displace the denture, causing soreness and limiting function, unless the flange is made parallel to the mylohyoid muscle when it is contracted.

Action of the Floor of the Mouth

The mylohyoid muscle arises from the whole length of the mylohyoid line, extending from 1 mm back of the distal end of the mylohyoid ridge to the lingual anterior portion of the mandible at the symphysis.

Medially they join fibers of mylohyoid muscle from the opposite side and posteriorly continue to the hyoid bone.

The posterior part of the mylohyoid muscle in the molar region affects the lingual impression border in swallowing and moving the tongue.

Mylohyoid Muscle and Ridge

An extension of the lingual flange beyond the palpable portion of the ridge, but not into the undercut has certain advantages:

1. Lack of direct pressure on this sharp edge of bone will reduce discomfort. If placed on the ridge, vertical and lateral stress cause pain.
2. Lingual border seal will be completed in the retromylohyoid fossa.
3. Flange guides the tongue onto the top of the lingual flange of the sublingual gland region.

Sublingual Gland Region

In the premolar region on the lingual side of the ridge, the sublingual gland rests above the mylohyoid muscle. When the floor of the mouth rises, the gland comes, close to the crest of the ridge and reduces the vertical space available for flange extension in anterior part of the mouth.

Lingual Frenum. Lingually attached close to the crest of the ridge.

Alveololingual Sulcus

The alveololingual sulcus[3] is a space between the residual ridge and the tongue, extends posteriorly from the lingual frenum to the retromylohyoid curtain. Part of it is available for the lingual flange of the denture. It is considered as three regions.

1. Anterior Region. It extends from the lingual frenum to where the mylohyoid ridge curves down to the level of the sulcus. Here a depression—premylohyoid fossa is seen. This fossa results from concavity of the mandible joining the convexity of the mylohyoid ridge.

2. *The Middle Region.* This extends from premylohyoid fossa to the distal end of the mylohyoid ridge curving medially from the body of the mandible. The curvature is caused by the prominence of the mylohyoid ridge.

3. *The Posterior Region.* This is the retromylohyoid space or fossa. It extends from the end of the mylohyoid ridge to the retromylohyoid curtain being bounded on the lingual by the anterior tonsillar pillar and on the buccal by the mylohyoid muscle, mandibular ramus and the retromolar pad. The support for the romylohyoid curtain is provided by part of the superior pharyngeal constrictor. The action of this muscle and the tongue determine the posterior extent of the lingual flange. The distal border should extend posteriorly to contact the retromylohyoid curtain when the tip of the tongue is placed against the front part of the upper residual ridge.

The Retromylohyoid Space

The retromylohyoid space is bounded medially by the anterior tonsillar pillar, posteriorly by the retromylohyoid curtain (which is formed posteriorly by the superior constrictor muscle) laterally by the mandible and pterigomandibular raphe, anteriorly by the lingual tuberosity and inferiorly by the mylohyoid muscle.

Lingual Flange

The lingual flange of the denture occupies the alveololingual sulcus. The distal end of the alveololingual sulcus ends at the retromylohyoid curtain.

The distal extent of the lingual flange is partly limited by the glossopalatine arch, which is formed by the glossopalatine muscle and the lingual extension of the superior constrictor. Anteriorly, the flange in the molar region is influenced by the mylohyoid muscle.

MICROSCOPIC ANATOMY OF SUPPORTING TISSUES

Crest of the Residual Ridge

Mucous Membrane. It is covered by a keratinized layer and is firmly attached by its submucosa to the periosteum of the mandible. In some patients, the submucosa is loosely attached to the bone and entire crest of the residual ridge and the soft tissue covering are quite movable.

The bone over the crest of the lower residual ridge is cancellous and is made up of bony trabeculae.

Buccal Shelf

Mucous Membrane. Along the buccal shelf is more loosely attached and less keratinized than mucous membrane covering crest of the lower residual ridge.

It contains a thicker submucosal layer and fibers of the buccinator run horizontally in the submucosa immediately overlying the bone.

Bone of the buccal shelf is covered by a layer of compact bone.

Limiting Tissues

Vestibular Spaces. Mucous membrane lining the vestibular spaces is similar to that in the upper jaw. Epithelium is non-keratinized and submucosa formed of loosely arranged connective tissue fibers mixed with elastic fibers. It is freely movable.

Alveololingual Sulcus. Anteriorly the submucosa contain components of the sublingual gland. In the molar region, the submucosa attaches to the mylohyoid muscle, and the mucous membrane covering the retromylohyoid curtain is attached by its submucosa to the superior constrictor. Posterior to the superior constrictor fibers is the medial pterygoid muscle running in a vertical direction.

Retromolar Pad

Mucosa is composed of a thin non-keratinizing epithelium. Submucosa contains glandular tissue, fibers of buccinator, superior pharyngeal constrictor, pterygomandibular raphe, and tendon of temporalis.

Further Reading

1. Kolb H.R. et al. Variable dentures limiting structures of the mouth. J Prosth Dent 1966; 16(2): 194-201.
2. Van Scotter D E et al. The nature of supporting tissues for complete dentures. J Prosth Dent. 1965; 15(2):202-207.
3. Brill et al. The dynamic nature of the lower denture space. J Prosth Dent. 1965;15: 365.
4. Edwards LF et al. Some anatomic facts of the masticatory apparatus. J Prosth Dent. 1955; 15:
5. Martone et al. Anatomy of the mouth and its related structures. J Prosth Dent. 1961; 12:1009.
6. Van Scotter OE et al. The nature of supporting tissue for complete dentures. J Prosth Dent.1965; 15: 485.
7. Chen M. Reliability of the fovea palatini for determining the posterior border of the maxillary denture. J Prosth Dent. 1980; 43 :133.

MULTIPLE CHOICE QUESTIONS

1. **Regarding the buccal shelf**
   a. It is the primary stress bearing area of the mandible
   b. It is bounded anteriorly by the labial frenum and posteriorly by the buccal frenum
   c. Bone in this area is very dense
   d. a and c alone are true
   e. All are true

2. **The masseteric notch is formed by**
   a. Masseter muscle acting on buccinator
   b. Buccinator acting on the masseter
   c. External oblique ridge
   d. Masseter alone

3. **Structures seen in retromolar pad include**
   a. Fibres of masseter
   b. Fibres of superior pharyngeal constrictor
   c. Fibres of buccinator of
   d. b and c

4. **_____ is a triangular soft pad of tissue at the distal and of the mandibular ridge.**
   a. Retromolar pad
   b. Maxillary tuberosity
   c. Retromolar papilla
   d. Buccal shelf

5. **The retromylohyoid space is seen in**
   a. Anterior region of the alveololingual sulcus
   b. Middle region of the alveololingual sulcus
   c. Posterior region of alveololingual sulcus
   d. None of the above

6. **The coronoid contour is an anatomic landmark seen in the**
   a. Maxillary impression
   b. Mandibular impression
   c. Seen in the buccal shelf area of the mandible
   d. None of the above

7. **The denture should be relieved over the incisive fossa because**
   a. It may affect retention and stability
   b. It may cause discomfort to the patient
   c. It may cause burning symptoms
   d. b and c

8. **_____ does not have any muscle attachment**
   a. Maxillary labial frenum
   b. Mandibular labial frenum
   c. Maxillary buccal frenum
   d. None of the above

9. **The primary stress bearing area of the mandible is**
   a. Crest of the residual alveolar ridge
   b. Slope of the residual alveolar ridge
   c. Buccal flange
   d. Buccal shelf

FAQ's

1. **Biologic considerations for maxillary impressions.**
2. **Biologic considerations for mandibular impressions.**

6

OBJECTIVES OF IMPRESSION MAKING

INTRODUCTION

The factors in impression making include retention, stability, support, esthetics and preservation of remaining tissue.

Complete denture retention[1] is a complex phenomenon. Till the early part of the 19th century, the prospect of retention without mechanical aid was not seriously considered. It was only later the awareness came that denture bases could be and should be retained by non-mechanical means.

DEFINITIONS FOR RETENTION

According to Glossary of Prosthetic Terms, "That quality inherent in the prosthesis acting to resist the forces of dislodgement along the path of placement."

According to Boucher "Retention for a denture is its resistance to removal in a direction opposite that of its insertion."

According to Grant and Johnson "Retention is defined as the resistance it posses to withdrawal from its planned position in the mouth."

Retention is the means by which the dentures are held in position in the mouth. It is the quality inherent in a denture that resists the force of gravity, the adhesiveness of foods and forces associated with the opening of the jaws.

FACTORS AFFECTING DENTURE RETENTION

These can be divided into: (i) physical, (ii) mechanical, and (iii) physiologic forces.

Physical Factors

Physical factors include: (i) adhesion, (ii) cohesion, (iii) surface tension, (iv) viscosity, (v) gravity, (vi) capillarity, (vii) vacuum devices, and (viii) atmospheric pressure.

Mechanical Factors

Mechanical factors include: (i) undercuts, (ii) springs, (iii) friction, and (iv) magnetic forces.

Physiologic Forces

Miscellaneous Factors. These include: (i) neuromuscular control, (ii) border seal, and (iii) intimate tissue contact.

Anatomic Factors. Anatomic factors that affect denture retention include:

Size of the Denture-bearing Area. Greater the denture-bearing area, greater retention will be seen. It is because of this that more retention is generally seen in the maxillary arch than in the mandibular arch.

Relationship of Denture Base with Denture-bearing Area. If the tissues are displaced while making the impression, the same configuration will be recorded to the denture. The displaced tissue rebounds, displaces the denture and so loss of retention occurs.

Physical Factors

Adhesion

Definition. It is the physical force involved in the attraction between unlike molecules.[6] According to Boucher, adhesion is the physical attraction of unlike molecules for each other.

Effectiveness of Adhesion Depends Upon. **Close adaptation of the denture base to the supporting tissue**. Better the adaptation of denture base to the supporting tissue, better will be the retention.

Fluidity of Saliva

Watery saliva: Saliva should wet the denture base and should spread out in a thin layer. This will help in better adhesion.

Thick and ropy saliva: It is produced mainly by the palatal glands under the maxillary denture base and it builds up pressure and literally pushes the denture out of position.

Area Covered by the Denture. Amount of retention obtained by adhesion is directly related to the area covered.

Patients with small jaws cannot expect retention by adhesion to be as effective as patients with large jaws. Thus the dentures must extend to limits of health and function of oral tissues if they are to have maximum adhesion and retention.

Adhesion acts when saliva wets and sticks to the basal surfaces of dentures and at the same time to the mucous membrane of basal seat.

It is also the molecular attraction between surfaces of unlike bodies in contact. This type of adhesion is observed between denture bases and the mucous membranes of patients with xerostomia.

Wetting Characteristics. For adhesion to be accomplished between a solid and a fluid, wetting of the solid by the fluid must take place. The degree to which this occurs depends on their relative surface tension. The wetting characteristics may be described in terms of the contact angle formed with solid surface on which it is placed. A high contact angle indicates poor wetting.

Gardette in 1800 fitted a set of dentures without springs as a temporary expedient. He found later that there was retention and the dentures were functional. Richardson stated that adhesive forces retained the denture and that adhesion of solids to solids is illustrated by pressing together two plates of glass having perfect occluding surfaces. Perfect exclusion of air was required which suggested that denture bases should fit accurately if adhesive forces were to operate in their retention.

Howland in 1921 stated that adhesion was the greatest physical principle involved in denture retention. But he stated that adhesion present was in inverse ratio to viscosity of saliva which is not in accordance with the expectation from known principles.

Cohesion

Cohesion is the physical factor of electro-magnetic force acting between molecules of the same material.

It is a retentive force because it occurs in the layer of saliva between the denture base and mucosa.

Factors Affecting Cohesion

1. *Area covered by the denture*: Cohesion is directly related to the area covered by the denture if all other factors are equal.
2. Thickness of salivary film: For it to be effective in retention the saliva film should be thin.
3. Adaptation of denture base to mucosa: Close adaptation of the denture base to mucosa is needed so that only a thin film of saliva is present.

Interfacial Surface Tension

Definition. It refers to the forces involved in maintaining the attraction of two opposed ground solid plates with an intervening fluid film that resists displacing forces applied at right angles to the fluid film surface. According to Boucher it is the resistance to separation possessed by the film of liquid between two well-adapted surfaces.[7]

The intermolecular forces responsible for cohesion in a fluid act equally on all molecules within the bulk of the fluid. At the surface, one component of these forces is missing, thus resulting in a net attractive force towards the interior of the liquid. This directional energy gives rise to the phenomenon of surface tension which counteracts forces tending to break the surface of the liquid and also gives the fluid the smallest surface area.

Surface tension is found in the thin film of saliva between the denture base and the mucosa of the basal seat.

Factors Affecting Surface Tension

1. *Denture bearing area*: Surface tension is directly proportional to the size of the basal surface of dentures,
2. Capillarity,
3. Atmospheric pressure, and
4. Psychological factors.

In order to get maximum surface tension: (i) saliva should be thin and even, (ii) there should be perfect fit of the denture base without distortion, (iii) a perfect seal should be present, and (iv) denture bearing area must be large.

Page has described interfacial surface tension as a phenomenon similar to Wilson's adhesive contact (1949).

Under a dislodging force perpendicular to the fluid film, the pressure within the fluid decreases. Together with the surrounding atmospheric pressure, this creates a pressure gradient across the peripheral meniscus that has formed. The force needed to separate the glass plates is proportional to the degree of pressure gradient multiplied by the surface area involved.

The smaller the film thickness greater the pressure gradient and so more the force required to separate the glass plates.

Tyson in 1967 confirmed the importance of a thin fluid film between two plates in producing a pressure gradient maintained by surface tension. Immersing the entire system in water eliminated the pressure gradient and the effect of surface tension which in turn reduced, the required separating force. Page in 1941 developed the dubious concept of mucostatics.

Viscosity

Viscosity is the resistance to flow of a fluid resulting from intermolecular forces acting within the fluid.

When a fluid is set in motion the cohesive forces within the fluid act as a form of intermolecular friction to oppose the movement. If a fluid tends to move between parallel plates, the molecules nearest the plates move only slowly because of the adhesive forces acting, while the central molecules move the fastest.

The closer the two plates are together the nearer the fluid approaches the speed of fluid near the plates. A thin film of fluid resists flow more readily than a thicker film. Fluids having a high viscosity resist flow more effectively than those of lower viscosity.

The additional saliva will cause loss of retention of the denture, because of the resultant increase in distance between the denture and mucosa.

Gravity

The definition is self-explanatory and involves the mandibular denture mainly.

Gravity helps maintain the lower prosthesis at rest. Granewald suggested the use of gold base complete dentures of a weight similar to that of the lost teeth and alveolar process.

Capillarity

Capillary attraction or capillarity is the force (developed because of surface tension) that causes the surface of a liquid to become elevated or depressed when it is in contact with a solid.

When the adaptation of denture base to the mucosa on which it rests is sufficiently close, the space filled with saliva can act as a capillary tube and helps retain the denture.

If the contact angle is more than 90°, a differential capillary force is possible hence the result is a rise in liquid. If the contact angle is less than 90°, a differential depression of liquid occurs. The contact angle of saliva to acrylic denture base is 75°. Capillary forces resist horizontally dislodging forces and so are useful in function.

Factors influencing capillary attraction:
1. Closeness of adaptation of denture base to soft tissue. Greater the distance less is capillary force.
2. Greater the size of the denture-bearing area greater the retention.
3. Saliva that is thick and ropy decreases retention.

Atmospheric Pressure

Atmospheric pressure is the physical force of hydrostatic pressure due to the weight of atmosphere on the earth's surface.

At sea level, this force amounts to 14.7 psi. When the denture is placed in the mouth, closeness of the denture base and soft tissue expels the air. So, pressure in the impression surface is less than that of the polished surface.

The difference between these forces results in a positive force that retains the denture. When dentures are subjected to dislodging or tipping forces, it is resisted by the weight of atmospheric pressure, i.e. 14.7 1bs/inch². So, it is referred to as an emergency retentive or temporary restraining force.

Factors Affecting Atmospheric Pressure
1. Closeness of adaptation to keep air out
2. Peripheral seal.

First recognition of the possible role for atmospheric pressure is credited to Gardette in 1800, when he fitted a set of dentures without their springs as a temporary expedient but found months later that they were functional and had retention. Synder et al demonstrated in 1965 the effect of reduced atmospheric pressure on retention of maxillary complete dentures. Measurements made in a pressure chamber at 4.7 psi simulating a 30,000 foot ascent above the earth demonstrated a decrease in denture retention. With a 70% decrease in atmospheric pressure, a 50% decrease in retention was noted.

At sea level, the force of atmospheric pressure acts with approximately 14.7 psi against the external surface of the denture, provided no air or gaseous pressure exists between the denture base and tissue surface. In reality this is not possible. The effectiveness of atmospheric pressure is reduced proportionately.

Clinically, it has been observed that retention of maxillary complete dentures is reduced by inadequate posterior palatal seal or by small palatal perforation. Tyson in 1967 demonstrated the role of surface tension and atmospheric pressure in denture retention in a series of experiments. He used a bell jar that enabled atmospheric pressure to be varied. Immersing the entire system in water eliminated the pressure gradient and effect of surface tension which reduced required separating force. If the active forces involved in these phenomena were cohesive, immersion would not have reduced retention.

Intimate Tissue Contact

It is the biologic factor that refers to the close adaptation of the denture base to the underlying soft tissues. The degree of tissue contact obtained depends mainly on the impression technique used.

An impression material with adequate flow properties should be used to avoid uneven pressure during impression procedures that could result in a localized rebounding effect of the compressed tissues under the denture base.

At the same time an impression material that places slight generalized pressure on the soft tissues is preferred.

Use of a moderately viscous light bodied impression material with sufficient flow, elimination of full arch relief spacers in tray and use of a perforated tray can reduce pressure applied on the tissue. This will ensure slight displacement of the soft tissue and ensures intimate contact of denture base to the tissue.

Border Seal

Border seal is the biologic factor that involves intimate contact of denture borders with the surrounding soft tissue.

The seal encompasses the circumference of the denture and includes features such as beading and posterior palatal seal to enhance retentiveness.

Fry in 1923, stressed the necessity of perfect adaptation between palate and mucous membrane and the importance of maximum possible coverage.

Peripheral seal of a denture is defined as the area of contact between the mucus membrane and peripheral polished surface of denture base.

The seal prevents passage of air between the denture and soft tissues. This seal depends upon proper extension of the denture borders both in width and height so that they fill the mucobuccal space and contact the cheek tissues laterally. At the posterior aspect of the denture in the soft palate area, there are no cheek tissues to seal the denture border. Therefore, the posterior palatal seal commands special attention.

Hardy and Kapur in 1918, reported that horizontal forces and lateral torquing of the maxillary denture can be resisted only by adequate border seal. Terminating the denture borders on soft resistant tissues will allow the mucosa to move with the denture base during function and thereby maintain denture seal.

Padgett in 1993 advocated an impression technique that would ensure maximum adhesion by using custom trays and ensuring a tight fit all round the periphery with buccal flange extending to the full depth of the sulcus.

Neuromuscular Control. This refers to the functional forces exerted by the musculature of the patient that can affect retention. This is primarily a learned biologic phenomenon. Certain characteristics can be incorporated into the external contours of the denture base to promote neuromuscular control.

The biologic factors influencing retention were reviewed by Pendelton. According to him, quest for a solution to retention can be solved only by an understanding of the anatomy and physiology of those structures in contact with the denture which are stress bearing, valve producing, postdam, and relief areas. Brill et al asserted that as normal muscle activity was dependent upon different impulses originating in proprioceptors in muscles and tendons, and exteroceptors recording changes in the mucosa of oral cavity and tongue, were concerned with denture retention. He believed that these receptors are of great importance in precisely adjusted muscular coordination of cheeks, lips and tongue.

Certain patients are able to tolerate broken or ill-fitting dentures well whereas others find it difficult to adjust to well-prepared dentures.

This is attributed to neuromuscular control. The biologic factor of neuromuscular control becomes important as experienced patients learn to alter their muscular function to harmonize with the prosthesis. Individuals vary in their ability to develop motor coordination and conditioned reflexes necessary to manipulate intraoral prosthesis.

Additional Factors in Denture Retention

Mechanical Factors

Undercuts. These can be favorable or unfavorable

It should be evaluated by a surveyor and if required eliminated. In this situation vertical placement of a denture is not possible. If the denture is placed from the side, it will engage the undercut and will provide mechanical resistance to a downward directed force.

Springs. Mechanical devices such as springs are used rarely to assist the retention of complete dentures, e.g. in postsurgical rehabilitation.

Magnets. Magnetic forces[3] of repulsion have occasionally been used for retention of dentures. The like poles of permanent magnets are contained in opposite dentures so that the forces of repulsion act to seat the dentures when the dentures are at or near to contact. In certain situation magnets can be used in overlay dentures.

Suction Chambers. It is utilized only for maxillary dentures. This type of device aims at the production of a reduced pressure in the circumscribed area of the denture base. Older devices like rubber suction discs caused problems to the patient.

Now a days relief areas are used to compensate for unequal displacability of the tissues contacted by an overlying denture and to improve stability. Such areas increase the distance between the denture and tissues over the area relieved and so cause a reduction of the retentive force.

Relief areas may be supplemented by valves which are designed to enable the patient to evacuate the relief area by sucking on a valve. The effectiveness of this is doubtful as the relief area is quickly filled by saliva and later by tissue that proliferates into the area.

A functional vacuum system was proposed by Kubali. He stated that retention could be improved in the denture by building a packing ring into the denture like the packing ring in a piston.

Physiologic Forces

Physiologic forces relate to the musculature of the oral cavity. In this respect, the buccinator, orbicular oris and musculature of the tongue may be regarded as the most important.

Active muscle fixation of dentures may be obtained by careful attention to the form of those surfaces which contact their environmental tissues.

The tongue on the lingual surface and the peripherally placed muscles of the lips and cheeks may be considered to act as antagonists. So when dentures are constructed carefully, the simultaneous contraction of the two muscle groups may stabilize the denture and retain it against its foundation.

The accurate approximation of the tongue, cheeks and lip to a denture acts to impede flow of saliva about the denture, thereby increasing the effective area for retention.

When a small displacing force is applied to a denture, the reduced pressure which develops in the salivary film under the denture will cause the soft tissue to move inwards, thereby reducing potential flow of saliva under the denture.

Inaccurate extension of a denture may allow increased saliva and air to enter under a denture and cause loss of retention.

In the lower denture, surface area covered by the denture is less compared to the length of the border. So, potential for leak of air and saliva under the denture base is high.

In the upper denture, there is little or no movable tissue available at the posterior palatal border. So, breakdown of the seal in this region can occur with slight displacement. To avoid this a proper posterior palatal seal is required.

The Denture. Fish was among the first to discuss the determinants of retention. He emphasized that each of the three surfaces of a denture, i.e. the tissue surface, the polished surface, and the occlusal surface had a role to play in the retention of the denture. The proper design of the different surfaces helps the dentist develop the different factors of retention.

Polished Surface. The polished surface of a denture should possess certain contours to maximize the retentive potential of the functioning orofacial musculature. Craddock described the gripping action of the buccinator muscle on the buccal flange of the mandibular denture. Proper contour and design of the polished surfaces should harmonize with the function of the tongue, lips and cheeks to affect a seating of the denture.

Occlusal Surface. Schlosser and Fish believed that a balanced functional occlusion is critical in promoting denture retention. The occlusion developed must be free of interferences in the functional range of movement to avoid dislodging forces. The position of teeth in the arch and the level of the occlusal plane are important in maintaining the retention of the denture.

Tissue Surface. Several biologic and physical factors have been described as determining the relationship of the tissue surface of denture base to underlying soft tissues. These include adhesion, cohesion, intimate tissue contact, border seal, etc.

Saliva. Saliva is secreted by the three major glands and other glands located in the lips and cheek. One of the important functions of saliva is to maintain a good peripheral seal.

Denture Periphery

Maxillary Denture Periphery. The most anterior part of the periphery of the denture base is grooved by the labial frenum. Distally in the region of the lateral incisor the fibres of incisivus labii superioris arise from the alveolar border of the maxilla and arch laterally to form part of the muscle tissue comprising a portion of orbicularis oris muscle.

In the region of the canine fossa and inferior to the infraorbital foramen is the origin of levator anguli oris muscle.

The buccal frenum limits denture base extension in the premolar region. Distal to this the zygomatic process of maxilla (root of zygomatic arch) limits denture extension. Further distally the buccinator muscle that arises from the alveolar process in the molar region and from the pterygomandibular raphe limits denture extension.

Between the tuberosity of the maxilla and upper end of the pterygomaxillary raphe, a delicate tendinous band bridges the gap between the maxilla and hamulus of pterygoid bone. A few fibres of buccinator muscle arise from this band and form a concavity in the overlying mucous membrane known as hamular notch.

The buccal space or retrozygomatic space creates problems in developing a border seal. This space should be filled to avoid ingress of air beneath the denture base.

Mandibular Denture Periphery. The most anterior part of the mandibular denture base periphery is grooved by the labial frenum. Lateral to labial frenum and arising from the incisive fossa is the mentalis muscle.

Further laterally the denture extension is limited by the incisivus labii inferioris muscle which is inserted into the modiolus.

More distally, the depressor labii inferioris muscle and the depressor anguli oris muscle influence denture extension.

The buccal frenum which is present superior to the depressor anguli oris limits denture extension.

Lateral to the first molar tooth, the tissue overlying the buccinator delineates the buccal sulcus. The muscle is attached to the external oblique ridge and pterygomandibular raphe with the superior fibres arising from the maxilla.

Distally, the denture base covers the anterior third of the retromolar pad as the buccinator fibres are inserted into the posterior two third.

As the outline of the lower denture proceeds lingually, the attachment of the buccinator muscle to pterygomandibular raphe and the superior constrictor limit possible denture base extension.

The palatoglossal arch which moves forward during swallowing, limits the posterior lingual extension of the denture base.

The lingual extension of the denture base is influenced by tissues overlying the mylohyoid muscle.

Anteriorly the lingual frenum, then sublingual gland, and in the midline tissue overlying the genioglossus muscle at its attachment delineates denture base extension.

Deeper Anatomy. Anteriorly, the oral sphincter and associated orbicularis oris have a strong influence on the appliance placed in the maxillary arch.

The modiolus where a number of muscles are inserted exerts influence on denture design in the premolar region.

The mandibular denture generally provides poor retention because: (i) of a movable floor of mouth which causes difficulty in establishing a border seal, and (ii) lack of ideal ridge height and conformation.

During border molding, special attention should be given to the area of the buccal frenum where the triangularis attaches. By sound impression procedures, accurate tissue contact can be obtained.

The draping effect of the cheeks and lips helps in obtaining a border seal.

Posteriorly the denture base should cover the posterior extension of the firmly bound keratinized tissue of the pear-shaped pad (term coined by Craddock).

The contour and inferior extension of the lingual flange are dependent on the action and anatomy of the mylohyoid muscle. The lingual flange slopes medially away from mandible to allow action of the mylohyoid muscle. This inclination also enhances the ability of the tongue to control the mandibular denture, providing a seating force on the denture.

The attachment of the mylohyoid muscle extends anteroinferiorly along the molar region to genial tubercles at the midline. Posterior fibres extend vertically to the hyoid bone while anterior fibres extend horizontally to meet fibres of the contralateral side. It is because of this that the lingual flange can be made longer posteriorly.

Mandibular Anterior Lingual Influences. This is the region where border seal is difficult to obtain. The mylohyoid muscle acts anteriorly to raise the floor of the mouth and genioglossus muscle attach to the region near the lingual frenum. The superior fibres of the genioglossus muscle attach to the superior genial tubercle to depress the body of tongue. Activation of the inferior fibres of genioglossus protracts the tongue. There are two techniques to obtain seal in the anterior region:

1. Horizontal extension of anterior lingual flange sublingually. Here the flange is extended inferiorly to contact the highest part of the floor of the mouth. Then flange is extended posteriorly to contact sublingual fold without impinging on submandibular or sublingual glands.

2. Here the flange is extended slightly anteriorly to provide a seal when muscular floor of the mouth is at rest. This is done after border molding. It will cause slight displacement of the mucosa.

STABILITY

Complete denture stability[2] is the resistance to horizontal or rotational forces. It differs from retention in that stability resists forces in the horizontal plane whereas retention is the resistance to vertical dislodging forces. Stability ensures the physiologic comfort of the patient while retention contributes to psychologic comfort. The lack of stability often makes ineffective the factors involved in retention and support. A denture that shifts easily in response to laterally applied forces can cause a disruption in the border seal or prevent the denture base from correctly relating to the supporting tissues. The factors that contribute to stability include ridge height and conformation base adaptation, residual relationships, occlusal harmony, and neuromuscular control.

1. The relationship of the denture base to the underlying tissues.
2. The relationship of the external surface and border to the surrounding orofacial musculature.
3. The relationship of the opposing occlusal surfaces.

The relationship of the intaglio of the denture base to the underlying tissues is dependent on the impression procedures of the clinician.

Frieman described the contacting of the labial and buccal flanges with the labial and buccal ridge slopes as critical factors contributing to stability. Adequate extension of the denture border as limited by movable tissues not only allows the establishment of border seal and coverage of maximum supporting area but also provides maximum contact of the denture base with facial and lingual ridge slopes.

The nature of the overlying soft tissues determines the potential of a given region in tolerating stress. Maxillary, facial and mandibular lingual inclines may be less effective due to the thin alveolar mucosal covering.

Boucher noted that stability is obtained by incorporating the surfaces of the maxillary and mandibular ridges, which are at right angle to the occlusal plane. He further stated that stability requires "maximum use of all bony foundations where the tissues are firmly and closely attached to bone".

MANDIBULAR LINGUAL FLANGE

The most desirable feature of the lingual slope of the mandible is that it approaches 90 degrees to the occlusal plane. This enables it to effectively resist horizontal forces. The posterior lingual flange is usually able to be extended inferiorly more than the anterior lingual flange. Anteriorly, the mylohyoid muscle fibers are directed more horizontally to communicate with fibers of the opposite side along a midline. Tendinous extent of contact of the lingual flange with the lingual ridge slope is thereby dictated by the functional mobility of the floor of the mouth (Fig 6.1).

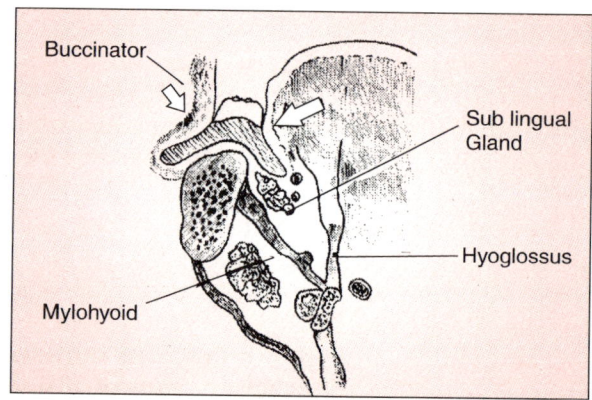

Fig. 6.1. Cross-section of the mandible and associated structures distal to the first molar.

Any flange extension[4] below the mylohyoid ridge must incline medially away from the mandible to allow for the mylohyoid muscle contraction. The degree of positive contact of firm ridge to flange may also be compromised by the presence of a thin mucosa overlying the bony ridge slopes that does not tolerate stresses effectively and, therefore may require relief (Figs 6.2a, 6.2b and 6.2c).

Large, square, broad ridges offer a greater resistance to lateral forces than do small, narrow, tapered ridges. Small rounded irregularities of the residual ridge also

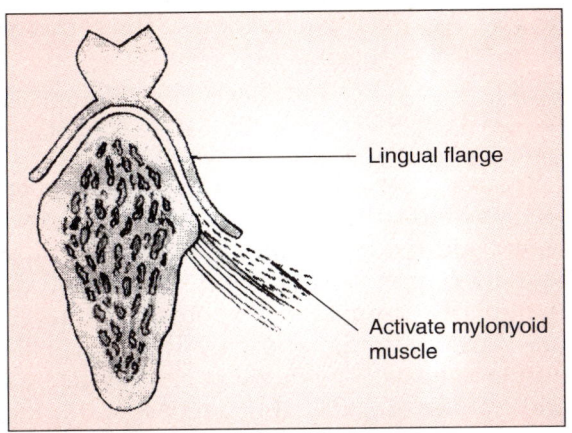

Fig. 6.2 A. The lingual flange of the mandibular denture should incline medially to allow for contraction of the mylohyoid muscle.

Lingual flange

Activate mylonyoid muscle

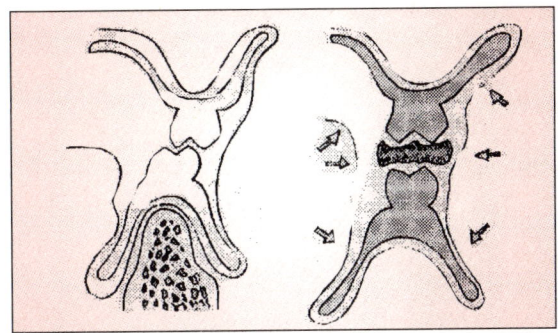

Fig. 6.2 C. The concave contours of the polished surface of maxillary and mandibular denture flanges permit the musculature to exert a seating action on dentures.

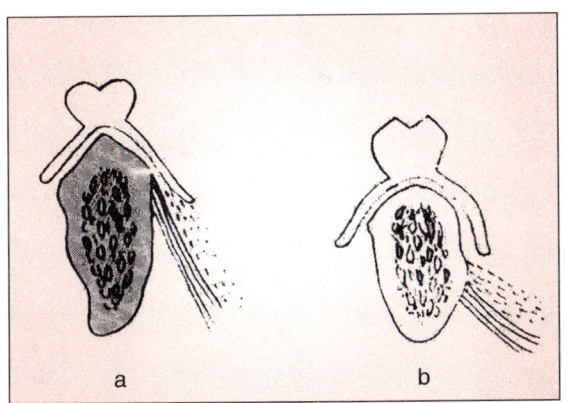

a   b

Fig. 6.2 B. Anteriorly the lingual flange inclines medially to allow for contraction of the mylohyoid, posteriorly due to a more vertical fibre direction, the flange may be extended vertically.

contribute favorably to stability. Removal of all irregularities to create a smooth, even ridge would diminish potential stability.

Square or tapered arches tend to resist rotation of the prosthesis better than ovoid arches.

The shape of the palatal vault contributes to stability as limited by the length and angulation of the palatal slopes. A steep palatal vault may enhance stability by providing greater surface area of contact and long inclines approaching a right angle to the direction of force.

Actions of the musculature on the denture base generally result in lateral and vertical dislodging forces.

The action of certain muscle groups must be permitted to occur without interference by the denture base so that they will not dislodge the prosthesis during function or compromise stability. Second, the dentist must recognize that normal functioning of some muscle groups can be used to enhance stability. Alterations in external denture base contours can lead to a dynamic seating and stabilizing action directed toward the prosthesis.

The denture border must be extended to contact the movable tissues. Actions of the levator angulioris (caninus), incisivus, depressor angulioris (triangularis) mentalis, mylohyoid, and genioglossus muscles can lead to dislodging forces if the denture base does not provide freedom for these muscles to function (Fig. 6.3 a and b).

The external surface should be developed to harmonize with the associated functioning musculature of the tongue, lips, and cheeks. It is believed that the contours of the polished surface provided the principal factor governing complete denture stability.

The basic geometric design of denture bases should be triangular. In a frontal cross-section,

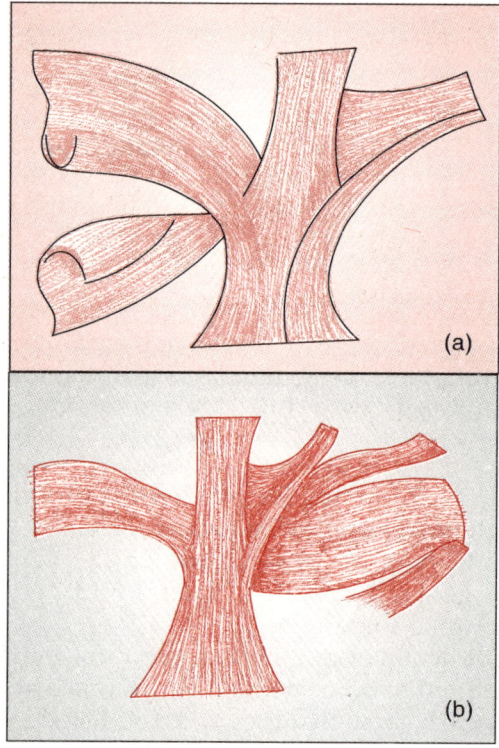

Fig. 6.3. Modiolus of cruculi

muscles. Anatomic landmark near the corner of the mouth is formed by the intersection of several muscles of the cheeks and lips. These include orbicularis oris, buccinator, caninus, triangularis, and zygomaticus muscles.

Because none of these muscles contains fibers that have more than one bony attachment, they depend on fixation of the modiolus to allow isometric contraction. Contraction of the triangularis, caninus, and zygomaticus muscles fixes the modiolus, allowing the buccinator muscle to tense, allowing it to control the food bolus on the occlusal table (Fig. 6.4).

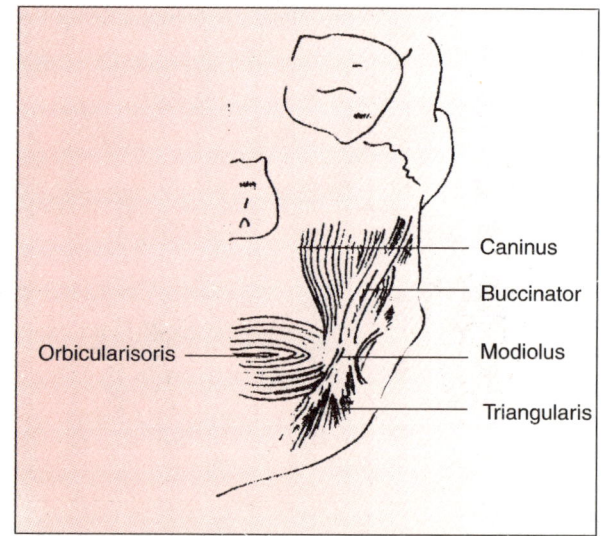

Fig. 6.4. Muscles of facial expression.

the maxillary and mandibular dentures should appear as two triangles whose apices correspond to the occlusal surface. The maxillary buccal flange should incline laterally and superiorly. The mandibular buccal flange should incline laterally and inferiorly, and its lingual flange should incline medially and inferiorly. Tongue should rest against a lingual range, incline medially away from the mandible and somewhat concave. Some authors recommend posterior extension of the lingual flange to fill the retromylohyoid space to permit the base of the tongue to contribute to the neuromuscular control of the prosthesis.

Generally, the buccal and labial flanges of the maxillary and mandibular dentures should be concave to permit positive seating by the cheeks and lips. The primary muscles of the lips and cheeks are the orbicularis oris and buccinator

The denture base must be contoured to permit the modiolus to function freely. In the premolar region the mandibular denture should exhibit both a shortened and arrowed flange to permit the action that draws the vestibule superiorly and the modiolus medially against the dentures.

The buccinator muscle may be divided into superior, middle, and inferior divisions. According to Fish, the superior fibers act to seat the maxillary denture, the middle fibers control the bolus of food, and the inferior fibers contribute to mandibular denture stability.

The idea of establishing harmony between the polished surface of the denture and the associated musculature has provided the basis for a number of techniques for complete denture construction. This "neutral zone" concept has been described with various modifications by a number of authors. The muscles should functionally mold not only the border but the entire polished surface. Even the teeth are placed within the neutral zone, where facial and lingual forces generated by the musculature of the lips, tongue, and cheeks are balanced. This functional rather than anatomic placement of the artificial teeth is believed to further enhance the stability of the dentures by minimizing active forces.

Harmony developed between the opposing occlusal surfaces also contributes to stability. Regardless of the type of posterior tooth form or occlusal scheme used, the dentures must be free of interferences within the functional range of movement of the patient. The functional range of movement refers to the positions through which the lower jaw moves horizontally during normal speech, swallowing, and mastication. During both function and parafunctional movements, the occlusal surfaces should not strike prematurely in such contacts causing uneven stresses to be transmitted to the dentures during function. This results in lateral and torquing forces that adversely affect stability. Bilateral, simultaneous, posterior tooth contact in centric relation is essential. Setting of anatomic or semianatomic artificial teeth to provide excursive balance is thought to minimize localized stress concentration and lateral dislodging forces by ensuring multiple points of contact to distribute functional occlusal forces. To minimize dislodging forces, the occlusion must be balanced throughout the functional range of movement of the patient. A balanced occlusion is limited by the buccolingual and mesiodistal width of the anatomic cuspal inclines.

Some authors recommend occlusal schemes that direct forces to minimize the unseating of the denture during unilateral excursive tooth contacts. Positioning degree teeth slightly lingual to the mandibular ridge crest may enhance denture stability. Zero degree teeth may reduce horizontal forces by elimination of the inclined planes introduced by the anatomic teeth.

The theories of lingualized occlusion provide both limited range of excursive balance and a directing force to the lingual side of the lower ridge during working side contacts. Such concepts minimize horizontal stress and enhance dentures stability by controlling the leverages induced by essential tooth contacts.

Woelfel et al showed that most functional closure of the complete denture patients occurred in close proximity to centric relation. In a study he demonstrated even force distribution regardless of tooth position in patients who chewed bilaterally. In another study, he further concluded that bilateral chewing contributed more to denture stability than to balanced occlusion.

Selection of cusp form and occlusal scheme involves the quality of the residual ridge in terms of height and conformation. Unfavorable ridges exhibiting severe resorption patterns may contribute to poor stability due to a poor denture base-residual ridge relationship. Anterior and posterior teeth should be arranged as close as possible to the position once occupied by the natural teeth with only slight modification made to improve leverages and esthetics.

A mandibular occlusal plane that is too high can result in reduced stability. First, lateral tilting forces directed against the teeth are magnified as the plane is raised. Second, the mandibular denture needs to be controlled by the musculature of the tongue, lips, and cheeks. An elevated occlusal plane prevents the tongue from reaching over the food table into the buccal vestibule. This compromises stability and makes control of the food bolus and denture more difficult.

Bisecting the interridge distance improves the mechanical advantage of the mandibular denture, but if excessive mandibular ridge resorption has occurred, the occlusal plane would be too low since less resorption usually occurs on the maxillae.

A problem of stability is the offset ridge relations seen in prognathic and retrognathic patients. Weinberg recognized the need to set teeth in crossbite when the ridges are in a severe crossbite relation.

Sufficient mandibular posterior occlusion must be developed so that contact against the maxillary denture extends posteriorly more than half the distance from the incisive papilla to the hamular notch. Without this contact the maxillary denture would tip anterosuperiorly, traumatizing the maxillary anterior ridge and loosening the maxillary denture.

The severe retrognathic or prognathic ridge relationship can be remedied only to a limited extent through prosthetic treatment.

Complete denture stability and retention are essential in providing successful prosthetic treatment. The factor of stability involves the tissue, occlusal, and polished surfaces of the denture.

SUPPORT

Complete denture support[5] is the resistance to vertical movement of the denture base toward the ridge. It counteracts those forces directed towards the ridge at right angles to the occlusal surfaces. Support involves a consideration of the relationship between the intaglio of the denture base and the underlying tissue surface under varying degrees and types of function. This relationship must be developed so as to maintain the established occlusal relations and to promote optimal function with a minimum of tissue ward movement and base settling.

Types of Support

The maxillary and mandibular dentures should conform to the underlying tissues so that the occlusal surfaces can correctly oppose one another at the time of insertion. Bilateral simultaneous contact should exist both at initial closure and under functional loading. The denture bases should maintain this relationship for a period of time. Without long-term support, complete denture retention and stability also become compromised.

Initial denture support is achieved by using impression procedures that provide optimal extension and functional loading of the supporting tissues, which vary in their resiliency. Long-term support is obtained by directing the forces of occlusal loading toward those tissues most resistant to remodeling and resorptive changes: (i) The denture is extended to cover a maximal surface area without impinging on movable or friable tissues, (ii) those tissues not capable of resisting resorption are selectively loaded during function, (iii) those tissues not capable of resisting vertical displacement are allowed to make firm contact with the denture base during function, and (iv) compensation is made for the varying tissue resiliency to provide for uniform denture base movement under function and maintain a harmonious occlusal relationship.

Maximal denture extension is essential in providing denture support. Denture should be extended to make positive contact with the soft, yielding peripheral tissues as limited by muscle function and bony or tendinous anatomic structures. The basic Snowshoe principle of maximal extension is that given a constant occlusal force, a broader denture-bearing area decreases the stress per unit area under the denture base, decreases tissue displacement, and reduces denture-base movement (Fig. 6.5).

Nature of Supporting Tissues

Ideally, the soft tissues should be firmly bound to underlying cortical bone, contain a resilient

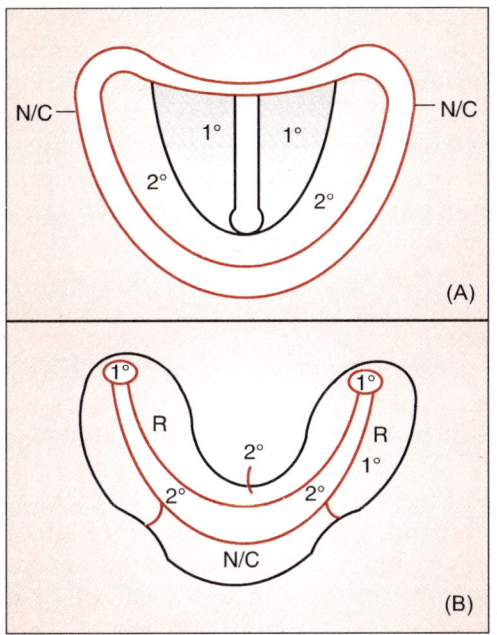

Fig. 6.5. Support areas of the: A, Maxilla, and B, Mandible.

keratin, localized hyperkeratosis, and epithelial ulceration or necrosis.

The presence of a layer of resilient submucosa moderates compressibility without mechanical impingement of the mucosa between the denture base and underlying bone. The fatty and glandular submucosa acts as a "hydraulic cushion" similar to the palm of the hand as described by Orban. Dense connective tissue of the lamina propria firmly binds the mucosa to underlying periosteum. Although not as effective in providing resiliency, this connective tissue layer serves as a protective base for the mucosa. The connective tissue bands firmly bind the masticatory mucosal covering of the edentulous ridges. Those regions, which possess a thin and/or less keratinized mucosa over bone without an intervening layer of submucosa, should be relieved or recorded without displacement.

Hard Tissues

Another requirement of ideal support is the presence of tissues that are relatively resistant to remodeling and resorptive changes. The problems associated with ridge resorption have been studied extensively by Tallgren et al. The rate and amount of bone loss and remodeling that occur in the anterior maxilla and mandible are of serious concern in prosthodontics. Consideration must be given to the maintenance of alveolar ridge height in the conventional complete denture patient. Minimizing the pressures in those regions most susceptible and directing the forces toward those regions relatively resistant to resorption can maintain healthy residual ridges.

Bone Factor

The response of bone to external forces is not completely understood. There seem to be some characteristics within the biologic make-up of the individual that determines the relative resistance of bone to resorption. This intrinsic bone factor is described by Glickman, Krol

layer of submucosa, and be covered by keratinized mucosa. The underlying bone should be resistant to pressure-induced remodeling. These characteristics minimize base movement, decrease tissue trauma, and reduce long-term resorptive changes.

Soft Tissues

Supporting soft tissues must be capable of withstanding the pressures induced through normal function of the prosthesis. The presence of keratinized firmly bound mucosa permits the tissues to better resist stress. Keratin is a scleroprotein present in the stratum corneum and is the end product of epithelial degeneration which protects the vital underlying epithelial layers. Generally, non-keratinized alveolar mucosa is not well adapted to tolerate the functionally generated stresses of a denture base. Excessive trauma to the mucosa beneath a denture base can lead to abnormal tissue changes such as the development of para-

et al and is unique to each individual. Bone factor can be determined only by studying the previous response of the patient's bone to stress. Such stress may be in the form of extractions, surgical trauma, or forces generated by a functioning prosthesis.

Although all bone responds to forces by remodeling as described by Wolff's law, it is interesting to note that the supporting alveolar bone may differ in its response to stress as compared to basal residual ridge bone. The response of bone to stress varies according to anatomic location.

The generally accepted pressure-tension concept appears to play an important role in the destruction or preservation of the bone of the residual ridges. This concept holds that pressure stimulates resorption whereas tension maintains the integrity or actually causes deposition of bone. Tension placed on bone is like that observed in the area of muscle attachment.

The retromolar pad is not a favorable denture-bearing area. The pear-shaped retromolar pad demarcates the distal border of a properly extended mandibular complete denture.

The pear-shaped pad area is associated with muscle and/or tendinous attachments of the buccinator, superior constrictor, and temporalis muscles. The deep and superficial tendons of the temporalis muscles insert medially and laterally in the mandible at the posterior border of the pear-shaped pad. Such muscle attachments and the overlying, firmly bound masticatory mucosa provide a stress-bearing region that is relatively resistant to resorptive changes.

Buccal shelf is the primary support area for the mandibular denture. It is usually covered by mucosa with an intervening submucous layer containing glandular connective tissue and buccinator muscle fibers. The buccinator muscle is attached inferiorly along the buccal shelf between the ridge crest and the external oblique ridge. The muscle fibers run along the shelf in a longitudinal anteroposterior direction, permitting the denture base to rest directly on a portion of the buccinator muscle without displacement. This buccinator muscle attachment extends posteriorly to include the pear-shaped pad area. These regions provide primary support for the mandibular denture base.

The role of the mandibular residual ridge crest in support depends on the nature of the ridge and the bone factor of the individual patient. Patients exhibiting broad square, well-developed residual ridges covered by tightly bound masticatory mucosa plus a favorable bone factor may rely on the ridges for support. Generally, the ridge crests are reserved as secondary support areas. The lack of muscle attachments and presence of cancellous bone usually result in resorptive changes occurring more rapidly than in the areas of primary support.

The remaining anatomic regions of the mandible are not usually essential in providing denture support. The less keratinized alveolar mucosa of the lingual and anterior labial ridge slopes lies directly over basal bone and does not tolerate pressure well. In fact, the lingual tissue over the mylohyoid ridge often requires relief to reduce impingement of the mucosa to effect border seal and not to promote support. In markedly resorbed mandibles, the genial tubercles provide a bony foundation resistant to resorption due to the genioglossus muscle attachments, but the friable overlying mucosa usually obviates its use as a primary stress-bearing area capable of resisting vertical forces.

The presence of pendulous, redundant, fibrous connective tissues over the mandibular ridge crest would preclude its use even for secondary support. Those genial tubercles covered by a skin graft would be considered as primary support regions.

Maxillary Anatomic Considerations

In the maxillae the horizontal portion of the hard palate lateral to the midline raphe should provide primary support for complete dentures. Van Scotter and Boucher describe the histology of the palate in detail. Keratinized masticatory mucosa overlies a distinct submucous layer everywhere but at the midline suture. The submucosa contains fatty tissue anterolaterally and glandular tissue postero-laterally. This resilient layer acts as a cushion for the functional stresses transmitted to the mucosa. Dense bands of connective tissue traverse the submucosa, firmly binding the lamina propria of the epithelium to the underlying periosteum. Over the midline raphe the mucosa is unyielding, has little or no submucosa, and must be relieved to avoid tissue impingement.

The cortical bone of the hard palate, composed of the palatine processes of the maxillae and the horizontal processes of the palatine bones, has been shown to resist resorptive changes in longitudinal studies of conventional complete denture patients.

The functioning tensor veli and levator palatini muscles of the soft palate may provide the sources of tension that counteract the pressure resorption normally expected beneath a denture base. In any event, the horizontal process resist resorption and is covered by keratinized mucosa and resilient submucosa. These properties indicate its essential function as primary denture-support area.

The crest of the maxillary edentulous ridge is also important in complete denture support. The soft tissue is often thick, keratinized, and firmly bound to the periosteum and underlying bone. A layer of dense fibrous connective tissue intervenes between the mucosa and bone and acts as a resilient liner for them. Despite this favorable soft tissue covering, the underlying cancellous bone is subject to resorptive changes.

Rapid Resorption Involving the Anterior Maxillary Ridge Beneath Denture

Resorption is usually more rapid when the lower anterior teeth are permitted to contact the maxillary denture without simultaneous posterior contact either in centric relation or during excursive movements. The appearance of loose, redundant tissue anteriorly together with fibrous, pendulous tuberosity is referred to as the "combination syndrome" by Kelly. Given proper attention, the maxillary ridge crest can remain relatively resistant to resorption and should be considered as a primary or, at the very least, as secondary supporting area.

Remaining facial slopes of the maxillary residual ridges are not essential in the denture support.

Relief Regions

Relief regions fall into three categories. First, tissues that are susceptible to resorption should not be subjected to functional pressures. These would include some maxillary and most mandibular ridge crests. Second are those regions that have a thin mucosa directly over hard cortical bone. These include the palatal midline raphe, tori and exostoses, and the lingual surface of the mandible, especially the mylohyoid ridge. Third, those regions of mucosa overlying neurovascular bundles such as the incisive papilla, and in some cases, the mental foramen.

PRACTICAL CONSIDERATIONS

One generally accepted principle of impression procedures is that the maximal allowable denture-bearing surface area should be incorporated. Many others recognized the need to record the different anatomic regions under varying degrees of pressure, depending on the nature of the tissue. The rationale behind these techniques is that certain tissues require slight placement while others must be recorded at rest or relieved.

A truly mucostatic or pressure-free impression is virtually impossible to achieve. The fluid impression material contained in a rigid tray inevitably causes some tissue compression. Even if it were possible to obtain a pressure-free impression of the tissues at rest, the mucostatic theory is based on the belief that oral tissues of the denture-bearing area behave as a confined fluid following Pascal's laws of hydrostatics. These laws state that pressure exerted on a confined fluid will transmit evenly throughout the fluid. Unfortunately, the fluid in oral tissues is not confined. The tissue fluids can move through the interstitial spaces in response to stresses placed on them. They also vary in their anatomic location and histologic make-up.

Ideally, the tissues beneath the denture base should be recorded in the shape and contour that they assume under a loading force. In this way, the more resilient tissues would be more displaced than those tissues that are unyielding, such as the maxillary midline raphe. Such an impression would provide an equalized distribution of pressure to the supporting tissues during function and avoid an unstable denture base rocking on a fulcrum point of unyielding tissue, such as the midline suture. The concept of equalized pressure distributed over the supporting areas will minimize localized stress concentration, which otherwise leads to pressure-induced resorption, mucosal irritation, and base instability.

Selective pressure impressions have some disadvantages and limitations. A denture base that records the functional contours of the denture bearing area displaces the more resilient tissues. At rest the denture base may rebound and pull away from the underlying tissues. Because no single technique can provide an equitable distribution of pressures both at rest and under function, the dentist must weigh the advantages and disadvantages in each situation.

Certain tissues should be recorded at or near rest while others should be subject to mild tissue displacement. Craddock has noted that an "automatic relief over hand to displace tissues can be obtained through the use of more viscous impression material. A study by Frank

was conducted to determine the effect of tray modifications and selection of impression materials on pressures exerted on the denture supporting tissues during maxillary edentulous impression procedures. The study concluded that: (i) differences in pressure were correlated to the use of different impression materials (irreversible hydrocolloid exhibited the highest pressures followed by thiokol rubber and metallic oxide-eugenol pastes, (ii) more pressures were measured at the crest of the ridge than on the palate when no relief was used; and (iii) generally, use of either escape vents or relief was equally effective in decreasing pressures and in equalizing the amount of pressure exerted on the ridge crest and the palatal areas.

ESTHETICS

Esthetics in dentistry is defined as the cosmetic effect produced by dental prosthesis which brings about beauty, attractiveness, charm and dignity to the individual.

- It starts from the stage of impression making.
- Esthetics in impressions refers to the development of labial and buccal borders so that they are in harmony with the labial and buccal sulcus.
- The borders must support lips and cheeks by filling the vestibular areas properly
- Insufficient development of labial and buccal borders causes loss of muscle tone resulting in lips losing their fullness and cheek collapsing.

IMPORTANCE OF SUBLINGUAL FOLD

The entire border of the denture[8] should be in contact with soft, displaceable tissue to obtain satisfactory retention. The anterior lingual border of the lower denture is related to mucosa that moves under the influence of adjacent muscles. So, the mucosa moves out of contact with the denture border. The sublingual folds may be used to obtain a seal in those regions. During tongue movement, the level of the floor of the mouth is continually altered. At rest, the floor of the mouth is at its lowest level. If the denture border is extended to contact the mucosa at this level, seal will be obtained at rest. But when the floor of the mouth is raised, a pressure is exerted through the mucosa against the denture border which may cause ulceration or displacement of the denture. If the denture border is ended at the highest level to which mucosa is raised, contact will be lost when the mucosa drops to a lower level (at rest).

The constriction of the anterior group of fibres of the genioglossus muscle depresses that part of the surface of the tongue to move upward and backward. This movement actively raises the floor of the mouth to its highest level displacing any denture base obstructing its movement. The sublingual fold overlies the genioglossus muscle and are raised and pulled away from the alveolar ridge when the tip of the tongue is raised. When the tongue is relaxed and its tip is allowed to rest in contact with the lingual surfaces of the lower anterior teeth, the sublingual folds also move downward and forward nearer to the alveolar ridge and denture border (Figs 6.6 and 6.7).

The **sublingual fold** may be utilized for improving retention. The denture border is extended horizontally backward until contact is made with the sublingual fold. Thus the seal is developed by the floor of mouth when the tongue tip is retracted and by the sublingual fold when the tongue is relaxed in a forward position.

Procedure. The special tray is extended downward with stick modeling compound while the tongue is retracted. Care should be taken to avoid overextension in this direction. Then the border is extended backward (with tongue retracted). The posterior border of this extension is trimmed until the sublingual fold

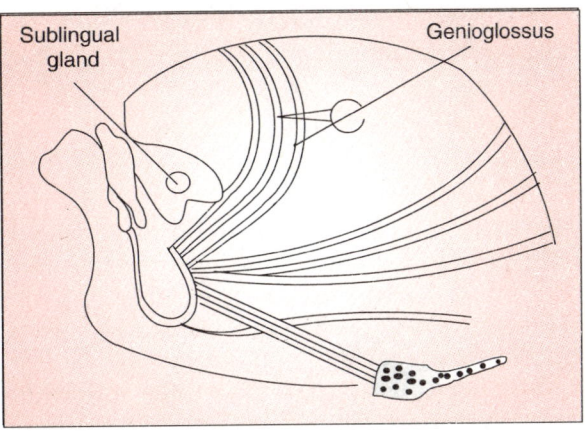

Fig. 6.6. Influence of sublingual fold in the retention of complete dentures.

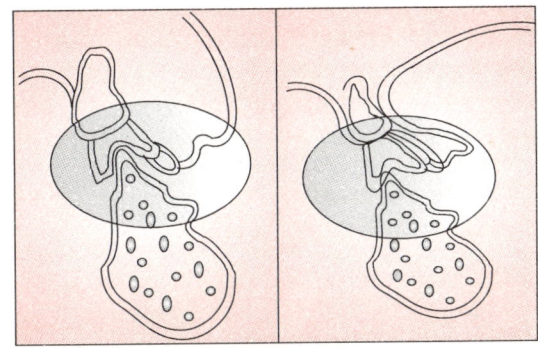

Fig. 6.7.

just makes contact with the border when the tongue is relaxed. The impression is then completed using zinc oxide-eugenol.

DENTURE ADHESIVES

History

The use of denture adhesives, fixatives and adherents began about the same time as the age of modern dentistry in the late 18th century. Adhesives or fixatives used in the 19th century were formulated by an apothecary who mixed vegetable gums to produce a material that absorbed moisture from the saliva and swelled to a mucilaginous substrate that adhered to the mucosa of the mouth and denture. The earliest patent pertaining to adhesives was issued in 1913.

Composition

The major constituents of denture adhesives may be divided into three groups: Group 1 consists of materials responsible for the adhesive properties, such as karaya gum, tragacanth, acacia, pectin, gelatin, methylcellulose, hydroxymethyl cellulose, sodium carboxymethyl cellulose and the synthetic polymers (polyethylene oxide, acrylamides, acetic polyvinyl); Group 2 contains antimicrobial agents such as hexachlorophene, sodium tetraborate, sodium borate, and ethanol; and Group 3 contains the additives, wetting and plasticizer agents.

Some of the flavoring agents used in denture adhesives are oil of wintergreen, oil of peppermint, and other agents similar in content.

Mode of Action

Denture adhesives are marketed as pastes, powders or creams. Adherent powders might include a vegetable gum such as acacia, tragacanth, or karaya. These materials are largely carbohydrates, swell to more than their original volume on the addition of water, and acquire viscous and retentive properties. Retention of dentures in the oral cavity is controlled by a complex interrelationship of adhesion, cohesion, atmospheric pressure, surface tension and viscosity. Denture adhesives provide an interface between the denture base material and the oral mucosa, and as such, interrelate these retentive forces between the denture and mucosa through an intermediary of a thin film of saliva.

Cream adhesives might derive their retentive properties from a polymer such as methyl cellulose, hydroxymethyl cellulose, or carboxymethyl cellulose. These cream adhesives spread laterally, excluding air and saliva from the tissue surface of the denture. The increase in viscosity of the cream layer compared with that of the saliva, is a factor for the increased retention.

Characteristics of an Ideal Denture Adhesive

- Non-toxic, non-irritating, and biocompatible with the oral mucosa.
- It should not promote microbial growth, and the product should be biocompatible.
- Odorless, tasteless, and easy to apply and to remove from the tissue-bearing surface of dentures.
- The adhesive should retain its adhesive properties for 12 to 16 hours before a need for application occurs.
- The ideal adhesive should provide comfort, retention (adhesion, cohesion) and stability to the denture, ensuring the patient's ability to function with security and effectiveness during speech, mastication yawning, and smiling.

USE OF DENTURE ADHESIVES DURING CLINICAL PROCEDURES

These may be used during the making of records with trial denture bases during denture fabrication, trial denture arrangement of teeth. Insertion of Dentures, immediate dentures.

Use of Denture Adhesives in Denture After Care

Reduction of tissue irritation. A study of 111 denture wearers revealed that the use of a natural gum or synthetic polymer denture adhesive over a 6-month period almost totally eliminated mucosal irritation.

Patients Who Need the Extra Security of Stable Dentures

Patients with Systemic Diseases. Certain systemic diseases may result in decreased or insufficient saliva flow. Denture patients experiencing hormonal and neurotransmitter changes and disorders in which muscle control is affected, such as myasthenia gravis, muscular dystrophy, Parkinson's and Alzheimer's diseases, and buccolinguofacial dyskinesia, may require denture adhesives to stabilize their denture.

Maxillofacial Surgery Patients. Maxillofacial prosthetic rehabilitation after ablative surgery, which leaves tumor patients with large maxillary or mandibular jaw defects, requires extensive prostheses with little or no retention. Particularly, edentulous patients with gross jaw defects may require the use of denture adhesives to retain large prostheses.

Administration of Drug Therapy. Frequently, the use of denture adhesives is a valuable adjunct to the retention of prostheses designed for the administration of drug therapy to oral tissues or to prostheses designed as radiation carriers or radiation protective prostheses.

Contraindications for the Use of Denture Adhesives

- Allergies of denture patients to denture adhesives or a component of the adhesive material preclude its use
- Dentures that are grossly inadequate in fit and function should not be continued in use with denture adhesives.
- Dentures that demonstrate excessive loss of vertical dimension because of extreme bone resorption and soft tissue shrinkage are beyond the use of denture adhesives. New dentures are indicated. Patients who have used denture adhesives without thoroughly cleaning the adhesive from the tissue surface of the denture, and has resulted in a sequential lining of a layered, caked deposit of hardened adhesive, should be instructed on a proper method of cleaning the adhesive from their dentures. If these patients are still not able to clean used adhesive material adequately from their dentures, they should

be discouraged from the further use of denture adhesives.
- Patients with broken dentures or dentures with missing flanges or borders or with sectional fractures should not use denture adhesives to retain their dentures. Repair of existing dentures or fabrication of new dentures is indicated.

Correct Application of Denture Adhesive

The correct application of denture adhesive to a denture is as follows

1. Clean and dry the tissue-bearing surface of the denture
   a. Remove residual adhesive material remaining in the dentures with tissue wipes and cotton applicators soaked with organic solvent
   b. Avoid scratching or mutilating the tissue-bearing surface of the denture
2. Wipe clean the epithelial tissue covering the denture-bearing regions from any previously attached denture adhesives, mucus, saliva, and food debris.
3. Apply small quantities of denture adhesive to the tissue-bearing surfaces of the denture.
   a. Wet denture before applying denture adhesive powder
   b. Apply adhesive to regions of the anterior alveolar ridge, centre of the hard palate, and posterior palatal seal for maxillary dentures.
   c. Apply adhesive to the sulcus of the denture over the crest of the alveolar ridge extending from the anterior sulcus to the distal extension for mandibular dentures.
4. Seat denture and hold it firmly by hand pressure for 5 to 10 seconds.
   a. Remove excessive adhesive (extruded beyond the denture borders) by gauze or tissue swipes.
   b. Instruct patient to close the jaw into centric occlusion several times to distribute the adhesive in an even thin layer between the mucosa and the denture bases.

Further Reading

1. Jacobson TE. A contemporary review of the factors involved in complete denture retention. J Prosth Dent. 1983; 49:5.
2. Jacobsen T.E. A contemporary review of the factors involved in complete dentures stability part II. Journal of Prosthetic Dentistry. Vol: 49, No.2, 1983, Pg. 165.
3. Behreman S J. The implantation of magnets to aid retention. J Prosth Dent. 1960;10(1): 807-11.
4. Wright C R. Evaluation of the factors necessary to develop stability. Journal of Prosthetic Dentistry. 1966; 16(3):414-29.
5. Jacobson T E et al. A contemporary review of the factors involved in complete dentures. Part III support. J Prosth Dent. 1983;49(3):304-12.
6. Tyson K W. Physical factors in retention of complete upper dentures. J Prosth Dent 1967; 18(2): 90-6.
7. Balhova Z. Physical factors in retention of complete dentures. J Prosth Dent.1971; 25(3): 230-35.
8. Lawson W A. Influence of sublingual fold or retention of complete lower dentures. J Prosth Dent. 1961;11(6):1038-49.

MULTIPLE CHOICE QUESTIONS

1. The following are mechanical factors in retention except
   a. Adhesion
   b. Springs
   c. Undercuts
   d. Friction

2. _____ is an emergency retentive force
   a. Capability
   b. Adhesion
   c. Surface tension
   d. Atmospheric pressure

3. The factors important in adhesion include all except
   a. The denture bearing area
   b. Consistency of saliva
   c. Undercuts in basal seat area
   d. Tissue contact of denture

FAQ's

1. Definition of
   a. Retention
   b. Stability
   c. Support

2. Factors influencing denture retention

3. Factors important for denture stability

COMPLETE DENTURES IMPRESSION

INTRODUCTION

Complete denture impression procedures are perhaps one phase on with much has been spoken about. Many methods and techniques have been suggested, claiming to give success irrespective of other factors. However, over the years, the knowledge of the anatomy, bone foundation, impression materials available has given us a much clearer insight to the impression theories and techniques. Whatever method is used, it is generally agreed that good impressions are basic to the fabrication of a good denture.

DEFINITIONS

Impression is the negative form of the teeth and/or other tissues of the oral cavity, made in a plastic material that becomes relatively hard and set while in contact with these tissues.

A complete denture impression is a negative registration of the entire denture bearing, stabilizing and border seal areas present in the edentulous mouth.

A preliminary impression is an impression made for the purpose of diagnosis or for the construction of the tray.

A final impression is an impression for making master casts. The master casts are used in fabricating the dentures.

Border molding: The shaping of the border areas of an impression, of the tissue adjacent to the borders to duplicate the contour and size of the vestibule.

The objective of complete denture impression procedure is to record all the available denture-bearing surfaces accurately such that stable and retentive prosthesis can be constructed.

Requirements for impression making include a knowledge of: (i) oral anatomy, (ii) basic and reliable technique, (iii) materials, (iv) skill, and (v) patient management.

OBJECTIVES

Five objectives of an impression as stated by Boucher in 1944 are:

1. Preservation of The Alveolar Ridges. This is achieved by an impression technique that covers the maximum supporting area as possible and using pressure within the physiologic limits of the tissue.

2. Retention. The factors of retention are adhesion, cohesion, interfacial surface tension, mechanical locking into undercuts, peripheral seal, atmospheric pressure, oral and facial musculature. Henry A in 1965 stated that primary retention depends upon close adaptation to the tissue and is proportional to the area covered.

3. Stability. Samuel Friedman in 1957 stated that stability is developed in the impression technique through more intimate contact of the labial and buccal flanges with the labial and buccal slopes of the ridges.

Boucher stated that stability required the maximum use of all bony foundations where the tissues are firmly and closely attached to the bone.

4. Support. It is provided by the maxillary and mandibular bones and their covering of mucosal tissue. It is enhanced by the selective placement of pressure. Maximum coverage provides the snow shoe effect which distributes applied forces over as wide an area as possible.

5. Esthetics. This refers to the development of the labial and buccal borders, so that they are not only retentive but also support the lips and cheeks properly. The vestibular fornix should be filled but not overfilled to restore the final contour.

Rules for making complete denture impressions (by RD Fisher in 1951).
- Roentgenographic, visual and digital examination of the oral cavity.
- Surgical removal of abnormal formations
- The required extension outlines
- The location and position for areas of variable tissue displacability
- Required retention outline
- The required adaptation.
- It should not distort the vestibular areas.

IMPRESSION MATERIALS

One or a combination of impression materials is not the panacea for making acceptable impressions in different situations. The character and the position of the tissues to be reproduced in the impression, the technique employed, and the purpose for which the impression is made dictate the choice of the material.

The type of **submucosa** and the relation of the supporting bone to the denture bases determine the method to be used to record the soft tissue and the properties the material should possess to make them desirable for use.

The oral mucosa with a tightly attached submucosa covers the crest and slopes of the residual alveolar ridges and the anterior two-third of the palate. If these tissues are recorded in their displaced form, and the denture is seated, the tissue will attempt to return to an undisplaced position. This effort of the tissues creates objectionable pressure to the supporting bone and dislodging pressure against the denture. Therefore it is not desirable to record this type of tissue in this displaced position and this advocates the use of an impression material that flows and allows the tissues to assume their undisplaced position before it sets. After setting, the material should remain dimensionally stable until the cast is made.

Oral mucosa that covers the soft palate and that which lines the vestibular fornix, has a loosely attached submucosa. When this submucosa is displaced with selective pressure procedure, the pressure is not directed to the supporting bone. The displaced tissue does not exert any appreciable force in an attempt to return to its undisplaced form. This type of tissue can be used for denture border seal. The impression material of choice is one that will displace the tissue and hold it in the displaced position as it sets.

Oral mucosa with a differentiated sub mucosa is located in the posterior one-third by the hard palate and in the retromolar pads. It is not desirable to displace the palatal mucosa in an impression as the pressure is directed at the bony support. A border seal can be developed in the anterior margin of the retromolar pad and the force can be directed in a horizontal direction, away from the supporting bone.

Gypsum Products

Plaster of Paris to which modifiers have been added to regulate the setting tissue and setting expansion are used in impression making.

Most frequently they are used in individualized trays of modeling compound or acrylic resin as a refining wash. If border refining is not required in the technique, it is used in a stock tray.

Advantages

- Minimal tissue distortion
- Accurate record of tissue details
- Quick flow
- Absorption of palatal secretions during setting
- Speedy handling
- Easy manipulation.

Disadvantages

- Pores in the plaster must be sealed before the stone is poured in the impression to form the cast
- Warpage in the palatal portion if the plaster is used in an impression tray that will not allow the plaster to expand in the flange areas during setting
- It is brittle and subject to breakage and is not suitable for reinserting into the mouth to adjust or check for accuracy of fit
- Saliva wets the material and distorts the surface when a mandibular impression is made
- Untidy to handle

- Dehydration of tissue allows the plaster to cling tightly to the tissues
- Separation of the stone cast from the impression is tedious and time consuming
- It will not record undercuts without breaking upon removal from the mouth.

Zinc Oxide-Eugenol Paste

Advantages

- Fluidity allows accuracy in recording the tissue details
- Minimal tissue distortion when the paste is allowed to flow with minimal pressure applied
- Ready flow
- Speed of handling
- Ease in beading and boxing
- Ease in separating from the cast
- Material not washed out by saliva
- No significant dimensional change after setting and can be preserved indefinitely without a change in shape
- It is used as a refining material in combination with other materials.

Disadvantages

- Setting time is not easily controlled
- Temperature and humidity influence the setting time
- Paste does not absorb secretions in the palate. Therefore if the secretions are profuse distortion results
- Untidy to handle
- Difficult to control at the borders
- May distort when removed from undercuts

Reversible Hydrocolloids

Advantages

- Tissue detail can be accurately recorded.
- Is used for the duplication of casts.

Disadvantages

- The reversible hydrocolloids can accurately reproduce detail of hard objects. This is not valid when reproducing soft tissue details. Any material that must be rigid until the material hardens or gels is capable of displacing soft tissues. If the tissues are to be reproduced in their undistorted position such distortion is not desirable

- Agar is subject to dimensional change by syneresis and imbibition and must be poured immediately
- It is easily distorted by movement during the gelation period
- Rapid cooling can cause stress concentration near the tray during gelation and release of these stresses after removal from the mouth can result in distortion
- Varying thickness of the material during gelation can also cause distortion
- They require special water cooled trays
- Gel is not easy to manipulate
- Beading and boxing are difficult.

The primary advantage of agar is that it will accurately reproduce undercut areas.

Irreversible Hydrocolloids

The soluble alginates dissolve in water and form viscous sols. The viscous sol is placed either in a perforated tray or in a rim lock tray and placed over the tissues. The gelation takes places first where the material is in contact with the tissue.

Advantages

- Simplicity of equipment
- Ease of manipulation
- Comfortable to the patient
- Short chair side time
- Accurate reproduction of undercut areas.

Disadvantages

- Not as accurate as reversible hydrocolloid in recording details of hard objects
- Composition affects its gel strength
- They deteriorate at elevated temperatures
- Powder should be weighed and not measured
- Alginates affect the hardness of the surface of stone. This can be overcome by immersing

the impression in hardening solution like 2% K_2SO_4 for 15 minutes.

Rubber Impression Materials

Rubber impression materials are shown in Colour Plate 2.

Advantages

- Accurately reproduce hard objects
- Remain dimensionally stable
- Do not affect hardness of stone
- Easy and tidy to handle
- Silicone base is pleasing in color and odor
- It records undercuts accurately.

Disadvantages

- Tray must be held rigidly for 8-12 minutes for setting
- Proper mixing is essential because if it is not homogenous, the impression will distort
- Ratio of materials is also critical
- Polysulfide base is untidy to handle and odor is objectionable.

Modeling Compound

Modeling compound is made either as tray material in the form of a cake or as impression material in stick form.

Impression materials are used for hard impressions of individual teeth and for border refining.

The trays that are made for modeling compound are refined at the borders and covered over the entire surface with other more fluid materials.

When the material is hardening, the tissue side is the last to be affected. The lower the temperature of the compound at the time of impression making, the less the error from the linear coefficient of thermal expansion.

American Dental Association (ADA) specification for compound for impression making allows a flow of 6% at mouth temperature. The compounds produced for tray material are allowed a flow of 2% at mouth temperature.

Modeling compound is subject to distortion during and after removal from the mouth.
- Warpage results when the mass is not thoroughly set prior to removal from the mouth.
- Warpage also results when the individual stresses are released.

Advantages of modeling compound
- Surface can be corrected
- Impression can be reinserted in the mouth to check the fit
- The surface does not have to be treated before pouring the stone cast
- The material can be beaded and boxed
- They are convenient for use and are tidy.

> The '3 Ms' of successful denture impression. This includes the **mold** (tray), **method** (impression technique) and **material**.

IMPRESSION TECHNIQUES

Table 7.1 gives classification of impression techniques.

Table 7.1. Classification of impression techniques
Classified according to:
(A) *Amount of pressure used*[1]
1. Pressure technique–based on pressure theory
2. Minimal pressure technique–based on mucostatic theory
3. Selective pressure technique–based on selective pressure theory.
(B) 1. Open mouth technique[6]
2. Closed mouth technique.
(C) 1. Hand manipulation or
2. Functional techniques.

Amount of Pressure Used

Pressure or definite pressure or mucocompressive technique is based on the pressure theory. The main objective of this group of impression techniques has been to attain better retention of the denture.

Advocates of this technique believe that the peripheries of the denture must be established during function. The pressure applied by occlusal loading during the impression making is comparable to the occlusal loading during function.

Technique (by Greene)

A preliminary impression is made in impression compound and a special tray is constructed using base plate with its periphery 1/8 inch shorter than the denture outline. With this tray, another impression with compound is taken. Well-fitting rims with uniform occlusal surfaces are made and the height of the bite adjusted against a similar bite rim on the lower ridge. Areas to be relieved like the median palatine raphe is softened and the impression is are again inserted in the mouth and is held under biting pressure for 1 or 2 minutes.

Peripheral muscle trimming is done by making the patient do various cheek and lip movements as in whistling and smiling. Posterior palatal seal is obtained by the swallowing movements of the patient, under biting pressure.

The claims made by the advocates of this group of impression techniques are that when muscle trimming is done, the border tissues are recorded in their functional position and not in their rest positions so that the dentures retain well and cannot be dislodged during any functional movements of the jaws. In addition, a positive peripheral seal is also obtained.

Demerits

1. Amount of pressure applied to the tissues is not only too great but is applied to the center of the palate and the peripheral tissues, which are not well suited to receive the maximum biting load. This interferes with the normal blood supply of these tissues resulting in transient ischemia and tissue breakdown. As soon as this change takes place, the excellent retention and peripheral seal are lost.
2. Dentures made over these impressions will fit well during mastication but will not be

closely adapted to the tissue when the patient is not chewing or at rest because the tissues tend to rebound.

3. The tissues may not maintain the shape they assumed on the day of the impression. The pressure applied can overstress the tissues. This often results in good retention initially but eventually by results in bone resorption and loose dentures.

Minimal Pressure Technique Based on the Mucostatic Principle

The term "Mucostatics" was coined by Dr. Carrol W. Jones. According to Christain G. Porter in 1953, in a brochure published by Mr. Page in 1946, he stated that all soft tissues are chiefly fluid since 80% or more of the tissue is composed of water, therefore they behaved according to "Pascal's law" which states that pressure on a confined liquid will be transmitted undiminished throughout the liquid in all directions. According to this concept, the mucosa will act like a liquid in a closed vessel and thus cannot be compressed. But this is not true as the tissue fluids can easily escape under the border of the denture. The mucosa is not a closed vessel.

According to the principle of mucostatics, the impression material should record without distortion every detail of the mucosa so that the completed denture would fit all minute elevations and depressions (so much emphasis was placed on recording detail that separating substances could not be used at any point in the procedure).

A metal base should be used rather than dimensionally unstable acrylics.

Adherents of the mucostatic principle considered interfacial surface tension as the only important retentive mechanism in complete dentures. Therefore they did not use conventional flanges because these did not resist vertical displacement which was the only movement capable of interrupting surface tension.

According to this concept, interfacial surface tension, the only major force in denture retention acts best when the surfaces are displaced at right angles to each other. The force is diminished as it approaches a parallel plane, so the flanges are kept short. For the lower denture, 2 mm or so below the crest of the ridge is said to be sufficient.

Impression Technique

A compound impression is made in a suitable tray and a cast is made on this. Baseplate wax is adapted which acts as a spacer. According to the denture outline, a special tray is made over this spacer. Postdam is obtained under light pressure. Spacer is removed and the impression is made with impression plaster with as minimum pressure as possible. No muscle trimming is advocated. Escape holes may be made for relief. Zinc oxide-eugenol paste/alginate can also be used.

Merits

- High regard for tissue health and preservation
- Suitable to areas where the residual ridges are sharp, thin and also flat flabby ridges.

Shortcomings

1. Page's application of Pascal's law to the field of denture impressions are only partly correct because the tissues involved are not wholly incompressible or static.
2. The claim that retention is only due to interfacial surface tension and not atmospheric pressure or border seal is not correct because this tensile force in itself is dependent upon adhesion and cohesion.
3. This theory overlooked the fundamentals laid down by Fisher RD in 1951 like: (i) maximum coverage of the basal seat area, (ii) periphery should rest on soft tissue at every given point, and (iii) there must neither be underextension nor overextension.
4. Presence of very short flanges affects retention and stability to a great extent. The

peripheral seal is not obtained and so when the dentures are not under function they lose stability.

5. Despite using methods for drying the mouth, it is difficult or virtually impossible to get an impression without a film of saliva and this prevents the securing of an impression with great accuracy.

6. Since stress from these dentures will not be distributed broadly over the basal seat, tissue health and retention may be compromised.

7. Tissues might have been different at the time of recording the impression and at the time of delivery of dentures. Such variations can possibly occur, and can affect the end results.

8. Minimal pressure dentures supply inadequate support to the face for the patient with severely resorbed ridge, as the denture would be small and it would be necessary to position the teeth over the crest of the ridge.

9. Stanley P Freeman in 1969 stated that this theory gave complete disregard for muscle coordination as a means of denture retention. The palate, the prime area of retention was often eliminated.

Muco-seal Technique

Muco-seal technique as stated by Pryor in 1946 was introduced as a variation to the mucostatic technique. The technique is similar to the mucostatic technique but the posterior lingual border covers just the retromolar pad. The anterior lingual border is molded by the floor of the mouth with the tongue in repose. The tray is extended horizontally backward over the sublingual glands towards the tongue to effect a border seal.

Selective Pressure Technique Based on the Selective Pressure Theory

This technique advocated by Boucher, combines the principles of both the pressure and minimal pressure techniques. The philosophy of the selective pressure technique is that certain areas of the maxilla and mandible are by nature

better adapted for withstanding extra loads from the forces of mastication. These tissues can be recorded under slight placement of pressure while other tissues must be recorded at rest or must be relieved.

Primary stress-bearing areas of the maxilla are the crest of the alveolar ridge and the horizontal plate of the palatine bone and for mandible is the buccal shelf area.

Secondary stress-bearing area of the maxilla is the rugae area and all the ridge slopes and of mandible are the retromolar pad area and all ridge slopes.

Areas requiring minimum pressure (relief) are the incisive papilla, midpalatine suture, tori, and crest of the mandibular ridge.

The selective pressure technique[2] uses custom trays constructed with less relief in the primary stress-bearing areas and greater relief and more impression material in the non-bearing areas. Thus greater amount of pressure is applied directly to the primary stress-bearing areas and less pressure is applied to the non-bearing areas. Thus this technique seeks to create a denture base that selectively loads the oral tissues during function of the prosthesis thus optimizing the stability and retention of the prosthesis.

Merits. Since the technique is based on the principle regarding both the biological as well as the physical factors concerning impression procedures, it is widely preferred especially in cases of well-formed healthy ridges.

Demerits
- Cannot be used in flabby ridge cases
- Opponents of this technique feel that it is impossible to record some areas with pressure different from that applied to other areas.

Making the Preliminary Impression

Preliminary Examination and Conditioning of the Patient. A complete case history of the patient and thorough clinical and oral examination is done. Evaluate the tissue forms, tongue position and the entire denture-bearing area. Dentures have to be kept out of the mouth for 48 hours prior to impression making to allow for recovery of the abused tissue.

Seating the Patient. The patient should be seated upright in a comfortable relaxed position with the occiput resting firmly in the head rest. Chair height and position are adjusted according to the comfort of the patient and dentist.

Selection of the Impression Tray. Beginning of a good impression starts with the selection of the correct stock tray. The tray should extend to cover the entire denture-bearing area and provide 5-6 mm space for the impression material.

If the tray is too large, it will distort the border tissues by pulling them away from the bone. If the tray is too small, the border tissues will collapse inward towards the residual ridge thus reducing support for the denture. Depending upon the type of the impression material used, either a perforated or non-perforated tray is used, e.g. compound or alginate.

Selection of the Impression Material. The material, the dentist selects should be one that has the characteristics and physical properties to achieve the goals that he desires from the impression. Manufacturer's instructions must be strictly followed to gain maximum advantage from the material.

Making the Preliminary Impression with Impression Compound

Maxillary Impression. Load the required amount of softened modeling compound into the selected tray, position and center it relative to the maxilla and the impression is made. Border molding is done within the functional limits, and the tray is held with a firm pressure till the compound sets. Chill it and remove the impression from the mouth. Examine the impression for proper extension and coverage. Refining of the borders is done if necessary (Fig. 7.1).

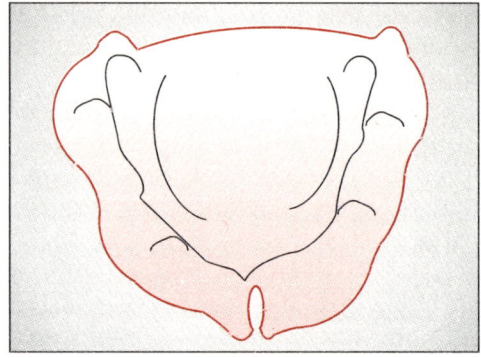

Fig. 7.1. Maxillary impression.

Mandibular Impression. This is made similar to the maxillary impression. The patient's tongue movements record the lingual borders (Fig. 7.2).

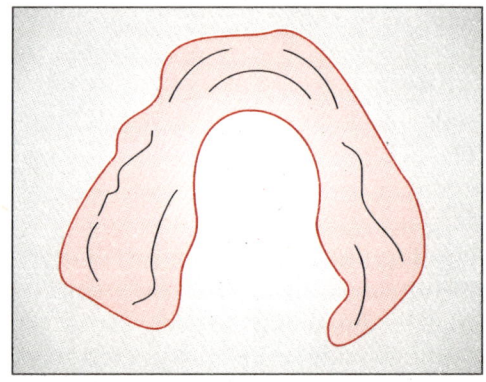

Fig. 7.2. Mandibular Impression.

Making the Final Impression

There are many ways of making the final impression:

1. As advocated by the **Greene Brothers,** the preliminary compound impression is separated from the tray and a final wash impression is made in this tray of compound impression.

Advantage. No extra appointment is necessary for the final impression.

Disadvantage. Bulk of compound tray cannot select areas of pressure and minimal pressure.

2. Preliminary impressions are made. The custom tray is constructed on the primary cast and the final impression is made in the custom tray. A key to obtaining a good final impression is a correctly extended and properly relieved tray.

Two contrasting techniques exist for providing relief within the custom tray for obtaining accurate border molding of the peripheral extensions: of the tray, and for making the master impression the Boucher technique and the Halperin technique. Both techniques require that the completed custom tray to be stable and extended properly during moderate function of the oral structures. Both philosophies advocate the selected pressure technique.

The technique advocated by Boucher suggests that the custom tray be provided with a 1 mm thick wax relief over the entire basal seat area within the outlined border on the cast. The posterior palatal seal area on the cast is not covered with the wax spacer. The completed custom tray will contact the mucous membrane across the posterior palatal border and additional stress placed here during the making of the final impression will help achieve a posterior palatal seal. In addition this part of the tray will act as a guiding stop to help position the tray properly during the impression procedure. A wax spacer will not be used if a metallic oxide impression paste has been selected for making the final impression.

Peripheral borders of the tray should be trimmed to within 2-3 mm of the anticipated peripheral extensions. After completion of the border molding procedures, the peripheral extensions are shortened by 1mm and the wax relief is removed completely to provide space for the impression material. Vent holes are advocated for both maxillary and mandibular custom trays and a master wash impression is made.

In direct contrast to this, the Halperin technique suggests that the custom trays be provided with 1mm thick wax relief over the peripheral extensions and buccal slope regions of the tray, including the posterior palatal seal region and that the custom trays be in intimate contact with the basal seat areas. The tray provides an internal finish line that forms a butt joint of compound to the tray after the border molding procedures are completed.

Border molding is completed when the peripheral seal is obtained with no border molding material extended into the internal aspects of the impression tray beyond the internal finish line. A master cast is poured directly into the border molded custom tray without using a wash impression.

Technique for Fabrication of a Custom Tray Using Light Cured Composite Resin. After identification and verification of the desired vestibular extensions on a preliminary cast, a pencil outline is scribed on the cast at the anticipated peripheral extent of the custom tray. A second line is scribed 2 mm inside the initial extension line. 1 mm thickness base plate wax is heated, adapted and trimmed back to the internal line of the cast. The exposed stone is coated with model release agent and a single sheet of triad trans sheet custom tray material is adapted to the preliminary cast. A handle is formed and the entire surface of the trial material is coated with air barrier coating. The assembly is placed in the trial curing unit. The material is light cured in increments of 1 minute for 4 to 5 cycles. The tray must be allowed to cool between the cycles to prevent the wax relief from melting. On removal the surface is scrubbed to remove the air barrier coating. The tray is teased from the preliminary cast and the peripheries are trimmed to remove sharp areas.

Border Molding Procedures

Different materials used for border molding are:
1. Modeling compound sticks—advocated by Boucher

2. Autopolymerising acrylic resins—by Jones
3. Tissue conditioning materials—by Chare
4. Polyether—by Smith E. Dale
5. Impression waxes adaptol—by Knapi
6. Perio pack—by Kirk and Holt
7. Metallic paste and elastomeric materials.

A stick of modeling plastic impression material is heated using a Bunsen burner to soften the material. It is then applied sequentially to the peripheral areas of the custom tray.

For the maxillary custom tray, a five-step addition of the modeling plastic is recommended during border molding procedures (Table 7.3). The posterior palatal seal is established initially, followed bilaterally by the retrozygomatic process and then buccal and labial flange areas.

For the mandibular custom tray, an eight-step addition of modeling plastic is recommended (Table 7.2). Bilaterally, the masseteric notch and the distal extension areas, the buccal shelf; buccal and labial flange areas and finally the retromylohyoid/mylohyoid/sublingual fold space areas are molded. After incremental addition of the modeling plastic to the custom tray, it is heated with an alcohol torch and then tempered in a water bath set to the appropriate temperature prior to insertion into the patients mouth. Prior to setting of the modeling plastic, the patient is instructed in functional tissue movements to mold the material.

Alternative Border-Molding Technique

An alternative border molding technique involves the recording all of the borders simultaneously. It has two general advantages.[5]

- The number of insertions of the tray are reduced to one
- Developing all borders simultaneously avoids propagation of errors caused by a mistake in one section affecting the border contours in another.

Requirements of a Material to be Used for Simultaneous Molding of all Borders

These should have sufficient body to allow it to remain in position on the borders during the loading of the tray

- allow some reshaping of the form of the borders without adhering to the fingers
- have a setting time of 3 to 5 minutes
- retain adequate flow while the tray is seated in the mouth
- allow finger placement of the material into deficient parts after the tray is seated
- not cause excessive displacement of the tissues of the vestibules
- be readily trimmed and shaped so excess material can be removed and the borders shaped before the final impression is made.

If the patient has excessive salivation, 2-3 minutes before making the impression gauze piece of catacaine is placed in the mouth.

The impression material is mixed according to manufacturer's instructions and tray is loaded with the material in an even 2 mm thin film. Tray is positioned in the mouth, seated firmly and border molding done within the functional limits of the tissues. Remove the impression, wash it and examine it for completeness. Final impressions are remade if: (i) voids are too large, (ii) excessive pressure spots are present, and (iii) incorrect border extension is present.

Spacers

In the upper tray escape holes (1-2 mm in diameter) are placed 1mm apart along the median palatine raphe beginning at the incisive fossa and ending just anterior to the PPS area. Escape holes are also placed in the presence of large tori and displaceable tissue.

In the lower tray escape holes spread 1/2 inch apart are placed along the crest of the ridge.

Frank has shown that the least pressure of 45% is produced when a tray with relief space and escape holes are used than when only relief space (40%) or only escape holes (65%) are used.

Table 7.2. Steps involved in border molding (mandibular)

Anatomic region	Tissues that influence extension	How to activate	What activation
	Mentalis muscle Incisive labi inferioris	Hand massage and manipulate the lip in a side-to-side motion	Activates the orbicularis oris muscle with its associated muscles of facial expression
Labial flange	Orbicularis oris with associated muscles of facial expression	Instruct the patient to evert the lower lip (pout)	Activates the mentalis muscles against the compound
	Labial frenum	Instruct the patient to lick the upper and lower lips with the tongue	Activates the orbicularis oris muscle and its associated muscle of facial expression
Labial frenum	Labial frenum and its associated connective tissue fibres	Elevate the frenum into the compound and then massage the lip with the side-to-side motion	Permits a seal to form by the molding of the area using the side to-side movement of the lip; therefore, maximum seal with freedom of movement
Masseteric notch	Masseter muscle	Instruct patient to close down on your fingers and the tray handle	Masseter muscle contracts against buccionator muscle
	Buccinator muscle Buccal fat pad	Manually manipulate the bucal fat pad by drawing the cheek	Buccal fat pad is elevated onto outer peripheral border to
		up to bring excess compound onto the tray	help seal and stabilize denture
Distal extension area	Pterygomandibular raphe Retromolar pad	Have patient open his mouth wide	Pterygomandibular raphe stretches, capturing the raphe and defining the most distal extension of the impression.
			Denture base covers the maximum amount of bearing area and is sealed on displaceable tissue.

Table 7.2. Steps involved in border molding (mandibular) *(Contd.)*

Anatomic region	Tissues that influence extension	How to activate	What activation accomplishes
Mylohyoid area	Mylohyoid muscle	Have the patient perform repetitive forced swallowing	Causes a forcible contraction of the palatoglasses fibers moves the compound inferiorly and medially. Raises the floor of the mouth through contraction of the mylohyoid muscle. The amount of movement of the floor of the mouth is often greater with tongue movement. The swallowing activity, therefore will sometimes allow the denture to extend further into floor of the mouth for a better seal and better stabilization. If different configurations to exist use the activity that provides it maximum extension compatible with function.
	Mylohyoid ridge and the medial body of the mandible.	Instruct the patient to move his tongue into the upper and lower vestibules on side each of his mouth	
	Tongue size, position, and amount of movement	Contour the border and the outer surface of the flange to pass under the tongue	
			The denture border can extend inferiorly and medially to the mylohyoid ridge so as to:
			Help prevent soreness the tissues over theridge.
			Have the tongue rest upon the outer, polished surface of the denture increase the stability of denture
Sublingual fold space (last area to be border molded)	Genioglossus muscle	Place additional compound into this area. Seal this area to its lowest level by massaging the compound downward with the index finger. Surface heat and gradually shorten this area by	Causes slight contraction of the genioglossus muscle, which pushes against the tissues superior to it. Only mild activation of the genioglossus muscle is accomplished, so that the lingual
	Tongue (with its associated intrinsic and extrinsic musculature)		
	Lingual frenum		

Table 7.2. Steps involved in border molding (mandibular) *(Contd.)*

Anatomic region	Tissues that influence extension	How to activate	What activation accomplishes
	Folds of mucosa covering the genioglossus muscle and sublingual glands	having the tongue just contact the handle of the tray to prevent reduction of the length too rapidly	flange in this area is gradually reduced until the most favorable level—that which provides for peripheral seal and tongue function—is reached. The mylohyoid muscle is activated when the tongue is elevated, but its effect is more limited in this area because it is inferior to the geniohyoid muscle and the soft tissues above it.
	Mylohyoid muscle	Instruct the patient to gently wet his upper and lower lips with his tongue.	
Lingual frenum	Lingual frenum with its intrinsic connective tissue fibers	Instruct the patient to protrude his tonguel slightly and move it from side to side. Make sure that the compound is warmed only in the area to be contacted by the lingual frenum.	Allows freedom of the lingual frenum connective tissue band to prevent the denture from being dislodged during normal tongue movements.
Buccal	External oblique	Manually manipulate the cheek with finger pressure upon the denture border in an anterioposterior direction	Moves the fibers of ridge the buccinator muscle and the soft tissues of the cheek in the direction of the muscle activity during patient function
		Look at the buccal flange internally to see that the cheek is not distended and the tissues of the cheek rest upon the outer surface of the dentures	Avoids overextension which can cause displacement of the denture base and soreness of the tissues
		Feel the edge of the flange with the ball of the index finger to check for	Avoids overextension which can cause displacement of the denture base and

Table 7.2. Steps involved in border molding (mandibular) *(Contd.)*

Anatomic region	Tissues that influence extension	How to activate	What activation accomplishes
		over extension	soreness of the tissues
			Provides detection of overextension of border and visualization of esthetics and facial form
Buccal frena	Buccal frena	Elevate the frena into the compound and then mold the cheek in an anterio-posterior direction	Allows for freedom of movement of the connective tissue band.
			Permits a seal to form by the manipulation of the cheek in a back and - forth motion; therefore, allows maximum seal and contact with freedom of movement.

Open Mouth Technique

Here the patient's mouth is partly open and the tray is held by the dentist. This technique is preferred because the operator can see whether muscle trimming is being done properly and the various muscle movements can be accomplished somewhat more easily.

Closed Mouth Technique

The rationale behind this technique is that the supporting tissues are recorded in a functional relationship. Vertical dimension is established before making the impression. The tray with occlusal rims are placed in the mouth and border molding and final impressions are made in a closed mouth position. A pressure similar to that of mastication is developed through the occlusal rims.

1. *Hand Manipulation/passive Method.* The contours of the denture borders may be obtained by the dentist with the use of manual manipulations of the lips and cheeks within functional limits. Patient's tongue movements record the lingual borders.

2. *Functional Movements/active Method.* The denture borders may also be formed by having the patient, make functional or physiological movements such as swallowing, sucking, grinning, licking, etc.

Toch's neuromuscular concept involves the functions of sucking and swallowing while making an impression and to bring the denture base into harmony with the physiological behavior of the muscles.

The only truly functional or physiological method of making impressions is the dynamic impression as described by Chase and Tryde et al. In this technique, the basal seat and borders are obtained with the use of impression material that continues to flow over an extended period of time (such as tissue

Table 7.3. Steps involved in border molding (maxillary)

Anatomic region	Tissues that mold	How to activate	What activation accomplishes
		Manually push softened compound into the retrozygomatic area with the halp of your index finger, the patient's mouth should be closed	Enables compound to occupy this space, which is often blocked by the coronoid process
Retrozygomatic area	Buccinator muscle fibers and overlying mucosa	Instruct the patient to pull in on your finger with his lips, and manipulate the cheek in an anterioposterior and downward direction.	Activates the buccinator muscle fibers and moves the overlying mucosa
Coronoid process area	Coronoid process	Instruct the patient to close firmly against your fingers.	Causes the masseter muscles to contract against the modeling plastic.
	Fibers of the temporal muscle attached to the coronoid process.	Instruct the patient to open wide then close and move his mandible to the opposite side	Activates the coronoid process and the attached fibers of the temporal muscle against the modeling plastic
	Buccinator muscle	Manually mold the cheek in a side-to side direction. Instruct the patient to pull his cheeks in on your finger. also instruct the patient to move his jaw from side to side to have the coronoid process mold the compound.	Simulates the movement of the buccinator muscle and associated soft tissues; the lip movement causes the buccinator muscle to contract. Improves esthetic form of lips and cheeks.
Zygomatic area of buccal flange	Zygomatico maxillary crest		
	Buccal frena and associated muscles of facial expression	Add or remove compound to allow the impression to fulfill esthetic requirements. Muscles do not exert a dominant role in the width of this dentureborder	Aids in the determining and limiting the flange length. Also improves esthetic form of lips and cheeks.
Buccal frena	Buccal frena with associated connective tissue fibers and the muscles of facial expression, particularly the caninus muscle and the orbicularis oris muscle which affect the frena movement.	Pull the buccal frena	Activates the connective tissue fibers of the frena while simultaneously causing movement of the associated muscles of facial expression (caninus and orbicularis oris muscles.

conditioning materials or wax). This material is placed in the patient's transitional denture and the patient's normal activities mold the borders over a period of time.

Functional reline-rebase technique and modified chew in technique as described by Robert C Vig is based on the same principle.

Disadvantages

This method cannot be used routinely. Some may use extreme movements, others less.

IMPRESSIONS BY THE USE OF CONTROLLED SUB-ATMOSPHERIC PRESSURE

Milo V Kubalek and Dert C Buffington developed a new concept of making impressions using the principle of vacustatics. Vacustatics describes subatmospheric pressure as a significant factor in the technique.

The object of **Vacustatic** technique is to reduce the stress on any given tissue by increasing the load-bearing area (mucostatic principle). The form of the tissue is recorded vertically and laterally (when a controlled partial vacuum is established). An impression tray specially built for the patient with attached small rubber hoses is maintained in the mouth without direct mechanical support of any kind. The difference between the subatmospheric pressure within the tray and the atmospheric pressure outside the tray is all that is needed to center the tray over the ridges in a static position. As vacuum develops between the soft tissue and the tray, a recording material in a fluid state flows from the border region into the evacuated space and envelopes the basal tissues. Border seal is determined by the readings remaining constant.

Disadvantage

Use of elaborate equipment.

IMPRESSION TECHNIQUES IN COMPROMISED PATIENTS

Impression techniques are modified in compromised conditions to achieve as much retention and stability as possible.

Impression Techniques for Restricted Access to the Oral Cavity

Patients may exhibit limited opening of the mouth following radical surgery or as a sequela to facial burns.

Walter described the use of sectional stock trays. Impressions of each side of the jaw was made one at a time and the 2 halves were joined and the cast was poured.

Impression Technique for Patients with Hyperactive Gag Reflex

Patients with hyperactive gag reflex can compromise the quality of treatment and may frustrate the dentist.

As Conny D J stated, the patient's problem whether iatrogenic, psychologic, anatomic or organic, disturbances must be identified and treated before making the impression.

Patient can be managed by: (i) clinical technique, (ii) prosthodontic management, (iii) pharmacologic measures, and (iv) psychologic intervention.

Impression Technique for Patients with Unsupported Movable Tissue (Hyperplastic or Flabby Ridges)

Impression technique for patients with unsupported movable tissue is done by recording the unsupported movable tissue with minimal displacement and the rest of the tissues with selective pressure. Many workers have suggested various techniques.

William H. Filler described a technique using two trays. The second tray is keyed on the first tray. Light bodied material is used in the initial tray as a corrective wash material and plastogum is painted over the areas not covered by the first impression in the second tray and impression is made. The two trays are held lightly together until the impression material sets and the impression is removed as a single unit.

Hobrik used a technique where only a single custom tray is used. Border molding is done in the usual manner and impression is made with heavy bodied addition silicone. The area of movable tissue is cut out and relief holes are made and a wash impression is made with light bodied impression material.

Zafarullah Khan described a technique where a window is cut in the custom tray where the unsupported area is present. The unsupported area is recorded in impression plaster, and the remaining area is recorded with thermoplastic impression material.

Splint method by Allan Mack is useful if tissues are exceptionally flabby. A loosely fitting tray or a special tray made with heavy relief over the flabby areas is taken. Plaster is mixed, applied over the flabby area to a thickness of about 2 mm and is allowed to set. Tray is filled with a second unit of plaster and the impression is made, the initial coating of the flabby areas thus acting as a splint while the impression is made and being removed with the impression.

IMPRESSION TECHNIQUE FOR PATIENTS WITH SEVERELY RESORBED MANDIBULAR RIDGE

The main aim of the impression procedure is to gain maximum area of coverage by obtaining a fairly long retromylohyoid flange, a better border seal for retention, and to educate and train the patient to maintain tongue position, i.e. forward and resting on top of the lower anterior ridge when the mouth is open.

Flange technique by Lott and Levin involves making impressions of soft tissues of the mouth adjacent to the buccal, labial and palatal surfaces and incorporating the resulting extensions or flange in the denture.

Flange is extended from the retromolar pad region to the sublingual region, large enough to restore the diameter of estimated resorption and patient is asked to forcefully perform functions of swallowing, etc. to give border extensions which cover the maximum surface area.

Tryde in 1965 used the dynamic impression method based on the same principle to obtain the sublingual flange.

Roberto von Krammack used modeling compound to record the extensions. The sublingual flange extension increases the tissue surface without interfering with the functions of mastication, deglutition and phonation.

Modified Fournet Tuller Technique Allan Mack used the principle of maximum coverage together with minimal pressure on the crest of the ridge to obtain retention and stability.

Impressions for Combination-syndrome Patients

Combination syndrome has been described as the characteristic features that occur when an edentulous maxilla is opposed by natural mandibular anterior teeth. These include loss of bone from the anterior portion of the maxillary ridge, overgrowth of the tuberosities, papillary hyperplasia of the hard palatal mucosa, extension of the mandibular anterior teeth, and loss of alveolar bone and ridge height beneath the mandibular removable partial denture. The impression should record the edentulous ridge with minimum distortion. This may be achieved by additional relief in the custom tray, verified clinically with pressure indicating paste, placement of additional vent holes to minimize hydraulic tissue displacement and the subsequent use of highly fluid impression material.

COMMON FAULTS IN PRELIMINARY IMPRESSION COMPOUND IMPRESSIONS

Lower Impression

Insufficient Depth in the Distolingual Pouch

Causes

- Flange of the tray short in this region
- Lack of impression compound in the tray
- Too little force used in seating the tray
- Tongue trapped by tray flanges because the patient failed to raise the tongue as the tray was seated. In some cases it is necessary to push the compound into the lingual pouch area with the forefinger just before tray is placed.

Insufficient Depth in the Lingual, Labial and Buccal Sulci

Causes

- Lack of impression material
- Not seating the tray with sufficient pressure.

Presence of Smooth Hollow in the Buccal Distal Periphery

Causes. Cheek was not released from beneath the compound border during functional trimming.

Edge of the Tray Showing Through the Impression

Causes

- Incorrect centering of the tray before seating
- In anterior lingual region, forward thrust of tongue not being countered by sufficient backward force on the tray
- Use of too large a tray for the mouth or failure to form flanges adequately.

Asymmetical Impression

Causes

- Failure to center the tray in the mouth
- More material on one side than on the other.

Correction to faults (1 and 2) are made by adding small softened pieces of compound to imperfect areas and then reseating and molding the impression; (3) error can by corrected by readaptation or with an entirely new impression.

Upper Impressions

A Crevice in the Midline of the Palatal Posterior 1/3rd

Causes

- Insufficient compound in the palatal area when filling the tray
- Insufficient pressure.

Excess Compound Extending Well Beyond the Posterior Palatal Tray Border

Causes

- Excess pressure, too prolonged pressure when seating the tray
- Too much compound in the palatal area when filling the tray.

Unsupported Compound Falling Away from Palate

Compound which is unsupported by the tray will fall away from the palate by its own weight dragging some of the supported compound with it producing an inaccurate impression.

Causes

- Insufficient material in the tray
- Failure to mold peripheral compound in this region when filling the tray
- Insufficient pressure
- Material too cold.

Tray Flange Showing Through the Compound

- Poorly selected or adapted tray
- Incorrect centering of the tray.

Excess Material in the Labial Sulcus

Causes
- Failure to locate the tray under the ridge
- Too much material in front of the tray.

Impression Technique by K Bhargara and Hardy[2]

Procedure. The edentulous mouth is surveyed clinically. A roentgenographic interpretation is made for any residual roots, or any spiny alveolar edges. Abused soft tissues should be allowed to return to health before the impression is made.

A stock metal tray that is oversized is selected. Impression compound is softened and loaded onto the tray. The impression is then made. The ridge and rugae areas of the impression are scrapped from 1-2 mm in depth depending upon the displaceability of the soft tissue and the prominence of the rugae. After this the plaster model is poured. After the plaster base set properly, the model is recovered and an outline is drawn for the extent of the special double thickness impression tray. This is kept 2 mm short of the sulcus. Compound is used to reinforce the tray. The compound is heated over a flame and rolled over the ridge area of the tray. It is also used to form the handle. The final impression is then made using low fusing compound zinc oxide-eugenol.

Dynamic Impression Methods

Dynamic impression methods[3,7] are useful in patients with advanced residual ridge resorption. In these patients, shape of the osseous structures, and presence of muscle attachments near the crest of the ridge make retention difficult to obtain. For these reasons, the range of muscle action as well as spaces into which the denture can be extended without dislocation must be accurately recorded in the impression. These are made using dynamic methods.[8]

Advantages
- Avoidance of the dislocating effect of the muscles on improperly formed denture borders.
- Complete stabilization because of the possibility of active and passive tissue fixation of the denture. These advantages are the result of the direct shaping of the impression material by functional movements of the muscle and muscle attachments that border the denture base.

Technique. Alginate is commonly used for this procedure because it can be mixed to the desired viscosity. In contrast to conventional techniques, the tissues to be included within the impression is covered with an abundant amount of irreversible hydrocolloid before the impression tray is inserted.

Impression Tray

Functions
- Tray should not interfere with muscle movements
- Tray must permit a proper thickness of impression material
- The tray should stabilize the mandible in a correct position to the maxilla. This requires a special design.

The individual tray of acrylic resin is made on the diagnostic cast and is perforated. The tray must be adjusted to conform to the movements of surrounding tissues.

The thickness of the tray periphery is critical. It should be adequate or the impression material may tear or loosen from the tray on removal from the mouth. The correct thickness of impression material against the denture-bearing tissue is secured by using "stops" made of a thermoplastic material. Those stops allow a correct orientation of the tray on the residual ridge during the making of the impression. One stop is placed in the central incisor region and one each in first molar region. The stops should extend for 3-4 mm along the residual ridge, 2-3 mm wide in a labiolingual direction and 2 mm high. The stops are made by melting the thermoplastic material onto the tissue surface of the tray and then pressing it against the preliminary cast until a space of 2 mm is achieved between the tray and the cast.

Then, the patient is asked to close his mouth slowly until the mandibular rests have obtained firm contact with the maxillae. The patient retains the position of the tray as the impression is being made. The patient is instructed to swallow 3-4 times at 10 seconds interval while the impression is in a moldable condition. The patient should protrude his lips and vigorously contract the buccinator muscle (in between swallows).

Characteristic's of Dynamic Dentures. The dynamic dentures differ from conventional dentures in that the borders are longer lingually and buccally.

Further Reading

1. Zinner ID et al. An analysis of development of complete denture impression techniques. J Prosth Dent 1981; 46(3):242-48.
2. Bhargava and Hardy. Journal of Indian Dental Association. J Indian Dental Assoc, 1959; 31: 141-44.
3. Levin B. Current concepts of lingual flange design. J Prosth Dent, 1981; 45(3): 242-52.
4. McCord et al. Impression making. Br Dental J. 2000; 188(9).
5. Solomon E G R. J Indian Dent Assoc. 1973. March 29.
6. Roberts AL. Principles of full dentures impression making and their application in practice. J Prosth Dent. 1951; 1(3):213-28.
7. Lott and Levin. Flange techniques. J Prosth Dent. 1966;1(16):394-00.
8. Tryde Gerd et al. Dynamic impression methods. J Prosth Dent. 1965;15(6): 1023-33.
9. Buckle G A. J Prosth Dent. 1955; 5(2): 149-61.

8

IMPRESSION TRAYS

INTRODUCTION

Impression tray is defined as a device or receptacle that is used to carry the impression material to the mouth, to confine the impression material in apposition to the denture-bearing area to record minute details, to control the impression material while it sets to form the impression, and to be able to support the impression when the models are being poured.

CLASSIFICATION

According to Levere and Freda in 1976 there are two types of impression trays:
1. Stock trays
2. Custom made trays/special trays/final impression trays.
   Stock trays can be
I. • Disposable—individualized tray
   • Non-disposable
II. • Metallic
   • Non-metallic

III. • Perforated
   • Non-perforated
   • Rim-lock trays—thickened flange edges for retention.
IV. Based on the type of dental arch
   • Edentulous
   • Dentulous
   The materials used in the fabrication of stock trays include:
• Metallic trays
   1. Tin-lead alloy   2. Stainless steel
• For non-metallic stock trays—plastic trays (Colour Plates 1 and 2).

Requirements of Stock Impression Trays

1. Tray must be rigid. Flexible trays cause distortion of the impression.
2. Dimensional stability. Tray should maintain its shape throughout the impression making.
3. It should be smooth to avoid injury to oral tissues.
4. It should provide uniform space for impression material.
5. It should not distort the vestibular areas.
   The first three are met by all the available commercial trays but the last two are not met by all stock trays. In stock trays the flanges may be overs or underextended. As a result uniform space is not available.

AUTOPOLYMERIZING RESIN IMPRESSION TRAYS

Autopolymerizing acrylic resin modified for trays and conventional autopolymerizing resin used for repairs, and baseplates are the materials frequently used for impression trays. Resin materials are easy to use, require no special equipment, and when manipulated properly make excellent impression trays. Resin impression trays can be made thin but reasonably rigid, modified easily by grinding with an arbor band or an acrylic bur and smoothed or polished readily. Properly constructed resin impression trays have sufficient dimensional stability to make an accurate impression.

The two methods of using these materials are the sprinkle-on method and the finger-adapted dough method (Colour Plate 1).

Sprinkle-on Method

1. Make an outline of the impression tray on the cast with a pencil. The borders usually are short of the vestibular reflections of the cast. Often the posterior border is determined by a line extending between the hamular notches, with the mid-point approximately 2 mm distal to the fovea palatina.
2. Block out the severe undercuts with wax, and adapt a layer of baseplate wax to the cast for relief. Trim the relief wax to the desired outline.
3. Paint tinfoil substitute on the stone cast and over the relief wax. The tinfoil substitute facilitates later removal of wax from the impression tray. If the tinfoil substitute does not wet the baseplate wax relief, often 1 or 2 drops of surface tension-reducing agent is added to the tinfoil substitute to increase the wettability and result in easier separation later.
4. Sift powdered polymer onto the cast and relief wax, and saturate it with liquid monomer from an eyedropper. Apply more powder and liquid until there is a uniform layer approximately 2 mm thick. The cast should be tilted during sifting to prevent unnecessary build-up of resin in the palatal region of maxillary casts or in the mucobuccal fold areas of mandibular casts.
5. Cure the impression tray under an inverted plaster bowl to reduce the porosity.
6. Mix more resin in a paper cup and, when it is in the dough stage, form handles and adapt them to the impression tray. Some dentists prefer only one handle in the anterior portion of the tray whereas others have suggested three handles or finger rests for mandibular impression trays. Position the handles in the first molar region and the anterior region of mandibular impression trays. Make the handles approximately 3 to 4 mm thick, 8 mm long, and approximately 8 mm high, place horizontal grooves across the facial and lingual surfaces of the handles to improve the grip. If necessary, the dentist can adjust the handles easily. Handles on the impression tray should approximate the position of the teeth on the finished denture.
7. Adapt the resin dough to the approximate size of the handle, and wet the resin tray at the point of attachment with liquid acrylic monomer in an eye-dropper or a cotton pledget saturated with it to facilitate chemical bonding.
8. After setting, remove the impression tray from the cast, and trim it with an arbor band or bur.
9. Examine the completed tray, and adjust and polish rough areas that can cause discomfort to the patient. Pumice the borders of the tray lightly to make the surface smooth.
10. Store the impression tray on the cast until needed.

Finger-adapted Dough Method

The finger-adapted dough method is used extensively for making resin impression trays. Specially modified resin tray materials can be formed into a dough that can be thinned readily or rolled to the desired thickness and adapted to the cast with finger pressure. The method is quick, and the resultant impression trays fit well and have acceptable dimensional stability.

Procedure

1. Place the outline for the resin impression tray on the cast, and bead the outline with a sharp instrument if desired. The resultant beading on the cured resin tray serves as a guide when trimming.
2. Place the outline for areas of relief on the cast.
3. Block out undercut areas with wax and adapt the relief wax to the cast. Removal of 4-mm squares of relief wax will expose the cast, thereby providing tissue stops.
4. Paint tinfoil substitute on the cast and relief wax.
5. Proportion the impression tray material according to the manufacturer's recommendations, and mix in a paper cup or other suitable container.
6. Check the consistency of the resin periodically, and remove it from the paper cup when it reaches the dough stage. Roll the resin to the desired thickness with a roller to make the impression tray uniformly thick.
7. Hand adapt the material to the cast carefully to avoid overthinning the resin on the convex portions of the cast. It is easy to overthin the impression tray by applying too much finger pressure. Light-colored impression tray resins offer an advantage, since it is frequently possible to see the relief wax through them and avoid overthinning.
8. Remove excess tray material from the cast borders.
9. Form the excess material into handles, and adapt them to the tray. Put more acrylic monomer on the impression tray with a cotton pledget or an eye-dropper at the point of attachment to improve bonding of the handles to the tray.
10. Make the handles small, so that they require only a minimal amount of time for finishing to the proper size.
11. Continue finger adaptation until the impression tray material remains adapted to the cast and does not rebound.
12. Cure the impression tray on the bench or under an inverted plaster bowl.
13. After setting, remove the impression tray from the cast, and trim the borders.
14. Smooth all rough areas and store the tray on the cast.

Vacuum-adapted Method

Vacuum or pressure-formed thermoplastic resin sheets can make good impression trays; the method is quick and easy, but it requires special equipment for adapting the resin sheet to the cast. The materials are available in a variety of colors and thicknesses as well as different degrees of flexibility.

Procedure

1. Place the outline of the impression tray on the cast with a pencil, or bead the outline with a sharp instrument if desired.
2. Block out the undercuts and place the relief on the cast with a material, such as a wet sheet of non-asbestos casting ring lining material, that will not melt during heating of the resin sheet.
3. Centre the cast on the vacuum-adapter plate.
4. Place a resin sheet of the appropriate color and thickness in the heating frame, and rotate the heating unit into position.
5. Activate the heating switch, and continue heating until the specified sag in the material occurs.
6. Lower the frame and resin sheet onto the cast, and start vacuum adaptation. After adaptation is complete, allow the resin sheet to cool, and then remove it from the vacuum-adapting unit.

7. Trim the excess material with a large bur and lathe.
8. Remove the tray from the cast, and trim the borders.
9. Add handles made of autopolymerizing acrylic resin or use preformed metal handles.
10. Store the tray on the cast until ready to use.

Shellac Method

Double-thickness shellac baseplate material is essential for fabricating an impression tray. An advantage of this method is the rapidity with which the shellac baseplate material can be adapted to the cast and the tray fabricated. The serious disadvantage is the lack of dimensional stability of the material, especially during the application of heat when border molding the tray with impression compound (Colour Plates 1, 2).

Procedure

1. Place an outline of the impression tray on the cast and bead if desired.
2. Block out undercuts on the cast with a plaster and pumice mix or with wet non-asbestos casting ring lining material.
3. Provide relief as required with a layer of wet non-asbestos casting ring lining material.
4. Centre a sheet of double-thickness shellac baseplate material over the cast, and melt it onto the cast with flame.
5. Fold the excess shellac material at the borders back onto itself to make them of the proper thickness.
6. Continue adaptation until the shellac material makes intimate contact with the cast and relief material.
7. Form a handle from scrap shellac baseplate material, warm it, and adapt it to the impression tray.
8. Allow the impression tray to cool, then remove it from the cast, and trim it to the border outline. If the cast has been beaded, use the beading on the tray as a guide when trimming. Remove the relief from the tray.
9. Perforate the shellac tray with a No. 8 round bur if using alginate impression material.
10. Store the impression tray on the cast until ready for use.

IMPRESSION TRAYS FOR IMMEDIATE DENTURES

When making trays for immediate dentures the considerations are different from making trays for conventional complete dentures because of the presence of teeth on the cast. The immediate denture treatment sequence used by many dentists consists of removing the posterior teeth; after a healing period making an impression of the relatively well-healed posterior ridges; completing the denture, and then removing the anterior teeth and inserting the denture. Therefore two areas of impression trays for immediate dentures that require consideration are (i) the impression of the edentulous ridges, and (ii) the impression of the remaining natural teeth.

Each of the three impression methods for immediate dentures requires a different type of tray. In one method, a one-piece full-arch impression tray covers the edentulous ridges and natural teeth. The disadvantages of this type of tray is its tendency to be bulky because it is necessary to have the relief over the natural teeth to block out undercuts. A second method of making an immediate denture impression is to use a custom-made impression tray for the posterior edentulous portion of the impression, and then make an over-all impression over the posterior tray and natural teeth. The third method is to use a two-piece tray. The first impression tray is made over the edentulous portion of the arch, and the second over the anterior portion of the arch and the anterior tray will join the first tray.

FULL-ARCH IMPRESSION TRAYS

Appleby and Kerchoff (1955) have described a method of making an overall acrylic resin impression tray for an immediate maxillary denture impression. Their method requires placing the tray outline on the cast, blocking out the natural teeth on the cast with wax, and adapting a layer of baseplate wax over the cast that extends to the border outline. The purpose of this relief is to provide space for the impression material. Autopolymerizing resin is used to make the overall impression tray. The procedure for making the full-arch impression trays involves the finger-adapted, vacuum-adapted, or the sprinke-on method. •

Finger-adapted Dough Method

Procedure

1. Outline the border of the impression tray on the cast with a pencil, and bead it if desired.
2. Block out the teeth on the cast with base-plate wax, so that the tray can be removed without breaking the teeth, adapt a layer of baseplate wax over the cast, and trim to the relief outline.
3. Paint tinfoil substitute on the stone cast and baseplate relief wax.
4. Proportion the autopolymerizing tray resin according to the recommendation of the manufacturer, and mix it in a paper cup. Immediately prior to reaching the dough stage, remove some material from the cup with a spatula, and place it in the border areas of the cast.
5. When the material reaches the desired dough stage, remove it from the cup, and roll it into a sheet of the proper thickness (2 mm).
6. Adapt the resin sheet over the relieved cast. Fold or trim the excess resin extending over the borders of the cast.
7. Continue finger adaptation until the resin begins to set.

8. Permit the resin to cure on the cast, and then carefully remove the tray from the cast.
9. Finish and polish the borders, and smooth rough areas to avoid discomfort for the patient. Perforate the tray with a No. 8 bur to aid in retaining elastic impression materials if desired.

The finger-adapted dough method is preferable to the sprinkle- on method for full-arch impression trays, but either is usable.

Vacuum-adapted Method

The principal advantage of this method is the minimal amount of time used in constructing a tray, and the principal disadvantage is the investment required for specialized equipment.

Procedure

1. Place the outline of the tray on the cast with a pencil or bead it with a sharp instrument.
2. Block out position undercuts and relief areas with a heat-stable relief material.
3. Centre the blocked out cast in the vacuum former.
4. Start the heater and, when the recommended amount of sag occurs, lower the heating frame and activate the vacuum.
5. After completing the adaptation, allow the resin to cool and trim the borders with a large bur in a lathe.
6. Remove the tray, and trim it to the previously established outline.
7. Smooth and finish all borders.
8. Extend the resin that projects over the anterior teeth as a handle for this type of tray.
9. Remove all traces of block out and relief material from the interior of the impression tray.
10. If specified, perforate the tray with a bur to improve retention of the impression material in the tray.
11. Store the completed tray on the cast until needed.

CUSTOM POSTERIOR TRAYS

A simple form of the sectional impression tray for an immediate denture is a tray made over only the edentulous portion of the cast. A second overall impression is made of the teeth and anterior vestibule with a stock tray. Making a custom posterior tray is quick and easy with tray resin and the finger-adapted dough method. It can also be made by the sprinkle-on or vacuum-adapted method.

Finger-adapted Dough Method

Procedure

1. Place an outline of the tray on the cast with a pencil.
2. Extend the impression tray outline to contact the lingual surfaces of the anterior teeth. This extension aids in positioning the tray in the patient's mouth and increases the accuracy of the impression. An alternate method is to use a wax ledge aproximately 2 mm wide anterior to the incisive edges of the teeth. It allows the tray to extend in front of the teeth and aids in positioning the tray.
3. Block out spaces between the teeth with wax to keep resin from entering the undercut areas and to prevent the teeth from breaking when removing the tray from the cast. After blocking out the spaces and undercuts, adapt one layer of baseplate wax for relief.
4. Paint tinfoil substitute on the cast and relief wax.
5. Using a paper cup, mix the resin according to the manufacturer's recommendations.
6. When the resin reaches the desired state, remove it from the paper cup and roll it into a sheet 2 to 3 mm thick, using a template mold or special roller. Adapt the resin to the cast, but do not overthin it on the cast prominences. Trim excess resin from the cast with a knife.
7. Continue adaptation of the resin until it begins to set. After setting, remove the impression tray from the cast and trim it to the previously established outline with an arbor band or an acrylic bur.

MULTIPLE CHOICE QUESTIONS

1. **Metallic trays are examples for**
   a. Stock trays
   b. Custom made trays
   c. Both
   d. None of the above

2. **In the sprinkle on method for making impression trays to reduce porosity, the following method can be used**
   a. Cure impression tray under water
   b. Cure impression tray under inverted plaster bowl
   c. Cure impression tray in open air
   d. None of the above

3. **The main disadvantages of shellac base plate trays are**
   a. Cost
   b. Fabrication procedure is lengthy
   c. Lack of dimensional stability
   d. Poor reproduction of detail

9

POSTERIOR PALATAL SEAL

INTRODUCTION

Retention in complete dentures (CD) is obtained by a combination of physical, mechanical and biologic factors. These factors of retention include adhesion, cohesion, interfacial surface tension, gravity, intimate tissue contact, peripheral seal, atmospheric pressure, and neuromuscular control. Among the biologic factors, border seal obtained by the intimate contact of the denture border with the surrounding soft tissue has got a tremendous influence. The border seal is continued across the palate at the posterior border to obtain the posterior palatal seal (PPS).

Schulze first observed the significant role of the thickness of fluid between two planes or surfaces on retention of dentures. He pointed out that the forces of adhesion, cohesion and surface tension are maximum when the thickness of the interposed film is minimum.

Synder et al (1945) demonstrated that presence of inadequate posterior palatal seal markedly reduced the retention of most of the maxillary complete dentures. Oslund demonstrated the necessity for intimate tissue contact and border seal for retention. However in cases where adhesion and cohesion were predominant, the lack of posterior palatal seal and border seal and presence of small perforations would not significantly alter the retentive properties.

DEFINITIONS

Glossary of prosthodontic terms defines the posterior palatal seal as the tissue along the junction of hard and soft palate on which pressure within the physiologic limits of the tissues can be applied by a denture to aid in the retention of the denture.

Functionally the PPS is similar to that of other areas of the periphery but it has got certain specific characteristics offered by the upward movement of the soft palate during function. All the other borders of the prosthesis are securely sealed by the soft tissue of the vestibular fornix and this seal is seldom broken except in conditions of extreme functional movement. The soft palate does not offer a similar seal because of its upward movement during function. Hence compressibility of soft tissue is utilized to obtain a seal at the posterior seal area.

115

Often during processing of the dentures, the dimensional changes of the acrylic resin will result in the formation of space between the tissue and the denture base. For this reason, a compensatory mechanism should be provided by establishing the posterior palatal seal. PPS compliments the border seal in utilizing atmospheric pressure to resist transient lateral thrusts whereas the forces like cohesion, adhesion and interfacial surface tension maintain the upper denture against vertical dislodging forces.

Some research workers maintain that the posterior palatal seal should be developed as a part of the impression procedure but differ in the materials and methods employed for the purpose. Others cater for the seal by suitably scraping the master cast but differ as to the manner of this scraping. Still others advocate combination of both these methods.

While the general consensus of opinion has been to place the seal over the compressible tissues along the vibrating line, controversial views have been expressed in placing the seal from the vibrating line to various locations as far back as 12 mm posterior to it.

The **vibrating line** is defined in the glossary of prosthodontic terms as "the imaginary line across the posterior part of the soft palate marking the division between the movable and immovable tissue". The fovea palatini are close to the vibrating line and are in soft tissue which make them useful as guides for the location of the posterior border of the denture. But their location in relation to the soft and hard palates and the vibrating line is variable.

The concept, location and placement of PPS for maxillary complete denture were first explained on an anatomic as well as mechanical point of view during 1900-1929.

FUNCTIONS OF THE POSTERIOR PALATAL SEAL[6]

1. To maintain contact with the anterior portion of the soft palate during functional movements of the stomatognathic system. Therefore the primary purpose of the posterior palatal seal is the retention of the maxillary denture.

2. A properly developed PPS will help reduce the gag reflex. There will not be any movement of the denture base and soft palate during normal functional movements.

3. Reduce food accumulation beneath the posterior aspect of the denture due to proper utilization of tissue compressibility.

4. Reduce patient discomfort when contact occurs between the tongue and the posterior end of the denture base as the posterior denture will closely approximate the soft palatal tissues.

5. Will compensate for the volumetric shrinkage that occurs during the polymerization of methylmethacrylate resin.

ANATOMIC AND PHYSIOLOGIC CONSIDERATIONS

The posterior palatal seal[1] is divided into two separate but confluent areas based upon anatomic boundaries. The postpalatal seal extends medially from one tuberosity to the other. Laterally the pterygomaxillary seal extends through the pterygomaxillary notch or hamular notch continuing for 3-4 mm anterolaterally approximating the mucogingival junction. This seal occupies the entire width of the pterygomaxillary notch.

The hamular notch is covered by the pterygomandibular raphae which extends from the posterior aspect of the tuberosity posteroinferiorly to insert into the retromolar pad. This fold of tissue gets activated when the mouth is wide open. So for the accurate recording of this area during the final impression procedure, the mouth should be partially closed.

There are two glandular openings called foveae palatini within the tissue of the posterior portion of the hard palate (usually lying on either side of the midline). The foveae are ductal openings into which the ducts of other palatal glands drain. Some investigators have advocated use of the fovea palatini as a guideline for the placement of the posterior palatal seal. But this may result in the posterior extent of the denture being short by a few millimeters (which will affect retention).

The median palatal raphe which overlies the medial palatal suture contains little or no submucosa and cannot tolerate any compression. This area should be carefully recorded during the final impression procedure.

Anterior and Posterior Vibrating Lines

The posterior palatal seal area lies between anterior and posterior vibrating lines.

The anterior vibrating line is an imaginary line located at the junction of the attached tissues overlying the hard palate and the movable tissues of the immediately adjacent soft palate. This line can be located by having the patient perform the Valsalva maneuver.

In this procedure both the nostrils are held firmly while the patient blows through the nose. This will position the soft palate inferiorly at its junction with the hard palate. The anterior vibrating line can also be approximated by visualizing the area while the patient says "ah" in short vigorous bursts. The anterior vibrating line will be curved due to the projection of the posterior nasal spine.

The posterior vibrating line is an imaginary line at the junction of the aponeurosis of the tensor veli palatine muscle and the muscular portion of the soft palate. It represents the demarcation between the part of the soft palate that has limited movement during function and the remainder of the soft palate that is markedly displaced during functional movements. This line can be visualized by instructing the patient to say "ah" in short bursts in a normal unexaggerated fashion. This line marks the most distal extension of the denture base.

Classification of Soft Palates

There are three classes of soft palate configurations. They are based upon the angle the soft palate makes with the hard palate. The more acute the angle of the soft palate in relation to the hard palate, more muscular activity will be necessary to effect velopharyngeal closure. So the more the soft palate is markedly displaced in function, the less that can be covered by the denture base (Fig. 9.1).

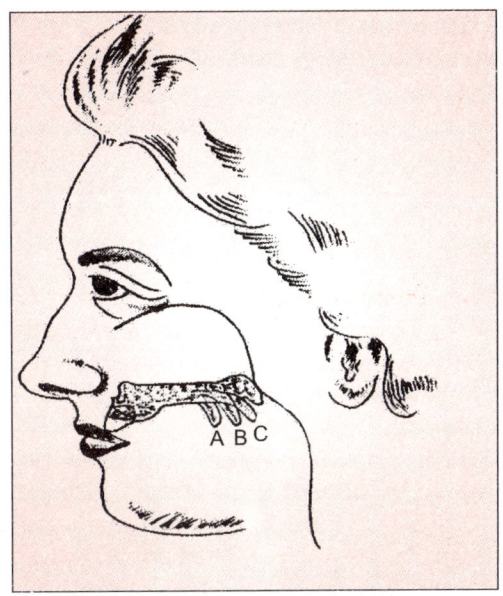

Fig. 9.1. Classification of soft palate.

Class I. Class I indicates a soft palate that is rather horizontal as it extends posteriorly with minimal muscular activity. The posterior palatal seal will be wide but not very deep. Class I palates are considered the most favorable configuration.

Class II. Class II designates palatal contours somewhere between a Class I and Class III.

Class III. Class III indicates the most acute contour in relation to the hard palate, necessitating a marked elevation of the musculature to effect velopharyngeal closure. It is seen along with a high V-shaped vault usually. The posterior palatal seal area will be smaller in width but deeper.

Techniques

Marc Apple Applebaum (1979) reported different techniques for the placement of posterior palatal seal:
1. Conventional approach by Hardy and Kapur.
2. Fluid wax technique by Nelson and Weintraub.[2]
3. Arbitrary scraping of master cast by Boucher.
4. Extended palate technique by Silverman.[3]
5. Adding PPS to an existing denture by Moghadam and Scandrett (1974)
6. Adding the posterior palatal seal by a technique avoiding the use of wax.

Conventional Approach[6]

1. After an accurate and fully extended final impression has been made and poured, a well-adapted resin tray is fabricated on the stone cast.
2. The posterior palatal seal area is then marked. The area is first dried with a gauze and then a T burnisher is used to palpate the hamular process. The hamular processes should not be covered by the denture. The anterior and posterior vibrating lines are then marked using an indelible pencil.
3. The resin or shellac tray is then inserted into the mouth and seated firmly to place. Upon removal from the mouth, the indelible lines should have been transferred to the tray. The tray is then returned to the master cast to transfer the line.
4. The area between the anterior and posterior vibrating lines is usually narrowest in the mid-palatal region because of the projection of the posterior nasal spine, and the outline will be in the shape of a cupid's bow. In the region of the pterygomaxillary seal, the vibrating lines will be confluent.

5. A Kinley scraper is then used to scrape the cast. The deepest areas of the seal are located on either side of the midline, one-third the distance anteriorly from the posterior vibrating line. It is scraped to a depth of approximately 1.5 mm. In the area of the median palatal raphe, the cast is scraped to a depth of 0.5-1 mm (as it cannot withstand heavy compressive forces).
6. On the cast there will be only a slight scraping as the seal approaches the anterior vibrating line, making this area shallower.
7. If the shellac tray is used, it is then replaced on the moistened master cast, reheated and readapted to conform to the scored palatal seal area. After the tray has cooled, it is placed back in the patient's mouth and its retentive qualities are evaluated.

Advantages

1. The trial base will be more retentive, which can produce more accurate maxillomandibular records.
2. Patients will be able to experience the retentive qualities of the trial base giving them the psychological security of knowing that retention will not be a problem.
3. The dentist will be able to understand the retentive qualities of the finished denture.
4. The posterior extension of the denture can be understood by the patient.

Disadvantages

1. It is not a physiological technique and so depends upon the accurate transfer of vibrating lines and careful scraping of the cast.
2. The potential for overcompression of the tissues is great.

Fluid Wax Technique (Physiologic Method).
The fluid wax technique is similar to the conventional technique except that in this technique the indelible transfer markings are recorded on the final wash impression. Corrective wax is used in this technique.

Patient position: The soft plate has to be recorded in its most functionally depressed position. This is essential for establishing a proper posterior palatal seal.

In order to obtain the maximum depression of the soft palate, the porionorbitale plane (FH plane) should be placed 30° below the horizontal, and the tongue should be firmly positioned against the mandibular anterior teeth.

Procedure

1. The wax is melted and painted onto the impression surface within the outline of the seal area.
2. The wax is then allowed to cool slightly below mouth temperature to increase its consistency and to make it more resistant to flow.
3. The impression is carried to the mouth and held under gentle pressure for 4-6 minutes to allow time for the material to flow.
4. Due to the position of the head and the tongue, the mandible will be translated anteriorly. The soft palate will then be passively brought downward and forward due to the indirect attachment of the soft palatal tissues to the body of the mandible and the insertion of the palatoglossus into the side of the tongue. The patient is also asked to periodically rotate the head so that all functional positions of the soft palate are recorded
5. After 4-6 minutes, the impression is removed from the mouth and the wax examined for uniform contact. Areas where contact is minimal will appear dull whereas areas where the tissue has been contacted will have a glossy appearance.
6. The secondary impression is reinserted and held for 3-5 minutes under gentle pressure followed by 2-3 minutes of firm pressure applied to the midpalatal area of the impression tray.
7. Final impression is then boxed and poured.

Precautions

1. The patient should not protrude his tongue beyond the approximated position of the incisal edges as this may foreshorten the posterior border of the final impression.
2. The patient should be cautioned against rinsing with cold water as this may contract the tissues and reduce the flow properties of wax.
3. The borders of the wax should terminate in a feather edge towards the vibrating line. If a butt joint is formed, proper flow may not have taken place.

Advantages

1. It is a physiologic technique displacing tissues within their physiologically acceptable limits.
2. Overcompression of tissues is avoided.
3. Posterior palatal seal is obtained increasing retention.
4. Mechanical scraping of the cast is avoided.

Disadvantages

1. More time is needed
2. Difficulty in handling the materials.

Arbitrary Scraping of the Master Cast. This technique involves scraping of the master cast arbitrarily by the dentist. This technique is the least accurate and is considered unphysiologic.

Silverman's Extended Palate Technique. In this technique, impressions are made with the head tipped at 30° displacement from the horizontal plane and with the tongue held in tension against the lower anterior teeth or tray handle. Silverman, stated that the dentures could be extended from 4-12 mm distal to the vibrating line.

Advantages

1. This technique can be used in patients who have lost excessive amounts of the anterior part of the residual ridge.

2. This can help overcome unfavorable leverages when the denture teeth are placed off the ridge in the same position occupied by the natural teeth.

Disadvantages

This technique can cause discomfort for the patient.

Adding a Posterior Palatal Seal to the Existing Denture (by Moghadam and Scandrett).[4] This technique is similar to the fluid wax technique except that in this technique wax is added to an already existing denture.

Procedure

1. After the wax has been placed in the PPS area, the denture is removed from the mouth. An indelible pencil is used to outline the anterior extent of the seal of the denture.
2. Utility wax is placed vertically across the palate separating the posterior two-thirds from the anterior region and extended across the posterior portion of the denture.
3. Stone is vibrated into the denture wax surface outlined by the utility wax. After the stone has set, wax is eliminated and the denture is cleaned.
4. The denture is then trimmed distal to the anterior vibrating line.
5. Lubricant is then applied to the unground areas including the polished surface of the denture and separating medium is applied to the cast.
6. Autopolymerizing acrylic resin powder is then added into the area created by the elimination of wax, and the cast is held firmly to the denture by rubber bands.
7. After the initial set has taken place, they are placed in a pressure pot with water (140° F) for 20 minutes under 30 psi pressure. After the cast and denture are separated, the excess acrylic is trimmed off and the denture is polished.

Calomini, Fieldman and Kuebker (1983). Described a technique for precise location and preparation of the posterior palatal seal on the master cast. This was a semiphysiologic method. In this technique, after finishing the final impression, both the hamular notch areas were palpated and located by means of a Landmore plugger No.3 or similar instrument and marked with an ink pencil or color applicator stick. The vibrating line was located by the phonation method and was marked on the palate. This line was connected with the ink mark in the hamular notches. Soft displaceable tissue, anterior to this vibrating line was palpated with the Landmore plugger and the area of displaceable tissue was marked. The maximum width between these two lines was 5-6 mm and in the midline was 2-3 mm. Dried impression was inserted into the mouth thus transferring the line to the impression. Impression was boxed and poured in dental stone. The ink mark on the impression was thus transferred to the cast. Posterior bead line was prepared on the cast to a depth of 1-1.5 mm and extended through the hamular notches. The other areas on the posterior palatal seal ware relieved with the scrapper. The depth of scraping varied.

Use of Light Cure Resin for the Intraoral Correction of the Posterior Palatal Seal. A high intensity white light is used. In this technique, light-cured resin is added in stages and cured.

Advantages

1. There is no extreme reaction to irritate the oral tissues.
2. There is minimal volumetric shrinkage during curing.
3. The technique closely approximates a physiologic technique.
4. Chair side time is less.

Troubleshooting

Underextension[5]

Causes

1. Some practitioners use the fovea palatini as a landmark for terminating the denture base. This may deprive the patient of 4-12 mm of tissue coverage.
2. Patient may be a gagger.
3. Failure of the dentist to carefully examine the hard and soft palates.
4. Lab technician may trim the posterior borders too short.

ESTABLISHING THE POSTERIOR PALATAL SEAL DURING THE FINAL IMPRESSION STAGE

Izharul Haque Ansari proposed this technique. Incorporating the PPS during the final impression stage has the following advantages over the conventional method of cast scribing:

1. The procedure places the entire responsibility of locating and incorporating the PPS into the hands of the clinician
2. The practitioner will then be able to assess the retentive qualities of the finished denture
3. Posterior palatal seal is incorporated into the trial denture base for added retention, thus increasing the diagnostic information and accuracy of record taking procedures
4. Overcompression of tissue is avoided.

The fluid wax technique is the method of choice for the establishment of PPS at final impression stage, but it has the following disadvantages

1. More time is required during the impression appointment
2. A heating unit is required to condition the wax
3. Difficulty may be experienced in handling the materials
4. Added care during the boxing procedure for cast formation is necessary to prevent distortion of the carefully added PPS wax.

PROCEDURE

1. Before the border molding procedure, trim and adjust the posterior border of the custom tray 1 to 2 mm distal to the vibrating line
2. Complete the border molding and make a final impression by using zinc oxide-eugenol
3. Remove the impression from the mouth
4. Mark the anterior and posterior vibrating line in the mouth with an indelible marking stick
5. Reinsert the maxillary impression in the mouth, transfer the location of vibrating lines to the impression. (If a minimal, unilateral undercut exists the ZOE impression can be reinserted). (In situations with bilateral undercuts, surgical correction may be required).
6. Redefine the transfer marking on the impression carefully and make criss-cross grooves with a hot instrument within the pencil outline. This will provide anchorage to the modeling compound to be use in the next step
7. Soften greenstick modeling compound over a flame, taper near the tip, and place within the outline of the PPS area. Alternatively use modeling compound heated in a plastic disposable syringe and place the compound precisely as previously described
8. Chill the compound after placing precisely within the pencil outline. Reheat the modeling compound with pinpoint flame or a Hanau alcohol torch. Quickly temper the compound in a waterbath and carry the impression into the patient's mouth and hold it in place under gentle pressure
9. For better control of pressure, place the wet impression in the mouth and slowly press in the midpalate region until it is firmly seated; observe the posterior border of the impression for escaping air-bubbles beneath the distal border. Add the greenstick modeling compound gradually until there is no leakage

10. Check the effect of PPS by upward pressure on the anterior region of the impression tray. An easy break of the seal indicates that further compression of tissue is required until an effective seal is attained. Excess modeling compound that flows anterior to the anterior vibrating line must be carefully removed with a sharp scalpel.
11. Remove the impression from the mouth; bead, box, and pour in stone.
12. Posterior palatal seal will be incorporated in the master cast, which allows the record base to be constructed and that accurately represents the finished denture base.

Under Post Damming

Under postdamming occurs when the patient keeps the mouth wide open during the trial impression.

This can be evaluated by placing the wet denture into the mouth and slowly pressing in the midpalatal region until it is firmly seated. If air-bubbles are seen escaping from beneath the distal border, then at that point, the denture is under postdammed.

Over Postdamming

Over postdamming occurs due to overscraping of the master cast resulting in excessive displacement of the palatal tissues.

Overextension

Overextension can occur due to overextension of the denture base. The patient may complain of difficulty in swallowing. This condition may be managed be removing those areas with a bur and repolishing.

Further Reading

1. Calomeni et al. Posterior palatal seal locations and preparations on the maxillary complete denture. J Prosth Dent. 1983; 49: 628-30.
2. Weintraub. Establishing the posterior palatal seal during the final impression procedure. J Prosth Dent. 1977; 94: 504-10.
3. Silverman S I. Dimensions and displacement patterns of posterior palatal seal. J Prosth Dent. 1971; 25: 470-88.
4. Moghadam, Scandrett. A technique for adding the posterior palatal seal. J Prosth Dent. 1974; 132: 443-47.
5. Landa J S. Trouble shooting in complete denture prosthesis. J Prosth Dent. 1959; 8: 978-87.
6. Hardy I R, Kapur K. Posterior palatal seal, its rationale and importance. J Prosth Dent. 1958; 8: 386-97.

MULTIPLE CHOICE QUESTIONS

1. **The Valsalva maneuver is used to determine the**
   a. Anterior vibrating line
   b. Posterior vibrating line
   c. Postpalatal seal areas
   d. None of the above

2. **The extended palate technique was introduced by**
   a. Boucher
   b. Hardy and Kapur
   c. Weintraub
   d. Silverman

3. **Under postdamming can be evaluated by**
   a. Direct examination
   b. By seating the wet denture and observing air bubbles escaping from underneath the denture.
   c. By placing the denture and doing the Valsalva procedure
   d. None of the above

FAQ's

1. **Definition of posterior palatal seal**
2. **Methods for recording posterior palatal seal.**
3. **Troubleshooting**

10

RECORD BASES AND OCCLUSION RIMS

DEFINITIONS

Baseplate (record base, temporary base, trial base). A temporary form representing the base of a denture. The baseplate is used for maxillomandibular (jaw) relation records, arranging artificial teeth, or trial placement in the mouth.

Stabilized Baseplate. A baseplate lined with a plastic or other material to improve its adaptation and stability.

Occlusion Rim. An occluding surface built on temporary or permanent denture bases for the purpose of making maxillomandibular records and arranging teeth.

The purposes of baseplates are: (i) to act as carriers for occlusal rims on which jaw relations are recorded, (ii) to hold the teeth in the wax set-up for the try-in stage, and (iii) to check the accuracy of the previously recorded records.

Dentists use the baseplates and attached occlusion rims to transmit important infor-

mation to the dental laboratory technician. Jaw relationships, the midline occlusal plane, high and low lip line, cuspid line, amount of horizontal and vertical overlap, and desired support for lips and cheeks can be indicated on the baseplate and occlusion rim.

REQUIREMENTS FOR BASEPLATES

1. The baseplate should adapt to the basal seat area as the finished denture base.
2. The baseplate should have the same border form as the finished denture base.
3. The baseplate should be sufficiently rigid to resist biting forces.
4. The baseplate should be dimensionally stable.
5. The baseplate as constructed should permit its use as a base for setting up teeth.
6. It should be possible to construct baseplates quickly, easily and inexpensively.
7. Baseplates should have no undersirable color.
8. The baseplate should not abrade the cast during removal and replacement.
9. It should take advantage of desirable undercuts and be of a material that bonds with that used to block out undercuts on

the cast so that it becomes part of the baseplate.

10. Baseplates should fit the cast accurately, be sufficiently rigid to resist closing forces, and has sufficient dimensional stability to maintain fit and rigidity throughout the clinical and laboratory procedures used in denture construction. Although they should satisfy these requirements, unduly thick baseplates might encroach on the space available for setting teeth.

11. They should be of an acceptable color, and the borders should be smooth, rounded, and similar to those of the prospective denture.

12. Removal of the baseplate from the cast or replacement should cause no damage to either.

BASEPLATE MATERIALS

Materials used singly or in combination for constructing baseplates are autopolymerizing resins, shellac baseplate material, thermoplastic resins, heat-curing resins, baseplate wax, and metal. Zinc oxide impression paste, elastomeric impression materials and hard or soft-curing resins are other types of materials used in combination to stabilize baseplates by improving their adaptation and rigidity. Lining the baseplates with self curing resins and elastomeric impression materials permits extension of the baseplate into moderate undercuts and removal or replacement of the baseplate on the cast without damage to either (Colour Plate 2).

Autopolymerizing Resin Baseplates

Autopolymerizing resins (cold-curing or self-curing resins) require an activator and a catalyst for polymerization and no external heat: (i) They are readily available at a reasonable cost, (ii) set hard and (iii) are rigid or soft and flexible according to the formulation, (iv) and take color satisfactorily, and (v) their handling characteristics are suitable for constructing baseplates that are both serviceable and economical. Therefore autopolymerizing resins, singly or in combination, are the materials used most frequently for baseplates.

Sprinkle-on Method

The sprinkle-on method is excellent. It consists of coating the cast with tinfoil substitute, sifting polymer powder on it, and saturating it with liquid monomer. Alternate applications of powder and liquid continue until the baseplate is of desired thickness. It is essential that this method be performed in a well-ventilated area to minimize exposure to resin fumes. Placing the baseplate in a pressure pot or under an inverted plaster bowl while it is polymerizing, results in less porosity.

Procedure

1. Carefully examine the cast and identify the undercuts that need relief.

2. Paint tinfoil substitute on the wet cast with extreme care, so that all parts contacting the resin receive coating.

3. Block out severe undercuts with baseplate wax to prevent the baseplate from extending into undercut areas.

4. Fill undercuts that are not severe with soft-curing autopolymerizing resin. Three methods of applying soft-curing resin are: (i) to mix the soft-curing resin powder and liquid in a dappen dish and applying it to the undercuts with a spatula, (ii) sprinkle on the soft-curing resin powder and saturate it with monomer from an eye-dropper, or (iii) paint the resin into the undercuts with a brush.

5. Occasionally, the soft-curing resin tends to flow out of the undercuts instead of remaining in place. It is posssible to prevent this problem by warming the surface of the resin with warm air from a chip blower or by dipping the cast into hot water. Warming produces a surface set on the self-curing resin, thereby assuring it will remain in place.

6. Sift the conventional autopolymerizing resin powder onto the cast and self-curing resin, and saturate it with liquid. Use an eye dropper to apply the monomer. Continue alternating applications of powder and liquid until the baseplate is of the desired thickness. Tilt the cast laterally while applying the resin to prevent pooling the liquid and powder in the palate of maxillary casts, which can cause an excessively thick palate. After completing the upward facing surfaces, tilt the cast in the opposite direction and build up the other surfaces in a similar manner. This procedure helps to prevent an undesirable build-up in the depth of the palate. An excessively thick palate requires reduction by grinding.

7. When the resin is of the desired thickness, (approximately 2 mm), it is ready to be cured. Cure the baseplate under an inverted plaster bowl or in a pressure pot under warm water for 20 minutes at 20 psi. The first method which requires no additional equipment produces an acceptable baseplate, though it often has more surface porosity.

8. Examine the cured baseplate on the cast to evaluate its adaptation. If blockout of the undercuts on the cast is adequate, directing a stream of air under the border will often lift the baseplate from the cast. It may be necessary to pry up the baseplate gently and lift from the cast, taking care not to break either one. If prying is necessary, do it on the side opposite the undercuts. When it is impossible to separate the baseplate from the cast, dip both in clear slurry water. This water will act as a lubricant and allows a the baseplate to be removed.

9. Trim the resin flash around the borders with an arbor band or a lathe, resin-cutting stone, or bur in a handpiece.

10. Smooth the borders and any rough spots on the baseplates with a wet rag wheel and a slurry of water and flour of pumice. A slow speed (1740 rpm) on the lathe with plenty of pumice slurry reduces the build-up of heat in the baseplate during polishing and speeds the procedure.

11. Store the finished baseplate in water until it is ready for use.

If a mandibular cast has an extremely flat ridge in the anterior region, the baseplate constructed on this cast will not be rigid, even after correct application of the resin. Reinforcing the baseplate with a stiff wire embedded in the resin and extending from premolar to premolar greatly improves its strength and increases its rigidity.

Finger-adapted Dough Method

Mix the powder and liquid together until the mixture is the consistency of dough, form it into a roll or sheet, and adapt it to the cast with finger pressure. A modification of this method is to roll the dough in a sheet of the desired thickness before adapting it to the cast.

Procedure

1. Identify the undercuts, and decide whether to use wax or self-curing resin for blockout.
2. Apply tinfoil substitute to the cast.
3. Put baseplate wax in severe undercuts and self-curing resin in moderate undercuts.
4. Proportion and mix the resin powder and liquid according to the manufacturer's recommendations. When the mixture is in the dough stage, form the resin into a roll, and adapt it to the cast. The resin baseplate should be approximately 2 mm thick. It is possible to make a convenient mold by impressing a double thickness shellac baseplate into a mix of artificial stone. After the stone has set, remove the baseplate and use the resultant mold to shape a resin sheet of uniform thickness into a baseplate.
5. Continue finger adaptation until the resin, being well adapted to the cast, does not spring away or rebound.
6. Place the baseplate on the cast under a plaster bowl or in a pressure pot for polymerization.

7. After curing, remove the baseplate from the cast, trim it, and smooth.

8. Replace the baseplate on the cast, and evaluate the adaptation and border thickness. Store the completed baseplate in water until needed.

Disadvantages

1. Unless using gloves, needless repeated contact with resin during adaptation may lead to contamination of the resin, or can result in contact dermatitis.

2. It is exceedingly difficult to achieve uniform thickness of the baseplate by hand adaptation. Invariably, the resin is too thin over the convex ridge portions and too thick in the less accessible areas.

3. Usually it is necessary to continue finger adaptation throughout polymerization to prevent rebound or lift-off of the resin, but this manipulation can cause distortion.

Confined Dough Methods

Stone-mold method

1. Adapt one layer of baseplate wax over the cast, and seal it around the borders to form a wax pattern for the proposed baseplate. Fill in the borders of the baseplate with additional wax to make them of the proper thickness. This pattern should duplicate the finished baseplate in thickness and contour; placing additional wax in undercut areas or over the midline on maxillary casts can increase the thickness.

2. Place index indentations on the land area of the cast at four widely separated points with a large round bur.

3. Paint separating medium on the stone and land areas.

4. Box the cast and pattern with boxing wax. This wax should extend above the cast to make the stone at least 15 mm thick.

5. Mix artificial stone with slurry concentrate to accelerate the set, and vibrate it onto the boxed cast and pattern.

6. Allow the boxed stone to set.

7. After setting, remove the stone index and lift the wax pattern from the cast.

8. Paint tinfoil substitute on the cast and stone index.

9. Reassemble the index and cast to check the fit.

10. Blockout undercuts on the cast with wax or self-curing resin.

11. Proportion the autopolymerizing resin, and mix according to the manufacturer's recommendations. When the mix reaches the dough stage, mold it onto the cast. Usually, 8 to 10 ml of monomer and 24 to 30 ml of polymer are enough; use excess resin to minimize voids.

12. Assemble the index and cast, and maintain closure with heavy rubber bands.

13. Cure the mold in a pressure pot in warm water at 2 psi for 20 minutes or bench cure it. Confinement and pressure from the stone index greatly reduces porosity.

14. After the resin has hardened, open the mold, remove the baseplate, and finish it.

Wax-confined Method. Among the advantages claimed for this method are that the wax pattern assures the proper thickness of the baseplate throughout, especially in the palate, and that the outer wax surface makes the record base neat and pleasing in appearance.

Procedure

1. Paint the cast with tinfoil substitute. Apply three coats, and allow the last coat to set for 10 minutes.

2. Blockout all undercuts on the cast with medium-hard baseplate wax.

3. Adapt one layer of baseplate wax over the blocked out master cast to make a wax form or tray. Trim the wax 2 mm short of the borders of the cast.

4. Make a thin mix of cold-curing acrylic resin tray material, using two parts polymer to one part monomer.

5. Put some of the resin mix in the borders of the cast and on the palate of the maxillary cast.
6. Pour the rest into the wax form and spread it evenly on the tissue side.
7. Invert the wax form, and carefully press the resin into place on the surface of the cast until it is 1 to 2 mm thick.
8. Mold the excess acrylic resin over the borders with the fingers until it is approximately 2 mm thick over the wax around the borders.
9. Cure the resin for 20 minutes in a pressure chamber at 20 psi or in warm water.
10. When cured, remove the baseplate from the cast, smooth it, and polish it. Do not overheat it. The blockout adheres to the inside of the resin base.
11. Fabricate occlusion rims on the record bases (Fig. 10.1).

This method results in a baseplate with a coating of baseplate wax on the exterior surface. The wax coating facilitates addition of a wax occlusion rim or setting of the denture teeth at a later time.

Shellac Baseplates

The principal advantage of shellac baseplates is the minimal amount of time required to adapt and make them. The main disadvantage is the chance of losing their initial adaptation.

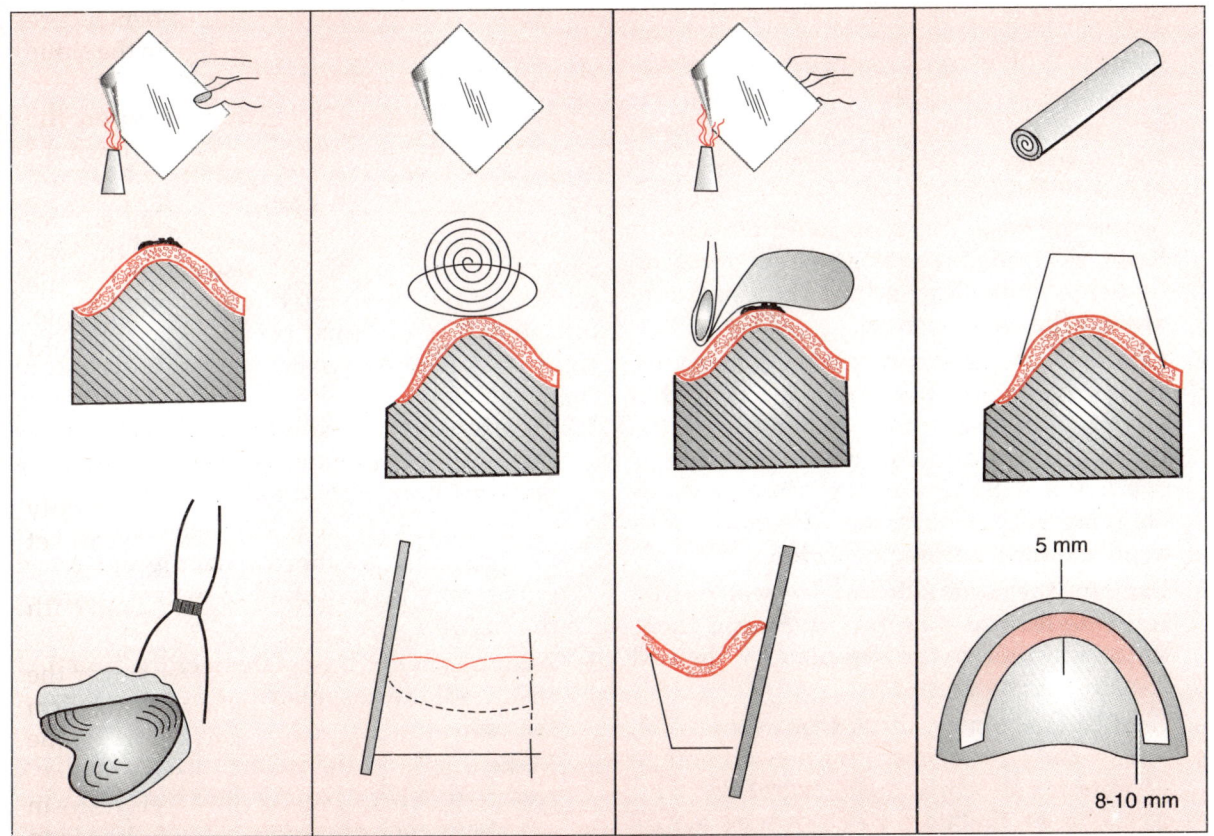

Fig. 10.1. Fabrication of a wax occlusal rim.

Procedure

The procedure is explained in the following step (Fig. 10.2 A–L).

1. Soak the cast in clear slurry water to keep the shellac baseplate from sticking to the cast when heated. An alternate method is to rub powdered talc onto the cast before adapting the baseplate. Failure to treat the cast or heating the baseplate too much will make them stick together and possibly damage the cast. Fill in several undercuts with a mix of one part flour of pumice to one part plaster, or soften the baseplate to make it withdraw from the undercut without breaking the cast. It is easy to remove the plaster-pumice mixture later.

2. Pass the baseplate through a Bunsen burner flame until softened, and place it over the cast, or place the baseplate on the cast and flame it with a Bunsen burner. When one shellac blank is not large enough to cover a cast, it is possible to add a piece of scrap shellac by flame softening both pieces and readapting them.

3. Soften the baseplate more with an alcohol torch, as needed, continue finger molding or use a spatula to adapt the baseplate around the entire border.

4. Cool the baseplate and remove it from the cast. If necessary, trim the borders with a arbor band, fast-cut stone, or bur. If the lathe turns too fast and too much pressure is exerted, it will gum up the trimmer. Non-clogging rubber abrasive wheels are also available for trimming baseplates.

5. Examine the tissue side for glossy areas that indicate lack of adaptation. Flame these areas, and replace the baseplate on the cast for more adaptation.

6. Shellac baseplates should be reinforced, Heavy-duty paper clips are a good source of wire for reinforcement. Adapt the wire to the casts. Embed a piece of wire across the posterior border of the maxillary baseplate. In the mandibular baseplate, embed it lingual to the crest of the ridge from premolar area to premolar area. The reinforcement significantly improves both the strength and rigidity of the baseplate.

7. After cooling, store shellac baseplates on the cast, to minimize warpage before use. Readapt them later if necessary. To prevent breakage of a shellac baseplate and/or cast, blockout undercuts on the cast, or warm the baseplate prior to separation if it extends into the undercut. Do not overheat or adapt it to a dry cast because it can stick to the cast.

Stabilized Shellac Baseplates

Baseplates stabilized with zinc oxide-eugenol impression paste. Shellac baseplates reinforced with zinc oxide-eugenol impression paste exhibit better adaptation and dimensional stability and have been in use for some time. Zinc oxide impression materials adapt well to the cast and can improve the dimensional stability of shellac baseplates. Their disadvantages are: (i) that the baseplates are thicker because of the thickness of the impression paste liner, (ii) their construction requires additional time, and (iii) blockout of undercuts on the cast is essential because the relatively rigid stabilized baseplates cannot extend into the undercuts.

1. Identify and blockout the undercuts on the cast with wax or a mix of one part plaster to one part flour of pumice.

2. Coat the cast with 0.001 inch (0.0025 cm) thick tinfoil. A toothbrush handle and pencil eraser may be modified to aid in adapting the tinfoil.

3. Adapt a shellac baseplate over the tinfoiled cast. Cool the baseplate and remove it from the cast.

4. Make a hole in the palate of the maxillary baseplate with a No. 8 round bur. Mix zinc oxide-eugenol impression paste, and place it into the baseplate. The hole will allow

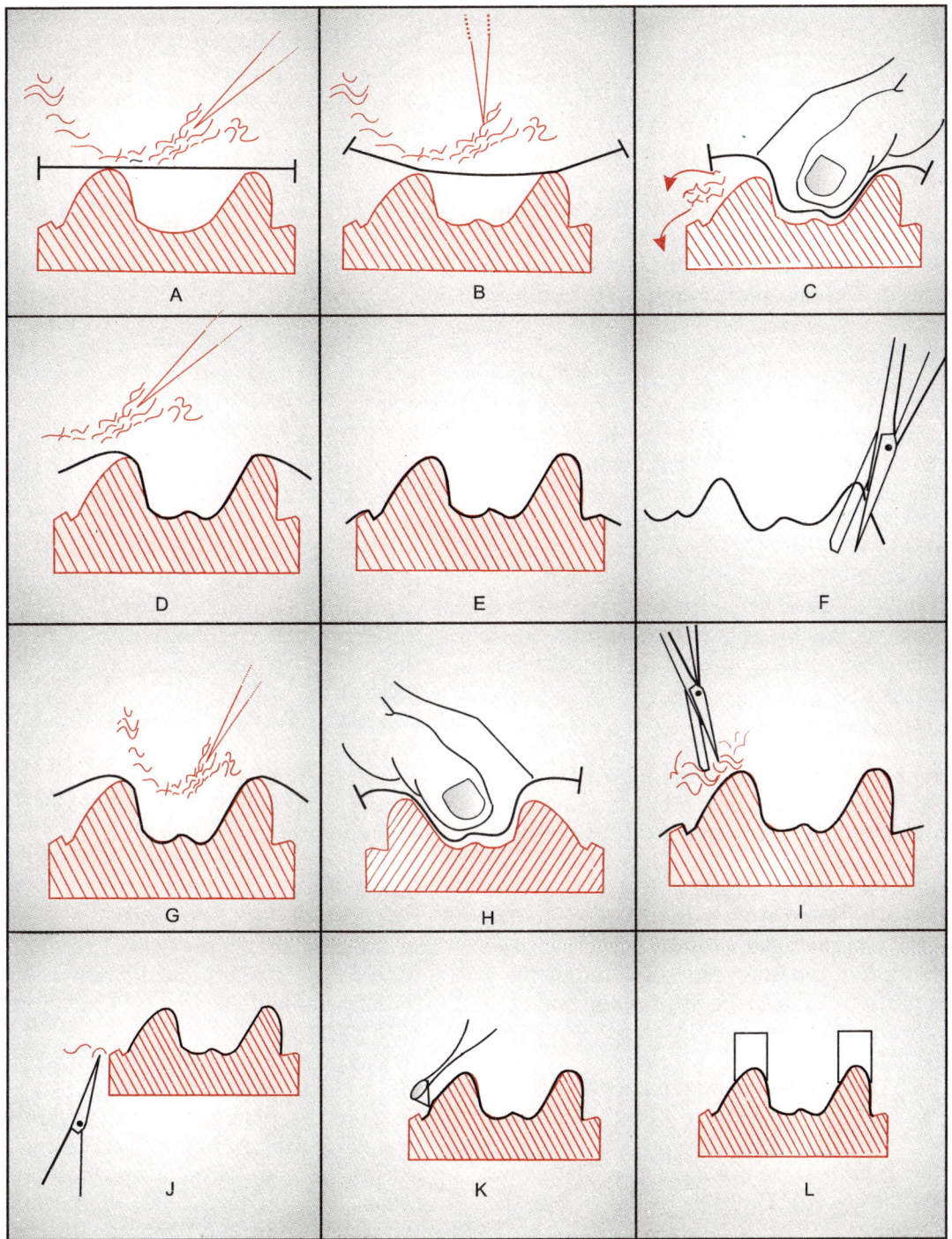

Fig. 10.2. Various steps in the adaptation of a shellac base plate.

excess impression material to escape and to minimize voids.

5. Replace the baseplate containing zinc-oxide impression paste on the tinfoiled cast in a position that will make the layer of impression material approximately 1 mm thick.
6. After it has hardened, remove the baseplate from the cast. The tinfoil is usually left in the baseplate but may be peeled off if desired. The baseplate is ready for use.

Baseplate Stabilized with Elastomeric Impression Materials

The advantages of using these materials as stabilizers are: (i) their inherent flexibility, and (ii) smooth surface. The flexibility of this type of material permits baseplate extensions into moderate undercuts and minimizes the need for blockout of the cast. The principal disadvantage of this procedure is the added thickness of the baseplate that results from using the elastomeric impression material liner.

Procedure

The procedures for constructing a baseplate stabilized with elastomeric imression material are similar to those using zinc-oxide impression material.
1. Apply tinfoil to the cast.
2. Make additional holes in the adapted shellac baseplate with a No.8 round bur to increase retention of the liner, and apply adhesive.
3. Proportion and mix the impression material according to the manufacturer's recommendations.
4. Apply the impression material to the interior of the baseplate, and seat it on the tinfoiled cast.
5. After it has set, remove the baseplate, and trim the excess. Peel the tinfoil out of the baseplate.
6. The completed baseplate fits the cast accurately and affords the patient con-siderable comfort during the jaw relation recording procedures.

Baseplates Stabilized with Autopolymerizing Resin

Autopolymerizing resin used as a liner improves both the adaptation and rigidity of the baseplate. The disadvantages of this method are: (i) the possibility of warping the baseplate as a result of internal stresses being released in the resin, and (ii) liner and the additional time required for fabrication.

Procedure

The technique for stabilizing a baseplate with autopolymerizing resin is similar to those described for zinc oxide-eugenol impression paste.
1. Identify undercuts on the cast, and block them out with wax. Since the resin liner is rigid, the baseplate cannot extend into undercut areas without risk of fracturing the baseplate or damaging the cast on separation.
2. Apply tinfoil to the cast, or coat it with tinfoil substitute.
3. Adapt the shellac baseplate to the cast, and trim it 2 mm short of the borders if using autopolymerizing resin borders.
4. If the cast is not tinfoiled, recoat it with a tinfoil substitute.
5. Place two holes in the canine area and two in the first molar regions of the baseplate with a No. 8 round bur. Place another hole in the palate when constructing a maxillary baseplate.
6. Mix autopolymerizing resin, and place it into the baseplate with a spatula.
7. Seat the baseplate on the cast. Exercise care in seating the baseplate on the cast to assure a thin uniform layer of autopolymerizing resin.
8. After it has hardened, remove the baseplate from the cast, examine it, and polish the borders.

Thermoplastic Resin Baseplates and Vacuum-adapted Resin Baseplates

A quick and easy method of making a usable baseplate is to vacuum mold a sheet of thermoplastic resin to a cast. The preformed resin sheet affords excellent thickness and reasonably good adaptation to the cast, particularly when using thinner sheets. The advantages of this method are: (i) simple technique; (ii) minimal amounts of time required; (iii) excellent control of thickness; (iv) choice of a variety of materials for baseplates, splints, trays, copings, and mouthguards; (v) satisfactory rigidity, particularly when using thicker materials; and (vi) excellent adaptation to the cast. The disadvantages are: (i) expense of the equipment, (ii) difficult in achieving an intimate adaptation to the cast in deep recesses and border reflections, and (iii) and the problem of forming smooth rounded borders from only one layer of a resin sheet.

Procedure

1. Examine the cast and identify the undercuts that require blockout: (deep undercuts and delicate creases or folds in the cast). Use a heat-stable blockout compound to preclude breaking the cast on separation. Do not use wax because it will melt at the temperature required for adaptation.

2. Select a resin sheet of the proper thickness, usually 0.060 inch. Thicker material is better for the mandibular baseplate, in which achieving adequate rigidity may be a problem.

3. Although the specific directions for molding vary with each manufacturer's equipment and materials, the principles are similar. Place the blocked out cast on the vacuum plate. Make certain that the cast bases are flat, and the sides are not undercut.

4. Position a resin sheet of the desired thickness in the holding frame, and align and activate the heating unit.

5. Watch the resin sheet while heating it, and when it sags approximately ½ inch below the lower edge of the hinged frame, lower the frame over the vacuum plate.

OCCLUSION RIMS

Definition: An occlusion rim is a wax form used to establish accurate maxillomandibular jaw relations and for arranging artificial teeth to form the trial denture. Its other uses include

1. It helps to determine the length and width of artificial teeth.
2. To determine the mid line of the arch for correct placement of central incisors.
3. To develop proper lip support.
4. To develop cuspid eminences (Colour Plate 2).

Dimensions of Occlusion Rims

The Maxillary Occlusion Rim: The anterior height is 21 mm from the depth of the labial sulcus and posterior height is 18 mm.

The Mandibular Occlusion Rim: The anterior height of the rim is 18 mm and the posterior height is determined by developing the rim parallel to the junction between the anterior two-third and the posterior one-third of the retromolar pad.

In clinical practice, dentists receive upper wax rims that are duly molded into the form of the upper denture at the chairside. The precise form of the upper wax rim or block depended essentially, on how the technicians were taught. In essence, considerable variation probably exists among technicians with regard to the positioning of the labial face of the rim. The consequence of this is that it is often a matter of chance that wax has to be removed or added to the upper rim. In an attempt to save clinical time and at the same time render the upper rims more appropriate in form for each patient, two techniques have evolved: (i) the biometric technique, and (ii) the Swissdent technique.

Watt and MacGregor outlined the principles of biometric guidelines to help compensate for facial changes following tooth loss, predominantly in the maxilla. In essence, they advocated that the replacement upper teeth be placed in mean pre-extraction positions. The 'fixed' points of reference taken for measurements were the remnants of the lingual gingival margin.

The Biometric Principle

The biometric principle has much merit in that: It helps to compensate for post-extraction bone loss by placement of the denture teeth in perceived pre-extraction positions. A further advantage of placement of the maxillary (denture) teeth labial/buccal to the residual ridge is that this promotes lower denture stability. The placement of the upper posterior teeth buccal to the maxillary ridge, in addition to compensating for the resorption pattern of the maxilla, also means that their palatal cusps may be placed over the mandibular ridge crest. In practice, the palatal cusps will therefore occlude into the central fossae of the lower posterior teeth, thereby directing occlusal forces onto the residual ridge. In addition this placement of the lower teeth over the lower ridge tends to avoid constriction of tongue space. Perhaps the principal deficiency of the biometric principle is that: (i) it does not necessarily customize the denture form for each patient, nor does it cater for biological ageing, and (ii) anatomical features not dissimilar to the remnants of the lingual gingival margin have been observed in patients suffering from anodontia.

Swissdent Technique

Swissdent technique, relies on close and unambiguous communication between the clinician and the technician. It uses two distinct measurements for each patient in order that the upper rim (termed the esthetic control base [ACB] may be customized for each patient. These two measurements are related to the patient's facial form and are taken immediately after the definitive impressions have been recorded and are despatched along with these impressions to the laboratory.

The first measurement is taken via the papillameter. The procedures to be followed for the papillameter reading are as follows:

- Place the papillameter inside the patient's upper lip and let it rest on the incisive papilla.
- Add addition-cured polyvinyl siloxane (PVS) putty to the papillameter and mold the upper lip to restore the vermilion border. In younger patient's the philtrum may be restored but this may not be possible in older patients.
- Determine how much of the upper incisor will be shown under the upper resting lip length.
- Level the PVS at the incisal level and record the reading from the graduated scale on the papillameter.
- The customized papillameter is sent to the laboratory and this enables the technician to have sufficient information to prepare an upper rim that provides upper lip support. Patient information, e.g. from photographs or via dentures favored by the patient may also be used to help determine the upper lip form which is well perceived by the patient. Equally, the alma gauge may be used to produce an upper rim ACB with equivalent dimensions labially to previous or current dentures that are considered adequate. The alma gauge comprises a graduated table and a spring-loaded pointer that is also graduated. The denture being 'templated' is placed on the graduated table and the pointer placed in the impression surface of the denture in the middle of the area occupied by the incisive papilla. The distance from the pointer to the incisal tip of the central incisors may be read off the graduated scale on the table. The vertical distance from the pointer tip to the incisal tips is then read off the graduated scale, giving a three-dimensional reading from the incisive papilla to the incisal tips of the central incisors.

The second measurement concerns the anterior width of the upper rim and for this a caliper-like device called an *alameter* is used. The alameter's usage is based on a reasonable clinical guideline, namely that the width between the alar cartilages in a patient. This reading enables the technician to evaluate the width of the upper rim, assuming that there is symmetry about the palatal midline.

Preparation of the Upper Rim

Upper rims comprise bases and rims. The bases may be made of wax, thermoplastic resin or of polymethylmethracylate (PMMA) while the rims are generally made of wax.

Technical Aspects of Rim Preparation

Using the papillameter and alameter readings, the anterior aspect of the rim may be customized, in wax to permit early visualization of the aesthetic form of the upper denture. The alameter reading further helps the technician customize the rim by establishing the intercanine distance customized for each patient.

The posterior aspect of the rim is also made of wax and resembles conventional record rims.

Figures 10.3–10.7 show the technical aspects of the procedure.

Clinical Stages in Determining the Form of the Upper Rim. There are eight clinical stages:

- Before immersing the rim in disinfectant material in keeping with conventional infection control procedures and prior to inserting the rim into the mouth, the clinician should ensure that the rim is well adapted to the master cast. Alternating finger pressure on each side of the rim should not elicit a rocking of the rim on the cast.
- When the rim has been inserted into the mouth and the clinician has ensured stability of the rim, the first clinical step is to ensure that the infranasal tissues are harmonious with the soft tissues of the middle third of

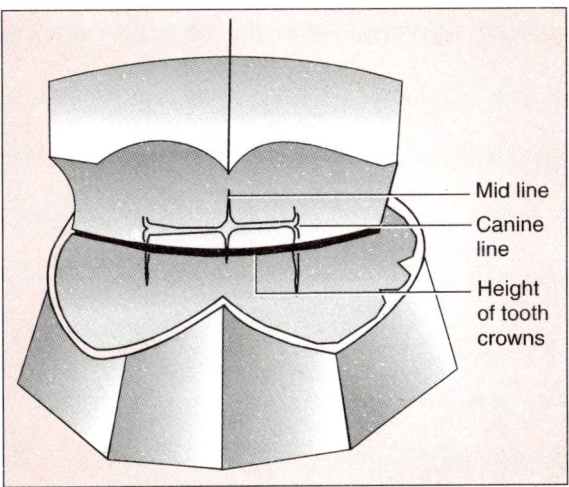

Fig. 10.3. Orientation marks on the occlusion blocks.

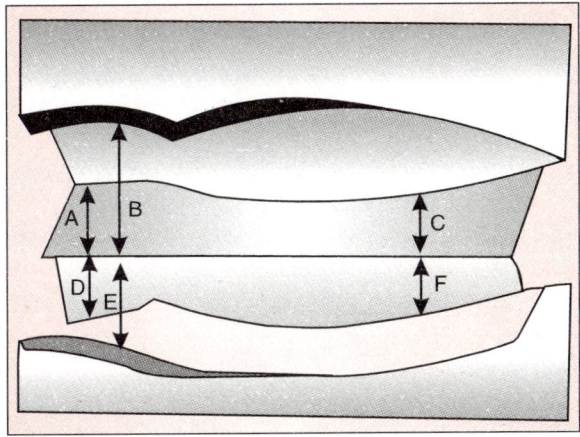

Fig. 10.4. Dimensions of maxillary and mandibular occlusal rims.

the face. Failure to do this may affect the form and length of the upper by raising the lip inappropriately.

Confirm that the upper lip is adequately supported. This should result in restoration of the vermilion border and may result in restoration of the philtrum although, this may not always be desirable or possible. Some clinical guidelines recommend that the vertical nasolabial angle should be 90°, although recent

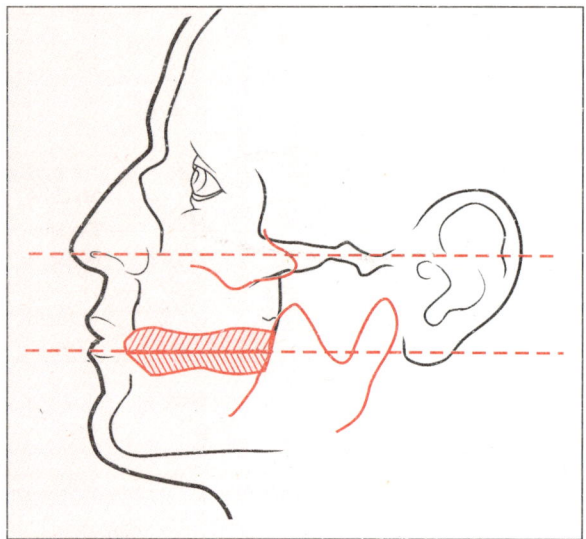

Fig. 10.5. Relationship of Camper's line to the plane of occlusion.

research casts doubt on the validity of this guideline.

• When the upper lip has been restored appropriately for the patient, it is then practical for the clinician to determine the position of the incisal point relative to the resting lip. Younger patients may reasonably be expected to show 4-5 mm of tooth beneath the resting lip, especially if the patient had a Class 2 division 1 profile. In contrast, a 70-year-old patient might be best suited by having the incisal point level with resting lip, or possibly 1 mm above this. Anteroposterior verification of the placement of the incisal point may be achieved by asking the patient to say a word containing a fricative consonant (labiodental sound), e.g. 'fish'; in general terms, the incisal point should correspond to the vermilion border of the lower lip.

• The next step in this clinical exercise is to determine the upper anterior plane. Given the position of the incisal point, the plane of the upper six anterior teeth is usefully determined by making it parallel to the interpupillary line. This may be done using a Fox's occlusal plane guide or any device giving a horizontal plane, e.g. a wooden spatula.

• When this has been performed, there is merit in determining the position of the mid points of the upper canine teeth. One useful way to record this is to use a photograph of the

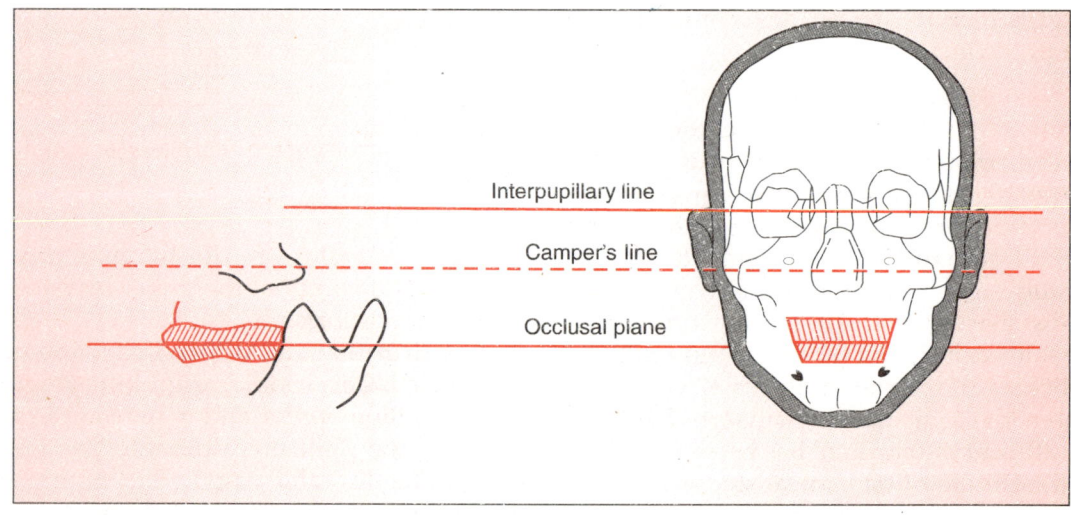

Fig. 10.6. The relationship of the interpapillary line, Camper's line and the occlusal plane.

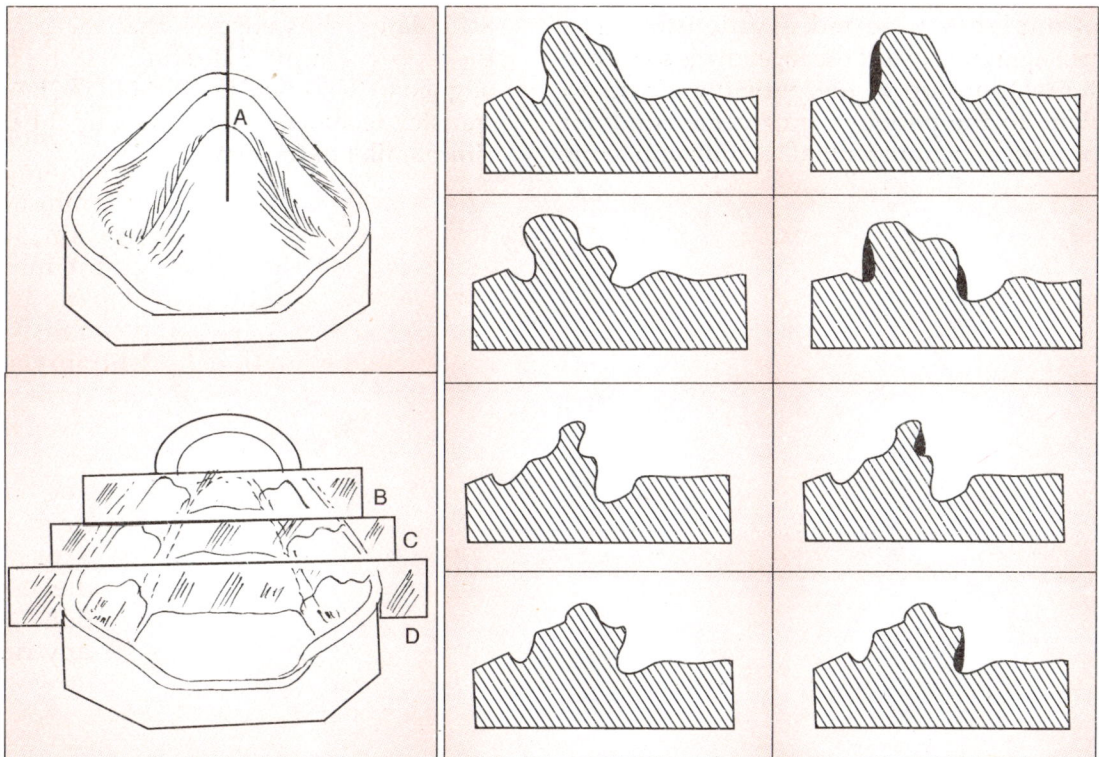

Fig. 10.7. Sections through anterior (A) Cuspid, (B) premolar, (C) and molar, (D) regions of edentulous mandibular cast showing undercuts before and after blockout.

patient when the patient was dentate. A clear, face-on photograph is required for this and regrettably these are not always available. Using the pupils as stable reference points, the clinician may determine the relative position of the upper canine teeth.

- Again using the mark on the rim corresponding to the canine tips as a reference point, the buccal form of the upper rim may be molded by reducing the inferior borders of the posterior rims by 3° to 5°. This procedure creates the buccal corridors and creates a more natural smile.

Before completing the customizing of the upper rim, the following should be scribed clearly on the anterior aspect of the rim: (i) center line, (ii) high smile line, and (iii) canine points.

- With the upper rim in situ ask the patient to smile; the upper rim should appear to be parallel to the lower lip line when smiling.
- The posterior border of the upper denture should displace the mucosa overlying the aponeurosis of tensor palati at the junction between the hard and soft palates. As the details of the displaceability of the tissues of the postdam are known only to the clinician, it is the sole responsibility of the clinician to scribe the appropriate extent and depth of the postdam using, e.g. a Le Cron carver or similar instrument. If not done so prior to this stage, the clinician should ensure that he/she scribes the postdam appropriately. Clinicians should consider the use of a facebow especially when a complete upper denture is opposed by a natural dentition or

an implant-supported overdenture. The principal purpose of the facebow is to record the relationship of the patient's maxillary plane to the patient's transverse condylar axis and then transfer that relationship to the articulator. This ensures that the plane of the upper complete denture will be better aligned to the condyles. Without the facebow transfer, technicians tend to set up the upper rim parallel to the bench top.

11

VERTICAL JAW RELATION

INTRODUCTION

It is imperative to mention that the objectives of complete denture service are to restore function, esthetics and to maintain health. In order to achieve these goals, it is essential that the jaw relations be accurately recorded and transferred.

Many a time failures of complete denture therapy may be attributed to the improper recording of maxillomandibular relationships.

CLASSIFICATION OF JAW RELATIONS

1. Vertical relations
2. Orientation relations
3. Horizontal relations (described in Chapter 12).

Vertical Jaw Relation

Vertical jaw relation refers to the length of the face. Vertical dimension has been defined as the distance between two selected points, one on a fixed, and one on a movable member.

The vertical dimension is maintained either by the occlusion of the teeth or by the balanced tonic contraction of the muscles of mandibular movements. There are two measurable length of the face. They are :

- Vertical dimension of physiologic rest position (Fig. 11.1).
- Vertical dimension of occlusion (Fig. 11.2).

Vertical Dimension

It is the distance between two selected points, one on a fixed and one on a movable member (GPT-7).

Vertical dimension is either maintained by the occlusion of the teeth or the balanced tonic contraction of the muscles of mandibular movements.

Vertical dimension of physiologic rest position is the vertical separation of jaws when the opening and closing muscles of the mandible are in state of minimal tonic contractive activities (Fig. 11.3).

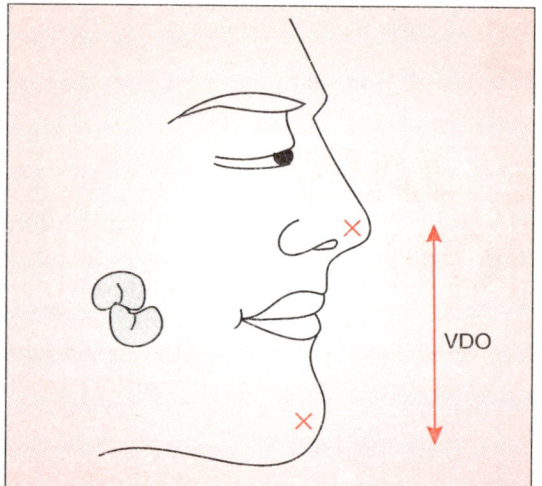

Fig. 11.1. Vertical dimension of physiologic position of rest.

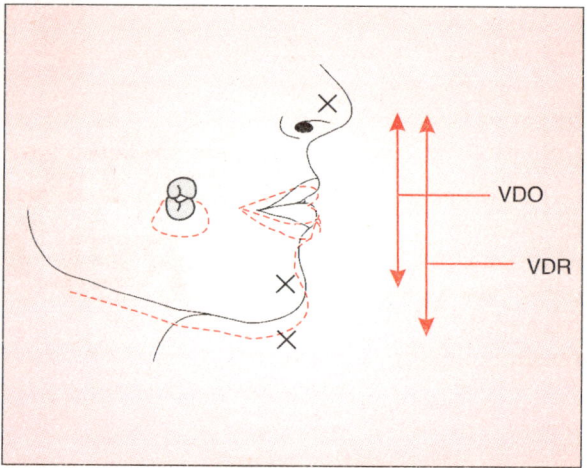

VDO (Vertical Dimension of Occlusion)
VDR (Vertical Dimension at Rest)

Fig. 11.3. VDO and VDR dimensions.

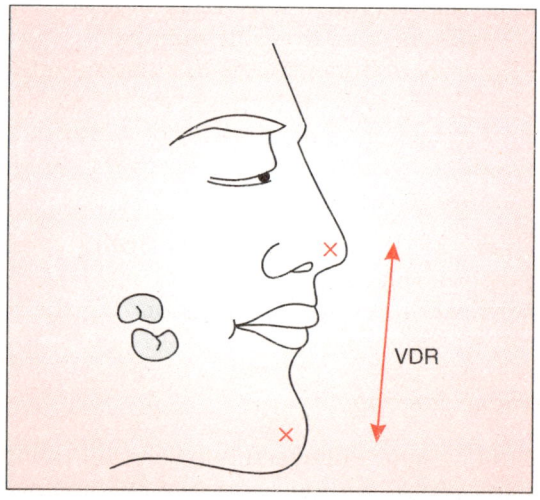

Fig. 11.2. Vertical dimension of occlusion.

Vertical dimension of occlusion is the vertical separation of the jaws when the teeth or occlusion rims are in occlusion (Fig. 11.3).

The interocclusal distance (free way space) is the distance between the occluding surfaces of the maxillary and mandibular teeth when the mandible is in its physiologic rest position. Hence, the interocclusal distance usually averages between 2 and 4 mm.

Rest vertical dimension = Occlusal vertical dimension + Interocclusal distance

During the fabrication of complete dentures, the centric relation record is made at the occlusal vertical dimension and transferred to the articulator.

An increased or decreased vertical dimension will have its drawbacks.

Effects of Excessively Increasing the Vertical Dimension

Discomfort. A patient acquires over a period of many years, habits which unconsciously and automatically control certain movements. Among these are the movements of the tongue and mandible while eating, talking, etc. By altering the vertical height there will be discomfort to the patient (to adjust for the new change).

Trauma. The jarring effect of the teeth coming into contact sooner than expected may cause apart from discomfort, pain owing to bruising of the mucosa by sudden and infrequent contacts.

Loss of Free Way Space. This may lead to annoyance[4] from the inability to find a comfortable resting position. Thus there will be rapid bone loss in the maxilla/mandible to find this needed rest.

Clicking of Teeth. At normal vertical height[1], teeth during speech help to produce sounds without coming in contact. However in cases of increased vertical dimension, opposing cusps frequently meet each other producing embarrassing clicking or clattering sound.

Appearance. There will be an elongation of the face but if it is only slight, it will usually pass unnoticed. Lips appear parted generally and there will be an expression of strain.

Effects of Excessively Reducing the Vertical Dimension

Inefficiency. The pressure that is exerted with teeth in contact decreases considerably in overclosure because the attachment of the muscles have been brought closer.

Cheek Biting. In cases where there is loss of muscular tone as well as reduced vertical height, the flabby cheek gets trapped between the teeth and gets bitten during mastication.

When overclosure is deliberate it is possible to avoid this cheek biting by setting the upper posterior teeth more buccally than normal producing greater overjet. Cheek biting often occurs because the buccal flange of the denture is too narrow and allows the cheek to fall.

Appearance. The general effect of over-closure[3] in facial appearance is of increased age. The lower third of the face is changed because the chin has the appearance of being too close to the nose and too far forward. The lips lose their fullness and the vermillion borders of the lips are reduced to approximate a line. The corners of the mouth turn down because the orbicularis oris and its attaching muscles are pushed too close to their origin with resultant loss of muscle tone. This gives the face an appearance of flabbiness instead of firmness.

Perleche. A reduced interarch distance often results in a crease at the corners of the mouth, which sometimes results in a disease known as perleche.

Pain in the Temporomandibular Joint (TMJ). The loss of posterior occlusion subjects the joint to a greater proportion of load and thus the meniscus is damaged resulting in clicking or crepitus which may be heard on movement. The temporalis and masseter muscles are affected by lack of posterior teeth contact which may be a source of pain and discomfort. In such cases, the patient has to protrude the mandible in order to occlude the teeth and the lateral pterygoid muscles become painful, and pain is centered on or anterior to the TMJ.

In these patients the vertical relation of occlusion should be built up gradually, in successive sets of dentures.

Impaired Hearing. Normally the tongue at rest completely fills the oral cavity. When a reduced interarch distance occurs, there will be a tendency to push the tongue towards the throat, with the result that adjacent tissues will be displaced and encroached on. This will result in closure of the opening of the eustachian tubes which causes impaired hearing. These claims are difficult to support.

RECORDING OF MAXILLOMANDIBULAR RELATIONS

Vertical Relations

Two recordings are done: (i) rest position, and (ii) occlusion position. Different methods for recording vertical dimension are depicted in Table 11.1.

Recording of the Rest Position

At present, no scientific mechanical methods of proven validity are available for extensive use in recording rest position. The different methods are as follows.

Table 11.1. Methods for recording vertical dimension

According to Boucher

1. Ridge relation
    a. Distance of incisive papilla from mandibular incisors
    b. Distance of incisive papilla from the crest of the ridge
    c. Distance of hamular notch from retromolar pad
    d. Parallelism of posterior ridges (open 5 degrees).
2. Measurement of former dentures
3. Interarch distance and physiologic rest position tests
4. Pre-extraction records
    a. Profile roentgenograms
    b. Casts of teeth in occlusion
    c. Facial measurements
    d. Acrylic resin face mask.
5. Park's theory of determining vertical relation
6. Vertical determination by means of power point
7. Wrights photographic method.

Heartwell classified the various methods for determining vertical dimension into those that are used for

1. Recordings for rest position
    a. Facial measurements
    b. Tactile sense
    c. Phonetics
    d. Facial expression
    e. Anatomic landmarks.
2. Recording of occlusion position
    a. Pre-extraction records
        i. Profile photographs
        ii. Profile silhouettes
        iii. Radiography
        iv. Articulated cast
        v. Face mask
        vi. Facial measurements.
    b. Phonetics
    c. Closest speaking space
    d. F,V, and S speaking anterior tooth relation
    e. Former dentures
    f. Wax occlusion rims
    g. Neuromuscular perception (by Lytle)
    h. Power point (by Boos)
    i. Myomonitor centric.

Facial Measurements. Instruct the patient to stand or sit comfortably upright with the eyes looking straight ahead. Insert the maxillary record base with the attached contoured occlusion rim. With either an indelible marker or a triangle of adhesive tape, place a point of reference on the end of the patient's nose and another on the point of the chin.

Instruct the patient to wipe the lips with the tongue to swallow and to drop the shoulders. When the mandible drops to rest position, measure between the points with a millimeter ruler. Repeat the procedure until the measurements are consistent.

Tactile Sense. Instruct patients to stand[1] or sit erect and open the jaws wide until strain is felt in the muscles. Then ask them to close slowly until the jaws reach a comfortable relaxed position. The distance is measured between the points of reference and compared with the measurements made after swallowing.

Phonetics. Two different methods are:
1. Have patients repeat the name "emma" until they are aware of contacting of the lips as the first syllable 'em' is pronounced. Repeat this procedure and ask the patient to stop all jaw movement when the lips touch. At this time, measure between the two points of reference.
2. Engage the patient in conversation so that their attention is diverted. A pause in speech, followed by relaxation as indicated by a drop of the mandible is indicative of another measurement.

Facial Expression. In normally related jaws the lips will be even anteroposteriorly and in slight contact. The lips of the patient with a protruded mandible will not be evenly related, the lower lip will be anterior to the upper lip and not in contact. The skin around the eyes and over the chin will be relaxed. Relaxation around the nares reflects unobstructed breathing.

Anatomic Landmarks[4]. The Wills guide is designed to measure the distance from the pupils of the eye to the rima oris and the distance from the anterior nasal spine to the lower border of the mandible. When these measurements are equal, the jaws are considered at rest. The asymmetry of the face makes the value of this method questionable.

Recording of the Occlusion Position

When the mandible is at rest it is hanging in space and is not in a completely static position but when the mandible is braced against the maxillae with teeth, the position is static and can be maintained for an indefinite time.

PRE-EXTRACTION RECORD MEASUREMENTS

Pre-extraction record measurements with former dentures and wax occlusion rims are used to determine the vertical dimension of occlusion. Neuromuscular perception and power point are methods for edentulous patients with no pre-extraction records/dentures.

Pre-extraction Records

Profile Photographs

Photographs should be made with teeth in maximum occlusion as this position can be maintained accurately for photographic procedures and then enlarged to life size. Measurements of anatomic landmarks on the photograph are compared with measurements using the same anatomic landmarks on the face. These measurements can be compared when the records are made and again when the artificial teeth are tried in.

Profile Silhouettes

An accurate reproduction of the profile in silhouette can be cut out in cardboard or contoured in wire. The silhouette can be repositioned to the face after the vertical dimension has been established at the initial recording and/or when the artificial teeth are tried in. Olsen painted a strip of plaster of Paris down the midline of the face from which a cut-out is made.

Radiography

The two types of radiographs advocated are the cephalometric profile and the condyles in the fossae. These methods are unreliable as inaccuracies exist.

Articulated Cast

The accurate maxillary cast is related in its correct anatomic position on an articulator with a face-bow transfer. An occlusal record in centric relation is used to mount the mandibular cast. After the removal of teeth the edentulous casts are mounted on the articulator and the interarch measurements are compared. This method is valuable in patients whose ridges are not sacrificed during the removal of the teeth or resorbed.

Face Mask

Swenson (1959) suggested the use of an acrylic resin face mask made before extraction Later when the patient is edentulous it is fitted on the face to check the vertical dimension.

Facial Measurements

Niswonger's Method. The patient is instructed to close the jaws into maximum occlusion after two tattoo points have been placed, one on the upper half and the other on the lower half of the face. The distance is measured, and these measurements are compared with measurements made between these points when the artificial teeth are tried in. Not commonly used because many patients would object to the tattoos.

Phonetics

Closest-speaking Space

Silverman[2] suggested this method which measures the vertical dimension.

The 'F' or 'V' and 'S' Speaking Anterior Tooth Relation

Incisive guidance is established by arranging the anterior teeth in the occlusion rims before recording the vertical dimension of occlusion (technique developed by Pound and Murrell). The position of the artificial maxillary anterior teeth is determined by the position of the maxillae when the patient says words beginning with 'f' or v'. The incisal edges should create a seal on the moist area of the vermillion border of the lower lip. The position of the mandibular anterior teeth is determined by the position of the mandible when the patient says words beginning with 'S' during which the incisal edges of the anterior teeth do not make contact ('S' position represents the protrusive phase of incisal guidance).

If the distance is too large, a vertical dimension of occlusion that it too small may have been established. If the anterior teeth touch when sounds like "ch", "s" and "j" are made, the vertical dimension of occlusion is probably too great.

Former Dentures

The most common method is a comparison of the measurements from former dentures with measurements made during the record making procedure. It is advisable to use other methods and establish the vertical dimension of occlusion in the occlusion rims and then compare the measurements between reference points with former dentures in occlusion.

The measurements made with former dentures are not acceptable because:

- Resorption of the ridges under the dentures may result in an increase in interocclusal distance
- Patients can shift the mandible/denture to accommodate for errors in occlusion
- Inaccurate adaptation of the denture base to the support results in displacement of the denture.

Wax Occlusion Rims

This technique is used for establishing both tentative vertical dimension of occlusion and the tentative centric relation of the jaws. The final evaluation uses facial expression and esthetics as a guide for teeth arrangement. Technique is as follows:

1. Establish the vertical dimension of rest and measure the distance between the points of reference on the nose and chin.
2. Make the interocclusal distance approximately. 3 mm less than the interocclusal distance at rest position.
3. Thinly coat the maxillary occlusion rim with petrolatum and seat the maxillary record base with the rim securely in the mouth.
4. A soft roll of baseplate wax about one-third the diameter of a lead pencil is attached to the occlusal surface of the mandibular occlusion rim. Contour it in a triangular shape with the base on the occlusion rim. Resoften the baseplate wax in a water bath or with an alcohol torch flame.
5. Seat the mandibular record base and hold it with the index fingers placed on the buccal flanges in the second premolar area bilaterally.
6. Request the patient to retrude the mandible and to close on the back teeth but to stop closing the jaw when they feel that the closure is sufficient (tactile sense). An experienced dentist can feel with his fingers and see, when the contraction of the elevator muscles begin to diminish. This should coincide with the patients perception of adequate closure.
7. Allow the wax to harden before removing the tentative record. Reinsert and have patient close to maximum occlusion. Measure the distance between points and compare with the measurements made at rest position. If the measurement is less than the measurement at rest and the baseplate wax was not penetrated through to make occlusion rim contact, the record is acceptable.

Neuromuscular Perception (by Lytle)

In this method a central bearing device is used.

- After mounting the casts, mount central

bearing plates on the record bases, adapting the plates to the patient's interarch distance.

- Adjust the bearing pin until the mouth is opened beyond the physiologic rest position. Lower the pin half a turn at a time having patients make two sharp contacts each time, until the patient indicate that he has closed too far. Turn the pin back a half turn and record the number of turns on the pin.
- Repeat the procedure, starting from an overclosed position. Open the pin a half turn have the patient make two sharp contacts of the pin after each adjustment. When the patient's signal is that he has reached excessive opening, turn the pin back a half turn.
- Recheck the record by repeating the initial steps.
- Instruct the patient to close (in centric relation) until the central bearing pin is in contact with the metal plate. Inject the fast setting plaster to secure the relation.
- This tentative record is transferred to the articulator.

According to the study of McGee, when this method was used patients tended to register a reduced vertical dimension of occlusion because they felt more comfortable in that position.

Power Point (by Boos)[5]

Attach the bimeter to an accurately adapted mandibular record base. Attach a metal plate in the vault of an accurately adapted maxillary record base to provide a central bearing point. Adjust the vertical distance by turning the cap. The gauge indicates the pounds of pressure generated during closure at different degrees of jaw separation. When the maximum power point is determined, lock the set nut. Make plaster registrations.

This theory is based on the assumption that maximum closing force can be exerted when the mandible is at vertical dimension of rest position. A correlation of results with bimeter and those by clinical and electromyographic methods showed that the use of bimeter produced increased vertical dimension.

Myomonitor Centric

Jankelson myomonitor is a solid state electronic instrument which delivers a small DC current via electrodes which are placed over the coronoid notch of the ramus of the mandible. It is intended to simultaneously stimulate all the muscles involved in mandibular movements and it positions the mandible in "myomonitor centric", i.e. centric occlusion by the "Jankelson myomonitor". According to study by Wander H it was found out that "myomonitor centric" was anterior to centric relation but was slightly retrusive to centric occlusion. Also myomonitor centric recordings were variable from the left and right sides of the same patient and varied on the same side of the same patient. Myomonitor centric position is not reproducible with repeated registrations on the same patient.

EVALUATING THE VERTICAL DIMENSION OF OCCLUSION

Following are the methods for evaluating the vertical dimension of occlusion.

Patient's Tactile Tense

Place the trial denture in the patient's mouth and ask him to open and close until the teeth contact. Ask the patient if the teeth appear to touch too soon, if the jaws seem to close too far before they touch or if the teeth feel just right. This method is not very effective with senile patients or in patients with impaired neuromuscular co-ordinations.

Swallowing Followed by Relaxing

With the denture in the mouth, instruct the patient to wipe the lips with the tip of the tongue, swallow and let the shoulders drop into a relaxed position. Watch the reference points and ask the patient to close the teeth together. If the teeth are together, it may indicate that no interocclusal distance exists.

Another method is based on the theory that teeth make contact at or near centric occlusion. Two small cones of a soft wax are placed one in each central sulcus of the mandibular first molars. Encourage the patient to swallow several times. If the vertical dimension of occlusion is correct, the wax will be penetrated and reduced to tooth contact.

Phonetics

The use of speech in evaluating vertical dimension of occlusion for patients receiving their first denture is of dubious value. But in patients for whom subsequent dentures are fabricated, phonetics is a useful aid.

In using phonetics, the enunciation of words is not of primary interest. The position of the tongue and the relation of the teeth are important.

Have the patient repeat these words:
- "Three thirty-three"—there should be enough space for the tip of the tongue to protrude between the anterior teeth.
- "Fifty-five"—incisal edges of the maxillary central incisors should contact the vermillion border of the lower lip at the junction of the moist and dry mucosa.
- "Emma and Mississippi"—the teeth should not contact.

With the Occlusion Rims

Following are the some of the tests:
1. Judgement of the overall facial support. When the patient closes the jaw slowly until the lips just touch, at this point mandible is at rest position.The lips are in unstrained contact. Next ask the patient to close the jaw so that in closing through the interocclusal distance, there is little or no movement of the lips. If the patient has decreased vertical relation (that is increased interocclusal distance), the lips close excessively, fold together and the vermillion tends to disappear.
2. Visual observation of the amount of space between the rims when the jaws are at rest.
3. Measurements between dots on the face when the jaws are at rest and when occlusion rims are in contact.
4. Observation made when sibiliant-containing words are pronounced to ensure that the occlusion rims come together but do not contact.

OTHER METHODS OF RECORDING VERTICAL DIMENSION

1. According to Niswonger, the patient must be seated with the ala-tragal line parallel to the floor. Then two marks are made, one on the upper lip and one on the chin. The patient is told to swallow and relax. The distance between the points are measured. Then occlusion rims are constructed so that the measured distance is 4/32 inch less than the original measurement. This method has the disadvantage that the points on the chin move and sometimes it is difficult to obtain two constant measurements.
2. Willis believed that the distance from the pupil of the eye to the rima oris should be equal to the distance from the base of the nose to inferior border of the chin when the occlusion rims are in contact.
3. Some observers also believed in equal thirds concept according to which the face can be divided into three equal parts. Generally it is very difficult to choose the exact point because of the variations.
4. Some clinicians have advocated parallelism of ridges as a method of determining proper vertical dimension. It may not hold true where severe or irregular resorption of the ridges have occurred.
5. Physiologic method of Shanahan (1955) : This is used to determine both vertical dimension and centric relation. According

to this method, the pattern of mandibular movement for an edentulous infant is the same as that for an edentulous adult. When the jaw reaches its highest point during deglutition, the point is likely to be the vertical dimension of occlusion. Other authors who concurred with this idea were Powell and Zander (1965) and Boucher (1955).

6. Pyott (1954) calculated rest vertical dimension in edentulous patients by making cephalometric radiographs at the physiologic rest position produced by swallowing. He then measured the distance between the nasal and frontal bones and the most protrusive point on the symphysis of the mandible. Occlusion rims were adjusted till a 3 mm difference existed between the rest vertical and occlusal vertical dimension.

7. Atwood (1966) found the cephalometric method to be the most accurate method of determining vertical dimension. He also reported variations between the sittings, in the same sitting and between readings with and without dentures.

8. Mc Grane (1949) established a 40 mm occlusal vertical dimension for his patients. Hundreds of patients with completed orthodontic treatment were measured. The basis for measurement was the mid maxillary and mid mandibular labial freni. He speculated that the distance from the incisal edge of the maxillary central incisors to the labial vestibule adjacent to the maxillary labial frenum was 2 mm. The corresponding for mandibular incisors was 18 mm.

9. Fayz et al (1987) reported the measurement slightly less than McGrane. The distance between the depth of the mucolabial reflection in the maxilla and mandible was 34.2 mm in right incisor region and 34.06 mm in the left incisor segment. The corresponding distances for the right and left canines were 36.7 and 36.94 mm. The distance from the depth of the vestibular fornix to the incisal edge of the anterior teeth was 21.24 and 21.28 for right and left maxillary central incisors. For mandibular central incisors it was 16.54 and 16.78 mm respectively.

10. Hurst (1962) devised a method based on the correlation between lip length, vertical position of the maxillary central incisors and the interocclusal distance in individuals with natural dentition. He classified upper lip length into five groups from extrashort to extra long. In extra long lip types, 2 to 5 mm of the lip extended beyond the incisal edges with 6 to 10 mm of interocclusal distance whereas for extra short lips all of the teeth might be exposed with approximately 1 mm of interocclusal distance plus 3 mm of gingivae.

11. *Pleasure's technique (1951).* Place a dot or a crossmark on the nose, and on the chin: A measuring device is kept ready. One has to ensure that the patient is not tensed or nervous. Patient should sit upright with the eyes looking directly forward. Insert the contoured maxillary rim in to the patients mouth. Instruct the patient to say 'm' and hold the lips when they first touch. Record the distance between the reference points. Several measurements are done and if it is not consistent an average is used.

Lower recording base is then inserted into the mouth. It is trimmed and contoured until it meets the maxillary rim evenly approximately 3 mm less than the distance previously recorded for the rest vertical dimension. As a general rule, a greater amount of vertical dimension is provided as the age of the patient increases.

12. *Pound and murrell's (1971) technique.* They described a technique wherein incisive guidance is established by arranging the anterior teeth in the occlusion rims before recording the vertical dimension of occlusion. The position of the artificial maxillary teeth when the patient says words beginning with 'F' and 'V' and mandibular

anterior teeth by the position of the mandible when patient says 'S' are used. Initially stable record bases are made. Occlusion rim is constructed on the maxillary base and labiopalatal and buccopalatal contours are adjusted. On the mandibular base initial 2-3 mm of the rim is built with baseplate wax. In the estimated location of anterior teeth, 3/4 inch thickness of bees wax is placed. This section is called "speaking wax". When the maxillary occlusion rim is in place it is adjusted for proper lip support. When 'F' and 'V' sounds are made the incisal edges create a seal on the moist area of the vermillion border of the lower lip. Then the midline is recorded with central incisors on either side. After this, base is removed and the lateral incisors are placed.

The incisal edges of the laterals and cuspids must be at same level as the central incisors. Return the record base to the mouth and make any changes necessary for natural appearance. The incisal edges should follow the curvature of the lower lip. Seat the mandibular base and adjust to the 'S' position. When 'S' sounds are articulated the mandible moves forward.

The incisal edges of the anterior teeth do not make contact. The midline is recorded on the mandibular rim, coinciding with the maxillary midline. The mandibular record base is taken out and speaking wax is removed from one side of the centre line. Then the remaining wax is removed and the artificial central incisors are arranged. The maxillary occlusal rim is made parallel to Camper's line. Place notches in it to aid in repositioning (Figs 11.4 and 11.5).

According to pound and Murrell this technique was successful in at least 80 percent of the patients. When the patient bites in retruded relation then there must be firm contact of the upper and lower anteriors. To assure that the record does not incorporate excess pressure, the patient

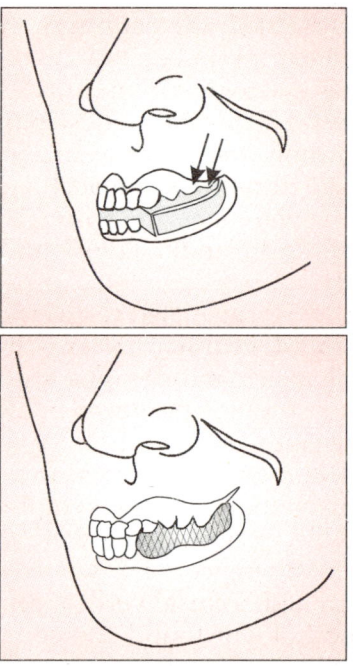

Fig. 11.4. Recording of the mandibular rim.

must be instructed to return to retruded position again, to close into the record with pressure and then open and close lightly. One may face problems in a patient with severe Class II jaw relations.

An alternative technique is to use base plate wax made passive by applying dry heat, plaster, impression compound (softened) or zinc oxide-eugenol as the recording material.

13. *Ridge relation.* The incisive papilla is a landmark that is least affected by resorption. The distance of the incisive papilla from the incisal edges of mandibular anterior teeth on diagnostic casts is around 2 mm. The incisal edge of the maxillary central incisor was found to be an average of 6 mm below the incisal papilla. The average vertical overlap was 4 mm. The mandibular incisors would average 2 mm from the crest of the maxillary anterior edge. For totally edentulous mouths the

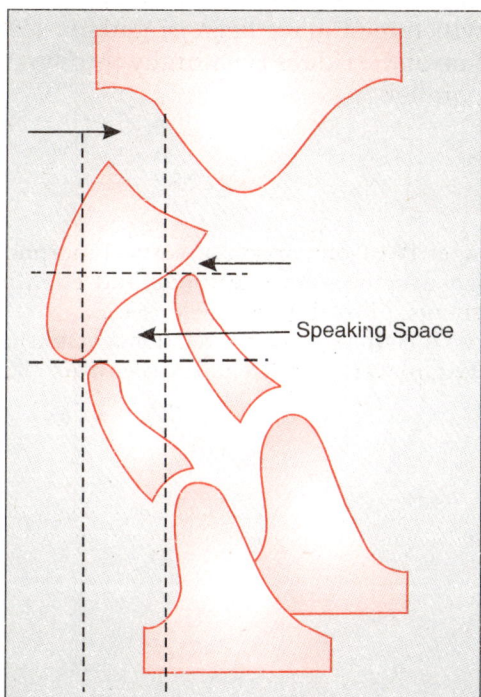

Fig. 11.5. Defining speaking space.

indicate the correct amount of jaw separation for the establishment of occlusion (Fig. 11.6).

This theory was found to be incorrect by Hanau and others who stated that the hinge axis of the mandible is on a line through the condyles for the first part of the opening movement of the mandible.

16. *Paralleling posterior ridges.* Paralleling the maxillary and mandibular ridges plus a 5 degree opening in the posterior region (as

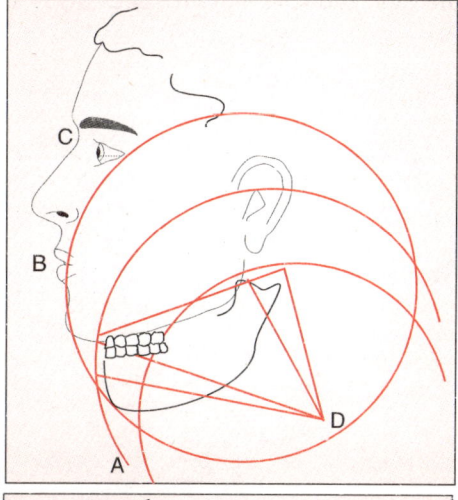

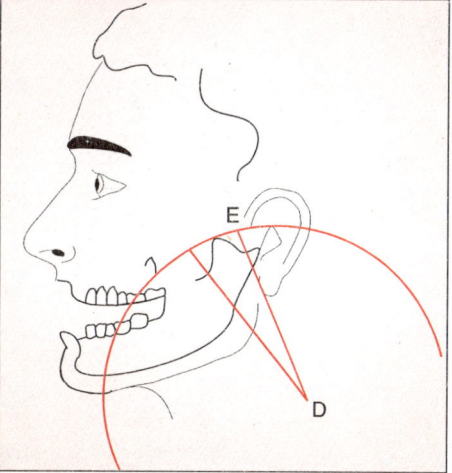

Fig. 11.6. Arcs showing opening and closing muscles of the mandible in the state of contractive activities.

distance between anterior ridges would be 12 mm. (6 + 4 + 2).

14. *Measurement of former dentures.* Dentures that the patient has been wearing are observed and are correlated with the patient's face to determine the amount of change required. These measurements are made between the borders of the maxillary and mandibular dentures by means of a Boley gauge.

15. *Park's theory of determining vertical dimension.* According to Park, the mandible closes on a rotational center that is away from the condyle and is below and behind the angle of the mandible. This rotational center is held until the point of the former occlusal plane is reached, and then upon further closure, the mandible rotates around the condyle. These two movements would scribe two different arcs and the point of intersection of these two arcs would

suggested by Sears) often gives a clue of the amount of jaw separation. In ridges that have undergone severe restoration or in which teeth have been irregularly lost the line of the ridges is naturally thrown out of parallel.

Further Reading

1. Swerdlow H. Vertical dimension. A literature review. J Prosth Dent. 1965; 15(2): 241-46.
2. Silverman M M. The speaking method in measuring vertical dimension. J Prosth Dent. Vol: 85; No.5.
3. Pound E. Controlling anomalies of vertical dimension and speech. J Prosth Dent. 1976; 1 36: 124.
4. Unger JW. Comparison of vertical morphologic measurements on dentulous and edentulous patients. J Prosth Dent. 1990; 64:232.
5. Boss R H. Intermaxillary relations established by biting power. J Am Dental Assoc. 1940; 27:

12

HORIZONTAL JAW RELATION

INTRODUCTION

The relation of the mandible to a horizontal plane of reference is the horizontal jaw relation. These are basically of two types: (i) centric relation (CR), and (ii) eccentric relation.

Centric relation is a classical reference and treatment position. Over the years a number of definitions have been put forward for centric relation (CR).

1. The most retruded relation of the mandible to the maxilla when the condyles are in the most posterior, unstrained position in the glenoid fossa from which lateral movement can be made at any given degree of jaw separation.

2. The most retruded physiologic relation of the mandible to the maxillae to and from which an individual can make lateral movements.

It is a condition that can exist at various degrees of jaw separation. It occurs around the terminal hinge axis.

3. The jaw relation when the condyles are in the most posterior, unstrained position in the glenoid fossa at any given degree of jaw separation from which lateral movements can be made.

4. The maxillomandibular relationship in which the condyles articulate with the most avascular portion of their respective disks with the complex in the anterosuperior position against the slopes of the articular eminences. This position is independent of tooth contact.

5. The maxillomandibular relationship in which the condyles articulate with the thinnest avascular portion of their respective disks with the complex in the anterosuperior position against the slopes of the articular eminence. This position is clinically discernible when the mandible is directed superiorly and anteriorly.

FEATURES AND SIGNIFICANCE OF CENTRIC RELATION

1. Centric relation is the horizontal reference position of the mandible that can be

routinely assumed by the edentulous patients. This makes it possible for the dentist to verify the relationship of the casts on the articulator, when they are mounted in centric relation. The patients cannot routinely close their teeth into centric relation when it is established on the articulator in some other position.

2. Edentulous patients use centric relation closure in mastication and in other mandibular activities (e.g., swallowing). The casts must be mounted on the articulator in this position so that opposing teeth on the complete denture will meet evenly when the patient closes in centric.

3. Correct registration of centric relation is essential in the fabrication of complete dentures. Many dentures fail because the occlusion is not planned or developed in harmony with this position.

4. It is the ideal arch to arch relationship and hence optimum position of the jaws for the health, comfort and function of the temporomandibular joint (TMJ).

5. Centric relation is related to the terminal hinge axis. In centric relation, condyles exhibit pure rotation without any translation. In this position, the mandible moves in a hinge motion to a distance of 15-25 mm at the incisal in the sagittal plane.[4]

6. It serves as a reference position for the institution of occlusal rehabilitation in dentulous conditions.[4]

7. It serves as a reference position to relate and nomenclate several occlusal positions of the upper and lower teeth.[4]

8. The terminal act of the masticatory stroke terminates in centric relation.

9. During deglutition, upper and lower teeth are braced against each other in centric.

10. It is a posterior border position and the posterior limit of the envelope of motion.

11. It is a repeatable, recordable position and physiologically acceptable for deglutition and mastication.

12. It is a starting point for the arrangement of the artificial teeth to develop maximum intercuspation in complete dentures.

MUSCLES INVOLVED IN CENTRIC RELATION[6]

The muscles that move and fix the mandible in its most retruded position relative to the maxillae are:
1. Posterior and middle fibers of temporalis.
2. Suprahyoid muscles mainly the digastricus and the geniohyoid.
   The lateral pterygoids have little activity.

CENTRIC RELATION AND CENTRIC OCCLUSION

Centric relation is a bone to bone relationship whereas centric occlusion is a relationship of the upper and lower teeth to each other.

In the Natural Dentition

The centric occlusion[5] is usually located anterior to the centric relation. The average distance is approx. 0.5 –1 mm. When the patient closes in centric relation, natural tooth interferences will initiate impulses and responses that will direct the mandible away from the deflective occlusal contacts into centric occlusion. This will create memory patterns that will permit the mandible to return to this position without interferences.

In Edentulous Patients[5]

The lack of teeth will make it necessary to use the centric relation as a reference position, when the natural teeth are lost. Therefore the edentulous patients cannot control mandibular movements or avoid deflective occlusal contacts in centric relation (as dentulous patients). Therefore in these patients, centric relation must be recorded. Centric occlusion can be developed to be in harmony with centric relation.

CONCEPTS OF RECORDING CENTRIC RELATION

Minimal Pressure Concept

According to this concept, records should be made with minimal closing pressure so that the tissues supporting the bases will not be displaced while the records are being made. Silverman has stated that the advantage of this concept is that the opposing teeth will touch uniformly and simultaneously at their first contact. The uniform contact of teeth will not stimulate the patient to clench (and relax) the closing muscles in periods between mastication.

Heavy Pressure Concept

Records are made with heavy closing pressure so that the tissues under the recording bases are displaced while the record is being made.

This concept will produce the same displacement of the soft tissues as would exist when heavy closing pressures are applied on the denture. The occlusal forces will be evenly distributed over the supporting residual ridges when the dentures are under heavy occlusal forces. However if the distribution of the soft tissue is uneven, the teeth will contact unevenly when they first touch. This uneven contact can stimulate nervous patients to clench and relax their closing muscles.

METHODS FOR ASSISTING PATIENTS TO RETRUDE THE MANDIBLE WHILE RECORDING CENTRIC RELATION

There are seven methods.

Stretch and Relax Movements

The patient is instructed by the dentist to move the mandible into a strained forward position and then relax followed by immediate backward movement. The patient can also be asked to place a finger on the chin to feel the mandibular movements. This procedure is repeated until the patient and dentist can feel the retruded position. This is also known as Boos exercise–in addition to retruding the mandible, it has the added advantage of muscle strengthening and coordination.

Retrusion of the Tongue

The patient is instructed to keep the tip of the tongue in contact with the posterior border of the maxillary record base and is then asked to close until the rims come into contact. The disadvantage of this technique is that the mandibular denture may be displaced by the tongue.

Swallowing

The patient is asked to swallow and conclude the act of swallowing with the occlusal rims in contact with one another. This method is considered as unreliable as people can swallow when the mandible is not completely retruded but is 1-7 mm anterior to the maxilla.

Head Position

Tilting the head backwards results in retrusion of the mandible because of the tension of the inframandibular musculature.

Disadvantages include: (i) position can be uncomfortable for the patient, and (ii) insertion and removal of occlusal rims from the mouth is very difficult.

Rapid Tapping of Occlusal Rims

Rapid and repeated tapping of the occlusal rims retrudes the mandible because the center of muscle pull will gradually work the mandible back.

Disadvantages

- Patient can be uncomfortable.
- Patient can easily close in a slightly protrusive or lateral position.

Temporalis Muscle Check

Muscles tend to show decreased function when the mandible is protruded. Therefore its contraction can be felt when the mandible is in the most retruded position.

Generalized Relaxation of the Patient

Total relaxation of the patient on the dental chair can help in retrusion.

THEORIES REGARDING CENTRIC RELATION

The anatomic mechanism responsible for centric relation is unknown because several different theories have developed.

Muscle Theory

Centric relation is the product of a defense reflex which causes the external pterygoid muscle to contract and thus halt the jaw every time the condyles approach the posterior depths of the glenoid fossa.

The opponents of this theory have stated that:

- This theory does not explain the fact that centric relation is the same at any vertical level.
- No explanation has been provided for the posterior hinge movement.

Woefel and Hickey found that the external pterygoid muscles are relaxed when the mandible is in centric relation.

Meniscus Theory

The articular disk has four definable zones, the thinner central bearing area and thicker anterior and posterior bands. Anatomic dissections have indicated that the central bearing area of the intra-articular tissue remains interposed between the condylar articular surface and the articular eminence during simulated jaw movements.

The thinner central bearing area is composed of densely woven collagen fibrils having no vascularity or innervation which indicates that this zone is adapted to accepting pressure.

The posterior movement of the condyle on the eminence has been attributed to wedging of the thickened posterior band of disk between the distal surface of the condyle and the roof of the articular fossa. The innervated posterior band possibly protects by sensory feedback, the thin roof of the articular fossa from heavy pressure and provides a biomechanically stable relationship.

It appears that any position posterior to this limit cannot be functional as the condylar articular surface cannot engage the central bearing area of the eminence nor can the position be biomechanically stable.

Ligament Theory

Ferrin was the first to present the ligament theory. He found that in cadavers, the temporomandibular ligament became tense, when the jaw was in the terminal retruded position. The opponents of this theory stated that the anatomic arrangement of the temporomandibular ligament is not well suited to halt the retrusive condylar movement.

Osteofiber Theory

This theory was introduced by Meyers. This involves a retrusive terminal stop formed by the soft tissue of the posterior part of the roof of the glenoid fossa.

Difficulties encountered in retruding the mandible may be:

- Biologic
- Psychologic
- Mechanical

Biologic. The lack of coordination in groups of opposing muscles (e.g., the protruding and retruding muscles) can influence mandibular movement. This lack of synchronization between the protruding and retruding muscles may be caused by habitual eccentric jaw positions adapted by the patient. This is seen more in

- Patients who have been edentulous for a long period.
- Patients with missing posterior teeth
- Denture wearers with marked attrition of teeth which permit sliding movement because of flat occlusal surface.

Mechanical. This occurs mainly because of poorly fitting denture bases which interfere with each other.

Psychological. It involves both the dentist and the patient. This may be due to

- The patient's inability to follow the dentist's instructions.
- Irritation of the dentist towards the patient because of the patient's inability to protrude the mandible.

FACTORS THAT INFLUENCE RECORDING OF CENTRIC RELATION

- Resilient action of supporting tissues.
- Fit of the denture bases affecting their retention and stability.
- TMJ and its neuromuscular mechanism.
- Pressure applied in making records.
- Technique employed in making records.
- Ability of the operator.

Historical Review

Myers ML[3] in 1982 gave a historical review on centric relation records. According to him the records are classified into

Direct Checkbites (Interocclusal Records)

These are the oldest records. Philip Phaff, the dentist of Frederick the Great of Germany in 1756, was the first to describe this technique of taking a bite. This was also known as mush, biscuit or squash bite. In this non-precision technique, small amounts of impression wax compound plaster or zinc oxide eugenol were placed between the edentulous ridges and the patient closed the jaws into centric relation.

Static Methods

Static methods involve placing the mandible in centric relation with the maxilla (at a static position) and then making a record of the relationship of the two occlusion rims to each other. Proponents of these methods have claimed that there is minimum displacement of the recording bases in relation to the supporting base.

Requirements of Ideal Interocclusal Records

According to Berman
- No resistance to closure
- Have true fluidity
- Should permit the masticatory mechanism to operate free from strain.

Indications

- Abnormally related jaws
- Extensively displaceable supporting tissue
- Large awkward tongue
- Uncontrollable or abnormal mandibular movement
- Correction of the occlusion of existing dentures.

Factors Influencing Interocclusal Records

- Amount and equalization of pressure[2] depends on the uniform consistency of the recording material.
  The accuracy of the vertical component of the record is in direct proportion to equalization of pressure exerted on displaceable supporting tissues and joints.
- Comfort of the patient depends on the stability, compatibility of record base and attached recording surfaces.

  Artificial teeth arranged in correct antero-posterior, mediolateral and vertical position in relation of the lips, tongue, cheeks and basal seat are more compatible to physiologic mandibular movement than occlusal rims.

- Record with multiple points of reference made by styli or cusp tips is more satisfactory than one using occluding surfaces of wax or non-cusp teeth.

Materials Used. Wax, zinc oxide-eugenol, elastomer, acrylic, plaster of Paris, eugenol free zinc oxide, modeling compound.

Dental Wax

Advantages

- Inexpensive
- Ease of manipulation. So, it can be used in incoordinated patients
- Hardens very quickly, so can be used whenever there is difficulty to retrude the mandible backwards and maintain in that position.

Dental waxes can be:

- Hard or soft
- Thick or thin

Disadvantages

- Difficulty in obtaining uniform softening.
- Difficulty in obtaining uniform wax thickness.
- Difficulty in obtaining uniform pressure in the wax
- Distortion
- Are subjected to being scraped, blunted, distorted, or compressed.

Zinc Oxide-eugenol

This is considered by many as a reliable interocclusal record.

Advantages

- Can be mixed to true fluid consistency
- Offers resistance to closure
- Adheres to its carrier
- Sets to a hard non-compressible consistency
- Sharp and record can be easily read.
- Articulation of casts can be achieved accurately without fear of distortion or compression of the record.

Disadvantages

Time factor. The position of the mandible must be held static until the zinc oxide-eugenol sets. If the mandible moves it can result in an improper centric relation. A study was conducted to determine the dimensional stability of eugenol free zinc oxide paste and ZnOE paste. It was concluded that eugenol free paste can be used effectively and can be stored indefinitely.

Techniques for Making Interocclusal Records

The record bases are placed in the patient's mouth and trial closures are made until the procedure is familiar for both the patient and the dentist. Vertical reference lines are then drawn extending from the buccal surface of the maxillary occlusal rim to the buccal surface of the mandibular rim. The interocclusal record is then made.

1. V-shaped notches are cut on both the maxillary and mandibular occlusal rims. Then a recording material of zinc oxide eugenol, plaster of Paris or wax is placed over the area of the notches and the patient is instructed to close in to centric relation. The disadvantage of this technique is that the occlusal rims may get displaced.

2. 2 mm of wax is removed from the occlusal surface of the mandibular rim. V-shaped notches are cut on the maxillary occlusal rim in the premolar and molar area to help in repositioning and to serve as a key for the recording material.

   The occlusal recording material is placed on the mandibular rim and the patient is instructed to close into it and to stop at the established vertical dimension.

3. Softening, the entire occlusal surface of one of the rims. The patient is then asked to close in centric. The disadvantages of this technique are that: (i) compression of the soft tissue might occur, and (ii) established vertical height is lost.

4. Softening the posterior surface of the wax rim by deep heating (preferably the lower rim) and leaving the anterior portion intact to maintain vertical dimension. Maxillary occlusal rim is also left intact.

5. Deep heating/pooling is done: The hot spatula is inserted down into the center of the lower occlusal rim on one side and then on the other allowing time for the inner hot portion of wax to soften the outer portion enough so that the outer walls will collapse readily under closing pressure.

Advantages

- Maintain vertical dimension
- Achieves a seal at the same time.

Graphic Methods

Graphic methods record a tracing of the mandibular movements in one plane. It indicates the horizontal relationship of the mandible to the maxilla. A graphic representation of the lateral border movements on a horizontal plane describes a figure known as a gothic arch tracing, arrow point tracing or needle point tracing.

Gothic Arch Tracing. The pattern obtained on the horizontal plate with a central bearing or tracing device.

Central Bearing/tracing Device. A device that provides a central point of bearing or support between the maxillary and mandibular dental arches. It consists of a contacting point that is attached to one dental arch and a plate attached to the opposing dental arch. The plate provides the surface on which the tracing of mandibular movement is recorded. It may be used to distribute occlusal forces evenly during the recording of maxillomandibular relationships and for the correction of disharmonious occlusal contacts (Fig. 12.1).

To make a needle point tracing, one condyle moves forward and inward during a lateral movement followed by movement in the opposite direction, with rotation occurring

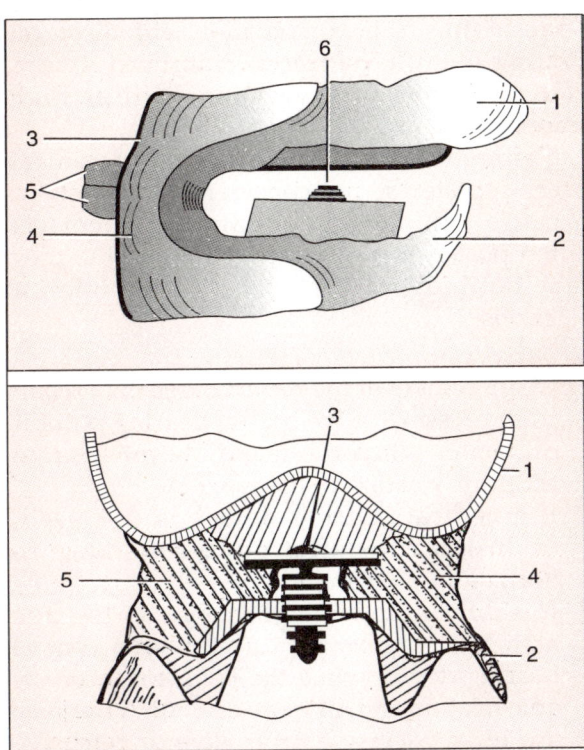

Fig. 12.1. Maxillary and mandibular record base with the central bearing device attached.

around the opposite condyle. The direction of lateral movements, produced by the patient is determined by the external pterygoid on the balancing side and the deep capsular ligament of the condyle on the working side. These lateral movements cut lines in the form of "V" with the point of the tracer resting in the apex of the tracing when the heads of the condyles are in their most retruded position.

Historical Review of Graphic Recordings. The earliest graphic recordings were based on studies of mandibular movements by Balkwill in 1866. The first known needle point tracing was by Hesse in 1897. This technique was then improved and popularized by Gysi in 1910.

Types of Tracing Devices

Extraoral. Extraoral tracing devices may be used in combination with wax or compound occlusal rims or in combination with a central bearing point (Gysi tracer, Stansberry tracer, Hall tracer, Sears trivet, and Phillips high tracer).

Extraoral tracings made without central bearing plate are not considered satisfactory, because although they indicate the correct anteroposterior position of the mandible they may not indicate the correct superoinferior relations.

Factors influencing a graphic tracing

1. Displacement of the record bases may result from pressure, if the central bearing point is off center when the mandible moves into eccentric relation to the maxillae.
2. If a central bearing device is not used, occlusion rims offer more resistance to horizontal movement.
3. It is difficult to locate the center of the true arch to centralize the forces with a central bearing device when the jaws are in favorable relation and far more difficult if the jaws are in an excessive protrusive or retrusive relation.
4. It is difficult to stabilize a record base against horizontal forces on tissues that are pendulous or otherwise easily displaceable.
5. Difficult to stabilise a record base against horizontal forces on residual ridges that have no vertical height.
6. Difficult to stabilize a record base in patients who have large awkward tongues.
7. Recording devices are not considered compatible with normal physiologic stimulation in mandibular movements.

Intraoral Tracers.
Examples are Siedel tracer, Ballard tracer, Messerman tracer, Needles technique.

Extraoral Tracings

1. The casts with the occlusal rims are attached to the articulator with the tentative centric relation record at the predetermined vertical dimension of occlusion.
2. The central bearing device is mounted. The central bearing plate is attached to the

Table 12.1. Differences between extraoral and intraoral tracings

Intraoral	Extraoral
1. Intraoral tracings are not visible during the tracing	Visible when the tracings are made
2. Tracing are small. So, in certain cases it may be difficult to locate the true apex	Tracings obtained are larger and so apex is more discernible
3. Tracer must be definitely rested in a hole at the point of the apex to ensure accuracy when plaster is injected between the occlusal rims.	Stylus can be observed in the apex of the tracing during the process of injecting plaster (so no hole is required)
4. If the patient moves his mandible before the occlusal rims are secured, the records shift on their basal seat. This destroys the accuracy of the record.	The patient can be guided more accurately.

maxillary occlusion rim (it should be flushing with the occlusal rim). 2 mm of wax is then removed from the mandibular occlusal rim. Then the central bearing plate with point is attached to the mandibular occlusal rim. The central bearing screw is turned upwards so that the point contacts the upper central bearing plate. The central bearing point and plate should be parallel to each other and should be centered in relation to each other (for the equalization of forces).

3. The tracing table is then mounted. The devices are securely attached to the occlusal rims, the stylus is attached to the maxillary rim and the tracing table to the lower rim.
4. The patient is then trained to move his jaw forwards, backward and to the right and left while gently applying guiding pressure with the thumb. When the patient becomes proficient in executing movements, the tracing table is prepared. It is coated with a

thin layer of carbon, wax or chalk powder dissolved in denatured alcohol.

Ney Excursion Guide. This is an aid in training the patient. Place the guide in a convenient position for the patient to see. Some patients respond more readily to the request to move the lower jaw to right, left forward and backward than to positions 1, 2, 3, 4, 5 and 6. Home is the most retruded comfortable position (Fig. 12.2).

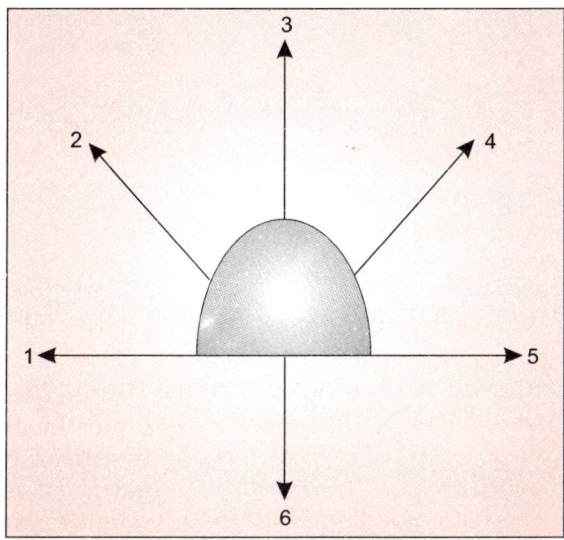

Fig. 12.2. Ney excursion guide.

Factors to be Kept in Mind During a Graphic Tracing

1. Displacement of the record bases may result (from pressure) if the central bearing point is off center when the mandible moves into eccentric relations with the maxillae.
2. If a central bearing device is not used, occlusal rims offer more resistance to horizontal movement.
3. It is difficult to locate the center of the true arches to centralize, the forces, when the jaws are in a favorable relation (and

even more difficult in abnormal jaw relations).
4. It is difficult to stabilize a record base on tissues that are pendulous or easily displaceable.
5. It is difficult to stabilize a record base against horizontal forces on residual ridges that have no vertical height.
6. It is difficult to stabilize a record base in patients—who have large awkward tongues.
7. Tracing is not acceptable unless a pointed apex is obtained.
8. Graphic recording is made at a predetermined vertical dimension of occlusion.
9. Graphic methods can record eccentric relations of the mandible to the maxillae.
10. Graphic methods are the most accurate means of making a centric relation record with mechanical instruments.

Explanation of Gothic Arch Tracing

A gothic arch tracing with a sharp apex can only be obtained by a pivoting of the mandible on one condyle first, and then the other as right and left lateral movements are made. If the condyles do not pivot or do not have centers from which lateral movements are made, a double tracing or one with a rounded apex will be obtained. A rounded apex is also caused by a shifting of record bases on their basal seats.

Many patients have developed faulty condylar positions because of malocclusions (either natural or due to faulty prosthesis or orthodontic treatment). Some patients can accommodate the muscular positioning of the mandible by tactile sensation from the teeth and periodontal membranes thus apparently conditioning the muscles away from the natural action. After the natural teeth are extracted, the condyles can assume a faulty position without the patient being aware of any strain. Gothic arch tracing can be misleading for such patients, unless much care and judgement are used.

Most of the proponents of the needle point tracing method assume that a correct tracing with a sharp apex is indicative of condyles being properly situated in the glenoid fossa. Unfortunately, the tracing merely indicates pivoting condyles; not whether the pivoting occurs in normal retruded or protruded positions in the glenoid fossa.

Intraoral Tracing: Hardy's Technique

Involves two steps: (i) fabrication of stabilized base plates, and (ii) development of tracing.

Fabrication of Stablised Base plates. Gross undercuts on the casts are filled. Single thick shellac baseplates are then adapted over the upper and lower casts and whenever feasible they are trimmed short of the undercuts. Tin foil was then burnished over both upper and lower casts with the aid of cotton roles so that no wrinkles are left in the tin foil. A metallic oxide impression paste is then placed inside the base plates, placed on the tin foil and allowed to harden. When hardened, it is removed from the cast and excess foil and metallic oxide paste are trimmed away.

Developing the Tracing. A horizontal line is drawn along the outside of the mandibular cast parallel to the flat bearing area in the region of the bicuspid molar teeth. A rim of modeling compound is constructed on the lower stabilized base plate so that its occlusal surface is parallel to this line. Vertical height is approximated to that of the final position of the lower anterior teeth.

A stiff brass plate is contoured to the size of the rim and luted to modeling compound so that it is also parallel to the marked line. A central bearing point is attached to the upper stabilized base plate with modeling compound. It is positioned as closely as possible to the centre of supporting areas of both the upper and lower residual ridge arches. In cases where centralization to both upper and lower arches is not possible the lower is favored. The tracer must be perpendicular to the tracing table.

The central bearing point is then adjusted to touch the lower plate at the previously determined vertical dimension. The occlusal rims are checked in the mouth to ascertain that no interference exists between them during lateral excursions.

The patient is instructed to exert light pressure and move his mandible to right, left and forwards (Fig. 12.3).

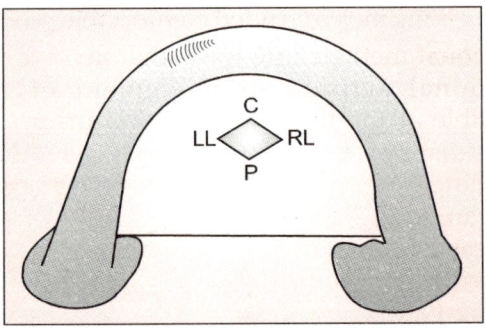

Fig. 12.3. Envelope of motion: An intraoral gothic arch tracing.

When a definite apex is observed, a disk with a small hole punched in the centre is placed over the tracing so that the apex of the tracing falls in the centre of the hole. This was luted in position with sticky wax and the occlusal rim is placed back in the mouth.

The patient is then requested to engage this small hole in the disk with the central bearing device and to hold the two base plates together as lightly as possible.

Soft impression plaster is injected between the base plates with a syringe. On hardening, the rim is removed as one unit.

According to Troppazzano, check bite record is the technique of preference in recording and checking centric relation. Its accuracy is far greater than is possible to obtain with the central bearing point. The central bearing point is based on the fallacious assumption that central bearing point will produce equalization of pressure. But this occurs only if two factors are present:
1. If normal ridge relations are present and central point of bearing can be placed in the

centre of the maxillary and mandibular foundational bases.

2. If mucosal resiliency is extremely slight. In the absence of these two conditions, it is impossible to register the equalization of pressure with the central bearing point.

FUNCTIONAL METHODS

Functional methods are those that involve the functional activity or movement of the mandible at the time the record is made.

The disadvantage is that displacement of the recording bases in relation to the supporting base can occur when the record is being made.

These include:

• Needles-House method
• Essig-Patterson method.

They also include methods that make use of swallowing for positioning and recording the centric jaw position. Functional methods of recording centric relation require stable record bases for accurate records. Displaceable basal seat tissue, resistance of the recording medium and the lack of control of equalized pressure contribute to inaccuracy.

Patients should have good neuromuscular coordination and must be capable of following instructions to obtain accurate records. The Needle-House and Essig-Patterson techniques are based on the same principle. The patient produces a pattern of mandibular movements by moving the mandible in to protrusion, retrusion and right and left lateral.

Both methods require tentative interocclusal wax records of centric relation at the tentative vertical dimension of occlusion to prepare the recording devices. Both methods adjust the recording medium at a height of vertical jaw separation which is in excess to the pre-determined dimension of occlusion.

Needles-House Method

Needle-House method uses a compound occlusion rim with metal styli placed in the maxillary rim. When the mandible moves with the styli contacting the mandibular rim, the styli cut 4 diamond shaped tracings. The tracings incorporate the movements in three planes and the records are then placed on an articulator (to receive and duplicate the records. (Fig. 12.4)

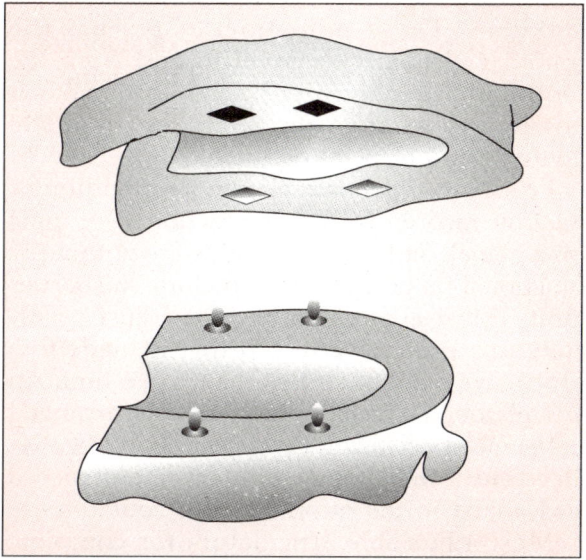

Fig. 12.4. Needle-House technique of recording centric relation

Patterson Method

Patterson method uses wax occlusion rims. A trench is made in the mandibular rim and a mixture of half plaster and half carborundum paste is placed in the trench. Mandibular movements generate compensating curves in plaster and carborundum. When the plaster and carborundum mix are decreased to the predetermined vertical dimension of occlusion, the patient is asked to retrude the mandible and the occlusal rims are joined with metal staples.

Eccentric Relation Records

An eccentric maxillomandibular relation is any relationship of the mandible to the maxillae other than centric position.

When an articulator that adjusts to protrusive and to right and left lateral movements is used, the purpose in making an eccentric relation record is to adjust the horizontal and lateral condylar inclinations so that the articulator jaw members perform eccentric movements equivalent, but not identical to the relative movements of the mandible to the maxillae. These adjustments permit the condylar elements to travel to and from the centric and eccentric positions and make it possible to arrange the teeth for complete dentures in balanced occlusion.

Protrusive and lateral maxillomandibular relation records made by functional, graphic (one plane), and tactile methods are within the functional range and do not include the border limits. Most articulators do not adjust accurately to a protrusive record that is made to a protrusive position of less than 5 to 6 mm. An articulator on which the teeth are to be arranged in balanced occlusion must accurately receive, an eccentric maxillomandibular relation record and adjust to the information it contains.

Most adjustable articulators for complete denture procedures will receive a protrusive interocclusal relation record, and the horizontal condylar inclination will adjust so that the instrument jaw members perform lateral and protrusive movements equivalent, but not identical, to the relative movements of the mandible to the maxillae.

Extraoral tracings with a central bearing device offer several advantages over other graphic methods if the bases to which the recording devices are attached are stable. The same vertical jaw separation and the same horizontal relationship is repeatable. The recording medium is injected with a syringe to eliminate any resistance factor of the medium that might influence the accuracy of the record.

The methods for eccentric maxillomandibular relation records may be -classified in a manner similar to the methods for centric maxillomandibular relation records.

1. Functional or chew-in procedures are exemplified by the Needles-house and Patterson techniques. After the record has been used to mount the mandibular cast in centric relationship to the maxillary cast, the articulator is adjusted to the eccentric records.
2. Graphic methods are exemplified by the extraoral arrow point or Gothic arch tracings made on one plane.
3. Tactile or interocclusal records are basically the same. The recording materials are different. Wax, compound plaster, and zinc oxide and eugenol paste used on the wax occlusion rim before the teeth are arranged for try-in are considered tentative records. The preferred time to make ecentric maxillomandibular relation records is after all the teeth have been verified. Seat the patient in a comfortable up-right position: (a) Verify the vertical dimension of occlusion; (b) verify the relationship of the maxillary and mandibular casts with a centric relation record; (c) check he plane of occlusion; (d) check the anteroposterior and mediolateral positions of the teeth for compatibility with the lips, tongue, and cheeks; and (e) determine the patient's acceptance of the esthetics of the teeth.

Technical Procedures

The graphic method of making eccentric maxillomandibular relation records is performed at the same sitting and with the same equipment used to make the centric relation record.

After the mandibular cast has been mounted on the articulator in centric relation, reseat the recording devices in the patient's mouth. Proceed as follows:

1. Measure a distance of 5 or 6 mm from the apex of the arrow point tracing on the protrusive tracing and mark this point.
2. Instruct the patient to protrude until the point of the stylus rests in the marked point.

3. Inject quick-setting dental plaster between the occlusion rims, allow the plaster to harden, and remove the case from the mouth.

4. Free the horizontal condylar adjustments on the articulator by releasing the locknuts.

5. Raise the incisal guide pin about 1/2 inch from the top of the guide table.

6. Carefully seat the record bases on the cast. An accurate seating of both condyles must be secured.

7. Secure the locknuts with positive finger pressure.

8. Record the right and left calibrations of the horizontal inclinations on the plaster mounting. This record is useful if the settings are accidentally moved.

The most common method to make a protrusive relation record is the tactile or interocclusal record method using a soft wax.

1. Seat the patient in a comfortable up right position.

2. Having ascertained that the teeth are set in an acceptable arrangement, rehearse the patient in the procedure. Seat the dentures and support the mandibular base with the tips of the index fingers and the thumb under the mandible in the same way as when the centric relation record was made. Instruct the patient to protrude the lower jaw for approximately 5 or 6 mm. Do not use any recording medium at this time. Observe the midline between the maxillary central incisors to determine if it coincides mediolaterally with the midline of the mandibular central incisors. It is often necessary to guide the patient's mandible until a protrusive movement is learned. Gentle pressure is usually all that is needed to guide the mandible.

3. When the patient has learned the protrusive position, remove the mandibular trial denture.

4. Place four layers of soft wax over the mandibular teeth and seal the wax on the lingual and buccal surfaces of the posteriors and the lingual and labial surfaces of the anterior teeth.

5. Soften the wax with a controlled open flame or water at 135°F.

6. Reinsert the trial denture and instruct the patient to protrude the lower jaws and to close into the wax. Allow the wax to harden before removing the trial denture and attached record.

7. Set the condylar post of the articulator at 0° on the lateral calibrations.

8. Inspect the wax record for evenness of contact. Records that lack contact in isolated areas or have uneven contacts are recontoured, and new records are made.

9. Release the horizontal condylar adjustments by freezing the locknuts. Raise the incisal guide pin 1/2 inch from the incisal guide table.

10. Place the maxillary and mandibular trial dentures in their respective mounting casts in the articulator.

11. Carefully relate the maxillary teeth to the wax protrusive records.

12. Examine the condylar elements to see that protrusion was 5 to 6 mm.

13. Manipulate the horizontal condylar housings while all the teeth are accurately seated in the record. Do not use force.

14. Secure the horizontal condyle adjustment locknuts with finger pressure.

15. Record the horizontal right and left inclinations on the plaster mounting. This record is useful if the settings are accidentally moved.

Lateral Relation Records

When an articulator accurately receives and adjusts to a lateral mandibular relation record the additional points of references are valuable. The more accurate the points of reference supplied in adjusting the articulator; the more harmony will exist between mandibular movements and cusp inclines.

Technical Procedures

Execute the graphic methods in the same manner as the protrusive relation record with the following exceptions. Two records are required-one of right lateral and one of left lateral. The articulator is adjusted as each record is made. When an interocclusal record of wax is made, additional layers of soft wax are placed on the balancing side to accommodate for the difference in the vertical jaw separation between the balancing and working sides.

Although the mechanics of making lateral jaw relation records appear simple, it is recognized that in complete denture con-struction the procedure is difficult and many inaccuracies occur. Hanau held the opinion that the setting of a lateral inclination by an anatomic record offers no particular advantages and that the required lateral protrusion can be determined on the finished case in the mouth by records, observation, and interpretations of symptoms on the ridges. He recommended the following formula to arrive at an acceptable lateral inclination.

$$L = H/8 + 12$$

L = Lateral condyle inclination in the frees;
H = Horizontal condyle inclination in degrees as established by the protrusive relation record.

Further Reading

1. Avant. Using the term 'Centric'. J Prosth Dent. 1971; 25(1): 12-15.
2. Kaper, Yurkstas .An evaluation of centric and relation records obtained by various techniques. J Prosth Dent. 1957; 7(6):771-85.
3. Myers M L. Centric relation records- A historial review. J Prosth Dent. 1982; 47(2):141-44.
4. Gilboe D B. Centric relation, A treatment option. J Prosth Dent.1983; 50(5):685-88.
5. Levin B. A reevaluation of Hanau's laws of articulation. J Prosth Dent. 1978; 39(3):254-58.
6. Becker C M. Mandibular centricity; centric relation. J Prosth Dent. 200; 83: 158-60.
7. Lucia V O. Centric relation the and practice. J Prosth Dent.1960; 10(5):849-56.
8. Dawson Peter. Centric relation its effect on occluso-muscle harmony. Dental Clin. North Amer. 1979; 2(2): 169-80.

MULTIPLE CHOICE QUESTIONS

1. _____ is an example for an extra oral tracer.
   a. Siedel tracer
   b. Masserman tracer
   c. Needles
   d. Philips high tracer

2. **Statement that is false regarding an intraoral tracing is**
   a. Tracings obtained are small.
   b. Stylus can be observed in the apex of the tracing during the process of injecting plaster.
   c. Tracings are not visible
   d. a and c

3. **An example for a functional method for recording centric relation**
   a. Interocclusal method by using wax.
   b. Interocclusal method using dental plaster.
   c. Gothic arch tracings.
   d. Essig-Patterson method.

4. **In the Essig-Patterson method for recording centric relation,**
   a. A mixture of half plaster and half carborundum paste is placed in a trench in the mandibular rim.
   b. Metal styli are placed in the maxillary occlusal rim.

c. Metal styli are placed in the mandibular occlusal rim and a tracing table is attached to the maxillary rim.
d. None of the above.

5. **The muscles that play a major role in centric relation position include all except**
a. Posterior fibres of temporalis
b. Middle fibres of temporalis
c. Genio hyoid
d. Lateral pterygoids.

6. **According to the osteofibre theory of centric relation,**
a. The temporomandibular ligament becomes tense when the jaws are in the centric relation position.
b. A retrusive terminal stop is formed by the soft tissue of the posterior part of the roof of glenoid fossa.
c. Centric relation is the product of a defence reflex which causes the external pterygoid muscle to contract.
d. None of the above.

7. _____ is a pattern obtained on the horizontal plate with a central bearing device.
a. A gothic arch tracing
b. An arrow point tracing
c. A needle point tracing
d. All the above

8. **The first needle point tracing was by**
a. Gysi   b. Hesse
c. Balkwill   d. Philips

9. **The effects seen in excessively reducing the vertical dimension include all except**
a. Trauma and discomfort
b. Clicking of teeth
c. Cheek biting
d. Poor appearance

10. **The true instrument regarding the use of phonetics for recording vertical dimension is**
a. When words starting with "f" and 'v' are pronounced, the incisal edges of the lower anterior teeth should create a seal on the upper lip.
b. When words starting with 'f' are pronounced, the upper and lower teeth do not contact one another.
c. When words starting with 'm' are pronounced, anterior teeth should barely touch each other.
d. None of the above

11. **The power point technique by Boos is based on the theory that**
a. The maximum closing force can be exerted when the mandible is at the vertical dimension of rest position
b. The minimum closing force is exerted when the mandible is in the vertical dimension of occlusion position.
c. Both
d. None of the above

12. **The neuromuscular perception method for determining vertical dimension was determined by**
a. Boos   b. Lytle
c. Silverman   d. Jankleson

13. **The muscles involved in centric relation include all except**
a. Medial pterygoids
b. Lateral pterygoids
c. Digastric
d. Temporalis

14. **Boos exercise involves**
a. Retrusion of the tongue
b. Stretch and relaxation
c. Swallowing
d. Alternation of head position

15. **The most advocated theory for centric relation is**
a. Muscle theory
b. Osteofibre theory
c. Meniscus theory
d. Ligament theory

16. The first needle point tracing was by
    a. Bonwill   b. Blakwill
    c. Hesse   d. Gysi

17. The most accurate method for recording centric relation is
    a. Interocclusal check record
    b. Gothic arch tracing
    c. Needle house method
    d. Patterson method

18. _____ is an aid in training the patient
    a. Needles tracer
    b. Siedal's tracer
    c. Ney excursion guide
    d. Intraoral tracer

FAQ's

1. Define centric relation

2. Importance of centric relation

3. Method for recording centric relation

4. Gothic arch tracing

5. Definitions of
   a. Vertical dimension of rest
   b. Vertical dimension of occlusion
   c. Freeway space

6. Methods for recording vertical dimensions

13

HINGE-AXIS

INTRODUCTION

According to the glossary of prosthodontic terms, a hinge-axis is defined as an imaginary line between the mandibular condyles around which the mandible can rotate without translatory movement or an imaginary line around which the mandible may rotate through the sagittal plane.

Terminal hinge position[1] is the most retruded hinge position. This position is the learnable, repeatable and recordable position of centric relation. The limits of hinge movement in this position have been determined to be about 12-15° from maximum intercuspation or about 19-20 mm at the incisal edges. The condyles are in a definite position in the fossae during the terminal hinge movement.

Establishing the maxillomandibular relationships in edentulous individuals, has engaged the attention of practitioners and prosthodontists alike, ever since the profession began to understand and interpret the various dynamic and static positions of the condyles in the glenoid fossa.

When the mandible moves as it does in carrying out the functions of mastication and speech, the various movements it makes and the relationship it assumes defy description because of their complexity. However, when the mandible is motionless, definite relationships to the cranium or maxilla can be established.

After the establishment of an acceptable denture space and restoration of facial contour, the positional relationship of the denture space to the condylar axis or kinematic axis has to be registered. The resultant records are then transferred to the articulator which is a techno-mechanical equivalent of the jaw. The articulator has a mechanical hinge-axis that has a fixed horizontal position parallel to its base and perpendicular to its midsagittal plane. When a face-bow record is used in conjunction with an articulator, the maxillary cast is mounted in relationship to the axis, (which now becomes the mechanical equivalent of the patient's anatomic hinge-axis). In this way the articulator is programmed to duplicate the patient's mandibular arc of opening and closing in the terminal hinge position (Fig. 13.1).

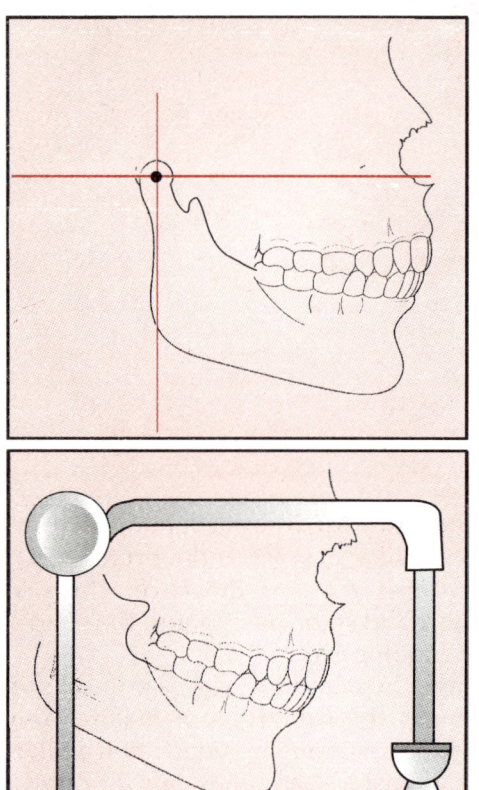

Fig. 13.1. Superimposition of transverse axis of mandible over opening axis of articulator.

In order to program a dental articulator to duplicate the hinge opening and closure of the mandible, it is necessary to make a hinge-axis record and transfer this information to the articulator. The face-bow is a reliable gadget to transfer the above relationship.

Different methods[5] have been used to locate and transfer the hinge-axis to the articulator. These techniques are divided into the two main groups of arbitrary and true or kinematic.

Either the anatomic or the kinematic hinge-axis face-bow transfer is the first step in recording the relationship of the maxillary arch to the condylar paths. These two methods of maxillary cast orientation differ basically only

in accuracy. Once the maxillary cast is oriented on the articulator, the centric relation record completes the static, or starting relationship between the maxillae and the condyles in the temporomandibular fossae. From this static starting position, dynamic eccentric condylar movements are initiated by means of eccentric interocclusal records or extraoral tracings.

Thus, the centric relation record and the kinematic face-bow transfer record combined together allow the clinician to anatomically orient casts of the patient's dentition to the articulator to simulate mandibular function.

IMPORTANCE OF HINGE-AXIS

***1. Determines Terminal Hinge Position.*[2]** The most posterior position that the mandibular musculature can achieve is the hinge position and one way of training the patient's musculature to assume this position is by the determination of the hinge-axis.

The proprioceptive neural patterns in the normal automatic and in the learned hinge movements are radically different. In the learned hinge movement, the proprioceptive sensations in the capsule are consciously felt while they exert their leading influence during the closing movement, at least in last phase, it is a true hinge movement. Thus the newly learned closing movement is in contrast with that in the average dentulous patient, which is automatic and directed by the signals of the periodontal sensations and is felt only at the end of the movement. This point is of great importance because it invalidates many findings on individuals in whom, the hinge-axis had previously been determined and who, therefore, are conditioned to perform conscious, as against automatic movement.

2. It helps in Locating Centric Relation. The location of the hinge-axis during face-bow transfer helps in the fixating anteroposterior relation of the mandible to the maxillae at the terminal hinge position which is the same as the centric relation. During the fabrication of the centric relation record, the condyles are properly positioned and mandible is restricted to pure rotation around the terminal position of the transverse horizontal axis of the mandible, so the clinician is able to obtain accurate, reproducible records that can be transferred to the articulator.

3. It Represents Occlusal Vertical Dimension. It represents to the occlusal vertical dimension what the needle point tracing does to centric relation.

4. It Records the Static Starting Point of Functional Mandibular Movements. In numerous patients investigated, the reference point representing the hinge-axis appeared with frequency in the region of the neck of the condyle at the posterior border in a region corresponding to the centre of the mandibular articulation. In some patients the hinge-axis was slightly forward at the centre of the neck of the condyle.

Thus we can pinpoint and say that the location of the transverse hinge-axis serves only to orient the maxilla and to record the static starting point for functional mandibular movements.

5. Cohen in 1960 mentioned the following advantages of location of the hinge-axis:

- Study casts may be mounted to determine if the patient's centric occlusion is in harmony with centric relation.
- Working casts can be mounted in the best relationship for the teeth or the denture bases.
- Since the hinge is a definite fixed component of every closing position of the mandible, it is necessary to reproduce it on the appropriate instrument if the occlusion is to be rehabilitated.
- It is possible to increase or decrease the vertical dimension on the instrument, without disturbing the centric relation.

6. Hinge-axis Expresses the Relation of Border Movements. The hinge-axis expresses a relation of border movements which involve or include the limits of all physiologic movements. Thus, with artificial teeth arranged in accordance with the reproduction of the border movements, the patient's out jaw movements are within the same field of action as he could with his own teeth.

HISTORY AND DEVELOPMENT OF THE HINGE-AXIS CONCEPT

The first actual kinematic location was evolved through the California Gnathological Society under the leadership of BB McCollum, and the credit for the idea of the mechanical location of an axis was given to Robert Harlan.

The first locations employed a modified snow face-bow and consumed as much as 8 hours. Current devices have evolved from this first crude mechanism and its attendant theories and observations. Many present day concepts and fallacies may also be traced to its origin.

History of Hinge-axis

1. The written story of the mandibular hinge-axis goes back to the time of Gray and his followers who recognized that the mandible moves on a hinge-axis as well as by means of the forward and lateral movements of the condyles in the glenoid fossae. Until, the time of Bonwill, the scientists treated the joints as if they had only a hinge action.

2. Balkwill in 1865, called the attention to the sliding actions of the joint. However, his article received little attention. He stated that the mandible turns on an axis that runs through both condyles during opening and closing motions. The horizontal condylar axis has played an integral part in duplicating the mandibular movements on the articulator.

3. Bonwill in 1860 assumed that forward motion of the joint was on a straight line and in a forward direction. This idea held

precedence until Walker around 1890 proved that the motion was forward and downward.

4. Snow in 1899 recognized the importance of the hinge-axis and he contrived the face-bow for transferring this axis to the articulator.

5. In 1905 Campion concluded from his studies of mandibular movements that dental casts should be mounted on the articulator in such a way that the rotational axis of the articulator coincides with the opening axis of the mandible.

6. The scientific basis for the hinge-axis theory and a practical method for locating the terminal hinge-axis came about through the work of McCollum and Stuart in 1921, and the Gnathological Society of California, was based on earlier studies of Balkwill, Bennett and Campion.

The credit for the idea of the mechanical location of an axis was given to Dr Robert Harlan.

In its purest form, the transverse horizontal axis is usually thought of as exhibiting a two-dimensional effect and as being independent of the vertical and sagittal axis. This may not be true, for this hypothesis assumes a situation which complies with the tenets of solid-body mechanics and pure rotation.

METHODS FOR LOCATING HINGE-AXIS

There are different methods for locating hinge-axis which can be broadly classified into arbitrary and kinematic.[3]

Arbitrary Methods

Arbitrary methods employ only tentative methods of locating the hinge-axis. The following points are commonly used. They are average, anatomical landmarks considered reasonably accurate for most clinical situations.

1. *1 cm in Front of the Line.* from the apex of the trague of the ear to the outer canthus of the eye.

2. *Beyron's Point.* 13 mm anterior to the posterior margin of the centre of the tragus of the ear on a line extending to the corner of the eye.

3. *Bergstrom Point.* 10 mm anterior to the centre of the spherical insert for the external auditory meatus and 7 mm below the Frankfurt Horizontal plane.

4. *Dawson's Palpatory Method.* This method uses palpation for locating the hinge-axis (advocated by Dawson). From a position behind the patient, the index finger was placed over the joint area, and the patient was asked to open wide. By asking the patient to repeat an opening-closing arc, it was possible to feel the condylar rotation and to locate the axis.

5. *Gysi Point.* Located 13 mm in front of the most upper part of the external auditory meatus on a line passing to the ectocanthion. This method was proposed by both Gysi, Hanau, Snow and Gilmer and is the most common point used today.

6. *Lejoyeux Point.* Located 10-11 mm in front of the ear on a line to the canthus and 5 mm below it.

7. *Laritzen-Bondner Axis.* This is determined by the use of specially constructed disks 10 mm in diameter and a plastic ruler. This point is located 12 mm anterior and 2 mm below the porion on the F-H plane.

8. *Abdal-Hadi Point.*[4] Abdal-Hadi's point is based on the high correlation between the width profile of the face and the X coordinate of the kinematic point. Thus the use of the linear regression formula permits prediction of the anteroposterior site of the kinematic point. This equation is

$$Y = 9.5 + 0.95\ (X)$$

Y = Width profile of face measured from the ectocanthion to the centre of the external auditory meatus.

X = Anteroposterior position of the kinematic point.

A constant distance equal to 0.5 mm was used above the line passing from the centre of the external auditory meatus to the canthus to locate the superoinferior position of the proposed method. Abdal-Hadi point is close to Lejougeux point.

Kinematic Methods

The kinematically determined axis point of rotation of the mandible is the most accurate of all present methods of estimating hinge-axis location. Its determination observes the motion of the stylus on an axis bow, as created by jaw movement, in relation to a flag fixed over the patient's condylar area. The axis point is accepted when the stylus no longer translates, but simply rotates. Various designs of recording equipment have been developed, some of which include use of multiple stylus and even of recording of accurate paths on radiographic film.

Geometric Principle for Locating Hinge-axis Through the Use of Stylus (double)

When a hinge-axis bow is used with a modified flag to record jaw movements, extended arcs of rotation are produced by the opening movements of the mandible.

Two theories of geometry are used in this technique:

• A line drawn through the centre of a circle perpendicular to a chord meets it at its midpoint, besides the arcs determined by the cord and secondly, the line joining the centre of a circle to the midpoint of a chord is perpendicular to the chord.

• Using these theorems, it should be possible to locate a rotation point by drafting perpendicular lines at right angles to the chords of arcs produced by a rotating mandible. Lines drawn from the midpoint of the chords, and at right angles to them, will intersect at the centre of the circle represented by the arcs. This centre is the true axis point.

Buhnergraph Instrument (1970)

Long at al offered the first recorded use of the geometric principle using a Buhnergraph instrument. The accuracy of the technique resulted from the location of centric relation at 2 degrees of jaw opening and plotting the position of the axis.

Pantograph

The pantograph is an apparatus consisting of two face-bows, one fixed to the maxilla and the other to the mandible. One holds writing devices, the other recording tables. In practice six writings or records are made at three places on each side of the head. One is anterior for an arrow point tracing, one is near the condyle to trace the horizontal movement path of a point near the condyle, and the last is usually fixed perpendicular to the second to record the vertical movement path of a point near the condyle.

There are presently three appliances available: One designed by Stuart, one by Granger and the third by Guichet. There are slight differences in the three:

For example, all the writers in Guichet's instrument are on the upper bow and are pneumatically controlled by one button. Thus, the apparatus can be used easily and speedily by one man. On the other hand, Granger's and Stuart's instruments have the condyle writers on the lower member and arrow point writers on the upper. The clutch preparation in these two techniques is tedious, and the chairside procedure is two or three times longer than the technique used by Guichet.

There is considerable value, however, to having the condyle writers on the lower bow because visualization of condylar movement is immediate. In addition, Stuart's and Granger's instruments record the centre of rotation for each condyle because their horizontal pen is set to the terminal hinge-axis. Guichet does not consider this necessary (unless the vertical dimension is to be changed) and thus his pen is slightly forward of the terminal hinge-axis.

Regardless of these differences, the pantograph affords us an excellent view of lateral mandibular movement.

Transograph

This was introduced in 1952 (which is essentially a hinge-axis-face-bow modified later to serve as an articulator). Transograph means 'a writing of jaw movements carried over to an articulator'.

The theory of transographics was postulated by Bererly McCollum and the Gnathological Society in collaboration with HL Page and Albinson. In this instrument, the patient's intercondylar distance ultimately formed the intercondylar distance in the articulator.

Transographics is based upon the split axis theory.

The theory behind transographics is that the condyle is an asymmetrical body and its sagittal, vertical and transverse axis do not intersect and therefore a common point of rotation does not exist.

The assets of transograph are:
- The registering device becomes a part of the articulator in which are incorporated the hinge-axis, bennett movement, and the cranial plane for each individual patient. Thus the individual functional movements of the mandible can be brought to bench without the need of any transfer which

eliminates the discrepancies common to most of the articulators.
- It has no mechanical connection (solid axis) between the two condylar bearings as seen in the conventional articulator. The transograph has its condylar bearings joined only by means of maxillary and mandibular arches. Thus each axial center is independent of the other.
- The intercondylar distance is adjustable thereby the distance between the rotating centers and the teeth are same in the articulator as observed in the patient's mouth.

Other Methods

Electromathematical Method

Electromathematical method determines a point of minimal translatory movement (Steady point) during the rotatory opening movement of the condyle. This method calculates mathematically, the 3D coordinates of the condylar rotation centers automatically. This technique is very precise, the reason being in the mathematical approach towards these methods.

Stereognathography

Using this method, the joint axis can be located in the articulator with an accuracy of 0.6 mm. In individual cases, errors may be upto 1.5 mm.

Moire Fringe Method

This method localizes the centre of rotation by defining two primary fringes, each of which is found by the intersection of three lines. The primary fringes intersect at the centre of rotation at 90° to each other, the angle least likely to produce an error in measurement. This method is extremely accurate and reproducible to within 2 mm of the real centre for angular changes as small as 3°.

This technique is useful in evaluating whether a joint is a simple hinge, or whether the joint moves about a changing axis of rotation referred to as a locus or centrode.

Digital Recording System Computerized Axiograph

Axiotron is an computerized axiograph used for determining the THA. This is attached to the mandible by means of the "Axiodapt" clutch system.

TECHNIQUE FOR LOCATING THE HINGE-AXIS ON THE PATIENT

The location and transfer of the hinge-axis are not very difficult procedures, but they must be carried out with great care because they are the foundation for many other procedures.

Preparation of Clutches

The technique for locating the terminal hinge-axis position is essentially the same for the dentulous and edentulous patient, but the method of attaching the clutch to the mandible are quite different.

The clutch is a mechanical device made to be rigidly attached to the mandibular teeth or the mandibular residual ridge to which a hinge-axis bow is attached.

The construction of the clutch for dentulous patient is done in the following way.
1. Make an accurate impression of the mandibular arch and pour a stone cast.
2. Construct a two-piece custom built metal clutch to fit the mandibular cast, or use a stock clutch fitted to the cast.
3. Parallel to the sagittal plane, attach a stud or stem to the centre of the labial surface of the clutch. The hinge bow will later be attached to the stud.

4. Attach the clutch firmly to the teeth with zinc oxide-eugenol impression paste.

The clutch for the edentulous patient is prepared in the following way:
1. Make an accurate impression of the mandibular basal seat and pour an accurate stone cast.
2. On the cast, make an accurate record base of self-curing or processed acrylic resin.
3. Attach compound occlusion rims firmly to the record base and secure a specially designed bite fork to the rims with the stem extending forward parallel to the sagittal plane.
4. Attach this assembly to the mandible with chin clamps or chin straps.

Instruction to Patient in Hinge Type of Movement

The patient must now be instructed in the hinge type of movement. The patient must be coached to let his mouth drop open, thus causing the relaxation of external pterygoid muscles, some patients may have difficulty in comprehending this movement.

Use of Trainer. Dr Raymond Cohen has designed a "trainer" which is an improvement over the Hickot retruder. By means of this trainer, the patient learns the rhythmic opening and closing that is essential for the location of the axis. The trainer is left on the patient for five to 10 minutes and then removed. The patient seems to cooperate better after this training. This trainer can be used for the centric interocclusal records.

Determining the Hinge-axis

1. Locate the approximate axis point by palpation and mark the spot in the patient's face with a soft pencil.
2. Adjust the flag to the appropriate axis point and mark it with a soft pencil.
3. Seal the mandibular clutch and check the patient's ability to properly open and close.

4. Attach the modified axis bow so that the mounting tube of the stylus assembly is opposite the approximate axis mark. The upper and lower style should be placed forward and equally above and below a horizontal line of orientation.

5. Adjust the stylus so that they will leave marks in the proper areas of the flag.

6. Train the patient to close in centric relation and practice opening movements. A controlled smooth movement is desirable.

7. Engage the style by forcing with a ¼ turn in the positioning tube.

8. After recording arcs, the patient should hold steady at the terminus until the style can be retracted.

9. Retract the style and lock them with a counter rotation of 1/4 turn. Procedures on both sides of the patient should be performed simultaneously by the assistant and operator.

10. Remove the stylus from the tubes.

11. Remove the flags and complete the geometric solution.

12. Return the flag to its proper position but do not alter any adjustments.

13. Place a pointer stylus in the mounting tube and advance it until it touches the flag, and adjust the pointer to coincide with the axis point determined by intersection of the plotted radii.

14. Retract the stylus and carefully remove the flag.

15. Ink the tip of the stylus and advance it until it leaves a mark on the patient's face.

SCHOOLS OF THOUGHT REGARDING HORIZONTAL AXIS

The story of the horizontal axis, sometimes called the transverse, intercondylar or hinge-axis goes back to the time of Balkwill. McCollum generally conceded to have given us our modern technique for its location, tells that Bennett, Gysi, and other early investigators recognized that the mandible opened and closed on an axis. From these early experiments they have evolved four main schools of thought regarding horizontal axis. They are:

Absolute Location of the Axis

These people believe that there is a definite transverse axis and should be located as accurately as possible. According to them:

1. With the aid of the face-bow, it is possible to relate the maxillary cast to the transverse axis of the articulator in the same relationship as the maxillae are related to the anatomic mandibular axis through the condyles.

2. The mandibular hinge-axis is coincident with and related to the maxillary hinge-axis by means of a centric relation record.

3. The path of closure on the terminal hinge, will be the same on the articulator as in the mouth.

4. The cusps of the teeth can be placed so that they will not collide during this border mandibular movement.

5. The hinge-axis relationships of the articulators must be a duplicate of the hinge-axis relationships of the jaws, or mechanical reproduction of jaw motions on the articulator are impossible.

Arbitrary Location of the Axis

This group includes those who believe that an accurate location of the terminal hinge position would be of some value, but do not believe that it has enough value over an arbitrary location to be worth the added effort necessary to locate it.

Cradrick states, the search for the axis in addition to being troublesome, is of no more than academic interest, for it will never be found to lie more than a few millimeters distant from the assumed centre in the condyle itself.

Non-believers in the Transverse Axis Location

The third group believes it is impossible to locate the terminal hinge position with accuracy. This group believes that the transverse axis is theoretical, but not practical. Kurth and Fainstein using an articulator and working models to locate the hinge-axis, found any number of points with a range of 2 mm that could be considered a point of rotation. Borgh and Posset could not record the axis on a modified Hanau articulator without errors, which mounted to 1-1.5 mm at a 10-15° opening. Boucher commented, the test seemed to be one of the accuracy of the machine work on the instrument rather than one of the validity of a hinge-axis registration. On the other hand, Lawritzen and Woford's findings were within an area of 0.4 mm in diameter in more than 95% of the attempts using the same range of opening.

Berk has proposed that there can be many compensating movements of the condyle other than pure rotation, and these compensating movements are movements of translation and side shift that are integrated with the movement of rotation. He concluded that the opening and closing hinge movements of the mandible, together with its fragmentary movements cannot be repeated by the opening and closing movements of an articulator which is about one axis only. Therefore, an arbitrary terminal hinge position would be just as accurate as one located with a kinematic face-bow.

Trapozzano and Lazzari found that in 57.2% of the subjects more than one condylar axis point was located on either one or both sides of the face. They concluded that these findings indicate that, since multiple condylar hinge-axis points were located, the high degree of infallibility attributed to hinge-axis points may be seriously questioned.

Split axis Rotation of Non-colinear Concept

A major challenge to the traditional concept of a single "intercondylar" axis was hurled by Harry Page in his proposal of the transographic[6] concepts. He postulated the existence of two mutually independent, noncolinear axis, or simply that each condyle had its own axis of rotation. Page theorized that since the mandible is flexible, such independence from a mutual axis is mechanically possible and anatomically allowable.

Since most observers have verified Stuart and McCollum's original work regarding the asymmetry of axis points, then two axis pins asymmetrically placed, rotating at right angles to their respective contralateral axis, would serve as proof that these axes are parallel but nonintersecting, i.e. noncolinear.

Alavans stated by definition, an axis is always a line never a point. Again by definition, an axis is invariably perpendibular to the path or plane of rotation it controls. That means that the transverse axis of each joint is a line and both of these are perpendicular to the same plane of opening and closing rotation.

The significance of the fact that these two transverse axis, are never symmetrically positioned in the same head now becomes inescapable; being perpendicular to the same plane of rotation, they are parallel to each other even though asymmetrically positioned and, by definition, parallel lines never meet. Again the single, intercondylar axis is proved to be an impossibility.

HINGE INTEROCCLUSAL CLEARANCE (HIC)

Hinge interocclusal clearance is that portion of the functional interocclusal space generated by the rotatory component of movement of mandible arching around the mandibular hinge-axis.

All the functional movements of the human mandible are comprised of both rotatory and translative movement, and are extremely variable from one cycle to the next.

If properly developed, it decreases the horizontal vectors of arcing paths of the mandibular teeth because of pure hinge rotation of the mandible and increases the vertical clearance between the maxillary and mandibular teeth when not in occlusion. These modifications will result in uprighting the chewing cycle, avoiding deflective occlusal contact on posterior teeth or reduce the potential for developing it, and improving the efficiency of the opening and closing of the mouth, especially during the initial phase of opening and near the end of closing. In other words, the five factors of occlusion are compensating factors in facilitating hinge rotation of the mandible, which is the primary mechanical physiologic function of the mandible.

Variables Affecting Hinge-axis Location[7]

If a single terminal hinge-axis exists, then centric relation registrations can be made at an increased vertical dimension of occlusion on a patient. But consideration of the mechanics of hinge-axis location indicates that the investigators could not prove the existence of a single axis common to both the condyles. They have shown existence of multiple terminal hinge-axis and suggest that the concept of one terminal hinge axis is fallacious.

The skill to accurately record the terminal hinge-axis depends on variables of the patient, dentist and the recording apparatus.

Patient Variables Affecting the THA location

Condyle Asymmetry. Sufficient evidence has been gathered to dispel belief that the condyle follows solid body mechanical principles. It is capable of displacements in true dimensions, and such displacements cannot be empirically discounted even during operator manipulation. The condyle is not a sphere contained within a controlling channel. Condyles are asymmetric bodies confined only to certain limits of questionable exactness by muscles and ligaments. The condyles are asymmetrically positioned in their relationship to the cranium and to one another. The mandible functions as a unit in spite of these asymmetries, and the resultant movement may be or resemble an arc. The operator seeking an axis either can or cannot locate the arc centre of the clutch. There is no logical justification for feeling that one is locating any other point.

If the condyle is asymmetric, it may not be capable of simple rotation but will act as an arc with a moving centre of rotation. This may well be the phenomenon observed when the stylus tip moves up and down and no rotation centre can be found. If such a camming occurs, then either the mandible flexes to compensate the distortion or movement will occur in the frontal as well as the sagittal plane, i.e. there will be a lateral bodily shift. This is more likely in a rigid system when the transverse horizontal axis does not parallel the frontal plane.

Inability to Locate a True Hinge-axis. In any system of kinematic axis location, an essential prerequisite is the attachment of the clutch to the mandibular teeth. An anterior crossbar which holds the stylii is anchored to this clutch. These stylii can only locate the arc centre of the rigid components of the combined mechanism, i.e. the crossbar, the clutch, and those teeth firmly grasped by the clutch. What is occurring at the condyles and the adjacent soft or hard tissues may or may not be in concert with the observations of the anterior components. No conclusions can be drawn that could infer that such an arc could have more than one centre of rotation. If it is an arc, there is one arc centre. It is not a pure arc, then a moving centre exists and no 'true' hinge-axis can really be found.

Myoplasm or Joint Pathosis. In the presence of myoplasm or joint pathosis, the mandible will not be free.

Emotional Condition of the Patient. Trapozzano and Laxxari stated that the ease with which the hinge-axis registrations can be made depend on the emotional condition of the subject.

Occlusal Interferences. Occlusal interferences cause incoordination of masticatory muscles and muscle splinting. If such a muscle splinting exists, the bracing of the mandible or condyle was possible. When trying to locate axis close to the terminal hinge-axis position, the splinted muscles could produce a point where an arc should register. When dealing in tenths of millimeters, such distortions are probable unless preventive measures are taken.

FACTORS OF THE RECORDING APPARATUS AFFECTING TMA LOCATION

Right Angle-nonright Angle System of the Bow

All typical hinge-axis locating devices employ a right-angle system within the device itself. However, when that device is placed on the mandible with the clutch, then the right angled system may be lost in relation to the axis, since there is little probability of placing the anterior crossbar parallel to an axis which is not yet located. The only locator that does not consist of a series of right angles is that described by Gregory and associates and commercially available as the "Loma Linda hinge-axis locator".

But Page felt that anybody can only rotate at right angles to the axis. But this does not relate to hinge-axis location. The axis locator is not an axle, a determiner of motion–but it is a seeker of a centre of motion. It does not

matter if the points located are connected to the side arms by a right angle, any other angle, as long as the connection is rigid. Only the point of termination (the tip of the stylus) has validity, and it only has validity in relation to the overall apparatus and its movement.

Length of Stylus Arms and Sharpness of Stylii

Trapozzano and Lazarri may be attributed to the evasiveness of a single arc centre when the traditional axis location apparatus is used. During translation very little is actually seen of the stylus tip during its non arcing movement. They concluded that short stylus arms and bluntness of the stylus detract from accuracy, short stylus produces short arcs which are too small for accurate plotting.

Factors of Operator Affecting THA Location

Visual Acuity. The skill to accurately record the terminal hinge-axis is determined by the visual acuity to discern small distances. When a subject's mandible is opened and closed 10 mm at a distance of 100 mm from the terminal hinge-axis, it is relatively easy to see the movement, when the stylus approaches within 1 mm of the terminal hinge-axis, this same subject will scribe a 0.1 mm arc. Inside of 1 mm concentration, visual perception and skill are demanded of the dentist to approach the terminal hinge-axis.

Thus, we can see that so many factors are dependent on the success of determining the true hinge-axis which are very often overlooked by the operator. Therefore the validity of the hinge-axis location is highly questionable.

Further Reading

1. Jack. D, Preston. A reassessment of the mandibular transverse horizontal. Axis theory. Journal of Prosthetic Dentistry. June 1979, page; 41-46.

2. Beard and Clayton. Studies on the validity of the terminal hinge axis. Journal of Prosthetic Dentistry. Aug 1981; Vol; 46, pg: 185.

3. Robert.G, Schallhorn.A study of the arbitrary centre and kinematic centre of rotation for face-bow mountings. Journal of Prosthetic Dentistry Mar, 1957, pg: 162.

4. L.Abdul Hadi. Evaluation of current arbitrary hinge axis determination methods. Journal of Prosthetic Dentistry. October, 1989, Vol: 63; Pg: 463.

5. J.F. Bowley. Evaluation of variables associated with the transverse horizontal axis. Journal of Prosthetic Dentistry. 1992; Vol: 68; Pg: 537.

6. Mortimer.C. Davis. Compete dentures and transographics. Journal of Prosthetic Dentistry. February, 1960; Vol: 10, Pg.62.

7. Weinberg L A. The transvere hinge axis. J Prosth Dent. 1959; 9(5):775-87.

MULTIPLE CHOICE QUESTIONS

1. _____ point is located 13 mm anterior to the posterior margin of the centre of the tragus of the ear on a line extending to the corner of the eye.
   a. Bergstrom's
   b. Gysi
   c. Beyron
   d. Abdal-Hadi

2. **The Abdal-Hadi point is**
   a. Located 10-11mm in front of the ear on a line to the canthus.
   b. 1 cm in front of the line from the apex of tragus of ear to outer canthus of eye.
   c. Is based on the high correlation between width profile of the face and X-co-ordinate of the kinematic point.
   d. None of the above

3. **The following are used as anterior reference points except**
   a. Orbitale minus 23 mm
   b. Orbitale minus 7 mm
   c. Nasion minus 23 mm
   d. Orbitale only

4. **The Quick mount face bow is used with**
   a. Denar 5A aritculator
   b. Whip mix articulator
   c. Denar SE articulator
   d. Dentatus

5. **Of the following, the most accurate method for determining hinge axis is by using**
   a. Beyron's point
   b. Gysi point
   c. Pantograph
   d. Arbitrary method

6. **The hinge axis helps in recording the following except**
   a. Centric relation
   b. Vertical dimension
   c. Starting point of functional mandibular movement
   d. All of the above

7. **The facebow was first contrived by**
   a. Snow
   b. Walker
   c. Bonwill
   d. Balkwill

8. _____ is the most accurate of all present methods of estimating hinge axis
   a. Arbitrary
   b. Kinematic
   c. Beyron point
   d. Gysi point

9. **Instruments used to determine true hinge axis include all except**
   a. Behnergraph instrument
   b. Pantograph
   c. Facebow
   d. a and b

10. **Transographics is based upon**
    a. Arbitary hinge theory
    b. Split axis theory
    c. Transverse hinge axis theory
    d. None of the above

11. **The theory of transographics was postulated by**
    a. Gysi
    b. Bergstrom
    c. B. McCullum
    d. Snow

FAQ's

1. **Definition and importance of hinge axis**
2. **Arbitary and kinematic methods**

14

FACE-BOW

INTRODUCTION

The face-bow is an instrument used to record the spatial relationship of the maxillae to some anatomic reference and transfer this relationship to an articulator. Customarily this reference is a plane established by a transverse horizontal axis and a selected anterior point.

The face-bow[1] is a caliper-like device used to record the relationship of the jaws to the temporomandibular joints or the opening axis of the jaws and to orient the casts in this same relationship to the opening axis of the articulator (Fig. 14.1).

A face-bow is used to record the three-dimensional relation of the maxillae to the cranium. The face-bow record is used to orient the maxillary cast to the articulator. This procedure is called the face-bow transfer. Mandibular opening and closing movements are reproduced when the transverse horizontal axis is coincident with the articulator hinge-axis. In order to create precise occlusion, the casts should be oriented correctly which depends on an accurate face-bow transfer.

The study of hinge-axis opening of the mandible and the need to accurately locate it has occupied many distinguished workers over the years.

Locating the transverse hinge-axis was first discussed by Campion (1902), who felt that the axis of the articulator should coincide with that of the patients. Other important workers in this field were Bannet (1908, 1924), Needles (1923, 1927), and Wadsworth.

Stansberry (1928) was dubious about the value of face-bows and adjustable articulators. He though that since an opening movement about the hinge-axis took the teeth out of contact, the use of these instruments was ineffective except for the arrangement of the teeth in centric occlusion. In his opinion, the plain line hinge type of articulator was just as effective.

McLean regarding the satisfactory construction of full dentures, said that opening or closing the bite on an articulator with an incorrect hinge-axis location would result in unsatisfactory occlusion of the dentures when they were placed in the mouth. When the hinge-axis on the articulator was too far forward compared with its location on a patient, closing the interocclusal distance would result in the dentures meeting prematurely posteriorly. If the axis was too far

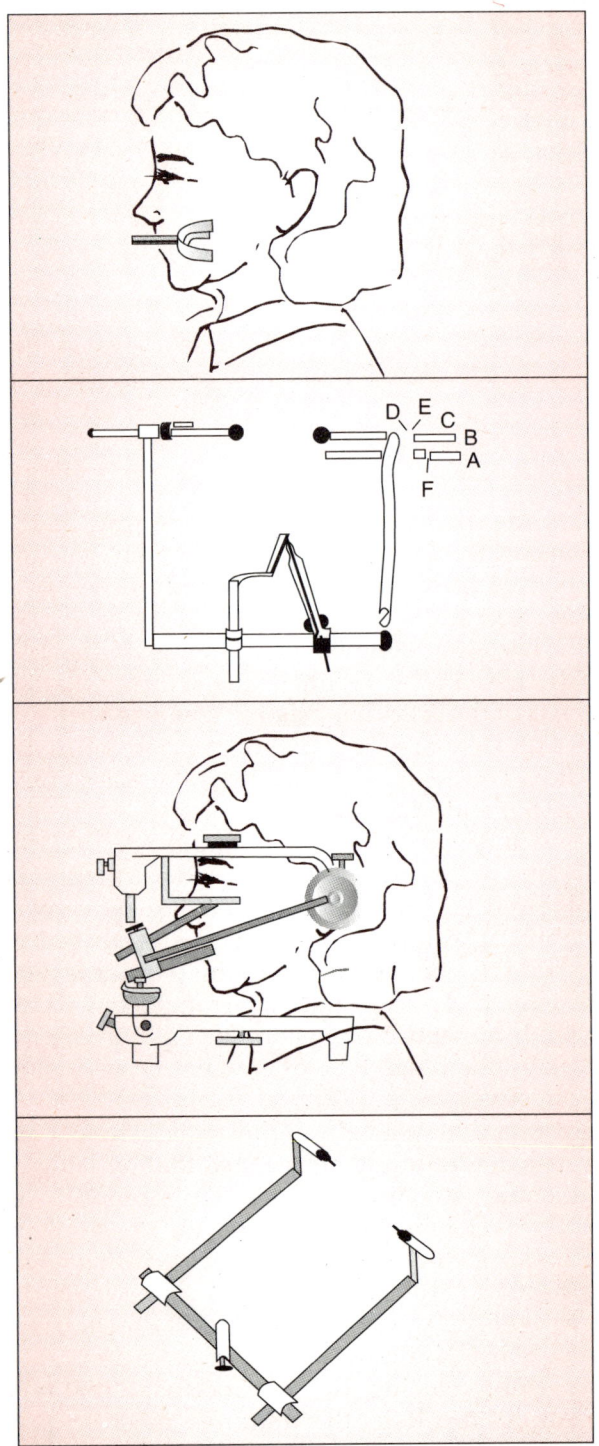

Fig. 14.1. Facebow and mounting.

posteriorly, premature contact would occur anteriorly. If the axis was too low, the lower denture would be forward of centric relation. If too high, the lower denture would be posterior to centric occlusion. The conclusion was that any alteration in the interocclusal distance must be made in the mouth or by the use of a hinge articulator. If the latter were to be used, then the hinge-axis must be determined as a stationary point (e.g., rotatory but not translatory) over the head of the condyle during hinge-axis movements and not by palpation or anatomical location.

McCollum (1939) was one of the leading advocates of the hinge-axis theory and published a very important series of articles concerning restorative remedies. He stated, "In 1921 I became convinced that the opening and closing centre of the mandible was the most important factor in dental articulation and that its determination was preliminary to transferring a record of jaw relations to an articulating instrument for a record of jaw relations.

In his articles he lauded Snow for his discovery of the face-bow and its use and at the same time he criticized Gysi on his views of the hinge-axis and for saying that changing vertical dimension is a chair side operation. McCollum also described how he came to demonstrate conclusively the existence of a definite opening and closing axis by using a face-bow rigidly attached to the lower teeth with an orthodontic appliance. He found wide variation in anatomic location of the points and between sides of the same individual. He said that the hinge-axis point remained constant throughout life.

Other important workers in this field were Highly (1940), Stuart (1947), Logan (1941), McLean (1944), and Branstad (1950).

Robert G Schallhorn (1947) studying the arbitrary centre and kinematic centre of the mandibular condyle for face-bow mountings concluded that using the arbitrary axis for face-bow mountings on a semiadjustable articulator is justified. He says that in over 95% of the subjects, the kinematic centre lies within a radius of 5 mm from the arbitrary centre.

Craddock and Symmons (1952) considered that the accurate determination of the hinge-axis was only of academic interest since it would never be found to be more than a few millimeters distant from the assumed centre in the condyle itself.

Posselt (1952) conducted extensive studies on the hinge-axis. He found that the extent of hinge opening between the upper and lower incisor teeth was 19.2 mm. Page (1952) described the "hinge bow" developed by McCollum in 1936 as one of the most important contributions made to dental science.

Lucia (1953) stated "the practical importance of the hinge and hinge-axis transfer to an articulator is of tremendous importance. " Without a hinge-axis transfer he thought it impossible to diagnose an occlusal problem.

Brandrup-Wognesen (1953) discussed the theory and history of face-bows. He quoted the work of Beyron who had demonstrated that the axis of movement of the mandible did not always pass through the centers of the condyle. They concluded that complicated forms of registration were rarely necessary for practical work.

Teteruck and Lundeen (1966) evaluated the accuracy of the ear face-bow and concluded that only 33% of the conventional axis locations were within 6 mm of true hinge-axis as compared to 56.4% located by ear face-bow. They also recommended the use of ear-bow for its accuracy, speed of handling, and simplicity of orienting the maxillary cast.

Thorp, Smith, and Nicholis (1978) evaluated the use of face-bow in complete denture occlusion. Their study revealed very small differences between a hinge-axis face-bow, Hanau 132-SM face-bow, and shipmix ear-bow.

Neol D Wilkie 1979 analyzed and discussed five commonly used anterior points of reference for a face-bow transfer.

He said that not utilizing a third point of reference may result in additional and unnecessary record making, an unnatural appearance in the final prosthesis and even damage to the supporting tissues. He suggests the use of the axis-orbitale plane because of the ease of marking and locating orbitale, and therefore the concept is easy to teach and understand.

Bailey JOJR and Nowlin TP in 1981 in their study concluded that face-bow transfer utilizing orbitale as the third point of reference does not accurately establish the relationship of the Frankfurt horizontal to the occlusal plane on the articulator.

Elwood H Staele et al 1982 evaluated esthetic considerations in the use of face-bow.

Goska and Christensen (1988) investigated cast positions using different face-bows. They concluded that it was not possible to establish clinical superiority between one type of face-bow and another because the casts are mounted in relation to anatomic landmarks that vary from subject to subject.

Brian D Monteith (1985-86) in a series of articles projected a cephalometric method to determine the angulation of the occlusal plane in dentulous patients. He prompted a hypo-thesis that the anterior cranial base acts as a template that govern the anteroposterior dimension of the nasomaxillary complex in which he studied the relationship between PONANS angle and orientation of occlusal plane. He found that an increase in PONANS angle had a flattening effect on orientation of occlusal plane, while a narrowing of the angle makes the occlusal plane steeper. He concluded that the value may be used to program an occlusal plane projector on the articulator and permit denture teeth to be setup directly against the plane in accordance with the orientation indicated. Accordingly Teledyne Hanau introduced a plane that can be attached to the lower member while mounting the upper cast, named as Hanau x P-117 Monteith adjustable plane.

HISTORICAL REVIEW

A short history of the face-bow and the period prior to its development will afford us a picture of the ideas that led to its development and the significance of its use.

About ninety years ago it began to be realized that in full denture prosthesis, it was important to mount the plaster casts in the articulator in a given positional relation to the condylar mechanism.

According to Bonwill, the distance from the centre of each condyle to the median incisal point of the lower teeth is 10 cm. He used this standard for mounting his casts in the articulator. Bonwill did not mention however, at what level below the condylar mechanisms the occlusal plane should be used. It appears that he mounted his casts with the occlusal plane in a horizontal position about midway between the upper and lower part of the articulator. It is evident that he considered this quite satisfactory.

Balkwill, an English dentist, devised methods that were an improvement on Bonwill's. Though these investigators were contemporaries, it is probable that they never heard of one another. Balkwill demonstrated an apparatus with which he could measure the angle formed by the occlusal plane of the teeth, and a plane passing through the lines extending from the condyles to the incisal line of the lower teeth. According to his investigations, this angle varied from 22 degrees to 30 degrees. He could also determine approximately the distance from each condyle to "the front of the gums". These were the measurements that he subsequently used for mounting his plaster casts in an apparatus that probably corresponded to an articulator.

It appears that the position of Balkwill's casts was much more correct than that which was obtained by Bonwill's method. Balkwill's theories were forgotten however, and it was only at the beginning of this century that they were rediscovered.

Another apparatus for localizing the plaster casts in the articulator was constructed by Hayes in the 1880's. This apparatus was known as the "caliper".

Caliper did not, however, represent any particular progress in the solution of these problems. Only the median incisal point was localized in relation to its distance from the two condyles. There was no control of the proper orientation of the occlusal plane.

Walker invented the "clinometer", a new type of instrument with which it would have been possible to obtain a relatively good value for the position of the lower cast in relation to the condylar mechanism, better than with all the previous apparatus, but it was an exceedingly complicated apparatus. Walker only used his instrument, however, for measuring the inclination of the condyle path; and he appears not to have utilized the possibilities of the instrument as a face-bow. He mounted his casts in the articulator in accordance with Bonwill's method.

A little later, at about the turn of the century Gysi constructed an instrument for registering the condylar path. Gysi, however, also employed his apparatus as a face-bow.

At approximately the same time as Gysi introduced his apparatus, Snow constructed an instrument which has become the prototype for all the later constructors of face-bows. Snow's face-bow, in spite of its very simple construction, was epoch making in prosthetic dentistry. Since then no fundamental changes have been made in the face-bow.

CLASSIFICATION

Face-bows may be grouped as:

1. Arbitrary face-bows
   a. Facia type
   b. Earpiece type
2. Kinematic face-bows/hinge-axis/adjustable axis face-bows.

Arbitrary Face-bows[2]

Arbitrary face-bows use arbitrary or approximate points on the face as the posterior reference points. The condylar rods are positioned on these predetermined points during the face-bow transfer procedure. Arbitrary face-bows are probably the most widely used type of face-bow and are sufficient for fabrication of most complete denture, Fixed partial, and removable partial denture prostheses. Many studies have shown that a small error in location will have only a negligible effect at the occlusal level. Furthermore, the resiliency and life effect (realeff) of the oral tissues make the exact transfer and location of the hinge-axis unnecessary.

Fascia Type. The fascia type of face-bow utilize approximate points on the skin over the temporomandibular region as the posterior reference points. These points are located by measuring from certain anatomical landmarks on the face. Various landmarks and measurements have been used for this purpose.

Earpiece Type.[3] The earpiece type of face-bow was first described by Dalbey. However, it was only during the 1960's that it gained in popularity. This type of face-bow uses the external auditory meatus as the arbitrary posterior reference point. For this a special earpiece is required instead of a condyle rod. The external auditory meatus is assumed to have a fixed relationship to the hinge-axis. Special condylar compensators on the face-bow or the articulator then compensates for this by positioning the condylar inserts at a prescribed distance behind the rotational axis of the articulator. Teteruck and Lundeen demonstrated the ear-bow to have more accuracy than the method using an arbitrary mark on the ala-tragus line. The ear-bow has gained in popularity because:

- It is simple to use
- Does not require measurements or marks on the face

- As accurate, if not more than arbitrary methods.

Kinematic Face-bow

The kinematic face-bow is used to determine and locate the exact hinge-axis points. The same face-bow is later used like the arbitrary face-bow to transfer these points on to the articulator. The kinematic face-bow is a more complex instrument requiring the fabrication of clutches which have to be attached to the lower jaws. It requires more chair side time and is rarely indicated for routine articulators with prosthodontic procedures. It also requires the use of articulators with condylar shafts which must be extended to meet the stylus of the face-bow. If the stylus is extended the true hinge-axis will be lost.

THE PLANE OF ORIENTATION

The maxillary cast in the articulator is the baseline from which all occlusal relationships start and it should be positioned in space by identifying three points which cannot be on the same line. The plane is formed by two points located posterior to the maxillae and one point located anterior to it. The posterior points are referred to as the posterior points of reference and the anterior one is known as the anterior point of reference.

Posterior Points of Reference

The position of the terminal hinge-axis on either side of the face is generally taken as the posterior reference points.

The hinge-axis is an imaginary line around which the condyles can rotate without translation.

Terminal hinge position is the most retruded hinge position. The limits of opening at this position has been determined to be around 12 to 15 degrees or 19 to 20 mm at incisal edges.

Location of the Posterior Reference Points

Prior to aligning the face-bow on the face, the posterior reference points must be located and marked. The posterior points are located by:

Arbitrary Method. Often the posterior points are located by measuring prescribed distances from skin surface landmarks. Some of the commonly used posterior points were shown by Beck to be clinically near the hinge-axis. He concluded that the Bergstrom point most frequently is closest to the hinge-axis. He identified the Beyron point as the next most accurate posterior point of reference. Studies by Weinberg show that a deviation from the hinge-axis of 5 mm will result in an antero-posterior displacement error of 0.2 mm at the second molar. An error of this size is usually of no consequence in removable prostheses with non-rigid attachments. With these prostheses, intended tolerances in the occlusion and the mobility of the supporting tissues may make a precise location of the hinge-axis an exercise with no advantage.

The following are some of the most commonly used methods

Method of Palpation. An alternative method of locating the hinge-axis arbitrarily is by a method of palpation
- From behind the patient, place the index fingertip over the joint area and ask the patient to open wide.
- As the condyle translates forward, the fingertip will drop into a depression where the condyle was
- The patient would then close. As the condyle translates back into centric relation position, its position can be located by the fingertip.
- By asking the patient to open and close, it will be possible to locate the axis within an average accuracy of 2 mm or less. The axis generally occurs near the centre of the depression felt by the fingertip.
- After locating the point it should be marked.

Kinematic Method. The most accurate method for recording the correct horizontal axis was developed by McCollum in 1921 using a kinematic device.

The technique for locating the terminal hinge-axis position is essentially the same for the dentulous and the edentulous patient, but the methods of attaching the clutch to the mandible are quite different.

Clutch Fabrication for Dentulous Patient

Several methods have been described for construction of clutches:
- Stock metal clutches which are attached to the teeth using quick setting stone or impression plaster.
- Two-piece custom-built metal clutch attached to the teeth using zinc oxide-eugenol impression paste
- Special clutches made with cold curing resin with the help of clutch forming molds (clutch formers)

Clutch Fabrication for the Edentulous Patient[4]

Firmly attaching a clutch to edentulous mandible presents a problem. Compound occlusion rims are firmly attached to an accurate record base of self-curing resin or processed acrylic resin. Specially designed bite fork is secured to the rims, with the stem extending forward parallel to the sagittal plane. Attach this assembly to the mandible with chin clamps or chin straps.

Once the clutches have been fabricated, the following sequence is followed:
- Place the patient in a semisupine position with the headrest tilted slightly backward.
- Connect the clutch to the face-bow.
- A graph or grid paper is placed adjacent to the skin over the TMJ region to help detect stylus movements (grid paper is held with the help of a headgear or another face-bow and clutch unit fixed to the maxillary arch).
- Guide the mandible to centric position and

assist the patient in making hinge openings and closing to a maximum of 1+ finger width or 10 to 13°.

- Check the movement of the stylus. The initial movement may be arc shaped.
- Adjust the stylus tip toward the centre of the arch until the tip rotates instead of arcing
- Remove the grid paper and record the point on the skin with the help of a dye.

Precaution. Care must be taken to record only the retruded hinge-axis. The mandible is capable of hinge-like motion at any point along the protrusive pathway.

When transferring the hinge-axis onto the articulator, the condylar shaft must be extended to meet the styli of the face-bow (in the Hanau series of articulators the extensible condylar shaft is indicated by a suffix X, e.g. Hanau H2-X). If the stylus tip of the face-bow is extended to meet the articulator's condylar axis, it will result in an erroneous hinge-axis transfer.

Anterior Point of Reference

Though snow determined the position of the plaster cast in the articulator, not only with regard to the distance of the median incisal point from the condyles but also all the other points on the occlusion plane, the whole problem was not solved. It was important to ascertain at what level in the articulator the occlusal plane should be placed. The selection of the anterior point of the triangular spatial plane determines which plane in the head will become the plane of reference when the prosthesis is being fabricated. The dentist can ignore but cannot avoid the selection of an anterior point. The act of affixing a maxillary cast to an articulator relates the cast to the articulator's hinge-axis, to the vertical axes, to the condylar determination to the anterior guidance, and to the mean plane of the articulator. The act achieves greater importance by the use of a constant third point of reference.

Reasons for Selecting an Anterior Point of Reference[5]

1. When three points are used the position can be repeated, so that different maxillary casts of the same patient can be positioned in the articulator in the same relative position to the end controlling guidances. With complicated and time-consuming recording techniques such as pantographic tracing, the dentist does not have the time, nor the means to repeat records each time. The technique calls for a new maxillary cast. For this reason it is important to identify the mark permanently or be able to repetitively measure an anterior point of reference as well as the posterior points of reference.

2. A planned choice of an anterior reference point will allow the dentist and the auxillary to visualize the anterior teeth and the occlusion in the articulator in same frame of reference that would be used when looking at the patient. For example, when using the Frankfort horizontal plane as the plane of reference, the teeth will be viewed as though the patient were standing in a normal postural position with the eyes looking straight ahead.

3. An occlusal plane not parallel to the horizontal in the beginning steps of denture fabrication may be unknowingly located incorrectly because of a tendency for the eye to subconsciously make planes and lines parallel. Therefore the dentist may wish to initially establish the restored occlusal plane parallel to the horizontal in order to better control the occlusal plane in its final position. The objective is to achieve a natural appearance in the occlusal plane. Mounting the cast relative to Camper's line best meets this objective.

4. The dentist may wish to establish a baseline for comparison between patients, or for the same patient at different periods of time. This is possible only through the use of a

three-point mounting that is constant from one patient to another or for the same patient.

Selection of an Anterior Reference Point

The various anterior reference points that may be used are as follows:

1. Orbitale. In the skull, orbitale is the lowest point on the infraorbital rim. On a patient it can be palpated through the overlying tissue and the skin. One orbitale and the two posterior points that determine the horizontal axis of rotation will define the axis-orbitale plane. The orbitale is transferred from the patient to the articulator with the help of an orbital pointer on the face-bow or by raising the face-bow itself to the level of the orbitale (Fig. 14.2).

Advantage

- It is easy to locate and mark the orbitale.
- The concept is easy to teach and understand.

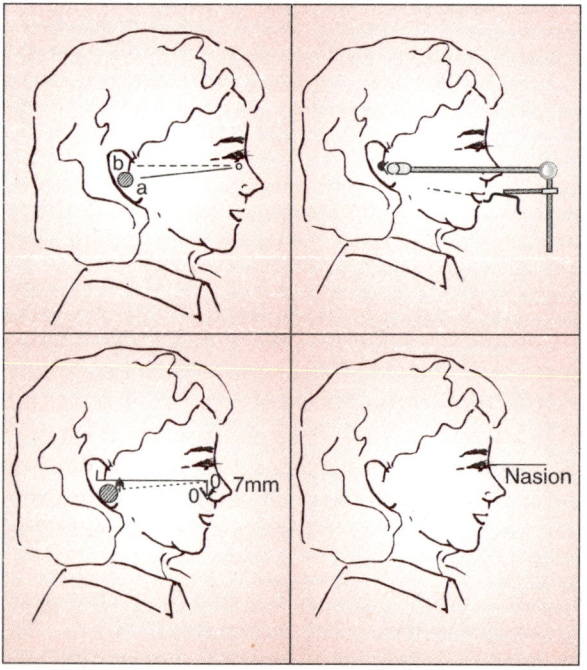

Fig. 14.2. Various anterior reference points.

Disadvantage

Relating the maxillae to the axis-orbitale plane will slightly lower the maxillary cast anteriorly from the position that would be established if the Frankfort horizontal plane were used.

2. Orbitale Minus 7 mm. The Frankfurt horizontal plane passes through both poria and one orbitale point. Because porion is a skull landmark, Sicher recommends using the midpoint of the upper border of the external auditory meatus as the posterior cranial landmark on a patient. Most articulators do not have a reference point for this landmark. Gonsalez pointed out that this posterior tissue landmark on the average lies 7 mm superior to the horizontal axis. The recommended compensation for this discrepancy is to mark the anterior point of reference 7 mm below orbitale on the patient, or to position the orbital pointer 7 mm above the orbital indicator of the articulator. Bergstrom's arcon articulator automatically compensates for this error by placing the orbital index 7 mm higher than the condylar horizontal axis. In either technique, the Frankfort horizontal plane of the patient becomes the horizontal plane in the articulator.

3. Nasion Minus 23 mm. According to Sicher, another skull landmark, the nasion, can be approximately located in the head as the deepest part of the midline depression just below the level of the eyebrows. The nasion guide, or positioner, of the quick mount face-bow, which is designed to be used with the Whip-Mix articulator, fits into this depression. This guide can be moved in and out, but not up and down, from its attachment to the face-bow crossbar. The crossbar is located 23 mm below the midpoint of the nasion positioner. When the nasion guide of face-bow is positioned anteriorly on the nasion, the crossbar will be in the approximate region of orbitale. The face-bow cross-bar and not the nasion guide is the actual anterior reference point locator. During the face-bow transfer, the crossbar of the face-bow supports the upper frame of the Whip-Mix articulator. The inferior surface of the frame is in the same plane as the articulator's hinge points. From this it can be concluded that the quick mount face-bow used with the Whip-Mix articulator employs an approximate axis-orbitale plane (Fig. 14.3).

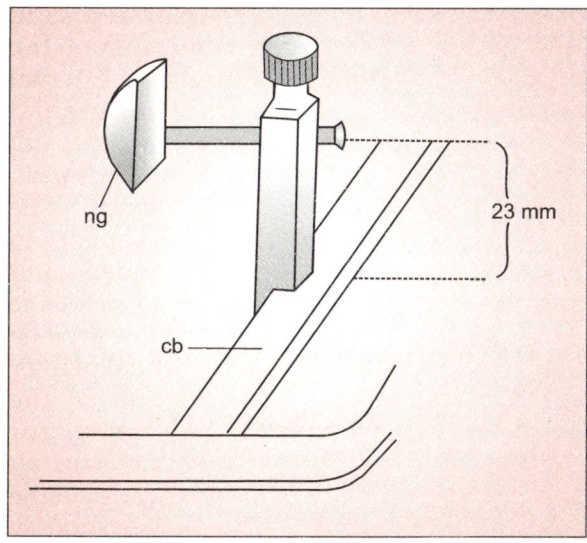

Fig. 14.3.

Incisal Edge Plus Articulator Midpoint to Articulator Axis-horizontal Plane Distance

Guichet has emphasized that a logical position for the casts in the articulator would be one which would position the plane of occlusion near the mid-horizontal plane of the articulator.

In accordance with this concept, the distance from the articulator's mid-horizontal plane to the articulator's axis-horizontal plane is measured. This same distance is measured above the existing or planned incisal edges on the patient, and its uppermost point is marked as the anterior point of reference on the face. This point can be recorded for future use by measuring vertically downward to it from the inner canthus of the eye and recording this measurement. The inner canthus is used because it is an accessible, unchanging landmark on the head.

With this technique, the face-bow transfer will carry the two predetermined posterior points of reference and this anterior point of reference to the articulators's mid-horizontal plane unless a subsequent decision raises or lowers them.

Alae of the Nose

A part of many complete denture techniques is to make the tentative or the actual occlusal plane parallel with the horizontal plane. This can be achieved in two ways: (i) a line from the ala of the nose to the centre of the auditory meatus describes the Camper's line—the dentist can transfer Camper's line from the patient to the articulator by marking the right or left ala on the patient, setting the anterior reference pointer of the face-bow to it, and with the face-bow, transferring the ala anteriorly, and the hinge points posteriorly from the patient to the articulator's hinge-orbital indicator plane, and (ii) a second method of establishing this relationship is to make a wax occlusion rim parallel to Camper's line on the face. This ensures that the tentative occlusal plane will not be too high or low.

Further Reading

1. Lawrence A. Weinberg. An evaluation of a face-bow mounting. J Prosth Dent. 1961; 11: 32-40.
2. Thorp et al. Evaluation of the use of face-bow in complete denture occlusion. J Prosth Dent. 1978; 39: 5.
3. Joyce Palik et al. Accuracy of an earpiece face-bow. J Prosth Dent.1985; 53(6):
4. Zuckerman G R. Practical considerations for using the face bow. J Prosth Dent.
5. Christensen R L. Rationale of the face-bow in maxillary cast mounting. J Prosth Dent. 1959; 9(3): 388-98.

MULTIPLE CHOICE QUESTIONS

1. **Extracted teeth can used for selection of all except.**
   a. Shade
   b. Form
   c. Size
   d. None of the above

2. **The truebyte tooth indicator can be used for determining**
   a. Length of upper central incisors
   b. Width of upper central incisors
   c. Length of lower central incisors
   d. a and b

3. **Among the Anthropometric measurements, the following are correct**
   a. The bizygomatic width divided by 3.3 gives width of the upper central incisor.
   b. The bizygomatic width divided by 3.3 gives the width of all upper anterior teeth.
   c. Both are true

4. **The typal form theory was introduced by**
   a. Frush and Fisher
   b. Leon williams
   c. Wright
   d. McCollum

5. _____ **is the amount of color per unit area of an object**
   a. Saturation
   b. Hue
   c. Value
   d. Translucency

6. **The squint test is used for determining**
   a. Form of the teeth
   b. Shade of teeth
   c. Size of the teeth
   d. Shape of teeth

7. **The first anatomic type posterior teeth was introduced by**
   a. Alfred Gysi
   b. Truebyte
   c. Victor Sears
   d. French

8. **The true statement regarding channel type posteriors is**
   a. The maxillary occlusal surface consisted of a central ridge that ran mesiodistally.
   b. The maxillary occlusal surface consisted of a deep channel that ran mesio-distally.
   c. It was introduced by Victor Sears.
   d. b and c are true.

9. **Scissor bite teeth were developed by**
   a. Mcgrane
   b. Victor Sears
   c. Avery brothers
   d. French

10. **Of the following, the non anatomic tooth is**
    a. French's mandibular pusteriors
    b. Avery brother's scissors bite teeth
    c. Hall's inverted cusp tooth
    d. Gysi's 33° posteriors.

11. **Advantages of nonanatomic teeth include all except**
    a. Better masticatory efficiency.
    b. Allow for greater range of movement.
    c. Lesser force will be directed to the denture bearing area.
    d. All are advantages.

12. **Wright's photometric method is based on**
    a. The observation that tooth length was in proportion to face length.
    b. Establishing a ratio by comparative computation of measurements of like areas of the face and photographs of a patient with natural teeth.
    c. Relating the interalar width to the space available for setting the upper anterior teeth.
    d. None of the above.

13. **A face bow is a device used to**
    a. Record the three dimensional relation of mandible to maxilla.
    b. Record the three dimensional relation of maxilla to the cranium
    c. Record the three dimensional relation of mandible to the cranium
    d. None of the above.

14. **The clinometer was introduced by**
    a. Walker   b. Hayes
    c. Snow   d. Balkwill

15. **The earpiece type of face-bow**
    a. Is a arbitrary type of face-bow
    b. Uses the external auditory meatus as the arbitrary reference point.
    c. Does not require measurements on the face
    d. All are true.

FAQ's

1. **Definition of face-bow**
2. **Types of face-bow**
3. **Posterior reference points**

15

TOOTH SELECTION

Introduction
Anterior teeth selection
Selection of posterior teeth
Methods used to select artificial tooth form

INTRODUCTION

The selection of teeth requires the consideration of biomechanical, psychological or esthetic factors.

Biomechanical Factors

There are certain mechanical limitations in the placement of anterior teeth that must be taken into account. The anteriors should generally be placed as closely in relation to the residual ridge as natural teeth. According to Fish the proper position of the teeth is the point where tongue and cheek pressures balance.

Psychological Factors

In esthetics, the patient's self-image is also important. For a patient, perception of his or her appearance may result in a broad smile or a tight-lipped, small, controlled smile (negative self-evaluation).

The Camper's line is thought of as a psychological plane of orientation. In the case of a vain person or a person who appears happy, the plane tends to rise; in a person who is depressed or discouraged it may slant downward.

ANTERIOR TEETH SELECTION

Anterior teeth selection is an important step in the fabrication of complete dentures. This can be verified only by the dentist utilizing the trial base and confirmed by the patient and family or friends.

If the patient has an old denture, the dentist should note it.

Pre-extraction Guides

Preextraction guides include photographs, diagnostic casts, radiographs, the teeth of close relatives and extracted teeth.

Photographs

- Provides general information about the width of teeth and possibly their outline form that is more accurate than information from any other source.

  An algebraic proportion can be established from the photograph. The known factors are interpupillary distance of the patient, the interpupillary distance on the photograph and the width or length of the central incisor on the photograph. The unknown factor is the precise width or length of natural central incisor.

Diagnostic Casts

Diagnostic casts of natural teeth are also reliable guides in both relating and arranging anterior teeth. The size and form of the anterior teeth can be determined on the diagnostic cast and comparable artificial teeth selected.

Intraoral Radiographs

These give information about the size and form of the teeth to be replaced. They may be slightly enlarged and can be distorted.

Son's or Daughter's Tooth Size

A sons or daughter's tooth size, color and arrangement can be used effectively in selecting and arranging artificial teeth for their parents.

Extracted Teeth

Some patients keep extracted anterior teeth which will provide excellent information as to the size and form of the artificial teeth, but cannot be used in selecting color.

Size of Anterior Teeth

- The size of the teeth should be in proportion to the size of the face and head. Generally larger people have large teeth. Variations are however possible.
- Women's teeth are often smaller than men's. This is true of the lateral incisors, which are more delicate in women than men.
- Seven anatomic entities are used as guides for the selection of anterior teeth for size.

Size of the Face

The average width of the maxillary central incisor is estimated to be one-sixteenth of the width of the face measured between the zygoma. The maxillary lateral incisors generally vary more in size, form and position than any other maxillary anterior tooth.

The *Trubyte tooth indicator* is useful in determining the size of the maxillary central incisors.

The combined width of the six maxillary anterior's is slightly less than one-third of the bizygomatic breadth of the face. The face-bow can be used as a caliper to record the bizygomatic breadth of the face.

Procedure. The indicator is placed on the patient's face allowing the nose to come through the central triangle. The pupils are centered in the eye slots and the center line of the indicator is held so that it contacts with the median line. The side indicator bar is slid in until it touches the face and the width of the upper central incisors is read in millimeter's. The bottom indicator bar is slid in until it reaches a position immediately beneath the chin with the lips at rest. The length of the upper central incisors is read in mm. The reading of the length of the central incisors will be accurate when the lips are at rest (Fig. 15.1).

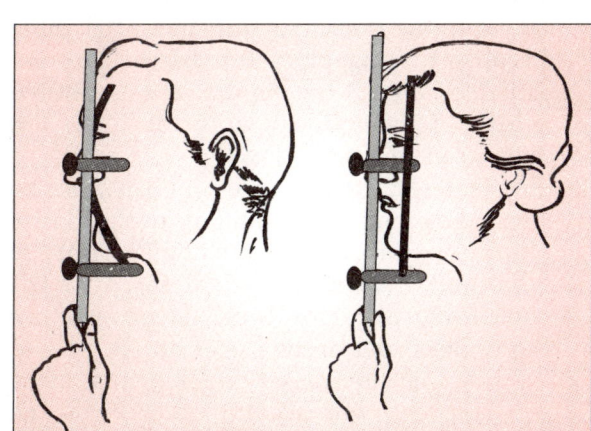

Fig. 15.1. Determining the facial outline with the Trubyte tooth indicator (profile view).

Size of the Maxillary Arch

The mold selector can be used to make measurements of the maxillary cast. For this accurately contoured occlusal rims are required. Measurements are made from the crest of the incisal papilla to the hamular notches, and from one hamular notch to another hamular notch. The combined length of the three legs of the triangle in mm is used on the selector.

The circular slide rule indicates the tooth sizes, anterior and posterior for both arches.

When discrepancies exist between face size and related arch size, the selection of anterior teeth should be governed more by face than by arch size, because of resorption.

Incisal Papilla and the Cuspid Eminence or the Buccal Frenum

There are two methods.
1. If the cuspid eminences are discernible, a line can be placed on the cast at the distal termination of the eminence. If they are not discernible, then attachments of the buccal frenum can be used.

   The distance from the distal of one eminence to the distal of the other is measured with a flexible ruler. It should follow the contour of the ridge and as it reaches the midline, it should be placed on the anterior border of the incisal papilla, because the maxillary central incisors are situated labial to the papilla. The combined width of 6 maxillary anterior teeth are measured in mm.

2. The distal of the cuspid eminencies can be located by using the maxillary occlusal rim. When the teeth are in occlusion and lips are together, the labial incisal third of the maxillary anterior teeth supports the superior border of the lower lip.

   In speech the incisal edges of maxillary anterior teeth contact the lower lip at the junction of the moist and dry surfaces of the vermillion border. This is best demonstrated when the letter "F" is pronounced.

An estimation of the position of the apex of the upper natural canine can be found by extension of parallel lines from the lateral surfaces of the ala of the nose onto the labial surfaces of the upper occlusion rim.

Anthropometric Measurements

Anthropometric measurements can help in selection of artificial teeth.

The greatest bizygomatic width divided by 16 gives an approximate width of upper central incisor, and that divided by 3.3 provides estimation of width of upper 6 anterior teeth. A face-bow is used to determine bizygomatic width.

Cranial Circumference to Width Ratio

The ratio of cranial circumference to the width of the upper anterior teeth is 10:1. As a general guide, upper anterior teeth whose overall width is less than 48 mm are relatively small and those listed over 53 mm are large.

Square, Tapering, Ovoid

The theory of matching teeth to face forms which are generally square, tapering or ovoid characteristics was advanced by J. Leon Williams.

Sketch of Anterior Teeth

The 6 anterior's are sketched out on the wax occlusion rim.

Tooth Width

Pound evaluated tooth width by measuring the distance from zygoma to zygoma, one to one and one-half inches back of the lateral corner of the eyes.

Tooth length is a measure of the distance from the hairline to the lower edge of the bone of the chin with the face at rest. These measurements are divided by 16 and indicate the length and width of the central incisor.

Dentogenics

Fisher has stated that the patient should be analysed first to sex—male or female, personality-vigorous or delicate, and then to age-young or old.

In general rounded, curved contours and delicate appearance indicate femininity. Prominent wider centrals, with incisal abrasion and worn cuspid tips indicate a personality of strength and vigor.

Form of Anterior Teeth

Three factors are used as guides for the selection of anterior teeth for form.

The Form and Contour of the Face[4]

The form of artificial anterior teeth should harmonize with the shape of the patient's face. The outline is viewed from a front view of the patient and from the labial of upper central incisor.

Shortly after the turn of the century dentistry found ranks in the mechanical march by adopting the theory of square, tapering and ovoid tooth forms, as a basis for denture esthetics. Countless measurements, charts, graphs and statistics firmly compressed all of humanity into this mechanical mold. So the mechanical theory of Williams replaced the temperamental theory.

Leon Williams claimed that the shape of the upper central incisor has a definite relationship to the face.

Thus if one of these teeth are enlarged, and the incisal edge placed above the eyebrow with neck of the teeth on the chin, the outline form will coincide with that of the face.

He classified the form of the human face into three types: square, tapering and ovoid, each type merging with the other without any clear line of demarcation. These are further subdivided on the basis of a combination of the characteristics of the three classes (Fig. 15.2).

In order to determine what type an individual belongs to, the operator imagines two lines, one on either side of the face, running about 2.5 cm in front of the tragus of the ear and through the angle of the jaw.

If these lines are almost parallel the type is square, if they converge towards the chin, it is tapering, and if it is diverging it is ovoid.

Leon Williams classification[4] is too limiting for sex interpretation in dentogenics.

The labial surface of the tooth viewed from the mesial should show a contour similar to that when viewed in profile. The three types of profiles are convex, straight and concave. The labial surface of the teeth should show a flatness similar to that seen when the face is viewed from under the chin or from top of the head.

Determination of Face Form. Tooth indicator is placed on the patient's face allowing the nose to come through the central triangle.

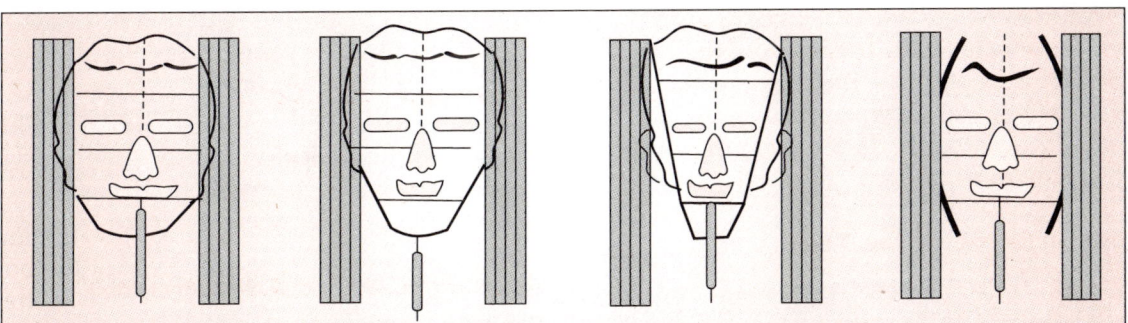

Fig. 15.2. Determining the facial outline with the Trubyte tooth indicator (frontal view).

Pupils of the eye are centered in the eye slots, and the indicator is held with its center line coinciding with the median line of the face. The form of the face is observed as it appears in comparison with the vertical lines of the indicator. In the square form, the sides of the face will approximately follow the vertical lines of the indicator.

In square tapering form, the upper third of the lower two-thirds will taper inward. In tapering faces, sides of the face from the forehead to the angle of the jaw will taper at an inward diagonal.

Determination of Facial Profile. Three points are checked, i.e. the forehead, the base of the nose and the point of the chin. If these points are in line, the profile is straight. If the points of the forehead and of the chin are recessive, the profile is curved.

Form refers to the outline of anything and shape is the quality of a thing that depends, on the relative position of all points composing its outline, e.g. facets, developmental grooves, and convexities.

Sex of the Patient

Curved facial features are associated with femininity, and square features are associated with masculinity.

Teeth of females are more ovoid or tapering than square.

Age

As features change with the ageing process, so does the form of teeth. The lips lose their curves and cupid's bow and the teeth wear at the incisal edges and interproximal surfaces. The labial surfaces seem flatter and outline form appears square.

Color or Shade of the Teeth

Color. It is the sensation resulting from stimulation of the retina of the eye by light waves of certain lengths.

Shade. It is the degree of darkness of a color with reference to its mixture with black. In a tooth yellow and gray are the two principal colors that are evident. The yellow is more prominent in the gingival third and gray is more prominent in incisal third.

Color has three qualities, all of which are involved in the selection of teeth. Hue is the specific color produced by the specific wavelength of light acting on the retina. It is the color itself, bluish green, yellow.

The hue of the teeth must be in harmony with the color of the patient's face.

Saturation (chroma) is the amount of color per unit area of an object, e.g. some teeth appear more yellow than others.

Brilliance (value). The lightness or darkness of an object. Variations in brilliance are produced by dilution of the color by white or black.

When yellow teeth are diluted with white, result is a light tooth. But if it is diluted with black, the result is a dark tooth.

Translucency. It is the property of an object that permits the passage of light through it, but does not give any distinguishable image.

The light rays are so broken up and diffuse that they cannot pass directly through the object as they would if the objects were transparent. Translucency has the effect of mixing the various colors of the tooth with the changing colors in the oral cavity.

Skin pigmentation has been classified from shallow to ruddy to olive and swarthy. In hair, there are black, brown square and blonde. In eyes, there are blue, gray, brown and black.

Age and Tooth Color. In some people the color of natural teeth darkens with age. This is because of the deposition of secondary dentin, or because of the wear of teeth. Extracted teeth can only be used to select the form of teeth.

Selecting Color of Artificial Teeth

Position of the patient- The patient should be in an upright position. The dentist should be in a position so that the teeth are viewed in a plane perpendicular to his plane of vision. The teeth should be viewed from different angles so that shadows do not influence the color. The patient's mouth should not be opened too wide.

Observation of the shade-guide teeth should be made in three positions: (i) outside the mouth along the side of nose, (ii) under the lips with only the incisal edge exposed, and (iii) under the lips with only the cervical end covered and the mouth open.

The first step will establish the basic hue, brilliance and saturation, the second will reveal the effect of the color of the teeth when patient's mouth is relaxed, and the third will simulate exposure of the teeth as in a smile.

The color selected should be such that it is inconspicuous. The color of teeth should be observed on a bright day when possible with the patient located close to natural light.

Squint Test. This helps in evaluating color of teeth with the complexion of the face. With the eyelids partially closed to reduce light, the dentist compares prospective colors of artificial teeth held along the face of the patient. The color that fades from view first is the one that is least conspicuous in comparison to color of the face.

Composition of the Material of Anterior Teeth

Normally porcelain or acrylic resin can be used.

Differences between porcelain and acrylic teeth

Acrylic Resin

1. The bonding of acrylic resin to denture base is by chemical means and no stresses occur in the region of the tooth.
2. High fracture toughness
3. Acrylic teeth wear to accommodate changes in occlusion but do not maintain vertical dimension of occlusion.
4. Produce a cushioning effect on chewing.
5. Silent on contact with opposing teeth.

6. Dimensional changes with water sorption.
7. Cold flow under stress and easily ground and polished.
8. Can be used when interarch space is diminished.
9. Crazing if not crosslinked and causes minimal abrasion of opposing dentition.
10. Acrylic teeth can be stained and filling inserted with ease in the laboratory.

Porcelain Teeth

1. The binding of porcelain to denture base is purely mechanical. The posterior teeth are held by acrylic flowing into diatoric holes in the teeth and anterior teeth are held by gold pins.
2. Brittle and may chip
3. Porcelain teeth do not wear to an even smooth articulation but do maintain vertical dimension.
4. They transmit the entire masticatory load to the ridge.
5. Sharp impact sound.
6. Dimensionally stable.
7. No permanent deformation.
8. Grinding difficult and glaze is removed.
9. Cannot be used in diminished interarch space.
10. Abrades opposing teeth and gold surfaces and staining is difficult.

Ceramic (composite teeth). It contains microfine particles of silica and has better bonding characteristics than porcelain.

Cosmetic Factor. The cosmetic factor involves personal grooming. When a person dresses neatly and keeps generally well groomed, the dentist should arrange the artificial teeth in positions that will complement these efforts. The teeth should harmonize with their settings. In case of patients who do not use cosmetics, exact reproduction of the arrangement of the natural teeth is not acceptable. Modifications of the natural arrangement may help to improve the patient's appearance.

Artistic Reflection

Artistic reflection is the arrangement of the teeth to reflect the dentist's concept of what he thinks appears natural for the patient. Many positions in which maxillary artificial anterior teeth may be placed will be harmonious with other facial features.

1. Vary the slant of the long axis.
2. Place the teeth so that the tip of the lateral incisors show while the patient speaks seriously, the amount depends on the age and sex and more for women than for men.
3. Create asymmetry in the divergence of the proximal surfaces of teeth from the contact points.
4. Use an eccentric midline.
5. Place one central and one lateral incisor parallel to the midline and rotate the other central and lateral incisor slightly in a posterior direction.
6. Move one maxillary central incisor slightly in an anterior direction to the other central incisor.
7. Place the neck of one maxillary central incisor in a posterior direction and neck of the other central incisor in an anterior direction.
8. Create asymmetry for the maxillary right and left cuspids. Rotate one in a more posterior direction than the other, place the neck of one in a more labial direction that the other.
9. Create a good smiling line by the proper placing of the maxillary posterior teeth medially in relation to the cheek. When the teeth are placed too far laterally the buccal corridor is eliminated, resulting in a harsh, ugly, and toothy appearance.

The esthetic appearance can be enhanced by:
1. Grinding the incisal edges.
2. Rotating and overlapping the teeth to give an irregular appearance.
3. Creating asymmetry in the divergences of the proximal surfaces of teeth from the contact points.

4. Creating a slight diastema between the lateral incisor and cuspid on the one side varying the direction of the long axis.

Facial features, mannerisms, facial expressions and tooth positions are inherited. The position of a daughter's or son's natural teeth can be an excellent guide when positioning the teeth for the parents.

SELECTION OF POSTERIOR TEETH

The selection of posterior teeth involves the selection of shade, size, number and form of the teeth.

Shade of Posterior Teeth

The shade of the posterior teeth should harmonize with the shade of the anterior teeth. The maxillary bicuspids are sometimes used for esthetics than for functional purposes. Bulk influences the shade of the teeth and for this reason, it is admissible to select a slightly lighter shade for the bicuspids if they are arranged for esthetics. They may be slightly lighter than other posterior teeth but not lighter than anterior teeth.

Size and Number of Posterior Teeth

Size and number of posterior teeth are closely related to usage. These characteristics are dictated by the anatomy of the surrounding oral environment and physiologic acceptance by surrounding tissues. The posterior teeth must support the cheeks and tongue and function in harmony with the musculature in swallowing, speaking and mastication. The buccolingual dimension of artificial teeth should be less than that of natural teeth to reduce the size of the food table. The occlusal table should be reduced to reduce the amount for occlusal forces on supporting tissues of the basal seat. The buccolingual width should not be great enough to embarrass the tongue or encroach on the buccal corridor. The anteroposterior or mesio-distal dimensions of the posterior teeth are determined by the edentulous area between the distal of the mandibular cuspids and ascending area of the mandible. It is better to choose a set of teeth shorter than this distance. The ascending area of the mandible is usually situated slightly anterior to retromolar pad. To place teeth at the ascending area of the mandible would be directing forces in an inclined plane. Forces directed to an inclined plane are more dislodging than forces directed at right angles to the support.

A ruler can be used to measure from distal surface of mandibular canine to the point that has been marked at the end of the available space. The total mesiodistal width in mm of the posterior teeth is often used as a mold number, e.g. mold 32L of the dentists supply company signifies that the four posterior teeth have a total mesiodistal dimension of 32 mm and a long occlusocervical length.

The height of posterior teeth is determined by measuring the interarch distance and then choosing the longest teeth that will fit the space without grinding. The shortest teeth will not fit the interarch distance. Acrylic teeth may be ground without worrying about retention because the bond is chemical rather than mechanical, but in porcelain care must be exercised with grinding, so that the mechanical retention is not obliterated by grinding.

The polished surfaces of the denture with the buccal and lingual flanges should slope away from the occlusal surfaces. The posterior teeth should have sufficient width to act as a table upon which to hold food during triturition.

The posterior teeth should not extend too close to the posterior border of the maxillary denture because of the danger of cheek biting.

If the posterior teeth do not extend far enough posteriorly, the forces of mastication would place a heavier load on the anterior part of the residual ridges. When the mandibular ridges slope up sharply at its distal end, the posterior teeth must not be placed on this slope.

This will cause the lower denture to slide forward when forces are applied to the posterior teeth over the slope.

Posterior teeth are not arranged over the retromolor pad. Because the histologic structure of the pad is too soft and too easily displaced that would allow the denture to tip during mastication. Because of this reason only three posterior teeth are used on each side of the denture for many patients.

The length of the maxillary first premolar should be comparable to that of the maxillary canines to have the proper esthetic effect.

Functional Requirements of Posterior Teeth

The posterior teeth bear the functional burden for the occlusion. By their arrangement, they serve to aid retention, preserve the health of the masticator tissues, masticate food and provide for patient's comfort.

The buccal position of the lower posterior teeth is determined by the needs of retention, and these teeth in turn determine the position of the upper posterior teeth. The buccal cusp or at least the anteroposterior central groove of the lower teeth should be located over a line drawn along the crest of or center of the lower ridge.

If they are located buccal to this position, the denture may be tipped upon the opposite side when the occluding teeth are engaged on the working side. If located too far lingually the tongue may be crowded and thus lift the denture during its movements.

The superoinferior position of the lower teeth is determined by the character of the residual ridges. If both ridges are equally strong, the occlusal plane is generally placed half way between them.

If, however the lower ridge is considerably flatter or in other respects weaker than the upper, the lower posterior teeth should be placed closer to the ridge in order to lessen the lateral torque on the ridge. They tend to preserve the health of the mandibular ridge. The lower ridge is more susceptible to trauma than the upper ridge for the simple reason that a given force is distributed through a maxillary denture with its greater basal area which result in less pressure per square millimeter on the maxillary mucosa than the same force distributed through the lower denture to the mandibular mucosa. In a low denture, force acts at the junction between 2nd premolar and first premolar.

History of the Development of Posterior Tooth Forms[6]

The search for an ideal artificial tooth that would provide maximum denture stability and masticatory efficiency and still provide adequate esthetics and wearing qualities has been going on for several centuries.

Anatomic Teeth or 33°C Teeth

Dr Alfred Gysi of Switzerland (1913) has been given the credit for designing the first anatomic porcelain tooth designed to function harmoniously with condylar and incisal function. He studied numerous dentitions and concluded that anatomic posterior tooth should have a cusp angle of 33°. This was marketed in the 19th Century and closely resembled natural unblemished teeth. They had transverse ridges and were intended for tight interdigitation in an angle class I occlusion. These teeth were called trubyte in the US. Disadvantage of the tooth was that it could not be used in crossbite situations.

In 1927 Gysi designed a modified crossbite posterior which was a definite departure from the universally accepted 33° posterior. In this type, the maxillary buccal cusp was almost eliminated resulting in a prominent lingual cusp that occluded into a lower anterior tooth.

The occlusal surfaces of all posterior teeth were reduced. Gysi described a mortar and pestle action for this occlusal scheme.

Pilkington-Turner Posterior Teeth

In 1932, Pilkington and Turner patented a new anatomic posterior tooth form having a slightly shallower cusp of 30° but closely resembling natural occlusal forms. These carvings were arrived at mathematically. All cusps are of tetrahedral form with transverse grooves having the buccal and lingual portions in alignment and apices of the cusps all lying on the surface of a sphere.

Unlike Gysi's, trubyte teeth which were tightly interlocked in all directions by transverse ridges and cusps, these posteriors were intended to provide a small degree of freedom in lateral excursion.

Modified Anatomic Form From 33° to O°

The first radical departure from anatomic posteriors was made by Victor Sears in 1922 in the design called chewing members and in 1928 he designed *channel type posteriors*.

The maxillary occlusal surfaces consisted of a deep channel than transversed mesiodistally the entire length of the 4 posterior teeth. The lower posteriors were approximately half the buccolingual width of standard anatomic teeth and were in effect, a single central ridge that ran uninterrupted the entire length of the occlusal table. They articulated with the central channel of the maxillary teeth and were designed or described by Sears to permit unlimited protrusive glide with inclines that limited lateral glide. These were the first non-anatomic tooth forms although they were not flat planes. They were intended to reduce the trauma to the ridge caused by an anteroprosterior shift of the bases during improper intercuspation.

In 1930, the *Avery brothers* introduced another modified form, the opposite of sears called the Avery brothers scissor bite teeth. The posterior occlusal surfaces were locked anteroposteriorly by grinding steps on the surfaces of the teeth, with the angle determined by the inclination of the condylar path. They were modified to be free in lateral excursion. The occlusion of these teeth scissors together was meant to shear food in lateral excursions.

In 1936, *Mcgrane introduced* "curved cusp" posterior teeth These were designed to lock anteroposteriorly and to be free laterally in an arc corresponding to an arbitrary radius from each vertical rotational axis of right and left condyle. The intent was to shear food in harmony with the lateral guidance of Bennett angle.

In 1935, *French* designed a severely modified tooth. The maxillary tooth was similar to Sears, as it had a central groove running mesiodistally but with very shallow buccolingual inclines to reduce lateral thrust. The mandibular teeth had a narrow mesiodistal food table moved to the lingual of the occlusal surface and a slopping buccal incline that was subocclusal.

He claimed that this design placed the axial occlusal forces lingually which favored stability of the lower denture.

The concept of modifying posterior teeth to direct force more lingually on the lower denture continued and Max Pleasure's scheme proposed in 1937 was to modify the lower posterior teeth occlusal surfaces to a reverse curve by tilting the tooth buccally. This does not provide for balancing contacts in lateral or protrusive excursions.

This scheme was later modified to provide balancing contacts. The reverse curve was set in the premolars, a flat occlusal surface in the first molar, and a Monson curve at the second molar for balance. The reverse curve was to direct forces of occlusion lingually to favor the stability of lower denture, while still retaining a balancing contact in the second molar.

John Vincent in 1942 introduced a change in materials by using metal inserts for resin posteriors. These inserts, originally of gold solder and later stainless steel were circles of metal that protruded from the middle third of the maxillary posterior occlusal surfaces with shallow buccal and lingual cusps protruding beyond the metal inserts. These teeth were set opposing French's mandibular posteriors.

The advantage was the self-adjusting quality of the resin teeth as they wore against the porcelain teeth.

In 1941 *Payne* described the modification of anatomic teeth set to a "lingualized occlusion" concept.

Sosin in 1961 replaced the maxillary second bicuspid and first and second molars with cleat shaped vitallium forms called crossblades. The dentures were brought to the try-in stage, the lower posterior teeth were removed and the case processed. At the time of insertion, wax was placed in this area, dentures inserted and the patient chewed the occlusal form into the wax. This was then converted to gold and cured to the existing lower denture. Levin modified this scheme by reducing the size of the crossblade to the maxillary lingual cusp. Myerson's FLX "freedom in lateral excursion" posteriors were developed to harmoniously balance as a result of the occlusal form.

Non-anatomic or O-degree Cuspless Teeth

Hall in 1929 was the first to design and utilize a cuspless tooth. He called it *inverted cusp tooth* and claimed that it eliminated the problems of denture instability due to the presence of cusps.

The tooth was flat with concentric cone-shaped depressions on the occlusal surface that were like inverted cusps.

In actual function the depressions became clogged with food and lost their efficiency because no escapeways were provided in this design.

Myerson designed a cuspless posterior tooth in 1929 which he called "True cusp". It had a series of transverse buccolingual ridges with sluiceways between them.

These were the first teeth to be commercially produced that provided for complete free gliding contact in all horizontal directions. They were of anatomic width and breadth.

In 1934 Nelson introduced teeth called "chopping block" posteriors which were flat occlusal surfaces with numerous ridges. The ridges on the mandibular teeth ran transversely and those on the maxillary teeth ran mesio-distally. Because they were perpendicular to one another in contact, an efficient shredding and cutting action was claimed.

Hardy in 1946 designed a metal insert upper and lower posterior which he called Vitallium occlusal (VO). These were produced in resin blocks of 3 posterior teeth simulating a buccal facade of 2 bicuspids and one molar. A narrow zigzag of vitallium ribbon was embedded on the occlusal surface and ran mesiodistally, establishing a narrow, flat convoluted metal surface that was raised slightly above the encasing resin. The articulating surfaces of these teeth were metal-to-metal ribbons that proved to be effective cusps.

In 1957, the *Myerson Tooth Corporation* introduced the first crosslinked acrylic tooth in a flat occlusal scheme called the "shear-cusp tooth".

Sears and Myerson proposed a combination of porcelain and acrylic occlusal scheme that would decrease the wear because the difference in the hardness of the two materials resulted in a decrease in friction between the two surfaces.

Coe Masticators designed by Cook in 1952 was one of the unusual non-anatomic posterior teeth. The second premolar and first molar were flat stainless steel castings with holes on the occlusal surfaces that exited diagonally to a port on the buccal surface. These teeth occluded with flat upper porcelain teeth to push the food through the holes and in a grinder-like fashion to break it into small particles. This action reduced the force necessary to masticate food by one-third.

Bader in 1957 introduced the cutter bar scheme to improve masticatory efficiency of flat teeth. Here upper porcelain cuspless teeth were opposed with a metal cutting bar replacing the second bicuspid, second molar and first molar.

In 1954, *Devan* formalized guidelines for using flat teeth in his neurocentric concept which stated that flat occlusal planes should have:

1. Flat planes in all directions with no inclination at all with respect to the underlying denture foundation.
2. Balance was considered unnecessary and undesirable, as the resulting inclines would create instability of the dentures.

In 1961, *Hughes* and *Reg* used a modified chew-in technique to determine a functionally generated path to which flat teeth would be set in order to achieve bilateral balance.

Types of Posterior Teeth According to Cusp Inclines

The cusp inclines for posterior teeth depend on the type of occlusion selected by the dentist. Posterior artificial teeth are manufactured with cusp inclines that vary from relatively steep to flat planes. Commonly used posterior cuspal inclinations are 0°, 33°, 20°.

The inclination is measured as the angle formed by the mesiobuccal cusp of the lower first molar with the horizontal plane.

Posterior teeth with 33° of cuspal incline offer the maximum opportunity for a fully balanced occlusion.

Posteriors with 20 degrees of cuspal incline are semi-anatomic in form and wider bucco-lingually than the corresponding 33 degree teeth. They provide less cusp height with which to develop balancing contacts in eccentric jaw positions than 33° teeth do.

Non-anatomic teeth with 0 degrees of cuspal incline are advisable when:

1. Only a centric relation record is being transferred from the patient to the articulator and no effort is directed in establishing a cross arch balanced occlusion.
2. They are also effective when it is difficult to record centric relations precisely from the patient or there are abnormal jaw relation-ships.

Advantages of Non-anatomic Teeth

1. When the teeth are contacting in non-masticatory mandibular movements as in

bruxism, the flat polished surface offers less resistance therefore less force is directed to the support.

2. These teeth will allow for a greater range of movement which is necessary in patients with malrelated jaws.

3. In the absence of residual ridges, there is no support present to resist dislodgement by horizontal or torquing force. Monoplane teeth offer less resistance to these forces, creating minimal horizontal pressure.

4. In cases where neuromuscular controls do not coordinate so that jaw relation records are not repeatable, the cusp form teeth cannot be balanced. Monoplane teeth are less damaging than cusp teeth not in balance.

5. Allow for easier servicing of the complete denture.

6. Allows construction of dentures with a simple technique and articulator.

7. Versatility of use, hence their employment in Class II and Class III relationships.

Disadvantages of Non-anatomic Teeth

1. Their anatomic form is inferior to that of cusp teeth.

2. Some patients complain of their inability to penetrate food effectively which renders the dentures mechanically inefficient.

3. They probably require the application of force in a nearly horizontal direction of jaw movement to shear food, and this results in lateral forces against the residual ridges.

Problems of Non-anatomic Teeth

1. Non anatomic teeth occlude in only two dimensions but the mandible has an arcuate dimensional movement due to its condylar behavior.

2. The vertical component present in mastication and non-functional movements is not provided for, so that this form loses shearing efficiency.

3. Bilateral and protrusive balance is not possible with a purely flat occlusion. Non-anatomic teeth set on inclines for balance require as much concern as anatomic teeth for jaw movements.

4. The flat teeth do not function efficiently unless the occlusion surface provides cutting ridges and generous spillways.

5. They cannot be corrected by much occlusal grinding without impairing their efficiency.

6. Non-anatomic teeth appear dull and unnatural to some patients and may create a psychological problem.

Advantages of Anatomic Teeth

1. They are considered more efficient in the cutting of food thereby reducing the forces that are directed at the support during masticatory movements.

2. They can be arranged in balanced occlusion in the eccentric jaw positions.

3. When the cusps are making contact in the fossae at the correct vertical dimension of occlusion with the jaws in centric relation, the position is comfortable. This point is a definite point of return, as through proprioception the jaws will return to this position.

4. They look more like natural teeth and are more acceptable esthetically.

5. The contours are more like natural teeth. They will be more compatible with the surrounding oral environment.

6. An attempted occlusion without cusps is disorganised because occlusion has depth.

Problems with Anatomic Teeth

1. The initial problem is the coordination of their cusps to harmonize with one another and the mandibular movements.

   An *unmodified cuspal tooth* for complete dentures can cause the following problems.
   - The use of an adjustable articulator is mandatory.
   - Eccentric records must be made for articulator adjustments.

- Mesiodistal interlocking will not permit settling of the base without horizontal forces developing.
- Harmonious balanced occlusion is lost when settling occurs.
- The bases need prompt and frequent refitting to keep the occlusion stable and balanced.
- The presence of cusps generate more horizontal force during function.

Monoplane and Polyplane Teeth Forms

1. Monoplane teeth were designed to occlude with the spherical plane of occlusion. These were set to bilateral balance as suggested by Pleasure.
2. Polyplane teeth were designed to balance on changing centers of rotation, which means that they can be set for bilateral balance.

A Historical Overview of Methods Used to Select Artificial Anterior Teeth for the Edentulous Patient

The upper central incisor is an important tooth in the dental arch and the width of this tooth dictates the width of the other anterior teeth. Various methods have been suggested for determining the form of the teeth (Table 15.1).

White in 1872 projected the concept of "correspondence and harmony". Here the temperaments called for a characteristic association of tooth form and color, while harmony called for a corresponding proportion and size of tooth to that of the face, and a tooth color in harmony with facial complexion: that both form and color were modified in harmony with sex and age. White considered the detailed line values of the teeth singly, and in the overall composition, and thought these were modified by age and sex. The goal projected was naturalness in form, appearance, and usability of restoration.

Hall in 1887 proposed the "Typal form concept". Hall stated that he worked out this

Table 15.1. Concepts for selecting teeth

Author	Year	Concept
Hippocrates	–	Temperamental
White	1872	correspondence and harmony
Hall	1887	Typal form concept
Berry	1906	Berry's biometric ratio method
Clapp	1910	Tabular dimension table method
Valderramma	1913	Molar tooth basis
Cigrande	1913	Finger nail
Williams	1914	Williams typal form method
Wilson	1914	Nasal index method
Warrin	1920	Warrin instrumental guide method
Nelson	1920	Maxillary arch outline form
Wright	1936	Photometric method
Meyerson	1937	Multiple choice method
Stein	–	Steins coordinated size technique
House	1939	House instrumental method
Sears	1941	Anthropometric cephalic method
Justi & Sons	1949	Frame harmony method
Dentists supply company	1950	Bioform technique
Austenal company	1951	Automatic instant selector guide

classification in 1865 and hence was presumably used before 1887. The basis of this classification was two fold, a major basis, which was the tooth's labial surface curvatures (transverse and gingival- incisal), outline form, and neck width, while the minor basis was the labiolingual inclination of the upper incisors in relation to profile types of straight, convex and concave. Hall gave the first definite measurements of typal tooth form in 1/48 inch, and the relative size of the teeth in an arch, using terms such as

- ovoid
- tapering
- square.

This classification exerted little influence on practice procedure of that time. It is of interest a quarter century before that of Williams.

The *"temperamental technique"* of selecting tooth form should be considered the pioneer technique from the point of view of influence and universal acceptance. It required several years to associate and establish dental characteristics of the temperaments, and to incorporate them in tooth forms. The basic items considered as indicative of tooth form for the edentulous patient were body and face size, form and function, complexion, and color of hair and eyes.

By 1838 teeth were being mass produced, and the tooth forms offered during the succeeding 25 years were conventional forms, or imitations of selected extracted teeth. During this period, a thousand or more differing forms were produced for sale, and they were selected by a "hunt and pick" method in dental depots. But in the decade of 1885 to 1895, the dental and facial characteristics of the temperamental classification had become quite uniform and stabilized by many publications in the dental journals. Thus, the common usage of the temperamental theory by tooth manufactures and dentists established this theory as basis for tooth selection.

Berry in 1906 projected the "Berry's biometric ratio method". In 1903, he said that the outline form of the inverted upper central incisor tooth closely approximated the outline form of the face. Therefore, the outline form of the edentulous face indicated the outline form of the anterior teeth to be chosen for a denture patient. Berry's continued investigation gave the correlation that the upper central incisor was 1/16th the face width and 1/20th the face length.

Clapp in 1910 suggested the "tabular dimension table method". This method was based on selecting tooth size from the overall dimension of six anterior teeth arranged on the Bonwill circle and the vertical tooth space present in the patient. Outline form was based on the operator's impression of harmony in face and tooth forms. This tabular method enabled the dentist to select and specify the mold of the teeth to be used by number, instead of delegating this function to the technician or a sales person.

Valderrama in 1913 presented the "molar tooth basis". Here varying measurements between combinations of cusp points indicated the size of the individual and overall tooth measurements. There is no indication that this technique ever received clinical use, principally because no molars are present in edentulous patients.

Cigrande in 1913 recommended the outline form of the fingernail to select the outline form to upper central incisor. The size was modified to meet the requirements of tooth space and other relationships. This technique did not find much acceptance by the dental profession.

Leon' Williams in 1914 suggested "williams typal form method". The basis of this method was nature's uninhibited plan in developing human face and tooth forms. This plan was interpreted by the geometric pattern created by the outline form of the skeletal face form, which he classified as square, tapering, and ovoid forms. The upper central incisor tooth was considered the model tooth of the arches. Modifying factors created by disease, development, physical forces and racial mixtures gave adulterated forms with a prevailing dominant form, but they were not considered significant to invalidate the theory. The theory and technique were widely accepted for many years, but later it has been questioned for its validity.

Wilson in 1914 introduced the "nasal index" method for selecting the width of upper anterior teeth. It related the interalar width to the space available for setting the upper anterior teeth. The interalar width gave an indication to the width of anterior teeth and recommended this index during selection of a tooth mold. Later Boucher et al in 1975 and Lee in 1962 concurred with Willson's "nasal index" method.

Wavrin in 1920 proposed the "wavrin instrumental guide technique". This was based on Berry's Biometric Ratio Method, and Williams' typal form teeth. While the instrument was quite satisfactory, its usefulness was mostly limited to a single manufactured product, hence it did not become popular as a regular method. Today this method is not used.

Wright in 1936 had put forward the "wright's photometric method". This was based on using a photograph of the patient with natural teeth, and establishing a ratio by comparative computation of measurements of like areas of the face and photograph. Then a mathematical formula was used to select the teeth.

Meyerson in 1937 suggested the "multiple choice method'. This was based on a need for a selective range in labial surface characterizations of teeth by time and wear. Harmony of tooth size and shape with face size and shape was associated with this technique, which was in use at that period.

Stein proposed the "stein's coordinated size technique". This was based on the coronal index, which was obtained by dividing the breadth by length of tooth and multiply it by 100. A coronal index of 70 to 100, was commonly used in prosthetics, as it represented the range of maximum frequency.

Sears in 1941 introduced the "anthropometric-cephalic index method". This was based on the observation that tooth length was in proportion to the face length. He found that the width of the upper central incisor could be determined by dividing the transverse circumference of the head by 13 or the bizygomatic width by 3.3. This technique has apparently received little attention and is no more in use.

Justi and Sons company in 1949 proposed the "frame harmony method". The basis of the method is that the size and proportions of the teeth are in harmony with the general bony proportions of the skeleton. The overall tooth size was selected by a mathematical formula, one-seventh the total dimension of the upper and lower bearing areas, with the dimensions of the individual anterior teeth correlated with a developed table of tooth dimensions to give the indicated overall dimension.

The *Dentists' Supply Company* in 1950 introduced the' Bioform Technique'. This was based on the geometric outline forms of face and teeth, the "House" classification of four basic and three-combination typal forms, and three dimensional harmony of tooth form and face form. It is associated with the tabular table and mold guide systems.

METHODS USED TO SELECT ARTIFICIAL TOOTH FORM

Simple Observation

Many studies have focused attention on the maxillary central incisor. Because of its prominent size, position, and shape in the natural dentition, central incisors can significantly influence facial appearance, and those that harmonize with the patient's features are of primary importance in successful esthetics lateral incisors and canines perform a subordinate role from an esthetic viewpoint but remain fundamental components in achieving optimum dentofacial appearance.

Temperament Theory. Prior to approximately 1915, the temperament theory was used extensively in medicine to classify illnesses and later in dentistry to aid in the selection of artificial teeth.

Hippocrates conceived the temperament theory in the fifth century BC based on a classification of illness according to the dominance of bodily fluids. Blood, phlegm, yellow bile, and black bile were translated into mental, physical, and functional characteristics. Resistance or susceptibility to certain ailments or conditions determined an individual's temperament classification. The four fundamental classifications were sanguine, phlegmatic, choleric, and melancholic. Twelve combinations of mixed temperaments, in which

1 temperament dominates another (e.g., nervosanguine), were also identified, for a total of 16 varieties.

In 1884, the use of the temperament theory was proposed in dentistry to aid tooth selection and improve esthetics. Sex and age were also considered factors that influence dental composition by either compromising or enhancing the esthetic effect. Formulation of these features determined the suitable tooth forms, sizes, colors, textures, and denture base contours for each temperament. Specific arch forms together with complementary palatal contours for each temperament were also described, e.g. a flat anterior arch that turned posteriorly to form two diverging lines was consistent with the bilious temperament. In cross-section, the palatal vault was almost square. The sanguine arch resembled a horseshoe in outline, while the palatal contour was semicircular. The nervous temperament had an arch that gently curved on either side to form a rounded point anteriorly. Likewise, the palate had a high vault, reminiscent of a gothis arch. An almost semicircular arch typified the lymphatic temperament, with a rounded, shallow palate.

Correlation Between Esthetic Factors

Relationship of Face Form to Tooth Torm.
Studies of esthetic factors have examined the possible correlation between various aspects of the head and anterior tooth size and position. One such study found an analogy between face and tooth form. In this study, facial outline was determined by drawing a line midway between the hairline and eyebrows to the zygomas on each side and down to the chin. The inversion of this outline form was purported to represent, almost without exception, the natural mold of the central incisor. It was also suggested that the original arch form could be assessed by using the inverted form of the cheeks and chin as an accurate guide. When viewed obliquely, the cheek outline revealed the labial contour of the

canines. It was suggested that incisors that complement this contour would produce a natural harmony between face and teeth. The inclination of the ascending ramus, when viewed from the front, dictated suitable canine eminence.

In 1960, Sears asserted that the total width of the maxillary anteriors can be determined by dividing the bizygomatic breadth by 3.3, however, concluded that the correlations between the breadth of the maxillary central incisor and the bizygomatic width were not consistent. The interalar nasal width has also been suggested as a guide for selecting anterior teeth. However, the absence of a static relationship between the facial soft tissues and anterior teeth precludes the accurate prediction of tooth size in relation to nasal width. The lack of a significant relationship between nasal measurements and anterior tooth size has also been addressed by Smith.

The Williams classification of anterior tooth forms probably represents the most significant contribution to denture esthetics. This series of publications examined natural teeth to discover features that provided a key to determining anterior tooth form and desirable esthetics. It was found that some teeth exhibited similar characteristics and therefore were grouped together. This resulted in three distinctive groups: square, tapering, and ovoid. Although a large number of teeth did not conform to any of these three categories, they nonetheless possessed dominant feature is of one of the typal forms, and this was the foundation of Williams' classification of tooth form. Square, tapering, and ovoid became Class I, II, and III, respectively, and the characteristics of each form were described accordingly.

Teeth that did not conform to a typal form were categorized into a combination form square, tapering or both, blended into ovoid, square or ovoid, or both; blended into tapering or finally, tapering, ovoid, or both blended into square. Combination forms were relationalized to make selection easier, resulting in

6 combination forms in both Class I and Class II and 4 combinations forms in Class III. From these classifications, lateral incisors and canines that harmonized with each classification were selected.

Relationship of Facial Contour to Tooth Contour

Sears described an alternative method of anterior tooth selection in which labial, incisal, and proximal outlines were the main considerations. According to this study, all three profiles should possess the same contour to achieve harmony of form, the degree of curvature being dependent on curves present in patient's face. This is referred to as harmony in degree of curvature and differs significantly from Williams' typal face form-tooth form classification.

Relationship between Facial Profile and Tooth arrangement

Facial angle has been cited as a determinant for inclination of facial profile as an accurate factor in the arrangement of anterior teeth. Anterior teeth that have been arranged to harmonize with protractive or retractive tendencies present in nature have been reported to provide continuity to dentofacial appearance.

Relationship between Arch form and Palatal Contour

Arch form has been proposed as a guide to the arrangement of anterior teeth. Based on the three typal arch forms: square, tapering, and ovoid. It was suggested that natural tooth arrangements should be simulated to improve esthetics.

Relationship between Arch form and Face Form

A continuous line drawn along the alveolar crest as far as the tuberosities and just posterior to the junction of the hard and soft palate, when inverted and superimposed onto the face, was found to correspond with the chin margin, jaw lines, cheek lines, and eyebrows. Artificial teeth selected to arch form, and therefore face form, produced an esthetically pleasing effect.

Influence of Alignment Form

Variations in alignment form using artificial teeth of the same mold illustrated the importance of alignment in achieving good esthetics. Maxillary dentures were fabricated to conform to square, tapering, and ovoid alignment forms.

Measuring Devices

A gauge for selecting tooth form, mold and length was developed to expedite artificial tooth selection. The Truebite Teleform gauge consisted of 1 flat bar and 2 rulers pivoted together to form three sides of a square. Placing the gauge on the patient's head, the 2 rulers were brought into contact with the sides of the face. For square and tapering facial types, the gauge was angled to extend from the zygomas to points midway between the chin and angles on either side. This resulted in an inclination of approximately 70 degrees to a horizontal line. Facial classification was determined via a pointer located on top of 1 ruler and scale on the horizontal bar above the head.

Face length, and thus tooth length, was arrived at by taking readings from the rulers on each side. However, the importance of considering soft tissue contours was stressed when using the device, since reliance on the skeletal framework might induce irregularities.

A device similar to that described above was assessed for the selection of anterior tooth forms. The tooth selector comprised 3 aluminum rulers resembling three sides of a rectangle. The longest bar incorporated a 1:16 and 1:17 scale. The 1:16 scale was intended for general use, the 1:17 scale specifically for female patients. One short arm remained fixed to one end of the longest bar, while the other short arm could be adjusted along a slot in the longest bar. Measurement of facial length and width taken from the longest ruler (in mm) translated into tooth forms analogous with face forms. Tooth form was identified by taking a measurement from hairline to symphysis across the zygomas. These measurements were converted into millimeters and combined with face form; anterior teeth of a suitable size and contour could then be selected. Compared with tooth form classifications derived using subjects methods on the same patients, a higher success rate was achieved using the tooth selector.

Combination Theories

Combination theories that encompass the best features of previously established methods reportedly result in a high success rate in achieving dentofacial harmony. An amalgam of the typal theory and dentogenics was described.

The combination of the influences of tooth form, size, shade, arrangement, and position, together with denture base contour and color, and functional elements such as vertical dimension, occlusal plane, and incisal guidance were studied. It was suggested that maintaining optimal phonetic function is a prerequisite in enabling total appreciation of the full esthetic value of lip support with arrangement, shade, form, and size of the teeth. The effect of including facial examination, smile analysis, determination of occlusal plane, and location of the upper midline on the selection of teeth was reported. The influence of heredity was noted to play a significant role in the relationship between face and teeth.

Mold Guide casts

The use of mold guide casts constructed from impressions of natural teeth has been described as an expedient method for determining harmonious form and composition. A selection of mold guides, made up of 6 maxillary anterior teeth, was placed intraorally until a satisfactory appearance was attained. Duplication of mold guide teeth or selective modification of stock teeth and their subsequent attachment to a temporary base allowed a more precise evaluation of size, form, rotation and inclination.

Computers and Formulas

Computer technology and formulas have been used to determine the precise degree of correlation between the factors discussed. These methods typically incorporated taking readings from anatomic landmarks on the teeth and face, digitizing these shapes, and using computer programs to derive shape plots.

A method for measuring the size and shape of maxillary central incisors incorporating the use of formulae was devised. The formula for determining tooth shape relied on the central incisor being regarded as a simple trapezium form by ignoring outline curvature. Three values for determining tooth shape were discussed: (i) surface area, an estimate of overall size; (ii) width index, a relation of the width to the height; and (iii) taper, a measure of the convergence of mesial and distal sides.

Further Reading

1. Frush.J.P and Fisher.R.D.How dentogenics interprets personality factor. J Prosth Dent. 1956; 6: 441.

2. Frush and Fisher. The Dynesthetic interpretation of dentogenic concept. J Prosth Dent. 1958; 8(4): 558-81.

3. Frush and Fisher. Age factor in dentogenics. J Prosth Dent. 1957; 7(l 1): 5-13.

4. Registration state III. Selection of teeth. J.F. McCord et al. Br Dental J. 2000; 188(12): 660-66.

5. Hardy I R. The development in the occlusal patterns of artificial teeth. J Prosth Dent. 2000; 85(3): 220-30.

THE DENTOGENIC CONCEPT

INTRODUCTION

The arrangement of artificial teeth to make them appear natural, requires study and training to differentiate between that which is natural and in good taste and that which is unnatural and in poor taste.

Dentogenics is the art, practice and technique of creating the illusion of natural teeth in artificial dentures and is based on the elementary factors suggested by the sex, personality and age of the patient.

The dentogenic restoration is designed to enhance the naturalness of appearance in the individual for whom it is made by its complimentary contribution of the beauty, charm, character or dignity observed in a fully expressive smile or in earnest conversation.

DEFINITION

Dentogenics was defined as the convergence of art, practice and techniques that enable a denture to add to a person's charm, character, dignity and beauty in a fully expressive smile.

THE DENTOGENIC MOVEMENT

The dentogenic movement as it was popularly called, began in the 1950s.

As proponents of dentogenics "Frush and Fisher" placed great emphasis on projecting a denture wearer's personality, sex and age. In collaboration with the Swissdent foundation, they stressed the need to avoid the "denture look". They added to face form and tooth form, the SPA factors: sex, personality and age.

They hypothesized[1] a personality spectrum ranging from vigorous to medium pleasing to delicate. Based on their experience, Frush and Fisher stated that 15% of the population is of the vigorous type. These individuals tend to be male. About 5% are delicate; and they tend to be female. The remaining 80% is the medium pleasing type, composed of both sexes.

Frush and Fisher placed great emphasis on the need for sculpting the tooth and for selecting the color and position in order to enhance the masculinity or feminity of the patient. They stressed the use of characterization to enhance age and sex.

Enhancing age means to make someone appear more youthful; enhancing sex means to make a "rugged" masculine type appear ruggedly masculine or a delicate feminine type appear more delicately feminine.

Hallaman has noted that the attempts to correlate tooth form with facial form, sex and patient personality profile do not stand up under scientific investigation.

Recent studies also do not support the belief that tooth shape and size have identifiable masculine or feminine characteristics. In a study of 300 diagnostic casts (equal number of male and female) judgements of sex were made by a layman, dental students, and dental faculty. The results shown an inverse relationship between correct judgement of the sex of the patient and the level of dental knowledge and experience of the judge.

However, from an artistic perspective the consummate delicacy of feminity and the ruggedness of masculinity remain as accepted guidelines reinforcing the dentogenic theory. The Swissdent corporation still strongly adheres to incorporating personality, age, sex and physiologic characteristics in the design of teeth.

Considering the matter of dentogenics, there are three basic factors in the denture esthetic concept. They include.

Age

In each individual,[2] age changes take place throughout the entire body, and the teeth are no exception. To arrange the teeth in disharmony with these changes is in bad taste, and the resulting appearance will be unnatural.

The objective of the age factor in dentogenics is to guide the prosthodontist in his efforts to maintain a high degree of conformity between his restoration and the patient's physiologic age structure.

For each patient, tooth shade is considered first. It is routine to consider light shades for young people and darker shades for older patients.

Age in the artificial tooth must also be accompanied by mold refinement. As we advance along the chronologic lifeline of an individual, normal wear plus trauma, and in some instances malocclusion makes inroads upon the original purity of tooth form.

We may reflect the appropriate age effects by creating the necessary age changes in the tooth.

Teeth tend to abrade with age. The central and lateral incisors abrade in a straight line. Whereas the cuspids abrade in a curve. The abrasion of the incisal edges of the anterior teeth flattens the arch. This is in harmony with the flattening of the lips as the cupid's bow of the upper lip disappears, and the fullness of the lower lip diminishes with the aging process (Figs 16.1 and 16.2).

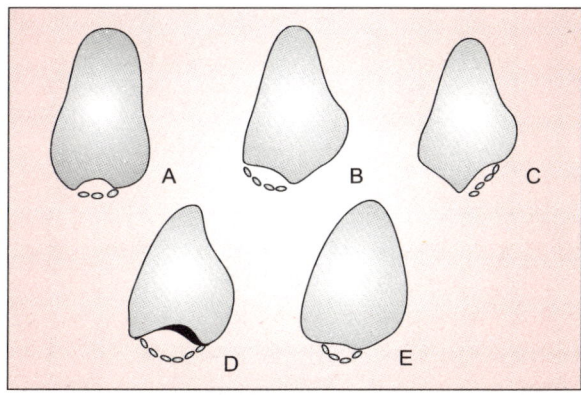

Fig. 16.1. Cuspids abraded to simulate age changes.

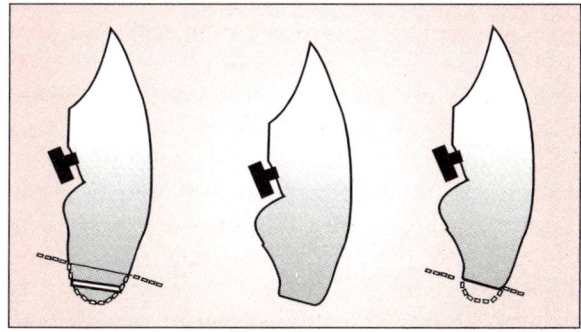

Fig. 16.2. Abrasion created on artificial teeth.

The interincisal distance tends to increase with age, therefore, the mandibular teeth become more visible. This is not an indication that the teeth have been positioned incorrectly in a vertical dimension. Increased visibility can result from loss of muscle tonus, allowing the lower lip to sag and the upper lip to drop.

The wearing away of the natural teeth at the contact points creates spaces between the teeth. The migration of teeth can also create spaces. Positioning the artificial teeth so as to simulate the wear creates a natural appearance.

In the natural teeth, we have seen the effects of erosion high on the gingival third and the necks of teeth. This erosion can be imparted to the artificial tooth, by careful grinding and polishing. This conveys the illusion of vigor and advanced age (Fig. 16.3).

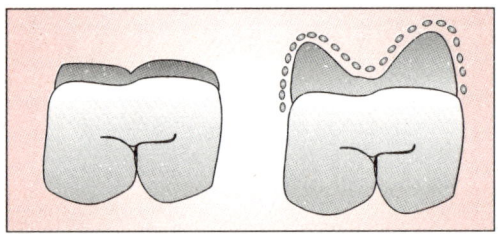

Fig. 16.3. An artificial tooth modified to simulate erosion.

Age Interpretation by Tooth Position. Tooth position[2] in the artificial denture becomes important in that imperfection is an **artistic** requirement in creating the illusion of natural teeth. This is opposed to the mechanistic alignment so frequently seen.

A condition so common in the natural teeth is the diastema. While occurring very frequently in youth, it is present even more often in the mouth of the adult in advancing years, because of drifting of the teeth resulting from premature loss of permanent teeth. The diastema places in the dentist's hands a splendid opportunity to create successfully the illusion of reality.

In the factor of age in the position of artificial teeth, the importance of planing the teeth in

the denture to convey the effect of variable long axis must be pointed out. The slightest rotation of tooth to convey the illusion of its own individuality totally separates it from its neighbor. In addition, the environment of the tooth is as important as the tooth itself. The matrix of the artificial tooth must be meaningful and not repetitive or inartistic. Colorwise, it is necessary to observe closely the color of the tissue in the mouth of the patient under consideration as here the physiology of the individual plays a more important part than the age factor. Massler has stated that as the age advances the attached gingivae lose their stippled appearance, appear edematous and smooth and the buccal mucosa becomes dry, inelastic and often wrinkled. Advancing age can be indicated appropriately by shortening the papillae, and by raising the gingival line to suggest recession.

Sex[3]

The sex of an individual influences the arrangement of the artificial teeth. The individual contours and the arrangement of teeth are different for males and females. Square features are associated with males and curved features are associated with females. The positions of the incisal edges, the prominence of the gingival portions of the necks of the teeth, and the positions of the body of the teeth reflect femininity, and masculinity.

Sex Interpretation by Tooth Positioning.[2] Positioning of the teeth is necessary, in conveying sex characteristics to a denture. However, definite position cannot be assigned to one sex or the other because factors other than sex must be taken into consideration.

A study of the position of natural teeth has revealed that
1. Roundness of the arch form denotes feminity and squareness denotes masculinity.
2. The incisal edges of the maxillary anterior teeth of females follow the curve of the lower lip.

3. The two central incisors set in perfect symmetry, are the starting positions for conventional tooth setups. By altering the tooth position, different facial patterns can be obtained:
   - By Bringing the incisal edge of one central incisor anteriorly, we can create a position which is evident but harsh. However, if we move one of the central incisors from the starting position out at the cervical end, leaving the incisal edges together, we can create a harmonious, lively position.
   - The second and more vigorous position is to move one central incisor bodily anteriorly to the other.
   - The third position is a combined rotation of the two central incisors with the distal surface forward, with one incisor depressed at the cervical end and the other depressed incisally.

Lateral incisors, being generally narrower and shorter than the central incisors, are less apparent; however, they can impart a quality of softness or hardness to the arrangement by their positions.

1. The lateral incisor rotated to show its mesial surface, slightly overlapping the central incisor gives softness or youthful coquettishness to the smile.
2. By doing the reverse, i.e. by rotating the lateral incisors mesially, the effect of the smile is hardened. We usually select the soft positions for the very feminine smile, and the hard positions for the vigorous male.
   - The cuspid teeth. The canine teeth can be placed in different positions.
     a. Out at the cervical end, as seen from the front.
     b. Rotated to show the mesial face
     c. Almost vertical as seen from the side
     d. It is evident that the prominent cuspid eminence gives to the cuspid greater importance and therefore gives to the smile a vigorous appearance more suitable to the masculine sex. The distal surfaces of the cuspids for females are rotated in a posterior direction; therefore, the mesial third of the labial surface is exposed when viewed from the front.
   - Maxillary first bicuspids. They are contoured and positioned to conform with the cuspids. Frequently the main concern in arranging the first bicuspid in a maxillary denture for a female patient is esthetics rather than functional because a woman normally exposes more maxillary teeth than a man, when speaking, smiling or laughing.

Depth Grinding: The Third Dimension

The denture look is mostly due to the flat appearance of the artificial upper anterior teeth, their lack of depth or of body (Fig. 16.4).

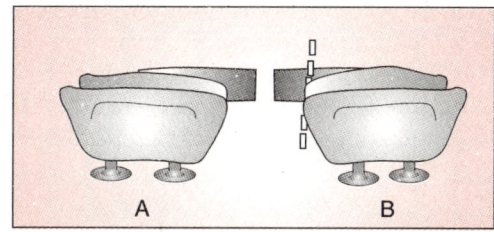

Fig. 16.4. A, Depth perception is limited because contact point is near the labial surface. B, depth of perception has been increased by depth grinding.

We always need that feeling of depth (the third dimension) for realism. Depth grinding is done on the mesial surface of the central incisor only. Central incisors are the widest, almost always longest and therefore, the most noticeable of the six anterior teeth, so they must be harmonized with the whole physical personality of the patient. The depth grinding procedure is as follows:

With a soft stone, the mesiolabial line angle of the central incisor is ground in a definite and flat cut, following the same curve as the mesial contour of the tooth in order to move the deepest visible point of the tooth further lingually. After this cut has been made a careful rounding and smoothing of the sharp angle made by the stone must be accomplished, and a perfect polish must be given to the ground surface so that it is indistinguishable.

A flat, thin narrow tooth is delicate looking and fits delicate women (little depth grinding) while a thick bony big-sized tooth, heavily carved on its labial face is vigorous and is to be used exclusively for men (rather severe depth grinding). In an average patient, i.e. a healthy woman or a less vigorous man, the depth grinding will be an average between delicate and vigorous.

Personality[4]

Sex identity in dentures is dependent upon personality and age factors in its final execution. The actual simplicity of the basic male or female tooth form is that it is a refinement of that tooth form which has its inception in the personality factor. Likewise, age is a refinement of the personality factor. Thus the foundation for dentogenic restoration is the personality of the patient (Fig. 16.5).

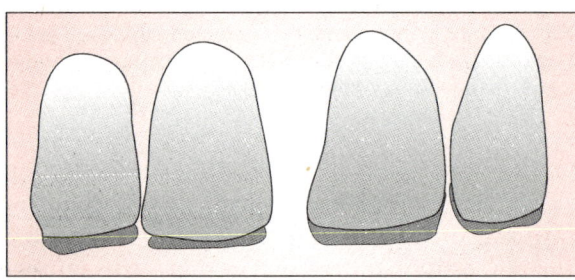

Fig. 16.5. A personality mold can be modified to make it appear more masculine or feminine.

The comprehensive use of personality depends upon our manipulation of tooth shapes (molds), tooth colors, tooth position, and the matrix (visible denture base) of these teeth;

The factors influencing personality include personal grooming and cleanliness, occupation, physical appearance and aggressive/regressive behavior patterns.

The precise prosthodontic application of this word lies in the three divisions of the personality spectrum:

1. Delicate—meaning frail, the opposite of robust
2. Medium pleasing—meaning normal, moderately robust, healthy and of intelligent appearance.
3. Vigorous—meaning the opposite of delicate; hard and aggressive in appearance, the extreme male, muscular type, almost primitive, ugly.

A small percentage of patients are delicate and a slightly larger percentage are vigorous. The remaining majority of patients fall into the medium section of the personality spectrum, but all of these have either vigorous or delicate tendencies.

Personality and Mold Consideration

Personality paves the path for further sex and age refinements, which are necessary to the dentogenic restoration. We consider the smile as the primary objective personality trait of the patient. We use this primary objective personality trait and personality spectrum for the selection of a mold category of the artificial teeth which we intend to place in that patient's denture.

The authenticity of patient personality and the implication of the personality spectrum in our esthetic interpretation transcend the necessity for commercial material consideration.

Wilhelm Zech has given us his concepts of the molds in the personality spectrum in vigorous, medium and delicate categories. Only about 10% of patients will be identifiable as truly vigorous and about 5% as truly delicate, the great majority of patients falling into the medium part of the personality spectrum.

THE DYNESTHETIC INTERPRETATION OF THE DENTOGENIC CONCEPT

The dentogenic concept of denture esthetics has been explained as the prosthodontic interpretation of three vital factors which every patient possesses: sex, personality and age. It is with a conscious consideration of these patient constants that the dentist has learned to apply his knowledge with the most effectiveness (Fig. 16.6).

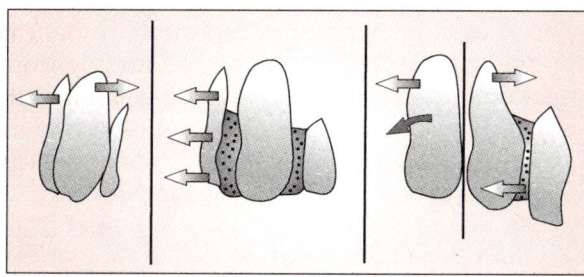

Fig. 16.6. Various dynesthetic positions of the central incisor.

Dynesthetic Theory

To apply the dynesthetic techniques in prosthodontics requires a knowledge of the dentogenic concept. The selection of artificial teeth, their subsequent sculpturing, the individual and detailed positions of these teeth, and the color and contour of the denture base are all part of the dynesthetic techniques and cannot be done in a comprehensive manner without reference to the patient's age, sex and personality as primary factors.

Dynesthetics is a compound word, 'dyn' from the Greek word dynamics, meaning power. The combining of the prefix 'dyn' with the word esthetics is necessary to the description of the philosophy and techniques of these supporting or working factors of the dentogenic concept.

The word dynesthetic has been applied to produce the effect of movement or progression. The dynamic value has been described as making the difference between an artifact and a work of art.

Areas of Responsibility

The dynesthetic techniques are rules which concern the three important divisions of denture fabrication:
1. The tooth
2. Its position and
3. Its matrix.

Dynesthetic techniques are not to be confused with the dentogenic procedures. The dentogenic procedure is the application by the dentist of these rules in the sequence of esthetic planning and are applied according to the sex, personality and age consideration. Therefore, it is important to make a delineation between the dynesthetic accomplishments of the dental technician in his laboratory procedure and the final dentogenic restoration as can only be created by a dentist.

Consideration in Dynesthetics

The following are the dynesthetic considerations which are necessary to the production of a dentogenic restoration.

Mold

The selection of an acceptable personality mold involves its subsequent treatment for abrasion, erosion, depth grinding, shaping and polishing.

Lip Support

Lip support is the bodily anteroposterior position of the teeth, which adequately supports the upper lip in a natural and pleasing manner. It is subject to slight modification and adjustments as work proceeds, but pleasing lip support is sacrificed only in the most extreme instances of old age or other circumstances where esthetics is of little consideration in the psychologic and physiologic comfort of the patient.

Midline

The features of a face normally slant one way or another and it is rather difficult to see a true midline in a dentition. Therefore, an eccentric midline in a denture, if not too exaggerated, is acceptable and may lend to the illusion of natural dentition. The mid- axis is important to the general composition and should be vertical to the incisal and occlusal plane (Figs 16.7 and 16.8).

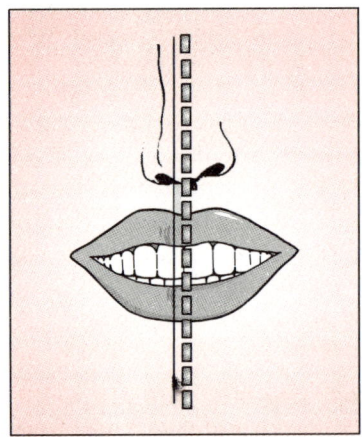

Fig. 16.7. An acceptable midline.

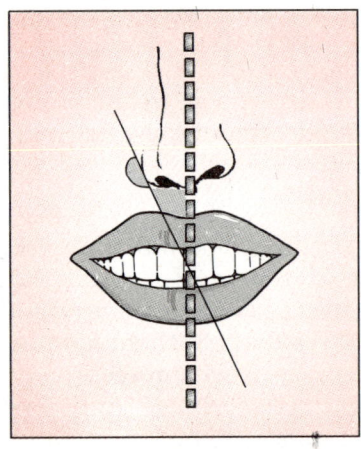

Fig. 16.8. An error resulting in an unacceptable midline.

Labioversion

Labioversion is necessary because the most pleasing effect is obtained when the long axis of the central incisors are either vertical or with slight labial inclination. This determination is made by observing the teeth in profile when the patient is standing in normal posture.

Speaking Line

The speaking line is the incisal length or the vertical component of anterior teeth. It is spoken of as speaking line because the final evaluation of incisal length is made when the patient is speaking.

A guide to vertical component using the incisal edges of the central incisors in their relationship to the lip line at rest as a measure is as follows.

- Young woman 3 mm below lip line at rest
- Young man 2 mm below lip line at rest
- Middle age 11/2 mm below lip line at rest
- Old age, senility 0 mm below lip line at rest to 2 mm above lip line at rest.

Smiling Line

The smiling line is a curve whose path follows the incisal edges of the central incisors up and back to the incisal edges of the lateral incisors and thence to the tips of the cuspids. It is determined by the age of the patient and decreases as the patient gets older (Figs 16.9 and 16.10).

Tooth Positions

Central incisors are the cornerstones of tooth position. If their positions are correct, then the positions of all of the other teeth will be more

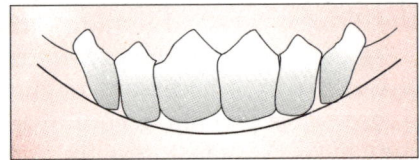

Fig. 16.9. Sharp curve of smile line indicates youthfulness.

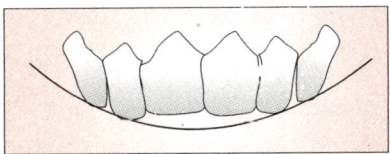

Fig. 16.10. Broader curve indicates older patient.

nearly correct. Their placement controls the midline, the speaking line, the lip support labioversion and the smiling line composition. The central incisors are also the basis of personality mold selection. Their importance lies in their primary forward position in the mouth, they are the first teeth to be seen in the smile. The relationship of the central incisors to each other is important. One central incisor is always placed bodily ahead or behind the other (Fig. 16.11). From this point, various degrees of rotation, labial inclination, and axial divergence will produce effects of additional strength, activity, and vigor to the entire dental composition.

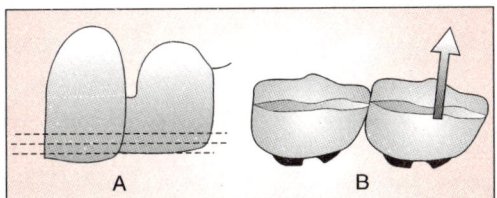

Fig. 16.11. A, Interincisal spacing. B, One central incisor can be placed bodily ahead or behind the other central incisor.

The central incisors should contrast sharply in size with the lateral incisors. The degree of contrast is subject to the experience and interpretation of the dentist. This can be accomplished easily by selecting a smaller sized lateral incisor and cuspid in the same mold as the central incisor.

The central incisors must be depth ground. The central incisors must dominate the lateral incisors in their positions within the general curve of the anterior dental arch. The lateral incisor should always fall within the line of the

arch, assuming the central incisors from the anterior limit of the arch form.

Lateral Incisor Position. The position of the lateral incisor is subordinated in importance to that of the central incisor. Its rotation, however, will either harden or soften the dental composition. The right and left lateral incisors should have asymmetric long axes. The lateral incisors should be positioned so that at least a portion is seen when the patient speaks seriously (speaking line determination). In dentogenics the lateral incisor is considered to be the personality tooth. The sex determination comes from either rounding the incisal edge for feminine effect or from squaring the incisal edge for masculine effect (Figs 16.12 and 16.13).

The Cuspid Position. The position of the cuspid tooth in the general arch form is important because it supports the anterior arch form in its widest part and controls the size of

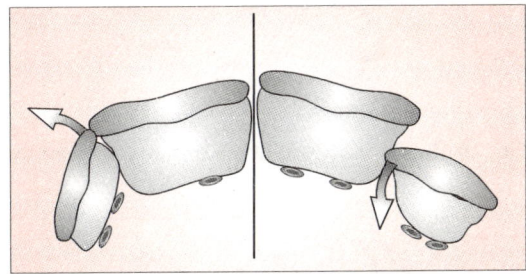

Fig. 16.12. S–Soft position of lateral incisor created by tipping the mesial aspect outward. H–is the hard position.

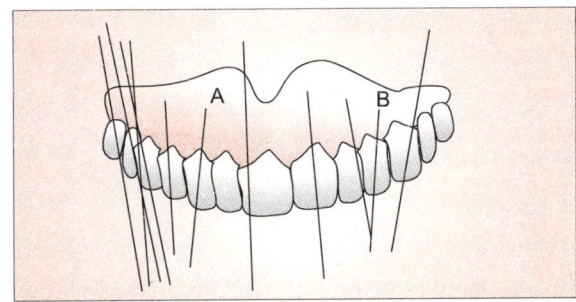

Fig. 16.13. Long axis of lateral Incisors (A) and (B) are asymmetrical.

the buccal corridor. The three basic requirements of the cuspid tooth position are: the tooth should be rotated to show its mesial surface; the cervical end should be out; and the long axis of the cuspid should be vertical (Figs 16.14, 16.15 and 16.16).

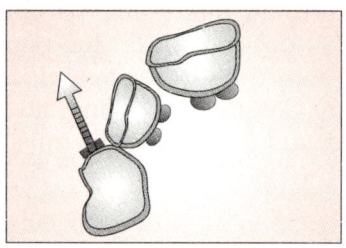

Fig. 16.14. Proper rotation of cuspid teeth exposes the mesial surface.

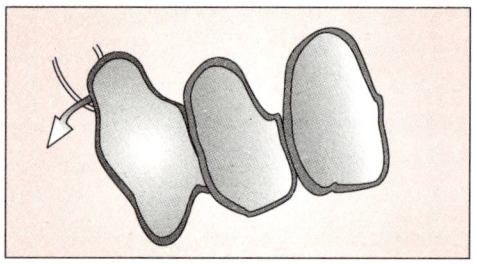

Fig. 16.15. Cervical end of the cuspid is moved out.

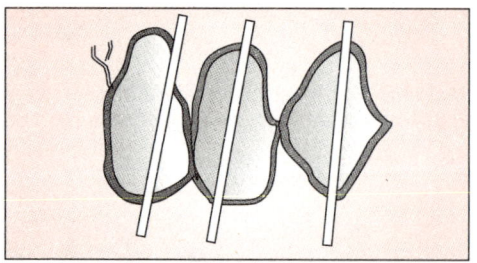

Fig. 16.16. Long axis of the cuspid is vertical when viewed from the side of the face.

Spaces

Spaces between the anterior or posterior teeth are extremely effective, but their size and position must be artistically and hygienically formed, or they will become unsightly repositories for food, bacterial plaque and calculus. There are certain rules to be observed with spaces. All spaces must be V-shaped to shed food, a diastema between the central incisors is unsightly and should be avoided; diastema should be controlled so as not appear unsightly at any instance.

Spaces placed between the posterior teeth serve as additional spillways for food through these spaces and creates additional cutting edges from the marginal ridges. These cutting edges are sharpened by grinding the proximal surfaces of the posterior teeth.

Embrasures

An embrasure gives freedom to the dental composition and differs from the diastema or spaces in that it represents a divergence of the proximal surface (since the contact areas are touching). An embrasure is employed in the same manner as the diastema or spaces but much more frequently (Fig. 16.17).

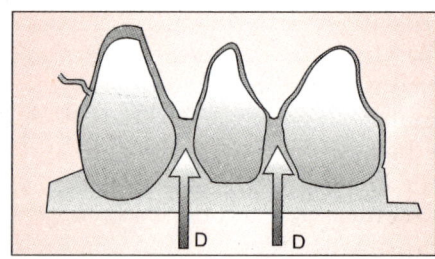

Fig. 16.17. V-shaped areas are the proper self-cleansing forms in all diastemas.

Buccal Corridor

The buccal corridor is a space created between the buccal surface of the posterior teeth and corner of the lips when the patient smiles. The buccal corridor begins at the cuspid, and its size and shape are controlled by the position and slant of the cuspid even though the actual corridor exists posterior to the cuspid tooth. The size of the buccal corridor is not critical and can be judged adequately by the eye in comparison with the natural dentition. The use of the buccal corridor prevents the molar to molar smile which is often characteristic of a denture.

Gum Line

The gum line at the cervical ends of teeth should vary in height. The generally acceptable rules for this are that the gum line should be formed: (i) slightly below the high lip line at the central incisors, (ii) lower than the central incisor gum line at the lateral incisors, (iii) higher than the central or lateral incisor gum line at the cuspid, and (iv) slightly lower, at the bicuspid than at the cuspid and variable for the bicuspids and molars.

Interdental Papilla

The interdental papilla forms the main part of the tooth matrix (visible denture base). Therefore, it occupies one-third of the total importance of the dental composition (the other two-thirds are occupied by the tooth and tooth position). In a dentogenic restoration, the esthetic consideration of the denture base lies in the matrix of the tooth. This is part of the denture base that is visible when the patient speaks or laughs. The balance of the denture base as seen on the articulator or in the hand is unimportant esthetically. Therefore, a dentogenic analysis is made with the denture in the mouth.

The correctly formed interdental papilla accomplishes four definite purposes: (i) it creates a hygienic, self-cleansing area, (ii) it is a complimentary factor in age interpretation, (iii) it determines the outline form of a tooth and makes the two-dimensional out line form of a tooth incidental to other esthetic requirements, such as the age interpretation in the papillae and the personality identification in the sculptured form of the tooth. The proper shape of the papilla can change a square tooth into a

tapering tooth or an ovoid tooth, and (iv) it brings a degree of color reflection to the interdental area which creates the illusion of natural dental composition.

The general rules for the formation of the interdental papilla are: (i) the papilla must extend to the point of tooth contact for cleanliness, (ii) the interdental papilla must be convex in all directions, (iii) the papilla must be shaped according to the age of the patient and they are classified as young, middle-aged or old-aged, and (iv) the papilla must end near the labial face of the tooth and never slope inward to terminate toward the lingual portion of the proximal surface.

Lingual Cutaway

The lingual cutaway is a groove in the lingual interdental surface which begins at the contact points of the teeth if they are together or at the tip of the interdental papilla if there is a diastema. It widens and deepens according to the natural divergence of the lingual proximal tooth surface. It fades away into the palatal surface of the denture.

The reason for the lingual cutaway is that food, when incised, will sweep through this polished channel and keep the area clean. It also prevents an unnatural exposure of plastic behind the tip of the papilla.

Labial and Buccal Denture Base Contour

We think of a natural base contour as being convex, vertically from the denture border to the tip of the interdental papilla in the anterior region. This necessitates a rather modest thickness of the border of the labial flange from buccal frenum to buccal frenum and eliminates the distortion of the mucolabial fold which appear too often as a bulge underneath the nose. A thickened anterior border of the wax occlusion rim distends the lip unnaturally outward and upward and should be prevented because this would disturb the proper recording of the low lip line. The denture base contour beyond the matrix (visible denture base) would provide a self-cleansing surface and therefore, would not be overaccentuated with depressions, grooves, wrinkles, folds, or any shape which would defeat the smooth cleansing action of the cheek or lips. Characterization for esthetics of the denture base beyond the visible portion is an impractical waste of time and effort.

Practical Application

The practical application of the dentogenic concept involves three separate educational phases. These include.

Education of the Dentist

The dentist who desires to excel in his work as a prosthodontist must strive to become exceedingly familiar with natural dentitions, particularly from the esthetic point of view. He must become so familiar with dentogenic principles that he may be able to apply them for the benefit of the patient whenever possible. It is important to adhere to the routine of photographing the mouth of every patient. Pictures of this type are invaluable as pre-extraction records and should be made before any work is begun.

A comparison of the photographs of natural dentitions to most artificial dentures will reveal striking conflicts. It should be possible to analyze the real and the artificial, to make comparisons and from what is learned, to avoid the pitfalls often found in the conventional denture tooth arrangement.

The task of arranging the visible teeth to reflect the personality of the patient, according to the dentogenic concept, is definitely the responsibility of the dentist. The utmost familiarity is necessary in order that the end result may be satisfying both to the dentist as well as to the patient.

Education of the Laboratory Technician

The dental laboratory technician may embody in the denture composition with relative success the dynesthetic subtleties and refinements necessary to satisfy the dentogenic requirements of the patient. Verifications by the dentist, by trial with the patient, are necessary before the denture is completed.

Since the patient is known to the technician only through the dentist, the ultimate success of the denture composition is in the dentist's hands.

Education of the Patient

The patient must be acquainted with nature. Obviously nothing else can succeed here as well as do pictures. The pictures should show natural teeth in the mouth in serious speech and during expressive smiling. Pictures should be selected to illustrate the dynesthetic phase of the dentogenic concept, such as the variable long axes of the central incisors, the 'soft and hard placement of the lateral incisors, and the canines in the desirable and less pleasing inclinations.

The pictures will assist in the re-establishment of nature's design in the mind of the patient and sharpen his recognition of the artificial. The preparation of the prosthodontist to accept the responsibility which is bound to follow such patient enlightenment is obligatory.

The dentogenic concept is an adventure into the realm of cosmetic art. It is esthetic philosophy. With the advent of dentogenics, a set of rules or guidelines, has been enunciated which can help the dentist by translating esthetic concepts into techniques. Although questions have been raised to the quantifiable scientific basis for the concept, few persons dispute its value as a very useful guideline in the selection of artificial teeth.

Further Reading

1. Frush J P, Fisher. Introduction to dentogenic restorations. J Prosth Dent. 1955; 5: 585-95.

2. Solomon E G R. Esthetics in complete dentures. (Notes).

MULTIPLE CHOICE QUESTIONS

1. **The proponents of the dentogenic movement are**
   a. McCollum and Sears
   b. Frush and Fischer
   c. Hallerman and Mathews
   d. House and Stein

2. **Changes in teeth with age include**
   a. Abrasion of teeth with the canines abrading in a curve.
   b. Decrease of interincisal distance with age
   c. Decreased visibility of teeth
   d. All are true

3. **Depth grinding is done on**
   a. Mandibular central incisor
   b. Maxillary central incisor
   c. Mandibular lateral incisor
   d. Maxillary lateral incisor

17

ARTICULATORS

INTRODUCTION

The academy of dental prosthodontics has defined the articulator as a mechanical device that represents the temporomandibular joints and jaw members to which maxillary and mandibular casts may be attached to simulate jaw movements.

DEFINITIONS

Articulator. It is a mechanical instrument that represents, the TMJ and jaw members to which maxillary and mandibular casts may be attached to simulate some or all mandibular movement.

Anterior Guide Pin. That component of an articulator, generally a rigid rod attached to one member, contacting the anterior guide table on the opposing member. It is used for the purpose of maintaining the established vertical separation.

Anterior Guide Table. That component of an articulator on which the anterior guide pin rests to maintain the occlusal vertical dimension and influence articulator movement. The guide table influences the degree of separation of the casts in all relationships.

Arcon.[5] A contraction of the words "Articulator" and "Condyle" used to describe an articulator containing the condylar path elements within its upper member and the condylar elements within the lower member.

Articulate. The relating of contacting surface of the teeth or their artificial replicas in the maxillae to those in the mandible.

Average Mean Articulator. An articulator that is fabricated to permit motion based on mean mandibular movements-class III articulator.

Condylar Articulator. Also called non-arcon articulator.

218

Adjustable Articulator. An articulator that allows some limited adjustment in sagittal and horizontal planes to replicate recorded mandibular movements.

Semiadjustable Articulator. An articulator that allows adjustment to replicate average mandibular movement–Class III articulator.

Fully Adjustable Articulator. An articulator that allows replication of 3-D movement of recorded mandibular motion–Class IV articulator.

Bonwill Triangle. Eponym for a 4-inch equilateral triangle bounded by lines connecting the contact points of the mandibular central incisor's edge to each condyle and from one condyle to the other, first introduced in 1858.

Curve of Monson. Eponym for a proposed ideal curve of occlusion in which each cusp and incisal edge touches or conforms to a segment of the surface of a sphere 8 inches in diameter with its center in the region of the glabella.

Curve of Occlusion. The average curve established by the incisal edges and occlusal surface of anterior and posterior teeth in either arch.

Fully Adjustable Gnathologic Articulator. An articulator that allows replication of 3-D movement plus timing of recorded mandibular motion–Class IV articulator.

FUNCTIONS

1. The primary function[1] of the articulator is to act as the patient in the absence of a patient.

   An articulator can be used to simulate the patient's TMJ, muscles of mastication, mandibular ligaments, mandible and maxilla and the complex neuromuscular mechanism, that programs mandibular movements.

   An articulator does serve as an extremely useful instrument in the absence of the patient, because the instrument can be programmed with certain patient records that allow the operator and the dental laboratory technician to fabricate a restoration that will be physiologically and psychologically successful.
2. Mounting of dental casts for diagnoses, treatment and patient presentation.
3. Fabrication of occlusal surfaces for dental restoration.
4. Arrangement of artificial teeth for complete and removable partial dentures.

ADVANTAGES

1. Properly mounted casts allow the operator to better visualize the patient's occlusion, especially from the lingual view.
2. When articulating teeth for complete dentures, the lingual view as provided with the articulator is essential if a proper occlusal scheme is to be developed.
3. Patent's cooperation is not a factor when using an articulator once the appropriate interocclusal records are obtained from the patient.
4. The refinement of the complete denture occlusion in the mouth is extremely difficult because of shifting of denture bases and resiliency of the supporting tissues. Interocclusal records can be obtained and complete denture occlusion can be refined outside the mouth on an articulator.
5. Considerably more chairside time and patient appointment time is required when utilizing the mouth as an articulator.
6. More procedures can be delegated to the auxillary personnel when utilizing an articulator for development of the patient's occlusion.
7. The patient's saliva, tongue and cheeks are not factors when using an articulator.

REQUIREMENTS OF AN ARTICULATOR

Minimal Articulator Requirements[2]

These are necessary for the fabrication of complete dentures to the patient's centric position. This position must be accurately refined for both monoplane or cuspless occlusion and cusp occlusion.

1. The articulator must accurately maintain the correct horizontal and vertical relationship of the patient's casts. In other words, it should accurately maintain centric position.
2. The patient's casts must be easily removed and attached to the articulator without losing their correct horizontal and vertical relationship.
3. The articulator should have an incisal guide pin with a positive stop that is adjustable and calibrated. This provides positive control over the patient's occlusal vertical dimension by the dentist and lab technician.
4. The articulator should be able to open and close in a hinge-like fashion. The articulator should accept a face-bow transfer utilizing an anterior reference point.
5. The face-bow transfer relates the maxillary cast to the horizontal axis of the articulator in the same manner that the patient's maxilla relates to the opening axis of TMJ. This allows minor changes in the patient's vertical dimension without grossly changing the patient's occlusion at the centric position. Also, the anterior reference point transfer facilitates the arrangement of the anterior teeth to the desired labiolingual inclination.
6. The construction should be accurate, rigid, and of a noncorrosive material. The moving parts should resist wear. The adjustments should be able to move freely and be definitely secured.
7. The design should be such that there is adequate distance between upper and lower members and that vision not obscured from the rear. The articulator should be stable on lab bench and not too bulky and heavy.

Additional Articulator Requirements

Additional articulator requirements are necessary if dentures are to be fabricated in balanced occlusion.

1. The condylar guides should allow right lateral, left lateral, and protrusive movements.
2. The condylar guides should be adjustable horizontally.
3. The articulator should have provision for adjustment of Bennett movement.
4. The incisal table should be a mechanical table that can be adjusted in the sagittal and frontal planes or a table that can be customized with autopolymerizing resin or grinding.

Optional articulator capabilities for fabrication of complete dentures would be an adjustable intercondylar distance and an immediate Bennett adjustment. These are of greater importance in fixed prosthodontics.

The immediate Bennett adjustment primarily influences the width of the central grooves of posterior teeth, whereas the intercondylar distance influences the character and inclinations of grooves and cusps. An average intercondylar distance of 110 mm is adequate for complete dentures.

LIMITATIONS

1. An articulator may have parts made from plastic material. It is subject to human error in tooling and errors resulting from metal fatigue and wear.
2. Articulators cannot duplicate the condylar movements in TMJ.
3. Articulators cannot reproduce border movements of the jaws or reproduce intraborder and functional movements.

The effectiveness of any denture depends upon:

1. How well the operator understands its construction and purpose.
2. How enthusiastic he is for a particular instrument.
3. How well the dentist understands the anatomy of the joints, their movements, and neuromuscular system.
4. How much precision and accuracy are used in registering jaw relations.
5. How sensitive the instrument is to these records.

HISTORY OF ARTICULATORS

The first instrument designs were attempts to duplicate anatomic relationships or to reproduce functional movements of the anatomy. More sophisticated articulating instruments evolved as more was learned about anatomy, mandibular movements, and mechanical principles.

Historically, some aspects of jaw physiology have been easy to duplicate mechanically on an articulator, such as the hinge movement, relation of casts to the hinge, and the inclination of the condylar path. These features, consequently appeared first on the instruments.

Other movements like Bennett movement, exact curvature of condylar path, and determination of intercondylar distance appeared later.

1. The Plaster Articulator.[3] The plaster articulator was first described by Philip Pfaff in 1756. A plaster extension on the distal portion of the mandibular cast was grooved to serve as a guide for a plaster extension of the maxillary cast. The extended casts together constituted the first articulator. This was the only means of relating the maxillary cast to the mandibular cast prior to 1805, when JB Gariot described the first mechanical articulator.

2. The Barn Door Hinge.[3] The barn door hinge is inexpensive and easy to obtain. A heavy duty hinge is modified by bending each arm 90° to form L-shaped upper and lower members.

3. The Adaptable Barn Door Hinge.[3] It is capable of opening and closing in a hinge movement. It has an anterior vertical stop which is usually a carriage or machine bolt. If the instrument is well manufactured and not flexible, lateral movement will be held to a minimum.

5. The New Century and Modified New Century Articulators.[3] This has been credited to George B Snow of the University of Buffalo. In 1906, he improved on the Gritman articulator of 1899 by converting the fixed condylar paths to adjustable condylar paths and adding a tension spring, which allowed a greater range of movement without compromising the stability of the frame. The rotation centers were placed 4 inches apart in accordance with Bonwill's theory.

6. The Gysi adaptable and Gysi Simplex Articulator.[3] The Gysi adaptable articulator was introduced in 1910, but it was beyond the technical ability and finance of most dentists. For this reason, Gysi simplex was introduced as a mean value articulator in 1914. It was competitively priced and did not require great technical ability to operate. The condylar guidance of the Gysi simplex is fixed at 33° and is shaped like the ogee path.

7. The Maxillomandibular Instrument. Designed in 1918 by George Monson, was based on the spherical theory. According to this theory, which evolved from the concepts of Monson, and a German anatomist, Graf Von-Spee, the mandibular teeth move over the maxillary teeth as over the surface of a sphere (Fig. 17.1).

8. The Stephan Articulator. The Stephan articulator developed in 1921, is similar in design to the Gariot hinge articulator of 1805, except that it has a fixed condylar inclination and allows for arbitrary lateral movements. A

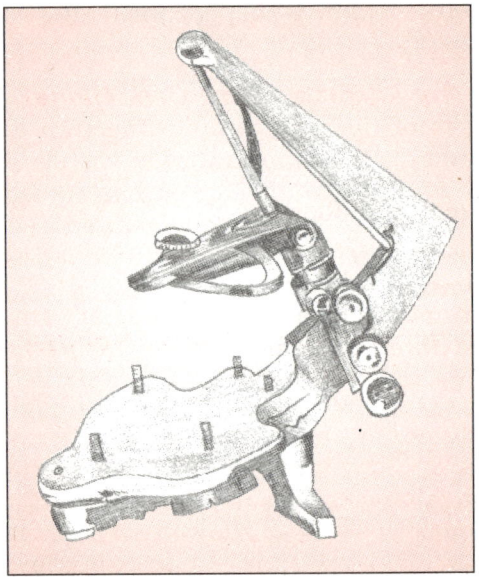

Fig. 17.1. Maxillomandibular instrument

posterior set screw holds the upper and lower members of the articulator at a fixed vertical dimension (Fig. 17.2).

9. Hanau Model H Kinoscope.[4] Rudolf C Hanau, an engineer was influenced by Dr Robert E Hall to study the design of articulators. Early in 1921, he developed a research model called the Hanau model C Articulator. In 1923,

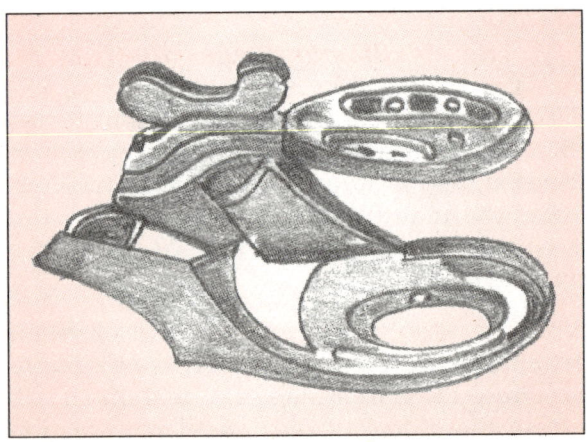

Fig. 17.2. Stephan articulator.

he developed another research instrument, the Hanau model H kinoscope articulator. It has double condylar posts on each side. The inner posts serve two purposes: (i) they act as the horizontal condylar guides, and (ii) they are moved inward or outward.

10. The Hanau Model H 110.[4] Evolved from the model H115 that was manufactured in 1922 and 1923. These instruments were developed because Hanau realized as had Gysi and others that the dental profession and lab industry would not accept the more complicated kinoscope instruments. It was designed to encompass mechanical averages of many previous concepts. It has individual condylar guidance adjustments in both the sagittal and horizontal planes. The lateral setting is calculated by dividing the horizontal condylar inclination by 8 and adding 12. This formula is given in the base of the articulator L = H/8 + 12.

11. The Hanau Model H 110 Modified. This instrument appeared in 1927 and introduced the incisal guide table. The improved table allowed for adjustment in three dimensions through a considerable range. The original incisal guide cup with its fixed curvature could be moved only as a unit.

12. The House Articulator. The Needles House articulator Chewin or other positional records can be used to set the House articulator, developed in the 1920's. Hooks that can slide along the intercondylar bar are used to vary the intercondylar centers of rotation without moving the lateral posts that support the condylar elements. The lateral condylar guidance is controlled by the Bennett guide, which is a wing attachment lateral to the condylar guide slot. There is a rotary milling device on the upper member that mills retrusively 0.02 inch, with the starting position being on the circumference of a circular milling movement (Fig. 17.3).

13. The Hanau Crown and Bridge Articulator. The HCBA 29-0 is a small

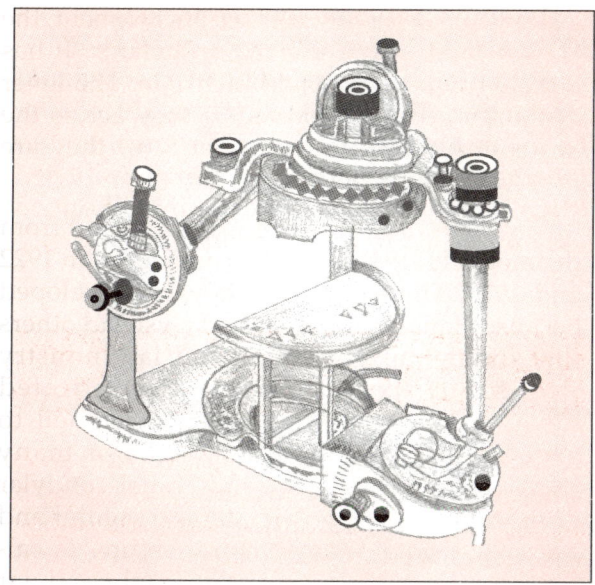

Fig. 17.3. House articulator.

articulator but unlike other hinge articulators, a posterior pin and cam guidance mechanism can be set to simulate working and balancing side excursions of 15°. The mechanism can be set to L for patient's left quadrant, R for restorations in the patients right quadrant, or A for anterior restorations or for equalizing right and left excursions.

14. The Stephan Articulator (Modified).
Introduced in 1940, it is a simple hinge joint articulator that has a fixed condylar path of 30°. It is similar in design to the 1921 model, except that the upper and lower mounting arms on this model are longer. An adjustable set screw in the posterior region holds the upper and lower members in a fixed vertical position.

15. The Stephan Articulator (Model P).
The additional features of the Stephan articulator model P are an incisal pin and a vertical height adjustment. Another version of this articulator was manufactured to include a fixed 10° incisal guidance.

16. The Pankey-Mann Articulator.[4]
It consists of base that holds a platform for the mandibular cast and a vertical post containing two movable assemblies.

The first assembly is made up of a horizontal rod that supports the face-bow and also has centers of rotation for measuring and cutting calipers. A second movable assembly holds the mounted maxillary cast.

17. The Dentatus ARL Articulator.
It is a semi-adjustable articulator, a shaft type of instrument with a straight condylar path and a fixed intercondylar distance. In mechanical design and principle, it is similar to the Hanau H2. An adjustable positioning mechanism in the upper member allows the use of a block that standardizes the upper member to the lower member. This allows the transfer of casts from one articulator to another articulator while the same relationship is maintained (Fig. 17.4).

18. The Improved New Simplex Articulator.
This instrument uses average movements. The condylar inclination is 30° with a Bennett movement of 75°. The incisal guide table adjusts from 0-30 degrees to accommodate various amounts of vertical overlap of the teeth to suit each patient.

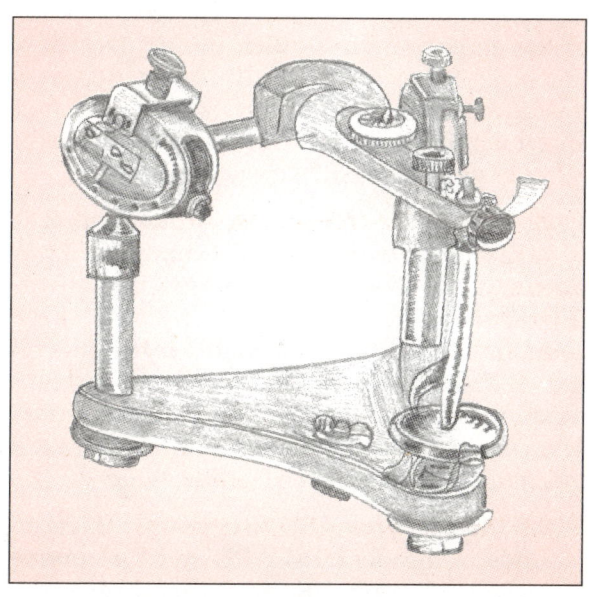

Fig. 17.4. Dentatous articulator.

19. The Verticulator. This consists of two rigid members that separate and close only linearly in the vertical dimension. It was developed to be used with the functionally generated path technique and Di-Lok quadrant trays. Another model introduced in 1968 accepts full arch casts.

20. The Ney Articulator.[4] It is an arcon instrument with no locking device between upper and lower members at centric position. The condylar elements are set to varying intercondylar distances. To facilitate mounting of the mandibular cast, the Ney articulator has a self- tripoding feature in its inverted position. A plastic incisal guide table or a metal incisal guide table that has a provision for making a region of freedom in centric position can be used.

21. The Whip-mix Articulator.[4] It is a simplified version of Stuart's fully adjustable articulator. It was designed for complete dentures and was intended to be useful as a diagnostic instrument and as a teaching aid. This is a semiadjustable arcon articulator and has three intercondylar adjustments: small, medium and large. These are selected by means of the accompanying quick mount face-bow that uses the external auditory meatus as a posterior landmark. This face-bow has a nasion anterior guide that establishes an anterior point of reference for maxillary cast positioning.

22. The Denar Model D4A Articulator. It is programmed from tracings made with a pneumatically controlled pantograph that was introduced and developed by the same company. It is a fully adjustable articulator. It has a definite centric lock and has accommodations to hold the casts in an open position. The curved incisal pin assembly can rest on a mechanical plastic incisal guide table.

23. The Dentatus ARO Articulator. It has all features of the dentatus ARL and the unique feature of a movable arm that holds the mandibular cast.

The universal joint and the locking device that attaches the movable arm to the base allow repositioning of the mandibular cast without remounting. The gauge block is used to center the lower member to the upper member, but once the mandibular cast has been repositioned articulator or casts cannot be interchanged without the aid of centric relation records.

CLASSIFICATION OF ARTICULATORS

At the international prosthodontic workshop on complete denture occlusion at the university of Michigan in 1972, an articulator classification was developed based on the instrument function, instrument capability, intent, registration procedure, and registration acceptance.

Class I. Simple holding instruments capable of accepting a single static registration Vertical motion is possible but only for convenience.

Instruments in this class accept a single interocclusal record, vertical motions may not be possible.
- The first articulators were called "slab articulators" and were formed by extending plaster indices from the rear of the casts. The casts were keyed to each other by means of their indices.
- The hinge joint articulator: JB Gariot designed the first hinge articulator in 1805. It consisted of a simple hinge with a set screw in the posterior against a metal plate to serve as a vertical stop.

Class II. Instruments that permit horizontal as well as vertical motion but does not orient via a face-bow transfer.
- Eccentric motion permitted is based on average or arbitrary values.
- Eccentric motion permitted is based on the theories of artribrary motion.
- Eccentric motion permitted is determined by the patient using engraving methods.

Class II A. A typical instrument of this class was designed by Grittman in 1800. The condyles are on the lower member of the articulator and their paths are inclined at 15°. The casts are mounted on this instrument according to Bonwill's theory (Fig. 17.5 a and b)).

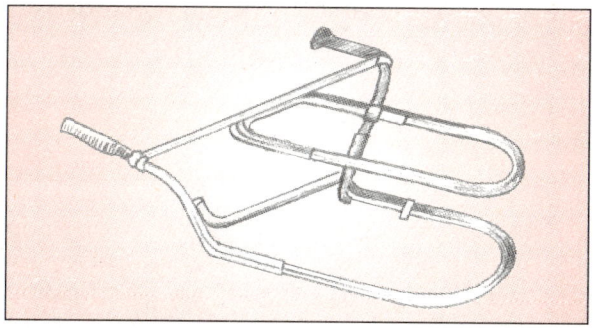

Fig. 17.5. (a) Bonwill articulator.

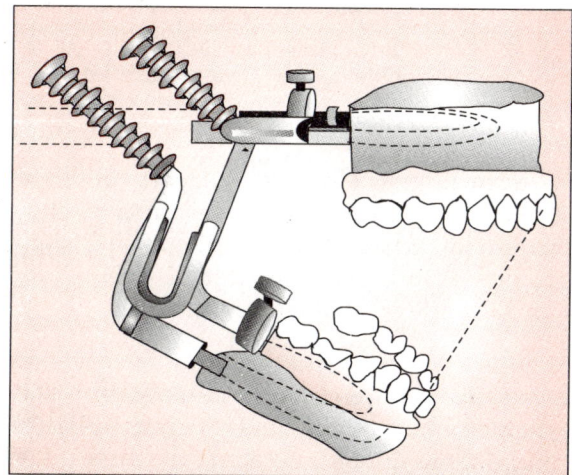

Fig. 17.5. (b) Bonwill's articulator with casts mounted.

Class II-B. Instruments in this class permit eccentric motion based on arbitrary theories of motion and will not accept a face-bow transfer. The maxillom mandibular instrument designed by Monson in 1919 is typical of this class.

Class II-C. Instruments in this class permit eccentric motion based on engraved records obtained from the patient and will not accept a face-bow transfer.

Class III. Instruments that simulate condylar pathways by using average or mechanical equivalent for all or part of the motions. These instruments allow for joint orientation of the casts via a face-bow transfer.
- Instruments that accept a static protrusive registration and use equivalents for the rest of the motion.
- Instruments that accept static lateral-protrusive registrations and use equivalents for the rest of the motion.

Class III A. Most popular was the Hanau model H designed by Rudolf Hanau, a mechanical engineer in 1923. His articulator accepts a face-bow transfer and the horizontal condylar inclinations are set by means of a protrusive interocclusal record. The condyles are on the upper member. The Bennett angle (L) was calculated from the horizontal condylar inclinations (H) by means of Hanau's equation.

$$L = H/8 + 12.$$

Dentatus was introduced in Sweden in 1944. This articulator is unique in that the relationship between the upper and lower members can be standardized with a gauge block, so that casts can be transferred from one articulator to another and still maintain the same relationship.

Class III B. Instruments in this class accept a face-bow transfer, protrusive interocclusal records and some lateral interocclusal records.
- In 1926, a fairly sophisticated articulator was introduced by Gysi called the truebite articulator.
- The Ney articulator was designed by De Pietro in 1960 and is a true arcon instrument. This was the first articulator to have condylar housings that contain adjustable rear, medial and top walls in one assembly.

Class IV. Instruments that will accept 3-dimensional dynamic registrations. These instruments allow for joint orientation of the casts via a face-bow transfer.

- The cams representing the condylar paths are formed by registrations engraved by the patient.
- Instruments that have condylar paths that can be angled and customized either by selecting from a variety of curvatures, by modifications or both.

Class IV-A. Instruments in this class will accept a 3-dimensional dynamic registration and utilize a face-bow transfer. The condylar pathways (or cams) are formed by registrations engraved by the patient. Instruments in this class allow for discriminatory capability of the condylar pathways.

The TMJ instruments was designed by Kenneth Swenson in 1965. An intraoral registration is generated by Studs in auto-polymerizing resin similar to the technique utilized with the House articulator. This is called a "stereographic" recording. The stereographic recording is then placed on the articulator and used to mold fossae in autopolymerizing resin.

All articulators in this class are arcon instruments with adjustable intercondylar distance (Fig. 17.6). The condylar housings can be adjusted in the horizontal, sagittal and frontal planes. Each has a Bennett guide adjustment. They all accept arbitrary or hinge axis face-bow transfers. They are often referred to as gnathologic instruments, because of their full adjustability.

- In 1968, Niles Guichet designed the Denar (D4A). Current fully adjustable model is D5A and is quite similar to D4A, except for refinements in machining and in the centric latch mechanism located at the rear of the articulator.

Class IV-B. In this class, instruments accept three-dimensional dynamic registration and utilize a face-bow transfer. The condylar pathways can be selectively angled and customized.

The 3-dimensional dynamic registration procedure utilized in this class is the pantographic tracing procedure. The tracings produced by the pantograph are called pantograms.

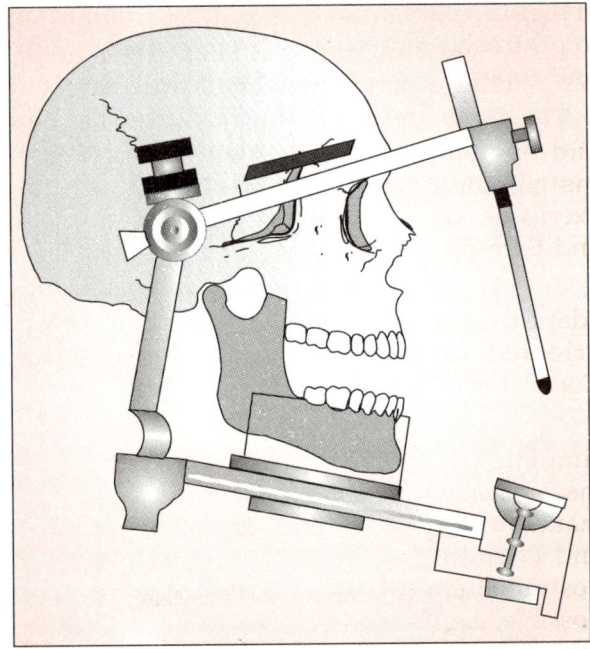

Fig. 17.6. An arcon articulator with its condylar guidance super imposed on the temporo mandibular joint

According to Charles M Heartwell Jr and Arthur O Rahn, a more descriptive classification of articulators for diagnosing dental problems and planning dental occlusion in natural and/or artificial dentures is:

Class. Instruments that receive and reproduce pantograms or stereograms. These articulators can be adjusted to permit individual condylar movements in each of the three planes. They are capable of reproducing the timing of the Bennett shift on the balancing side and its direction on the working side. These articulators are also referred to as four-dimensional instruments, e.g. Granger, Gnathorelater, Ney articulator, Stuart gnathogic computer, TMJ stereographic, Denar D5A and SE.

Class II. Instruments that do not receive stereograms. Articulators of this class are capable of being set to the individual timing and directions of the Bennett movement. Most of the articulators are capable of being adjusted to protrusive jaw records. This is divided into four types.

Type I (hinge). This type is capable of closing and opening in a hinge movement. A few instruments have limited non-adjustable excrusive like movements, e.g. Gysi simplex and Barn-door hinge.

Type II (arbitrary). This type is designed to adapt to specific theories of occlusion or are oriented to technique, e.g. Monson, the Correlator, Verticulator, Transograph.

Type III (average). This type is designed to simulate condylar pathways by average, or mechanical equivalents for selected aspects of mandibular motion. Adjustments of horizontal and lateral condylar guidance by means of positional jaw records or mini recordings is possible, e.g. Hanau, Dentatus, House, Whip-mix, Denar mark II.

Type IV (special). This is designed and used primarily for complete denture construction, e.g. Stansberry tripod, Kite dentograph, Irish duplifunctional.

Boucher classified articulators based on the design. There are articulators based on:

(i) theories of occlusion, (ii) types of records used for their adjustments, and (iii) the adjustments of which they are capable.

Articulators Based on the Theories of Occlusion

1. Bonwill Theory of Occlusion. This theory proposed that the teeth move in relation to each other as guided by the condylar controls and the incisal point. It was known as the theory of equilateral triangle in which there was a 4 inch (10 mm) distance between the condyles and between each condyle and incisal point, e.g. those designed by WGA Bonwill.

2. The Conical Theory of Occlusion. Proposed that the lower teeth move over the surfaces of the upper teeth as over the surfaces of a cone, with a generating angle of, 45° and with the central axis of the cone tipped at an angle to the occlusal plane, e.g. The Hall automatic articulator designed by RE Hall.

3. Spherical Theory of Occlusion. The spherical theory of occlusion (Fig. 17.7) shows that the lower teeth move over the surfaces of

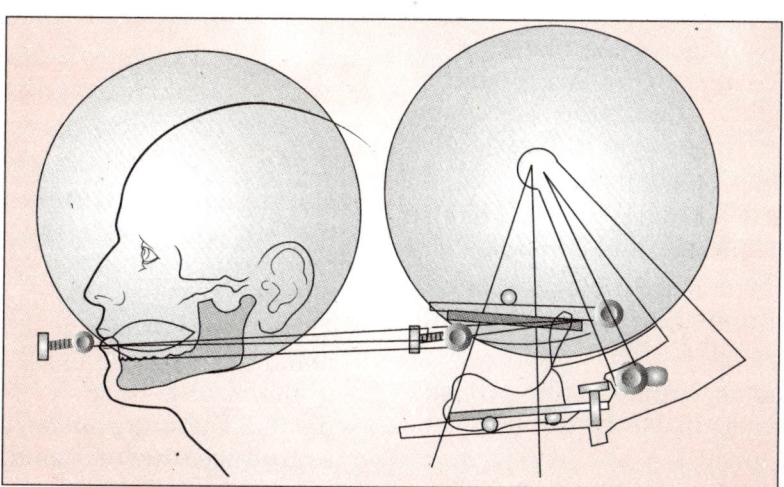

Fig. 17.7. Monson's spherical theory of occlusion.

the upper teeth as over the surface of a sphere with a diameter of 8 inches. The center of the sphere is located in the region of the glabella and the surfaces of the sphere passes through the glenoid fossa along the articulating eminences or concentric with them. This was proposed by Monson in 1918, e.g. maxillomandibular instrument.

Articulators Based on the Types of Records Used in their Adjustment

Three general classes of records are used for transferring maxillomandibular relationship from the patient to the articulator:
- Interocclusal records.
- Graphic records.
- Hinge axis records.

Some articulators are designed for use with only one type of record, whereas others use combinations of two or three types of records.

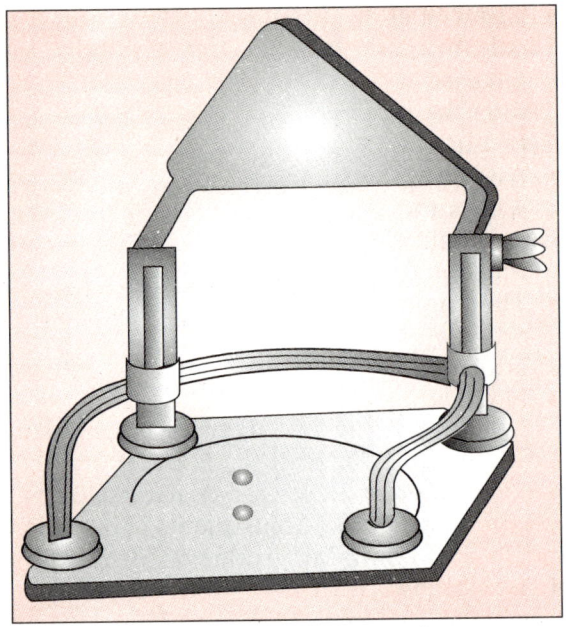

Fig. 17.8. A plain line articulator

Other Classifications

Posselt has classified articulators into three groups based upon their design:
- Plain line or simple hinge axis (Fig. 17.8)
- Mean value types with fixed condylar paths and incisal inclines.
- Adjustable articulators.

Primary disadvantage of the plane line or mean value articulator is the lack of individualized information concerning the spatial relationship of the patients joints to each other and to the terminal hinge axis.

Gillis, Boucher and Kingery (1936) classified articulators into adjustable and non-adjustable

Weinberg (1963) classified artculaters into: (i) arbitrary, (ii) positional, (iii) semiadjustable, and (iv) fully adjustable.

Beck classified articulators into: (i) suspension instruments, (ii) axis instruments, and (iii) tripod instruments.

Thomas (1973) classified articulators as: (i) arbitrary, (ii) positional., and (iii) functional.

Sharry (1974) classified articulators as: (i) simple hinge type, (ii) fixed guide type, and (iii) adjustable.

Filiani classified articulators as: (i) fully adjustable, (ii) semiadjustable, and (iii) non-adjustable.

SELECTION OF ARTICULATORS

Key Factors

- No mechanical instrument will reproduce the movements of the condyles in the temporomandibular fossae for all individuals.
- The accuracy of an articulator in reproducing mandibular movements is in direct relation to the records (made of mandibular movements. Therefore an articulator that will reproduce the movements recorded by natural teeth is not neccesarily the instrument of choice with the edentulous patients.

- Clinical evaluation of articulators particularly in complete denture constructions have so many variables that each dentist must be honest with himself in appraising results.
- An immediate side shift of the mandible without rotation is an anatomic and technical possibility. Individually controlled side shift must be molded for each patient.
- The single most important requirement of an articulator is to maintain centric relation. Next is to maintain vertical dimension of occlusion.
- No incisal guide can reproduce the arrangements of the anterior teeth.
- Sophisticated instruments require sophisticated methods to record mandibular movements.
- The sophisticated instruments are too expensive for students. When an articulator is used in the reconstruction procedures involving natural teeth, the articulator of preference is one that will accept pantograms in three planes, a 4-dimensional instrument.

When an articulator is selected for complete denture construction, the type will depend on: (i) type of occlusion to be developed, and (ii) kind of jaw relations records that will be made to adjust the articulator.

Further Reading

1. Weinberg L A. An evaluation of basic articulators and their concepts. J Prosth Dent. 1963; 13(4): 622-40.
2. Weinberg L A. An evaluation of basic articulators and their concepts. J Prosth Dent. 1963; 13(4): 644-63.
3. Mitchell D L. Articulators through the years. Part I. J Prosth Dent. 1978; 39(3): 330-38.
4. Mitchell D L. Articulators through the years. Part II. J Prosth Dent.1978; 39(4): 451-58.
5. Beck H.O. A clinical evaluation of the arcon concept of articulation. J Prosth Dent.1959; 9: 459.

MULTIPLE CHOICE QUESTIONS

1. **An arcon articulator is an articulator**
   a. Containing condylar elements in the upper member and condylar path elements in the lower member.
   b. Containing condylar path elements in the upper member ad condylar elements in the lower member.
   c. Containing both condylar elements and condylar path elements in the lower number.
   d. None of the above.

2. _____ **is an articulator that allows replication of 3-D movement of recorded mandibular motion.**
   a. Condylar articulator
   b. Semi adjustable articulator
   c. Fully adjustable articulator
   d. Average mean articulator

3. **Optimal articulator requirements include**
   a. Incisal guide pin and incisal guide table.
   b. Adjustable inter condylar distance and immediate bennett adjustment.
   c. Immediate bennett adjustment and incisal table that can be adjusted.
   d. Adjustable intercondylar distance and condylar guides that allow right lateral, left lateral and protrusive movement.

4. _____ **is the earliest articulator**
   a. Plaster articulator
   b. Barn door hinge
   c. Mean value articulator
   d. Gysi simplex

5. **The maxillomandibular instrument is based on**
   a. Bonwills triangle
   b. Curve of occlusion

c. Spherical theory

d. None of the above

6. _____ articulator was developed to be used with the functionally generated path technique.
a. Ney articulator
b. Pankey mann articulator
c. Hanau crown and bridge articulator
d. Verticulator

7. **The TMJ instrument is an example for a class _____ articulator**
a. II A   b. II B
c. III A   d. IV A

8. _____ **is an example for an articulator used primarily for complete denture fabrication.**
a. Irish Duplifunctional
b. Hanau

c. Dentatus

d. Denar mark II

9. **Statement that is true regarding Hanau articulator**
a. It was developed by Rudolf Hanau
b. It is a non arcon articulator
c. The bennett angle is measured by the equation $L = \dfrac{H}{8} + 12$
d. All are true.

10. **Hall's automatic articulator is based on**
a. Spherical theory
b. Conical theory
c. Bonwill's equilateral triangle
d. All of the above

11. **Example for a fully adjustable articulator**
a. Hanau   b. Dentatus ARO
c. Denar 4A   d. Ney

18

CONCEPTS OF OCCLUSION

Definition
Lingualized occlusion
Balanced occlusion
Non-balanced occlusion

DEFINITIONS

1. Anatomic Occlusion. An occlusal arrangement where in the posterior artificial teeth have masticatory surfaces that closely resemble those of the natural healthy dentition and articulate with similar natural or artificial surfaces/or anatomical occlusion.

2. Anterior Guidance. The influence of the contacting surfaces of anterior teeth on tooth limiting mandibular movements.

3. Anteroposterior Curve. The anatomic curve established by the occlusal alignment of the teeth, as projected onto the median plane, beginning with the cusp tip of the mandibular canine and following the buccal cusp tips of the premolar and molar teeth, continuing through the anterior border of the ramus, ending with the anterior most portion of the mandibular condyle.

4. Articulation. The state of dynamic contact relationship between the occlusal surfaces of the teeth during function.

5. Bull's Rule (acronym for buccal of the upper, lingual of the lower) applies to Clyde H Schulyers rules for occlusal adjustment of a normally related dentition in which those cusps contacting in maximum intercuspation are favored by adjustment of those cusps which are not in occlusal contact in maximum intercuspation.

6. Compensating Curve. The anteroposterior curvature (in the median plane) and the mediolateral curvature (in the frontal plane) in the alignment of the occluding surfaces and incisal edges of artificial teeth that are used to develop balanced occlusion.

7. Condylar Guidance. Mandibular guidance generated by the condyle and articular disk traversing the contour of the glenoid tossa.

8. Fischer's Angle. Eponym for the angle formed by the intersection of the protrusive and non-working side condylar paths as viewed in the sagittal plane.

9. Linear Occlusion. The occlusal arrangement of artifical teeth, as viewed in the horizontal plane wherein the masticatory surfaces of the mandibular posterior artificial teeth have a straight, long narrow occlusal form resembling that of a line, usually articulating with opposing monoplane teeth.

10. Lingualized Occlusion. This form of denture occlusion articulates the maxillary lingual cusps with the mandibular occlusal surfaces in centric working and non-working mandibular position (attributed to Earl Pound).

11. Mechanically Balanced Occlusion. A balanced occlusion without reference to physiologic considerations as on an articulation.

12. Monoplane Articulation. The arrangement of teeth by which they are positioned in a single plane.

13. Monoplane Occlusion. An occlusal arrangement where in the posterior teeth have masticatory surfaces that lack any cuspal height.

14. Non-working Side. That side of the mandible that moves toward the median line in a lateral excursion. The condyle in that side is referred to as the non-working side condyle.

15. Non-working Side Condyle Path. The path the condyle traverses on the non-working side when the mandible moves in a lateral excursion which may be viewed in the three reference planes of the body.

16. Physiologically Balanced Occlusion. A balanced occlusion that is in harmony with the TMJ and the neuromuscular system.

LINGUALIZED OCCLUSION

Lingualized occlusion, one of the more popular occlusal schemes was introduced by Alfred Gysi in 1927. The basic concepts of lingualized occlusion were suggested by Payne. It was Earl pound who first used the term "lingualized occlusion". This occlusal scheme should not be confused with the placement of mandibular teeth lingual to the ridge crest.

This occlusal scheme was introduced as an attempt to maintain the esthetics and food penetration advantages of the anatomic form while maintaining the mechanical freedom of the non-anatomic forms. It uses anatomic teeth for the maxillary denture and non-anatomic or semianatomic teeth for the mandibular denture. By definition, this form of dental occlusion articulates the maxillary lingual cusps with the mandibular occlusal surfaces in centric working and non-working mandibular positions. The maxillary buccal cusp is kept out of occlusion and only the maxillary lingual cusp will function in eccentric movements.

The mandibular posterior teeth are selected based on whether a balanced scheme is used. For a balanced scheme, the maxillary lingual cusp will oppose a mandibular tooth with an occlusal table having shallow inclines. For a non-balanced scheme, monoplane mandibular denture teeth are selected.

The lingualized occlusion concept allows a sharp penetrating cusp on the maxilla to occlude against a relatively flat occlusal plane. It works by a "mortar and pestle" action. The maxillary lingual cusps are free to move in all directions. These cusps can penetrates the bolus and then operate on the bolus in a holding and grinding fashion (as in a mortar and pestle.)

Lingualized occlusion (first described by S Howard Payne). This form of denture occlusion articulates the maxillary lingual cusps with the mandibular occlusal surfaces in centric working and non-working mandibular positions.

Linguo-occlusion. An occlusion in which a tooth or a group of teeth is located lingual to its normal position.

Indications

1. In a situation where the patient places a high priority on esthetics but the oral condition requires the use of non-anatomic teeth, e.g. severe alveolar ridge resorption, Class II ridge relationship.
2. When a complete denture opposes a removable partial denture.
3. Parafunctional habits.

Advantages

Payne stated the advantages as:
1. Can be adapted to different types of ridges
2. A solid maximum intercuspation
3. Absence of deflective occlusal contacts in lateral excursions
4. Esthetic arrangement of teeth
5. Balanced articulation can be achieved.

Types of Tooth Forms used

1. Semianatomic teeth
2. Non-anatomic teeth
3. Myerson lingualized integration tooth molds.

Principles of Lingualized Occlusion

1. Anatomic teeth are used for the maxillary denture. Teeth with prominent lingual cusps are helpful.
2. The buccal cusps are raised above the occlusal plane. They have no functional role. They improve esthetics and help prevent cheek biting.
3. Non-anatomic or semi-anatomic teeth are used for the mandibular denture. A narrow occlusal table is preferred where severe residual ridge resorption has occurred.
4. Modification of the mandibular posterior teeth is accomplished using selective grinding.
5. When the patient moves into a working relationship, the lingual cusp of the maxil- lary teeth functions against the mandibular teeth (hence the term lingualized occlusion).
6. Meyerson lingualized integration (MLI) molds have been introduced for use in lingualized occlusion.

Advantages of MLI Tooth Molds

1. Provide maximum intercuspation.
2. An absence of deflective occlusal contacts.
3. Adequate cusp height for selective grinding.
4. Natural and pleasing appearance.

MLI Teeth are Available in Two Posterior Tooth Molds (Table 18.1)

1. Controlled contact (CC)
2. Maximum contact (MC).

The mandibular teeth are same for both molds. (with lower cusp height and multiple sliceways). The difference between the two molds is in the maxillary posterior teeth.

The controlled contact molds are indicated for patients in whom uncertainity exists in reproduction and repeatability of centric jaw relation position. This is because this mold will provide for greater freedom of movement around maximum intercuspation.

Maximum contact molds are used for patients with good muscle control and easy reproducibility of jaw relation records.

Steps in Arrangement of Teeth

1. Mandibular teeth are set first to establish the occlusal plane.

Table 18.1. Differences between the molds	
Controlled contact	*Maximum contact*
1. Indicated for patients in whom uncertainity exists in reproduction of centric relation position	1. For patients with good muscle control and easy reproducibility of jaw relation records
2. Cusps heights are lower	Maxillary teeth are more anatomical in appearance with greater cusp height
More flexibility is permitted around maximum intercuspation	More exacting occlusion can be attained in maximum intercuspation
Bilateral balanced articulation is present but with lesser range of contact	Bilateral balanced articulation can be obtained over a range of movement (may require minor selective grinding)

2. Anteroposterior and mediolateral compensating curves are established in the mandibular arch.
3. Maxillary teeth are set.

BALANCED OCCLUSION

Types of Balance

Balance may be : 1. Unilateral
                  (i) lever
                  (ii) occlusal
          2. Bilateral
          3. Protrusive

Unilateral Lever Balance

Unilateral lever balance is present when there is equilibrium of the base and its supporting structures when a bolus is interspersed between the teeth on one side, and a space exists between the teeth on the opposite side. This is encouraged by
1. Placing the teeth so that the resultant direction of force on the functional side is over the ridge or slightly lingual to it.
2. Having the denture base cover as large an area as possible
3. Placing teeth as close to the ridge as possible

Unilateral Occlusal Balance. This is present when the occlusal surfaces of teeth on one side articulate simultaneously as a group with a smooth uninterrupted glide.

Bilateral Occlusal Balance

Advantages

1. Balanced occlusion facilitates the stabilization of the denture base. As one side comes into contact in a lateral eccentric excursive movement, bilateral contacts will prevent the rocking of the denture away from the underlying supporting structures. This movement can cause soreness and inflammation.

2. Swallowing. During the course of a day an average individual swallows approximately 1500-2000 times. During each swallowing cycle teeth come into contact. Bilateral balance allows these contact's to be made evenly without displacing, scuffing or shearing of the denture base against the oral mucosa.

3. Chewing. The axiom "Enter bolus-exit balance" is a frequently heard argument to refute balancing complete dentures. Brewer and Hudson demonstrated that during the masticatory cycle teeth make contact. Balanced occlusion will prevent the disruptive lateral forces that are generated against the basal seat during parafunctional activity. If balanced occlusion is not established, unequal pressure will be exerted against the basal seat during the terminal arc of closure of the chewing cycle. Nepola stated that balanced occlusion makes possible the greatest possible use of masticating power so that food may be properly prepared for digestion.

4. Para functional movements. During parafunctional movements, balanced occlusion will prevent the destructive lateral forces that are generated against the basal seat.

5. Christensen phenomenon. In Protrusive movement of the mandible a space is created by the downward and forward movement of the condyle riding along the articular eminence. This removes the posterior teeth from occlusion (the natural dentition) This shift of pressure to the premolars is known as **Christensen phenomenon**. In complete dentures if balanced occlusion is not provided in protrusive excursion, the resulting posterior disocclusion and pressure in the premolar area can cause dislodgement of the base (Fig. 18.1).

Disadvantages of Balanced Occlusion
- Difficult in Class II cases.
- Tend to encourage lateral and protrusive grinding habits
- Semi or fully adjustable articulator is required
- Trapazzano studied masticatory efficiency of balanced and non-balanced occlusion and concluded that masticatory efficiency was

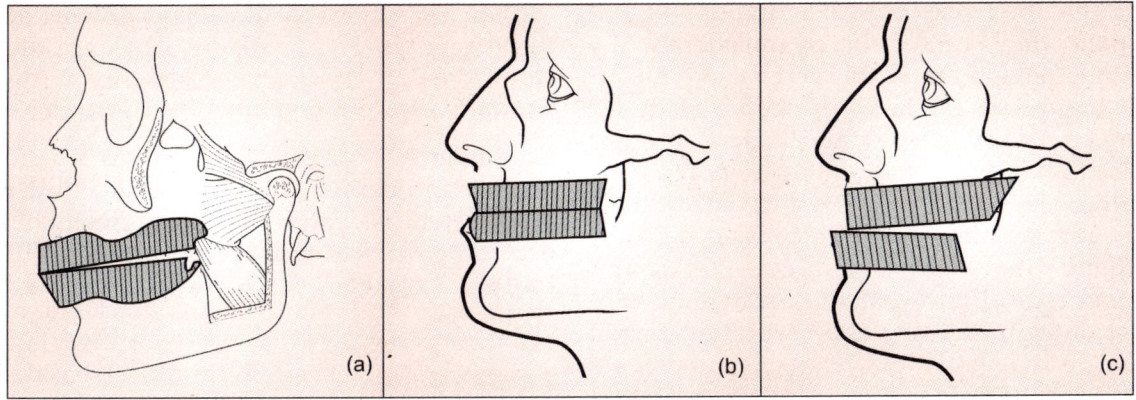

Fig. 18.1. Christensen phenomenon

only slightly greater but that stability was greatly enhanced

- Procedures involved in producing a set-up of dentures in balance occlusion are much more complex and time consuming than those producing dentures without balance.

Thielemann's Formula or Principle

Thielemann's formula and principle states non-mathematically that

Trapazzano stated that the degree of condylar inclination registered results from:
1. Shape of the bony contours of TMJ
2. Action of the muscle attaching to the mandible

$$\text{Balanced occlusion} = \frac{\text{Condylar guidance} \times \text{Incisal guidance}}{\text{Cusp height} \times \text{Curve of spee} \times \text{Plane of occlusion}}$$

3. Limitation of movements effected by the attaching ligaments
4. Method used for registration (displacement of tissues upon the which recording bases rest is referred to as realiff).

Condylar Guidance.[5] Dentist has the power to establish all factors except condylar path. It is the mandibular guidance generated by the condyles traversing the contours of the glenoid fossa.

It refers to the path that the transcranial rotation axes of the condyles travel during mandibular opening. This path may be measured in degrees from the FH plane. It is one factor which the edentulous patient presents and which in no way can be modified by the operators. Once the condylar inclination has been registered, no increase or decrease can be affected by the operator.

It forms one of the end controlling factors and is obtained by means of a protrusive registration.

Incisal Guidance.[2] Incisal guidance is defined as the influence of the contacting surfaces of mandibular and maxillary teeth on mandibular movements.[4]

It is the second end controlling factor.[4] Incisal guide angle is the angle formed in the horizontal plane by drawing a line in the sagittal plane between the incisal edges of maxillary and mandibular central incisors when teeth are in centric occlusion.

Limitations. Imposed on the selection of incisal guidance angle are:
- Ridge relation
- Arch shape
- Ridge fullness
- Inter ridge space
- Phonetic or esthetic requirements of the patient.

Within the range of these limitations, incisal guidance angle can be altered considerably by altering the horizontal and vertical overlap.

If the incisal guidance is steep, it calls for steep cusps and steep occlusal curve to effect occlusal balance. This is detrimental to the denture bases.

So for complete denture occlusions, incisal guidance should be as flat as esthetics and phonetics will allow. If the arrangement of anterior teeth necessitates a vertical overlap, a compensating horizontal overlap should be set to prevent dominant incisal guidance from upsetting posterior teeth balance.

To increase the incisal guidance, horizontal overlap and vertical overlap should be increased.

Orientation of Occlusal-plane

Average plane established by incisal and occlusal surfaces of teeth. If the soft tissues surrounding the dentures are to function as they did for natural teeth, the occlusal plane should be oriented exactly as it was when the natural teeth were present.

By positioning the anterior teeth correctly for esthetic appearance and locating the posterior end of the occlusal plane approximately 2/3 way up the retromolar pad, the dentist determines the orientation of the occlusal plane.

Cuspal Inclination[3]

Cuspal inclination refers to the angle between the total occlusal surface of the tooth and the inclination of the cusp in relation to that surface.

33-mesial slope makes 33° angle with a plane touching the tips of all cusps of the tooth

Tipping the teeth can produce an occlusal curve and make the effective height of the cusps greater or less. Even 0° teeth can be arranged to present inclined planes to their opposing teeth.

Cuspal inclination can be reduced when the distal end of the lower tooth is set lower than the mesial end or made steeper by opposite tipping.

Prominence of Compensating Curves

Prominence of compensating curves is defined as the anteroposterior curvature and the mediolateral curvatures in the alignment of the occluding surfaces and incisal edges of artificial teeth that are used to develop balanced occlusion.

Lateral Curve

Curve of Wilson. An imaginary line drawn mediolaterally to touch cusp tips of similar teeth on each side of the mandibular arch. When viewed in the frontal plane it appears to be concave.

Curve of Monson

Eponym for a proposed ideal curve of occlusion in which each cusp and incisal edge touches or conforms to a segment of the surface of a sphere 8" in diameter with its center in the region of glabella (Fig. 18.2).

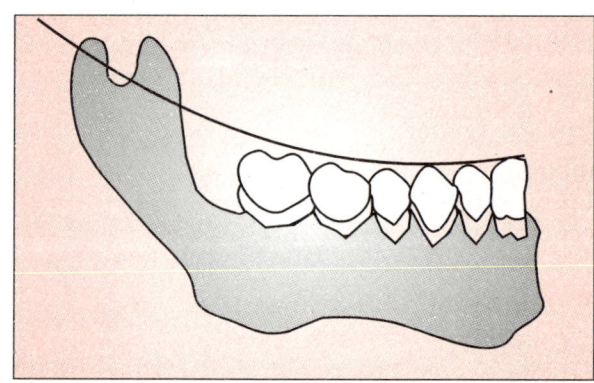

Fig. 18.2. Curve of Monson.

Curve of Pleasure/Anti-Monson/Frequency C/Probability C/Reverse Curve

In excessive wear of teeth, occlusion of cusps and formation of either flat or cupped-out occlusal surfaces is associated with reversal of the occlusal plane of the premolar, first and second molar teeth (III molars-unaffected) whereby the occlusal surfaces of the mandibular teeth incline facially instead of lingually and those of the maxillary teeth incline lingually.

So in complete dentures, the incorporation of mediolateral curves results from an inward inclination of lower posterior teeth.

Trapazzano (1963) reviewed Hanau's five factors and detected that only three factors were actually concerned in obtaining balanced occlusion (Fig. 18.3). He eliminated the need for compensating curves and called it triad of occlusion.

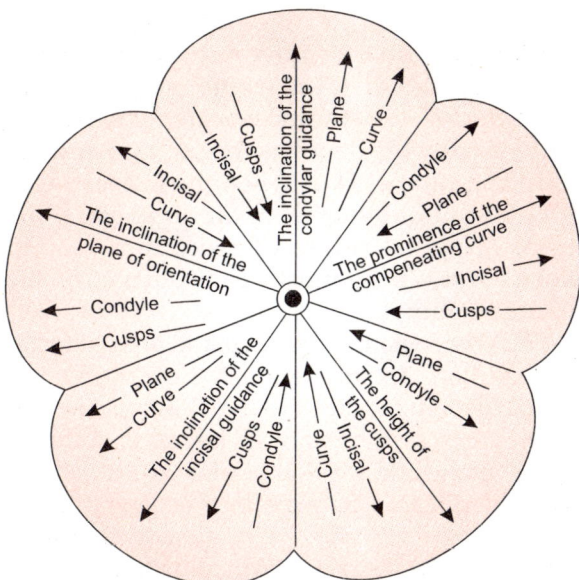

Fig. 18.4. Articulation quint by Hanau.

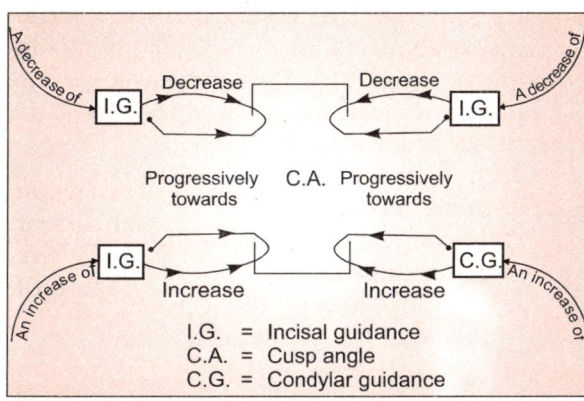

Fig. 18.3. Trappazano's triad.

Levin (1978) described the laws of articulation in a Quad (Figs 18.4, 18.5). However, Hanau's five laws were found to be more acceptable:

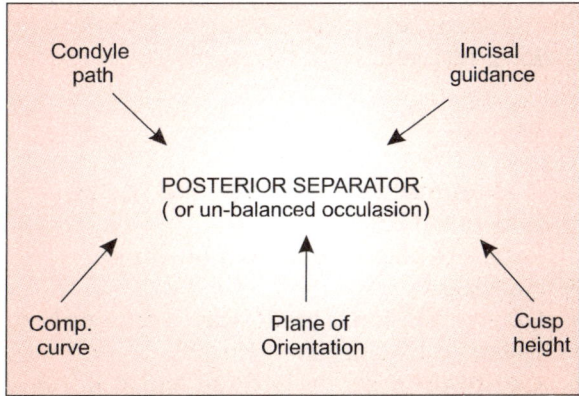

Fig. 18.5. Laws of occlusion (Lott).

Laws of Lateral Balance

1. Condylar inclination on the balancing side
2. Incisal guidance
3. Compensating curves on balancing and working side
4. Cusp height or inclination on balancing side.
5. Lingual inclines of upper buccal cusps on working side
6. Buccal inclines of lower lingual cusps on working side
7. Bennett shift on working side.

Balancing Ramps[1]

Balancing ramps built in the region of the retromolar pads greatly simplify the procedure of balancing the occlusion. This applies

1. When posterior teeth with zero degree cusps are used and when vertical overlap is considerable.

If esthetics is considered more important, posterior teeth will not contact in protrusive position resulting in tripping of dentures.

When balancing ramps are used, as the mandible begins to move into a protrusive excursion, the distal marginal ridges of the occlusal surfaces of the most posterior maxillary teeth (usually the II molars) begin to ascend the balancing ramps. Thus when the incisal edges of opposing anterior teeth are in contact, the distal marginal ridges of the upper second molars rest on the most distal portion of the balancing ramp.

Thus the incisors in protrusion are balanced by maxillary molars against the ramps. The same balancing ramps are made broad enough so that they will balance in lateral excursions of the mandible. Distobuccal margins of the occlusal surfaces of maxillary second molars glide along the ramps on the balancing side. Consequently, the patient can glide from centric occlusion to protrusive occlusion and from right and left lateral excursions without the discomfort of intercuspal interferences, diminished retention, tissue irritation and clicking of teeth.

Procedure

1. Wax is built up buccally and distally on lower trial base
2. Excess is placed to allow polishing
3. Acrylised
4. Centric relation is made, then a remounting, followed by selective grinding
5. Cavity preparation is done and it is filled with silver amalgam
6. Polished.

Grewcock (1953) suggested that the following factors must the considered in the establishment of balanced occlusion:
- True centric occlusion
- Free lateral guiding movements
- Equal distribution of stresses
- Retention or re-establishment of physiologic occlusal vertical dimension.

Teeth in true centric occlusion will be subjected to axial stress only, the maximum intensity of which is controlled by muscle tension reaching its correct physiologic degree of contraction at the normal occlusal vertical dimension.

Lateral stresses to the point of overloading can cause progressive destruction of the periodontium. Free lateral movement should be established by selective grinding to eliminate cusp interference.

Occlusal equilibrium is sought to ensure that all teeth will lie as uniformly stressed as possible during mastication. Certain conditions which render it advisable to change the vertical dimension are esthetic considerations, pathologic conditions such as periodontitis and its sequelae, functional requirements and disturbances in the TMJ resulting from vertical dimension abnormalities.

Grewcock put forth three principles in the establishment of balanced occlusion. They are:
1. Orthodontic treatment
2. Selective grinding
3. Prosthetic reconstruction
   - Without changing the height of occlusal vertical dimension.
   - Re-establishment of occlusal vertical dimension when possible.

NON-BALANCED OCCLUSION

Balanced occlusion involves the simultaneous, bilateral anterior and posterior occlusal contact of teeth in centric and eccentric positions. All other occlusal arrangements are considered as non-balanced occlusion. These include the arrangement of teeth according to the spherical theory, organic occlusion, occlusal balancing ramps for protrusive balance, and transographics and on a plane.

Spheric Occlusion

Spheric occlusion involves arrangement of teeth with anteroposterior and mediolateral inclination in harmony with a spherical surface.

Organic occlusion (organized occlusion). Organic occlusion calls for the alteration of the shape of the cusps of the teeth to provide prosthetic teeth that have cusps suitable for the individual patient. The ridge and groove directions of the posterior teeth are determined as a result of the movements of the condyles. The cusps height, fossa depth of posterior teeth and the proper concavity of the lingual surfaces of the maxillary anterior teeth are determined as a result of mandibular movements. The cusp-fossa contact relation is developed when the jaws are in centric relation.

When the mandible is moved in a protrusive direction, the incisors cause separation of the posterior teeth. When the mandible is moved in a lateral direction, the canine causes separation of the posterior teeth. The posterior teeth are altered by grinding and inclined to provide a lack of contact on the working and balancing side in eccentric mandibular movements. The cusps are related to a cusp for a centric relation in which the cusp can enter the fossae and escape without lateral or sagittal interferences. In centric occlusal position the posterior teeth should protect the anterior teeth.

Neutrocentric Concept (by Devan)

Neutrocentric concept embodies the centralization of occlusal forces that act on the basal seat when the mandible is in centric relation to the maxillae. This concept states that the anteroposterior plane of occlusion should be parallel with the plane of the denture foundation and not indicated by the horizontal condylar angle. Compensating curves will not be provided. In a mediolateral direction, teeth are set flat with no medial or lateral inclination.

Features of Neutrocentric Concept

1. Eliminates anteroposterior and mediolateral inclines of the teeth and directs the forces of occlusion to the posterior teeth
2. The posterior teeth are placed in as mediolateral a relation (in reference to the residual ridge) as tongue function will allow.
3. Patient is instructed to avoid incising with anterior teeth
4. As non-anatomic teeth are used, there will be no projection above or below the occlusal plane
5. The horizontal condylar guidance and lateral guidances of the articulator are set at zero
6. The buccolingual width of the teeth are reduced in order to direct force towards the center of the ridge and to reduce frictional forces
7. Number of teeth are reduced to avoid placing a tooth on the ridge in the second molar area.

Further Reading

1. Nepola S R. Balancing ramps in prosthetic occlusion. J Prosth Dent.1958; 8(5): 776-80.
2. Weinberg L A. Incisal and condylar guidance in relation to cuspal inclination. J Prosth Dent. 1959; 9(5): 851-61.
3. Christensen F T. The effect on change in incisal guide angle on cusp angulation. J Prosth Dent. 1971; 26(1): 93-8.
4. Schuyler C H. The function ad importance of incisal guidance in oral rehabilitation. J Prosth Dent. 1963; 13(6): 1011-28.
5. Pipko D J. Evaluation of validity of condylar path curvature. J Prosth Dent. 1969, 11(6): 626-38

MULTIPLE CHOICE QUESTIONS

1. _____ is the angle formed by the intersection of the protrusive and non working side condylar paths as viewed in the sagittal plane.
   a. Condylar guidance angle
   b. Incisal guidance angle
   c. Christensen's angle
   d. Fischer's angle

2. True statement regarding balancing ramps
   a. They are used for developing balanced occlusion,
   b. They are placed opposite the maxillary second molars
   c. Used with zero degree teeth
   d. All are true

3. _____ is the state of dynamic contact between the occlusal surfaces of the teeth during function
   a. Occlusion
   b. Articulation
   c. Mechanically balanced occlusion
   d. Anatomic occlusion

4. Bull's rule is used
   a. To set teeth to balanced occlusion
   b. For occlusal adjustment
   c. To perfect occlusal morphology
   d. None of the above

5. A physiologically balanced occlused is one in which
   a. Occlusion is not in harmony with physiologic factors
   b. Is the same as anatomic occlusion
   c. Occlusion that is in harmony with the temporomandibular joint and neuromuscular system
   d. Is the same as bilaterally balanced occlusion

6. The term lingualized occlusion was first used by
   a. Earl pound
   b. Gysi
   c. Payne
   d. Boucher

7. The true statement regarding lingualized occlusion
   a. Is the same as linguo occlusion
   b. It works by a "mortar and pestle" action
   c. Can be used in patients with parafunctional habits
   d. b and c are true

8. The "controlled contact molds" are used in situation
   a. Where good muscle control exists
   b. Reproducibility of jaw relation records is good
   c. Uncertainty exists in recording centric relation position
   d. All of the above

9. Christensen's phenomenon is seen during
   a. Protrustive movement in nature dentition
   b. Protrusive movement in denture-wearing patients
   c. In lateral movement in natural dentition
   d. In lateral movement in denture-wearing patient

10. The factor that cannot be controlled or modified by the dentist when developing balanced occlusion is
    a. Incisal guidance
    b. Condylar guidance
    c. Compensating curve
    d. Cusp height

11. The curve of pleasure is also referred to as
    a. Curve of Monson
    b. Reverse curve
    c. Probability curve
    d. b and c

FAQ's

1. Definition of
   a. Occlusion
   b. Balanced occlusion
   c. Nonbalanced occlusion

2. Hanau's quint

3. Lingualized occlusion

GNATHOLOGICAL CONCEPTS

INTRODUCTION

The term gnathology was originally coined by McCollum in 1926 to describe the study and treatment of the entire mouth as a functional unit. The term gnathology is derived from the Greek word 'Gnathes' which means 'jaws' (gnatho pertains to jaw or cheek).

McCollum believed gnathology as science that deals with the biologies of the masticatory mechanism that is the morphology, anatomy, histology, physiology, pathology and therapeutics of the oral organ, especially the jaws and teeth and the vital relations of these organs to the rest of the body. The use of the term gnathology was coined to call the attention of dentist to the importance of jaws without minimizing the importance of teeth. Gnathology deals with the masticatory apparatus as a unit and concerns with the function of this complex oral entity.

COMPONENTS OF THE ODONTOSTOMATOGNATHIC SYSTEM

Gnathology deals with the masticatory apparatus as a single unit. The three inseparable units are: the TMJ, occlusal surfaces, and neuromuscular components. These three function in harmony. Disorder of any one affects the other two. Problems of occlusion cannot be understood or treated without a knowledge of the TMJ, the muscles and the neuromuscular mechanism.

The Temporomandibular Joint

The area where craniomandibular articulation occurs is called the temporomandibular joint. The joint is formed by the mandibular condyle fitting into the mandibular fossa of the temporal bone.

The condyle, the portion of the mandible that articulates with the cranium has medial and lateral projections called poles. The medial poles generally is more prominent than the lateral. The total mediolateral width of the condyle is 15-20 mm. The articulating surface of the condyle extends both anteriorly and posteriorly to the most superior aspect of the condyle convex. The squamous portion of the temporal bone is made up of a concave mandibular fossa into which the condyle fits. This is also referred to as the articular or glenoid fossa.

Posterior to the mandibular fossa is squamo-tympanic fissure which extends mediolaterally dividing into the petrosquamous fissure anteriorly and the petrotympanic fissure posteriorly. Anteriorly, a convex bony prominence, the articular eminence exists. The steepness of the articular eminence determines the pathway of the condyle when the mandible is positioned anteriorly. The posterior roof of the mandibular fossa is thin, indicating that this surface is not designed to withstand stress.

The TMJ is considered as a ginglymoarthroidal joint as it allows both hinge and gliding movements. It is also classified as a compound joint (because it is made up of two bones and the articular eminence, which serves as a non-ossified bone).

Articular Disk. The articular disk is composed of dense fibrous connective tissue. It is devoid of nerves and blood vessels. In a sagittal section, it has three regions: a central area, which is thinnest and called the intermediate zone and anterior and posterior borders. The posterior border is slightly thicker than the anterior border. The articulating surface of the condyle is located in the intermediate zone. The precise shape of the disk is determined by the morphology of the condyle and the mandibular fossa.

The articular disk is attached posteriorly to an area of loose connective tissue that is highly vascularized and innervated. This is known as the retrodiskal tissue. Superiorly it is bordered by the superior retrodiskal lamina which contains elastic fibers. Inferiorly it is bordered by the inferior retrodiskal lamina that has collagenous fibers.

The articular surfaces of the mandibular fossa and condyle are lined with dense fibrous connective tissue. This gives it certain advantages. This tissue is less likely to breakdown over time and has a greater ability to repair itself.

The capsular ligament encloses the articular disk and divides the joint into two cavities. The superior cavity is bordered by the mandibular fossa and the superior surface of the disk. The inferior cavity is bordered by the mandibular condyle and the inferior surface of the disk. The internal surface of the cavities are lined by specialized endothelial cells that form a synovial lining.

These cells produce synovial fluid. This fluid helps in lubrication and provides metabolic requirements to these tissues. The fluid is produced by two mechanisms, boundary lubrication and weeping lubrication.

Accessory Ligaments of the TMJ

Sphenomandibular Ligament. This ligament arises from the spine of the sphenoid bone and extends downwards and laterally to a small bony prominence (lingula) of the mandible. It has only a limited effect on mandibular movement.

Stylomandibular Ligament. It arises from the styloid process and extends downwards and forwards to the angle and posterior border of the ramus of the mandible. It helps in limiting the excessive protrusive movements of the mandible.

Muscles of Mastication

Masseter. This is a rectangular muscle that originates from the zygomatic arch and extends downwards to the lateral aspect of the lower border of the ramus of the mandible. The posterior portion has fibers that run almost horizontally.

Functions
- When the entire muscle contracts, it elevates the mandible
- When the anterior portion contracts, the mandible is raised vertically

- Contraction of the middle portion will elevate and retrude the mandible.

The Medial Pterygoid. It originates from the pterygoid fossa and extends downward, backward and outward to insert along the medial surface of the mandibular angle.

Functions. When its muscles contract the mandible is elevated. This muscle is also active in protruding the mandible. Unilateral contraction can cause mediotrusive movement of the mandible.

The medial pterygoid is made up of two heads: A superficial portion consists of fibers that run downward and backward, the deep portion consists of fibers that run vertically.

Functions
- Elevation of the mandible
- The superficial portion helps in protruding the mandible.

The Temporalis. It is a large fan-shaped muscle that originates from the temporal fossa and the lateral surface of the skull. The fibers extend downward form a tendon and inserts into the coronoid process and anterior border of the ascending ramus.

It can be divided into three areas based on the fiber direction and ultimate function. The anterior portion consists of fibers that are directed vertically. The middle portion has fibers that run obliquely across the lateral aspect of the skull

Lateral (external) Pterygoids
The inferior lateral pterygoid. This muscle originates at the outer surface of the lateral pterygoid plate and extends backwards, upward and outward to its insertion on the neck of the condyle. When both the inferior lateral pterygoids contract, the mandible is protruded; unilateral contraction creates a mediotrusive movement of the condyle and causes a lateral movement of the mandible to the opposite side.

Superior lateral pterygoid. This muscle is smaller than the inferior lateral pterygoid. It originates at the infratemporal surface of the great sphenoid wing and extends backwards to insert on the articular disc capsule and near the neck of the condyle. This muscle is especially active during the power stroke (such as in chewing) and when the teeth are held together.

Bennett Movement

Bennett movement was described by Bennett in 1908 to indicate a lateral bodily side shift of the mandible taking place on the working side. Several terms have been introduced as an alternative to Bennett movement such as : (i) mandibular side shift, (ii) Bennett side shift , and (iii) lateral side shift.

Although Bennett has described about this movement which become popularly known as Bennett movement, the original discovery of this movement should go to Balkwill. As early as in 1870 Balkwill observed that the mandible opened and closed on an axis that runs through the condyles, that the condyles move downwards and forwards in protrusion and also the mandible moves bodily from side to side. His observation was forgotten and remained in the archives of London library. Without knowing Balkwill's work Bennett demonstrated that the TMJ permitted three kinds of movements.

Bennett side shift has two components, an immediate side shift which is straight outside bodily shift (laterotrusion) and a progressive side shift which occur at a rate which is directly proportional to the forward movement of the orbiting condyle of the opposite side.

Occlusal Philosophies and Concepts of Occlusion

1. Gnathological concept of occlusion, point centric concept of occlusion.
2. Long centric occlusion.
3. Cuspid protected occlusion.
4. Multiple contact position.
5. Group function.
6. Mutually protected occlusion.
7. Bilateral balanced occlusion, crossmouth balance.

8. Organic occlusion.
9. Myocentric occlusion.

MALOCCLUSION

Occlusion is also referred as contact position or occlusal position of teeth. If an occlusion which is defined as normal according to Angle's classification of malocclusion has a slide in centric, this is dangerous. The presence of a centric slide or any other form of occlusal disharmony in lateral movements has a pathological influence on the stomatognathic system, and this decides whether malocclusion is physiological or pathological.

The classical description of malocclusion by Angle seldom results in TMJ pain dysfunction. One of the reasons for this is because of the fact that in Angle's divisions of malocclusions, there is harmony between centric relation and centric occlusion and there is no cuspal interference that prevents the mandible from closing in centric position. In other words, in the Angle's classification of malocclusion, there is no condylar slide in centric position. Condylar slide is harmful as it can produce muscle spasm and TMJ dysfunction.

The orthodontica malocclusion is physiological malocclusion as it causes no detrimental influence on TMJ of muscle function. Contrarily, in a person with no apparent orthodontic malocclusion, the presence of a centric slide from the gnathological point of view is a malocclusion.

Classification of Malocclusion

1. Morphological malocclusion (developmental malocclusion, physiological malocclusion).
2. Pathological malocclusion (gnathological malocclusion, functional malocclusion),
   The Angle's system of malocclusion is based on key to occlusion, while the gnathological concept of malocclusion is based on occlusioneuromuscular harmony.

Morphological Malocclusion

The orthodontic classification of malocclusion is an esthetic oriented malocclusion. The orthodontic malocclusion refers to malaligned or malposed teeth which is a developmental and morphological condition presenting esthetic problems. It is a physiological occlusion for that particular individual and well within the limits of normal neuromuscular response. A malocclusion of this nature cannot cause a neuromuscular disharmony or TMJ dysfunction.

Pathological Malocclusion

A pathological malocclusion is a condition where there is a centric prematurity and deflective occlusal contact, which can trigger neuromuscular response to alter the neuromuscular behavior leading to plan of action or plan of inaction. It has been shown that one tenth of a millimeter displacement of the condyle ventrally due to deflective occlusal contact can give rise to muscle spasm and the consequences which follow it. Elimination of undesirable occlusal contacts relieves spasm and reveral occurs.

Types of Pathological Malocclusion

1. Centric prematurity. As a result of centric occlusion not being identical with centric relation, premature contact occurs when the jaws meet in centric relation. These cuspal interferences prevent the mandible from closing in terminal hinge closure. Mandible deviates medially, distally and laterally.

2. Working side (functional side) cuspal interferences and prematurity. Occlusal interference in the form of premature contact of the lingual cusps of functional side must be removed to permit the buccal slopes on the functional side to contact each other.

3. Parafunctional contacts. Parafunctional contacts are non-functional occlusal contacts which are harmful and it should be eliminated.

Balancing contacts. This is seen on the balancing side between the palatal cusp of the upper and buccal cusp of the lower.

Protrusive contacts. This is seen between the upper and lower posterior teeth when the jaw is in protrusion.

OPTIMAL OCCLUSION

Characteristics of Optimal Occlusion and Principles of Occlusal Rehabilitation

1. The direction of axial stress should be as nearly as possible to the long axis of the teeth. Avoid detrimental horizontal overloading of the teeth. Horizontal stress is not compatible to the periodontal membrame.
2. Distribute occlusal force simultaneously on as many teeth as possible in terminal hinge closure.
3. Optimum centric occlusion. Teeth should meet uninterfered in retruded closure.
4. The teeth should move in and out of centric occlusion without any slide or interference.
5. Canine should act as proprioceptive guard for lateral movement. It should separate all other teeth in lateral movement. There should be no lateral glides of other posterior teeth.
6. Anterior group contact should be possible. Anterior teeth should disclude the posterior teeth from coming into contact.
7. When canine-guided relation cannot be restored there should be group function between the buccal cusps on the working side. Avoid crossmouth balance which is detrimental.
8. If centric occlusion is slightly in front of centric relation, provide an unrestricted glide from CR or CO.
9. A cusp-to-fossa occlusion, tripoding of cusp elements (between cusp and fossa). Achieve tripodisation as far as possible.
10. Observe for clear, short, snapping sound when teeth are tapped in centric occlusion.

TMJ DISORDERS

Temporomandibular disorders comprise a wide range of clinical conditions involving the TMJ. There are several disorders affecting the joint which have an organic lesion in it. Diseases which affect the other joints of the human body are also common to this joint. These lesions form a very negligible proportion of persons seeking treatment requiring the expertise of our medical colleagues for its recognition and management. However, the more common TMJ problem which one sees today is not a disorder of the joint having a joint pathology, but rather a healthy joint manifesting certain symptom complexes. These are better understood by a dentist rather than the other specialists in medical profession.

Thus, the dental practitioner finds himself in an important position where his medical associates look upon him for the diagnosis, management and execution of necessary treatment of TMJ dysfunction. The functioning of TMJ is related to occlusion of teeth and there is no one justified or competent than the dentist who can understand and recognize this condition better. Initially persons having TMJ dysfunction seldom visit the dentist but rather seek consultations from their general physician, orthopedic surgeon, otolaryngologist or pain clinics before finally being referred to the dentist's office. Is the dentist properly equipped to take up the responsibility to identify the condition and provide relief ?

Classification of TMJ Disorders

Broadly, TMJ disorders can be grouped into two categories. There are conditions affecting the joint showing evidence of inflammatory, traumatic, congenital or developmental origin. There is yet another condition where there is no demonstratable clinical, radiographic or biochemical evidence to show the presence of any organic lesion in the joint. In other words, it is a healthy joint which manifests certain signs and symptoms of dysfunction.

Group A: Pathology in the Joint

Infective Arthritis
1. Very rare
2. Caused by specific organisms
3. Origin from an open wound, infection from ear or blood borne.
4. Acute pain, swelling, warmth, skin discoloration present.
5. Evidence of septicemia
6. Diagnosis confirmed by culture of joint fluid.

Rheumatoid Arthritis
1. Temporomandibular joint is never the site of onset of rheumatoid arthritis but may occur in those who have rheumatoid arthritis in other joints.
2. Characterized by inflammation of synovial tissues accompanied by infiltration of lymphocytes and plasma cells.
3. Results in destruction of angular surface of the joint and may be accompanied by fibrous ankylosis.
4. In early stage there is joint pain but in later stages there is restriction in movements of the lower jaw.

Degenerative Arthritis or Osteoarthritis
1. In non-weight-bearing joint such as TMJ, the incidence is low as compared to weight-bearing joints.
2. Rarely before middle age.
3. The cartilage covering the condyle thins out, later the condylar head is denuded of cartilage; rough bony surface comes in relation to the joint cavity.
4. The disk thins out and eventually perforates.
5. Cracking sounds and crepitus felt.

Traumatic Arthritis
1. Severe trauma produces synovitis accompanied with sharp pain, swelling and dysfunction.
2. Trauma due to careless extraction procedures, yawning and dislocation often cause the posterior part of the capsule to tear.
3. Deviation of the mandible to the affected side.
4. Tenderness on palpation through the external auditory meatus.

Lesions in the Disk
1. Perforation of disk.
2. Tearing of the posterior attachment of disc.

Metabolic Joint Diseases
(e.g. gout, osteomalacia, hyperparathyroidism, Paget disease.

Lesions in Group A are rare and not within the scope of a dentist to manage them. These disorders should be differentiated from a more frequently seen TMJ dysfunction which does not have any pathology in the joint.

Group B: No Evidence of Articular Pathology

There is no disease in the joint but only dysfunction.

1. Costen's Syndrome (Distal Displacement Theory). A collection of symptom complex of TMJ and ear disturbances described by Costen in 1934, which he attributed to overclosure of the jaws due to loss of posterior teeth. Some of the classical features he described were: intermittent impaired hearing, stuffy sensation in the ears, dizziness, tinnitus, dull drawing pain within ear, headache above vertex, occiput and behind ear, burning sensation in the throat, tongue and side of nose and snapping noise in the joint while chewing. Costen felt that consequent to decrease in the vertical height of the jaws, the condyle was displaced posteriorly against the posterior structures of the TMJ, thereby compressing the auriculotemporal, chorda tympani nerves and the other retrocondylar structures. Symptoms described by Costen were related to pressure on these structures.

The condylar distal displacement theory was later challenged by many research workers who proved conclusively that the symptom complex described by Costen are unrelated anatomically and clinically. Today, there is no clinical condition such as Costen's syndrome, since it has been disproved.

2. Anterior Displacement Theory: Ramjtord felt that the anterior displacement of condyle during centric closure is detrimental and pain is elicited from contacts in the anterior area of TMJ rather than the posterior region of the joint. This theory is supported by the observation that patients with TMJ dysfunction have preference to use the affected side for chewing. This can be explained as follows:

During mastication the condyle on the chewing functional side simply rotates without any forward translation, while of the non-functional side, the condyle translates medially and forward. Assuming rest is given to the affected side and chewing is done on the unaffected side, then in this case, the condyle on the unaffected side rotates while the condyle on the affected side translates forward. This advancing condyle could elicit pain in the sensitive anterior areas. To avoid this, the affected side is used for chewing.

The anterior displacement theory is further supported by the observation that persons with bruxism and wear facets in the tip of cuspids exhibit TMJ pain on the opposite side. This shows that on the bruxing side the condyle rotates, while the condyle on the non-bruxing side which advances forward causing pain from the anterior sensitive area.

Ramjford also stated that 1/10 mm of anterior displacement or slide of the condyle from its centric relation position during masticatory closure could produce muscle spasm and pain. This condylar slide from centric position occurring at the time of power closure is a recognisable cause for TMJ dysfunction. Elimination of centric slide can result in remarkable resolution of TMJ pain.

3. Temporomandibular Joint Dysfunction Syndrome [Myofacial Pain Dysfunction Syndrome (MPDS) Muscle Dysfunction Syndrome (MDS)]. These are synonymous terms used to describe the same condition. Schwartz in 1955 described a syndrome comprising painful limited movement of the jaw, accompanied by muscle tenderness and clicking which he termed as TMJ pain dysfunction syndrome. This is based on muscle dysfunction and relates the symptoms primarily to muscle spasm and psychic tension. Occlusion of teeth play a secondary rule.

This muscle dysfunction theory was later supported by Laskin who felt that the TMJ pain is muscular in origin and termed it as myofacial pain dysfunction (MPD) syndrome. According to him spasm of the muscle was the primary factor responsible for the symptoms of pain and dysfunction.

Diagnosis of TMJ Dysfunction Syndrome: Cardinal Features: Positive Characteristics

Pain

- Pain and tenderness of unilateral origin.
- Dull ache in ear or preauricular area.
- Pain may radiate to the angle of the mandible.
- Pain worse while awakening in the morning.
- Pain may be mild in the morning but gradually worsen as day progresses.
- More pain at meal time.
- Common areas of tenderness are the joint region, angle of the mandible and the temporal region.

Muscle Tenderness

Muscles of mastication exhibit tenderness on palpation. Lateral pterygoid is the most common muscle to be involved. Neck muscles may also be involved.

Limitation of Movement

The third cardinal symptom is limitation of jaw movement. This is seen as restricted mouth opening and deviation of mandible on mouth opening. Often a shift in the middle is also observed.

Clicking

Clicking sound and noises in the joint are also a common features in TMJ pain dysfunction. Sometimes clicking can occur alone as the only sign without the accompaniment of other symptoms.

Negative Characteristics

1. Absence of clinical, radiographic or bio-chemical evidence of any organic changes in the joint.
2. Lack of tenderness when palpated through the external auditory meatus.

Role of Emotional Stress and Psychic Tension

Emotional and psychic tension manifests in an individual in the form of sleep loss, depression, frustration, anxiety and fatigue, which result in spasm of the muscles of mastication. It is interesting to observe that persons with TMJ pain dysfunction syndrome have increased urinary levels of 17 OH steroids and catecho-lamines which are linked with stress. In severe cases of pain dysfunction, psychological counseling alone produced a marked regression of symptoms without the need for the execution of any other form of treatment.

Treatment Options of TMJ Pain Dysfunction

1. Since functionally it is a muscle dysfunction with no pathology in the joint, there is no justification for any radical forms of treatment such as joint surgery (condy-lectomy, mensectomy), intra-articular injections (steroids, sclerosing solutions) or extensive occlusal equilibration and grinding. These procedures produce irreversible changes.

2. Treatment should be directed towards emotional problems, if there is a need for it. Psychological consultations and psycho-therapy sessions are recommended.

3. *Occlusal disengagement.* This can be achieved by bite plane appliances and bite raising appliances which prevent the posterior teeth from contact. This prevents trigger from occlusal discrepancies reaching the CNS which cause abnormal mandibular positioning. Various types of appliances such as bite planes and bite raising Hawley's plates help in repositioning the condyle to its centric relation position.

4. *Correction of occlusal discrepancies.*
   - Correct disharmony between centric relation and centric occlusion.
   - Correct centric slide.
   - Treat bruxism.
   - Eliminate all forms of parafunctional occlusal contacts.

5. Eliminate non-functional teeth contacts on the balancing side–when the jaw is moved to one side for function, there should be contact between the upper and lower posterior teeth on this side only. There should not be any occlusal contact between this working side and TMJ of the other side (balancing side). If occlusal contacts are present on the balancing side, they then act as interferences between the working side and the TMJ on the opposite side. These interferences act as fulcrum points which could trigger TMJ dysfunction.

6. Eliminate postcanine fulcrums when the mandible is brought to lateral excursion. When the mandibular anterior teeth are brought to protrusive edge to edge contact during incision, there should be no other teeth contact between these groups of teeth and the TMJ points. Only the upper and lower anterior teeth should contact each other, leaving the posterior teeth out of occlusion. If there is posterior contact, then these contacts can also act as fulcrum between the anterior group of teeth and

TMJ to trigger TMJ dysfunction. If such parafunctional contacts are present, then eliminate them.

7. *Restore correct vertical dimension.* Reduced vertical dimension can cause overcontraction of the closing muscles of the jaw. Prolonged overcontraction of these muscles can cause spasm. Extract unopposed third molars–Unopposed third molars cause deflection of mandible during centric closure. This deflective closure in turn causes muscle spasm and pain. Extraction of these teeth gives a quick relief of symptoms.

8. *Replacement of missing teeth with dentures.* Neglected edentulous spaces cause a change in masticatory function. This faulty pattern of mouth closure gives rise to dysfunction of the muscles of mastication. Failure to replace edentulous spaces with restorations can also result in extrusion of teeth, which deviate the mandible during centric closure. Extract overerupted teeth.

9. *Medicaments.* Avoid antidepressant drugs for prolonged periods, avoid indiscriminate use of phenylbutazones, cortisone and indomethacins. Analgesics give only temporary relief. NSAIDS give relief, but symptom relapses on withdrawal of the drug. Tranquilizers and muscle relaxants are recommended and should be used only for a short time.

    Rule. Avoid excessive drugging, as drugs have limited value.

10. *Physiotherapy*
    - Ethyl chloride spray
    - Infrared short wave therapy
    - Retrusive reflex muscle exercise
    - Limited mouth opening exercise
    - Home and self-discipline.
    - Advise the patient to open and close in straight line in an up and down manner without protrusive or lateral movements. During this, patient holds his chin firmly with this forefinger and thumb, forcing the jaw upward as he opens the jaw.

- Do not open mouth too wide. Open the mouth to a point where clicking is about to occur.
- Advise back-sleeping.
- Recommend soft but properly nutritioned diet.

Management of TMD (Temporomandibular Disorders)

The majority of TMD patients achieve good relief of symptoms with conservative noninvasive management. A multidisciplinary model includes patient education and self-care, cognitive behaviour intervention, pharmacotherapy, physical therapy, orthopedic appliance therapy are advised for TMD patients.

Patient Education and Self-care

Instruction in a self care routine should include rest of the masticatory system through voluntary reduction of masticatory function, habit awareness and modification and a home physiotherapeutic program. A home physiotherapeutic program of moist heat and or ice to the affected areas, massage of the affected muscle and gentle range of motion and exercise can reduce pain and increase the range of motion.

Cognitive Behavior Intervention

This is an important part of the overall biopsychosocial treatment program for TMD patients. Persistent habits can be changed only by comprehensive stress management and counseling programs.

Pharmacotherapy

Non-steroidal, anti-inflammatory drugs (NSAIDs) are effective analgesics and anti-inflammatory agents. These are used for articular disorders. Intra-articular temporomandibular injection of corticosteroids has been recommended for severe articular pain. Tricyclic antidepressants have pain modification properties at therapeutic doses much lower than those used for antidepressant effects. These are indicated for patients with neuropathic pain, sleep disturbance and chronic muscle pain.

Physical Therapy

Physical therapy helps to relieve musculo-skeletal pain, restore normal function and promotes repair and regeneration of tissues.

Physical Agents Include

Electrotherapy and Ultrasound Devices.
Electrotherapy devices produce thermal, histochemical and physiologic changes in the muscles and joint and ultrasound devices produces deep heat to the joints to control pain, treat joint contracture and decrease muscle pain.

Vapocoolants.
Fluoromethane vapocoolant sprays followed by muscle stretching reduces muscle soreness and tightness.
- Local anesthetic injections and acupuncture. These are useful for myofascial pain.

Orthopedic Appliance Therapy

Orthopedic appliances or intraoral appliances, occlusal splints, orthotics, night guards, bruxism appliances have a 70-90% rate of success. Complications include major irreversible changes in the interocclusal\interarch relationships.

Types of Appliances
- Stabilization appliances
- Anterior positioning appliances

Stabilization appliances. Stabilization appliances provide:
- Stabilization of the joint
- Redistribution of forces at the tooth and/or joint level
- Protection of teeth from the effects of bruxism
- Relaxation of elevator muscles.

Anterior positioning appliances. These are also referred to as mandibular orthopedic repositioning appliances (MORAs).

Indications
- Acute joint pain
- Painful joint noise
- Closed lock
- Associated secondary muscle symptoms from inflammation and pain.

These appliances reportedly reduce or change the location of stress in the joint by subtly altering the structural relationships.

Occlusal Therapy

Occlusal therapy is undertaken in a patient with TMD after the patient's pain has been relieved and range of motion has improved. The maxillomandibular relationship, neuromuscular activity and psychosocial status of the patient must be stable before treatment is commenced. A proper treatment sequencing is essential including pretreatment with interocclusal appliance, auxillary dental treatment, appropriately timed appointments and prolonged provisional treatment and cementation.

Treatment of occlusion should be considered on an individual basis, on the basis of the specific structural and physiologic needs of the patient's masticatory tissue systems.

Specific treatment objectives include
- A maximum symmetrical distribution of intercuspal contacts
- Axial or near axial loading of teeth
- An acceptable occlusal plane
- Guidance contacts that allow freedom during closing, incursive and excursive gliding mandibular movements without deflection of the mandibular teeth
- An acceptable vertical dimension of occlusion.

Surgery

Temporomandibular surgery s indicated for patients with specific TMD articular disorders. Surgical management may vary from closed surgical procedures (arthrocentesis and arthroscopy) to subcondylar osteotomies (condylotomy).

MULTIPLE CHOICE QUESTIONS

1. **The term gnathology was coined by**
   a. McCollum   b. Bennett
   c. Costen   d. Ramjford

2. **The TMJ is considered as a**
   a. Hinge joint
   b. A compound joint
   c. A ginglymoarthroidal joint
   d. a, b, c
   e. b, c only

3. **The articular surfaces of the temporo-mandibular joint are lined by**
   a. Collagen tissue
   b. Fibrous connective tissue
   c. Hyaline cartilage
   d. None of the above

4. **The true statement regarding the articular disk**
   a. The articular disc is devoid of nerves and vessels
   b. It has a thin central area where the articulatory surface of the condyle is located.
   c. The articular disc is attached anteriorly to the retrodiscal tissue.
   d. a and b are both true.

5. **The _____ determines the pathway of the condyle when the mandible is positioned anteriorly.**
   a. The capular ligament
   b. Articular eminence
   c. Retrodiscal tissue
   d. The mandibular fossa

6. **Synovial fluid is produced by**
   a. The retrodiscal tissue
   b. Cells in the internal surface of synovial cavity.
   c. Dense fibrous connective tissue.
   d. The intermediate zone

7. **Bennett shift is _____**
   a. The lateral bodily side shift of the mandible taking place on the working side.
   b. The lateral bodily shift of the mandible taking place on nonworking side.
   c. The protrusive movement of the mandible.
   d. None of the above

8. **Mandibular orthopaedic repositioning appliances (MORAs) are**
   a. Stabilization appliances
   b. Anterior positioning appliances
   c. Help in stabilization of the joint.
   d. a and c are true.

20

TOOTH ARRANGEMENT

INTRODUCTION

Many factors enter into the arrangement of artificial teeth in a denture. It is not simply a mechanical procedure of placing teeth to follow the form of the arch but requires dexterity and a knowledge of biology.

The arrangement of teeth must be physiologically and esthetically acceptable. Physiologically, they must be compatible with the lips, tongue, and cheeks, whether the mandible is in a relaxed position or in a motion. The teeth function in harmony with the surrounding environment in masticating, swallowing, speaking, yawning and all parafunctional mandibular movements.

The physiology of the supporting tissues must also be considered. When the teeth are arranged to meet physiologic requirements, their positions will contribute to preserving the supporting tissues and they will appear natural in most situations.

FACTORS GOVERNING THE POSITIONS OF TEETH

The positions of the artificial teeth are influenced by:
- The functions of the surrounding structures
- Cellular structure of basal seat tissues.
- The anatomic limits
- The mechanical aspects.

The four principal factors that govern the positions of teeth for complete dentures are:
- The horizontal relations to the residual ridges
- The vertical position of the occlusal surfaces and incisal edges between the residual ridges.
- The esthetic requirements.
- The inclinations for occlusion.

Horizontal Positions

The horizontal positions of the teeth to residual ridges involve placing the teeth anteroposteriorly and mediolaterally: (i) to provide stability, (ii) to direct the forces of mastication to areas most favorable for support, (iii) to support the lips and cheeks for esthetics, and (iv) to be compatible with the functions of the surrounding oral structures.

To Provide Stability

It has been found that forces directed at right angles to the supporting tissues are more stabilizing than forces directed at an inclined plane. Protrusive and lateral movements involving tooth contacts result in forces directed towards inclined planes, and these forces are capable of dislodging the denture.

In normal situations, habit and comfort through proprioception and flexor reflexes guide the movements of the mandible. These movements result in tooth contacts at the position of greatest comfort. Protrusive and lateral movements are capable of dislodging the denture.

1. The patient may not be able to adjust. So, in order to avoid dislodging the dentures patients should be instructed to crush their food by closing up and down and not side by side and by cutting the food into small pieces.
2. The character of the mucosa and submucosa must be considered when the teeth are positioned. The forces of mastication should not be directed to tissue incapable of withstanding the force. Examples are retromolar pad and vestibular fornix.
3. The importance of positioning artificial teeth for physiologic compatibility is illustrated by acts of swallowing, speaking, masticating or moistening the lips with tongue.

In swallowing, tip of the tongue is placed against the palatal surfaces of maxillary anterior teeth and the anterior third of the palate. The teeth are clenched to prevent the food from escaping into the vestibular spaces. The rhythmic contraction of the tongue propels the trapped food up and backward. The orbicularis oris and attached muscles contract and force saliva and small particles of food from the vestibular spaces into the oral cavity and seal off the space distal to the last molar tooth. The artificial teeth must be placed in suitable horizontal positions to allow the muscle activity to occur naturally.

During speech,[5] the positions of the teeth influence speech as exemplified by 'ch' and 'sh' sounds. When maxillary anterior teeth are placed too far posteriorly as related to the lower lip, the 'f' sound may be muffled.

In mastication, the tip of the tongue reaches into the buccal and labial vestibules, gather's food and places it on the occlusal surfaces.

When teeth are placed too far in lateral or anterior direction, the vestibular spaces are obstructed to the tongue.

When teeth are placed too far in a medial or posterior direction, the tongue will dislodge the mandibular denture in order to reach over the teeth.

The positions of the natural teeth are not always compatible with the oral environment. The positions of the clinical crowns of natural teeth may or may not have conformed to the pressures of the soft tissues to occupy a place in the dental arch compatible with function or esthetics.

In all conditions, it may not be functionally or esthetically acceptable to place artificial teeth in the exact positions formerly occupied by natural teeth.

The crests of residual ridges aid in the positioning of teeth if natural teeth were recently extracted and the cortical plates of bone remain intact. The more the resorption, the further from the ridge the teeth are placed.

In the maxillary residual ridge, placing the artificial teeth over the crest of the ridge can be unesthetic. The artificial teeth should be placed labial to the ridge.

Anatomic landmarks aid in relocating the center of the mandibular alveolar ridge. These guidelines are placed on the mandibular cast and help in positioning the artificial teeth in horizontal relationship to the residual ridge.

Anatomic Landmarks

1. Retromolar Fossae. Are triangles formed by the external oblique line and mylohyoid line. These lines converge to form the apex at the base of the anterior border of ascending ramus of the mandible. The third molar forms the base.

The mylohyoid line is on a plane with the lingual surfaces of the mandibular posterior teeth. This point corresponds approximately to the middle of the retromolar pad in mediolateral directions.

2. Retromolar Papilla. Is a small pear-shaped area of gingival tissue that remains fused to the scar after the loss of the last molar tooth. This small, hard, pale pear-shaped tissue is situated at the base of retromolar pad near the center of residual alveolar ridge.

3. Retromolar Pad. Is a triangular or pear-shaped soft pad of tissue located at the distal end of the mandibular ridge. It contains glandular tissue, fibres of buccinator, superior constrictor and temporalis muscle. The pterygo-mandibular raphe enters the pad at the superomedial surface and the pad is dis-placeable.

The mandibular canine is the turning point in the arch. The distal surface of the canine is usually rotated in a posterior direction in line with the center of the posterior alveolar ridge. The position of the distal surface of canine is located by passing a marker parallel to the pupils of the eye, intraorally at the corners of the mouth.

These two points are located on the occlusal rims and transferred to the mandibular cast. With these landmarks, the crest of the alveolar posterior ridge is located.

Limits to Placing Posterior Teeth. The mandibular arch determines the posterior limit for placing posterior teeth. The mucosa considered capable of bearing stress terminates at the retromolar papilla.

The stress-bearing mucosa in the mandibular arch is usually anterior to the stress-bearing mucosa of the maxillary arch.

If the mandibular residual ridge has a steep ascent towards the anterior border of the ramus of the mandible, the distal of the most distal mandibular tooth is placed anterior to this ascent.

To support the cheek, it is often desirable in the maxillary arch, to place a posterior tooth in a more distal position than the last tooth in the mandibular arch.

The medial extension of the mylohyoid ridge determines the medial limit in placing mandibular posterior teeth. If teeth are placed more lingually, tongue may dislodge the denture. The lingual surfaces of the posterior teeth should be placed in a medial direction not to exceed the mylohyoid line. Then the teeth will not be placed in a medial direction more than the medial surface of lingual flange of the denture base. The actions of tongue and cheeks and esthetics primarily determine the lateral limits of the mandibular posterior teeth.

The shape, size and relation of the maxillary arch to the mandibular arch influence the position of the premolars. These are considered in the arrangement of teeth for esthetics.

The buccal surfaces are placed continuously with the arch of the anterior teeth. In normal ridge relation, the lingual cusps of the maxillary posterior teeth occlude in the central fossa of the mandibular posteriors. So, the buccal cusp of the upper posteriors is located lateral to the buccal cusp of lower posteriors, which helps in supporting the cheek and in reducing cheek biting.

When maxillomandibular relations are not normal, occlusal relation of teeth are different. When maxillary arch is broader than the mandibular arch, the maxillary posterior teeth should not be moved medially over the palate to meet the mandibular posterior teeth or vice versa. A limited alteration in the position of the teeth may be enough.

Residual Ridge Malrelation

When both residual ridges are protruded, the arrangement of teeth is basically the same as for normal ridges.

When the mandibular residual ridge is protruded or when it is retruded in comparison to the maxillary ridge, alterations in tooth placement will be required.

Limits to Placing Anterior Teeth. Placing anterior teeth in harmony with functional activity involves placing the teeth in an anteroposterior and mediolateral position in harmony with the action of the lips and tongue. The artificial anterior teeth should not be used to incise food.

The mediolateral and anteroposterior positions of the anterior teeth influence sounds in speech. To make the 'F' sound, the maxillary central incisors should barely contact the vermillion border of the lower lip at the junction of the moist and dry mucosa. The positions of mandibular anterior teeth affect the 'S' sound.

When the patient makes the 'th' sound, the tip of the tongue should make contact with the palatal surface of the maxillary anterior teeth.

When the anterior tooth are placed in normal positions to support the lips, the normal muscle tonus is maintained. Placing teeth too far in a posterior direction allows the muscles to be unsupported and the lips to sag. Placing anteriors in too far an anterior direction can overstretch the muscles.

When the maxillary anterior teeth are present, the incisal papilla is located on the palatal side and between the necks of the maxillary central incisors. The artificial teeth should also be placed anterior to incisal papilla.

When the natural teeth are present, inclinations of the anterior teeth as related to the crest of the alveolar ridge are downward and forward. This relationship is accentuated as resorption increases.

When the maxillary artificial teeth are placed, a common error is to place it near the crest of the residual ridge.

Definite anatomic landmarks that are used in arranging anterior teeth are: (i) incisive papilla, (ii) midsagittal suture, and (iii) canine lines.

The direction of resorption of the mandibular residual ridge causes the crest to become located more anteriorly. Compared to the maxillary residual ridge, the mandibular residual ridge is more favorable as a guide for locating artificial teeth. There are two factors for this:

1. The positions of the clinical crowns of the natural mandibular anterior teeth are more in line in a vertical direction with the alveolar process of the mandibular arch than the maxillary anterior teeth.
2. Direction of resorption of mandibular residual ridge.

The horizontal position of the posterior and anterior teeth follow the shape and form of the dental arch.

The size and shape of the head are reliable factors in determining arch form. Long narrow heads are associated with long narrow palates, tapered arches and a tapered anterior tooth arrangement. The arrangement of teeth for tapered arches places central incisors farther forward than the canines.

Round heads are associated with square arches and a broad flat arrangement of anterior teeth. The labial surface of central incisors are in full view and canines are prominent. Here central incisors are nearly horizontal with the canines. In an ovoid arch form, the 6 anteriors are placed in a gentle curve.

Vertical Positions

The arrangement of artificial teeth in the correct vertical position involves placing the anterior and posterior teeth in an acceptable position between the two residual ridges in a vertical direction. It should provide: (i) denture stability, (ii) favorable forces, (iii) support for lips and cheeks, and (iv) compatibility.

Vertical Positions of Mandibular Posterior Teeth

Two anatomic guidelines to establish the vertical position of the occlusal surfaces of posterior teeth are: (i) orifice of duct of parotid gland, and (ii) retromolar pad.

1. The occlusal surfaces of the maxillary first molar is measured approximately 1/4 inch below the Stenson's duct. This measurement is based on averages which are recorded on the lateral surface of the maxillary occlusal rim.
2. The occlusal surfaces of the last mandibular natural molars is on a plane approximately at the bottom of the upper third of retromolar pad. This position is compatible with the position of tongue and cheeks.

After casts are properly oriented on the articulator, a mark is placed on the cast on the top of the retromolar pad. This point is then extended onto the lateral borders of the cast.

The occlusal groove located opposite the occlusal plane of the natural mandibular posterior teeth can be used as a guide to positioning the posterior artificial teeth in a vertical direction.

Vertical Positions of Maxillary Anterior Teeth

Esthetics and phonetics are used to establish the vertical position of incisal edges of the maxillary anterior teeth. The patient is instructed to say 'fifty-five' and teeth are adjusted until the incisal edges of the maxillary central incisors contact the vermillion border of lower lip at junction of dry and moist mucosa. If this position is also esthetic, occlusal plane is established.

Aids in Establishing Vertical Position of Artificial Teeth

Impressions and Thickness of Labial Surface. The facial musculature should be supported with properly formed denture borders. These borders are formed by the functional position of labial and buccal vestibules at established width of final impressions. Overextension of the labial borders gives the patient the appearance of having a cotton roll beneath the lip.

A stretched appearance of the lip may result in distortion of philtrum, nasolabial and mentolabial folds. Too thin underextended flange does not support the lip well.

In patients, who have been edentulous for too long, significant alveolar ridge resorption would have resulted, which requires thicker borders to restore proper muscle tone. In patients with a prominent labial ridge, it may be possible to avoid a flange at all since the ridge itself gives adequate fullness.

Vertical Jaw Relations. The correct vertical dimension of occlusion is essential in the proper positioning of the orbicularis oris and associated muscles. These muscles function correctly if their physiologic lengths are maintained. They sag if the occlusal vertical dimension is insufficient, accelerating the unattractive edentulous ageing process.

Excessive vertical dimension made in an effort to eliminate age lines results in a stretched and strained appearance of the lower third of face affecting the muscle function, speech, and mastication.

Anterior Teeth Arrangement. Placing anterior teeth in harmony with functional activity involves placing the teeth in an anteroposterior and mediolateral position in harmony with the action of lip and tongue.

The artificial anterior teeth should not be used to incise the food. A sufficient horizontal overlap should be established to prevent the anterior teeth from contacting when the posterior teeth are in centric occlusion.

Phonetics in Placement of Upper Anteriors

1. To make the 'f' sound as in fifty-five, the incisal edges of maxillary central incisors should barely contact the vermillion border of the lower lip at the junction of the moist and dry mucosa.
2. When the patient makes 'Ch' sound, the tip of the tongue should make contact with the palatal surface of maxillary anterior teeth.

If teeth are placed too far in a posterior direction, contact is too great and the sound is muffled. When the teeth are placed in too far an anterior direction the sound will be distorted.

When anterior teeth are placed in favorable positions to support the lips, the normal muscle tonus is maintained. If the teeth are placed too far in posterior direction, muscle will be unsupported and the lips will sag.

Anatomic Landmarks to be used in Placing Maxillary Anteriors

Incisive Papilla. The labial surface of natural central incisor lies approximately 8-10 mm anterior to the center of incisive papilla. In south Indian populations, this distance was found to be 10-12 mm. As the papilla is affected very little by residual ridge resorption, it serves as an excellent guide to maxillary central incisor positioning. The incisive papilla is also a good reference point for midline placement. The lateral incisors and canines are placed so as to contact the upper lip as a guide after arranging the central incisors.

The tips of the canines lie on a line passing through the midpoint of the incisive papilla. A line connecting the canines and the papilla is designated as the C-P-C-line (Fig. 20.1).

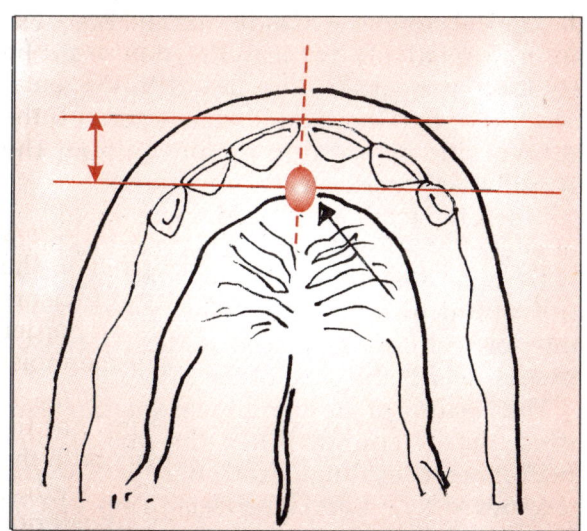

Fig. 20.1. Relationship of maxillary central incisors to the incisive papilla.

Horizontal Tooth Placement with Position Relative to the Labial Vestibule. The labial surfaces of natural teeth are found as far forward as the reflection of the labial vestibule. The artificial teeth should be arranged in this position with imaginary extension of their roots projected to the resorbed anterior alveolus. There is an obtuse angle between the labial surface of the central incisor root and the labial surface of the clinical crown of the tooth. The labial surface of the residual ridge can be used as a guide in determining the proper inclination of anterior teeth (Fig. 20.2).

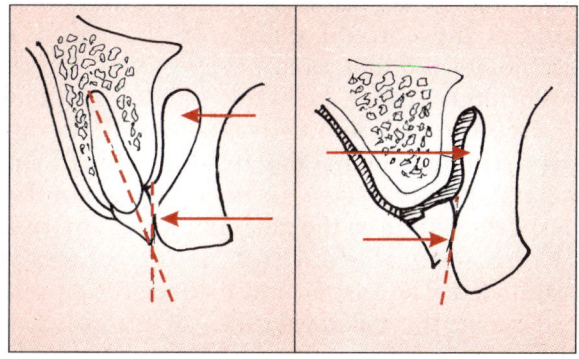

Fig. 20.2. Incisal two-thirds of the labial surface of incisors supporting the lip.

The artificial teeth should be placed in such a manner that incisogingival contour of maxillary anteriors are in harmony with the profile of the individual.

The upper lip is supported in the area of the philtrum by the labial surface of the maxillary anterior teeth and at corners of the mouth by the canines.

In normally related jaws, when the teeth are in occlusion, superior border of the lower lip is supported by the labial incisal third of the maxillary anterior teeth. If anterior teeth are placed too far in an anterior direction, the upper lip is stretched. The stretched lip is noticeable at the philtrum and commissures.

Horizontal Tooth Placement with Position Relative to the Rugae. The labial surface of the canines in south Indians is located 10 mm lateral to the lateral end of the first rugae. On extending the lateral end of the rugae, the lines pass just distal to the midpoint of canine cusp.

The incisal papilla and rugae are exposed on the waxed set up by cutting open a window on the trial base to utilize these landmarks for the set-up.

Horizontal Teeth Placement with Position Relative to Palatal Gingival Vestige.

The horizontal distance between the palatal gingival and the labial or buccal surface of the ridge (buccopalatal breadth) is 6 mm in the sagittal plane for the central incisors and 8, 10 and 12 mm in the coronal plane for the canines, premolars and first molars respectively. On an edentulous upper cast, the palatal gingival vestige can be identified as a raised fibrous band running along the residual ridge. The palatal gingival vestige occupies a similar vertical position as the palatal gingival margin of the natural dentition from which it originated. The vestige and the incisive papilla can be on the palatal surface of the residual ridge, on its crest or even labial and buccal to it depending on the amount of alveolar resorption that has taken place.

The Midsagittal Suture, the Incisal Papilla and the Labial Frenum.
These are guides to the median line.

The canine lines. The six maxillary anterior teeth occupy the space between the distal of the right canine eminence and distal of the left canine eminence. When the canine eminences are visible on the cast, a line coinciding with the posterior margin of the eminence coincides with the posterior surfaces of the canine.

When the eminences are not visible, points that are recorded at corners of the mouth using the mandibular occlusal rims are used as reference.

Individual Tooth Placement

The incisal edges of the central incisors and canines should rest on the occlusal plane whereas the lateral incisors are about 1 mm short of the occlusal plane.

Frontal view. The long axis of central incisor, are nearly perpendicular to the occlusal plane. The lateral incisors angle medially slightly. The canines usually angle more medially than lateral incisors. The tip of the canines should not be more labial than the necks.

Occlusal view. The central incisors face forward, whereas the canines are rotated distally, displaying more of their mesial surfaces. The incisal edges of canines parallel the alignment of the posterior ridges.

Sagittal view. The central incisors flare slightly in a labial direction, lateral incisors, flare more in this direction. The long axis of canines are nearly perpendicular to the occlusal plane in this view.

Placement of Mandibular Anterior Teeth

While the upper anterior teeth are important in smiling, the lower anterior teeth are important in speech.

The direction of resorption of the mandibular residual ridge causes the crest to be located more anterior. In natural teeth, the position of the clinical crowns of mandibular anterior teeth are in a relatively vertical direction with the alveolar process of the mandibular arch. Because of this the mandibular residual ridge is favorable as a guide for positioning the mandibular anterior teeth.

When the teeth are placed, there should be an overjet of at least 1 mm. This is determined by the anteroposterior relation of the maxillary and mandibular ridges. The mandibular anterior teeth are so placed to direct occlusal forces towards the crest of the ridge.

The position of the mandibular anterior teeth affect the 'S' sound. When the mandibular incisors are set in a lingual direction the 'S' sound becomes softened, and when set in a more labial direction, is sound becomes whistled.

In a frontal view, the long axis of the central incisors are perpendicular to the occlusal plane.

The lateral incisors are tipped medially, slightly. The long axis of the mandibular canines tip more medially than lateral incisors. In a sagittal view, the central incisors are tipped in a labial direction slightly. The long axis of the lateral incisors are nearly perpendicular to the occlusal plane. The mandibular canines angle forward slightly.

Placement of Posterior Teeth

There are different concepts regarding placement of posterior teeth.

According to Boucher. The preliminary arrangement of the posterior teeth involves the application of principles that are similar to the arrangement of anterior teeth. The artificial posterior teeth should be placed as close as possible to where the natural teeth were placed (Fig. 20.3).

Unlike in the placement of anterior teeth where certain guidelines are followed, in the placement of the posterior teeth guidelines are not available.

The factors that are considered important in placement of posterior teeth are:

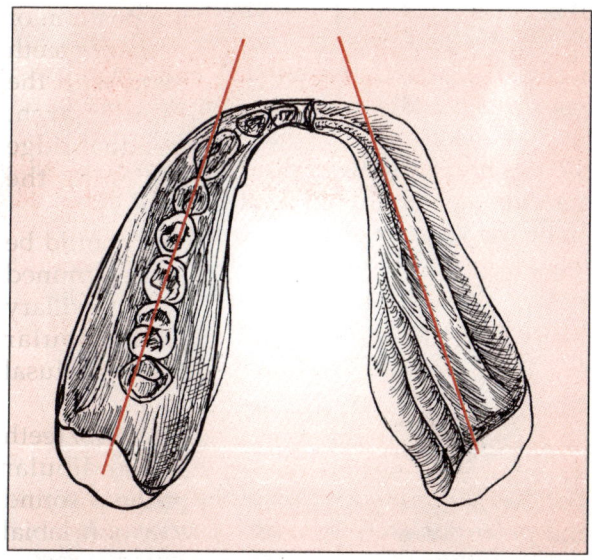

Fig. 20.3. The reference line for the setting of lower posteriors.

- Height and orientation of occlusal plane.
- The arch form.

After the casts are mounted on the articulator, guidelines are established to determine the position of the artificial teeth.

Maxillary Cast

1. A line is drawn parallel to the frontal plane that touches the anterior margin of the incisal papilla.
2. The midline follows the midpalatal suture and bisects the incisal papilla. The line is perpendicular to the first line.

When canine eminences are present, the most distal extent is recorded with a line on the cast.

Mandibular Cast

1. A line is drawn parallel to the frontal plane, bisecting the residual ridge. The direction of resorption of the residual ridge must be taken into consideration.
2. A point is marked in the mandibular occlusal rim designating the distal of the mandibular canines.
3. A line is marked that extends from canine point along crest of residual ridge to retromolar pad. This serves as a guide for buccolingual position of mandibular posterior teeth.
4. A line that bisects the retromolar pad designates the posterior vertical occlusal plane height (Fig. 20.4).

Setting Maxillary Anterior Teeth in Wax for Try-in. If the occlusal rims have been accurately carved to support the lips during the jaw relation procedure, they will act as a guide for the correct anteroposterior tooth position in dental arch. If they have not been adequately carved, alterations in tooth position may be required. For example, if the lips need more support when occlusal rims are in the mouth, the incisors should be set a little out of the labial surface of the wax rim.

A small section of occlusal rim is cut where the central incisor is to be placed. The wax is

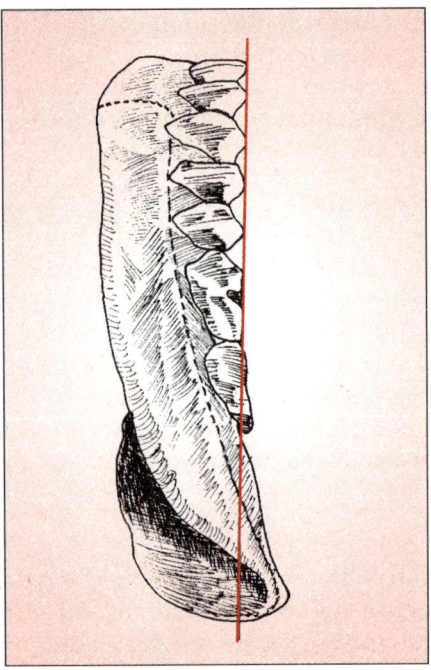

Fig. 20.4. Lower posteriors set with the compensating curve.

then heated until wax pools in that place. This will provide a socket for the artificial tooth.

The tooth is placed in molten wax and moved into desired position with its mesial surface on the midline and its incisal edge just overlapping occlusal surface of the lower occlusal rim.

The remaining teeth are placed. The lower anterior teeth are then placed in lower occlusal rim so that the mesial surfaces of two central incisors will be in the same sagittal plane as mesial surface of upper central incisors.

The imaginary roots of the mandibular anterior teeth must be so positioned that they would extend into the residual alveolar ridge. This often places the mandibular anterior teeth labial to the ridge.

Horizontal Overlap

The horizontal overlap of the maxillary over the mandibular teeth should be fairly uniform from one side of the dental arch to the other.

Orientation of the Occlusal Plane. The orientation of the anterior occlusal plane is determined by esthetics. The position at which incisal edges of the anterior teeth meet is the level of the anterior plane of occlusion.

The posterior (or distal) plane of occlusion should be so located that if it were extended it would be level with the junction between the middle and distal thirds of the retromolar pad.

If the anterior teeth are correctly placed, then the location of the posterior occlusal plane will place it at a level that is familiar to the tongue. If the plane is located higher or lower to gain leverage, the dentures will interfere with action of the tongue. The height of the occlusal plane in the anterior region of the dentures is influenced by the length of the lips, ridge height, incisal guide angle and amount of maxillomandibular space.

Inclination of occlusal plane is important to the stability or instability of dentures. If the plane is too low in the anterior region and too high in the posterior region, maxillary denture will tend to slide down under pressure. If the reverse occurs, the mandibular denture will slide down under pressure. Ideally, the plane of occlusion should parallel both ridges.

The vertical orientation and inclination of occlusal plane is determined by amount of bone lost from maxilla and mandible. If more bone has been lost from the maxilla than mandible, the occlusal plane should be closer to the mandible. It should not be at a level that would favor the weaker of the two ridges. The most reliable guides for occlusal plane are the height at the corners of the mouth and height of retromolar pads.

Tentative Buccolingual Position of the Posterior Teeth

The buccolingual position of the posterior teeth and posterior arch form are determined:
- Anteriorly by the positions of anterior teeth.
- Posteriorly by the shape of basal seat provided by the mandible.

The curvature of the arch of the anterior teeth should follow pleasingly towards the posterior teeth. The posterior teeth should continue this curvature in such a way that they are properly related to the bone that supports them and to the soft tissues that contact their lingual and buccal surfaces.

In final tooth arrangement, the posterior form of the arch will be determined by neutral zone between the cheeks and tongue. This is the space resulting from loss of bone from the residual ridges. Also, factors like cheeks, tongue also influence final arrangement of teeth.

Posterior teeth will have their most favorable leverage if they are placed close to the residual ridge and lingual to it. This is not practical. Posterior teeth placed buccal to the ridge can cause a denture to tip when pressure is applied to them in this bad leverage position. This is magnified as the occlusal plane is located further away from the ridge.

Tentative Arch Form for the Posterior Teeth

The basic principle for the buccolingual positioning of posterior teeth is that they should conform to the shape of the residual ridge.

A perpendicular drawn from the buccal side of the crest of the ridge should bisect buccal cusp of the lower first molar. This rule applies regardless of the differences in the widths of the upper and lower jaws. Therefore the arch form and buccolingual positions are keyed to the mandibular basal seat regardless of alterations that may be required if the upper arch is wider or narrower.

Generally, the posterior teeth will fall between two lines extending posteriorly from the distal surfaces of canines to the buccal and lingual margin of retromolar pad.

Guidelines for Centric Occlusion

There are three specifications for teeth in centric occlusion.

• The upper teeth should overlap the lower teeth.

• Long axis of each upper tooth should be distal to the long axis of the corresponding lower teeth.

• Each tooth except the lower central incisor and the upper last molar should be opposed by two teeth.

These are the specifications for tooth arrangement in testing the accuracy of CR records and mounting of casts.

There are two basic methods to arrangement of posterior teeth in occlusion: (i) one involves setting the maxillary teeth first in relation to a line drawn over the crest of the mandibular ridge and then setting the mandibular teeth to the maxillary teeth, and (ii) the other method involves placing each mandibular teeth or all the teeth before the corresponding maxillary tooth or teeth are set. The second method permits mandibular teeth to be set more accurately in relationship to the residual ridge than the first.

Procedure for Setting Posterior Teeth in Centric Occlusion Only

The height of the posterior segments of the occlusal rim are reduced on one side keeping the full height of the rim on the other side. This will make space for the tooth on one side and also maintain vertical dimension on the other side.

Wax is pooled distal to the maxillary canine to make a socket for the maxillary first premolar. The maxillary first premolar is placed with its long axis parallel to the buccal surface of canine and then the second premolar is placed.

Wax is pooled in mandibular occlusal rim directly under proximal surfaces of upper premolars. The cervical end of second premolar is placed and then articulator is closed, so that tooth is forced into the wax. Then lower first molar is placed, upper first molar and so on.

The lower first molar is placed bucco-lingually in relation to the ridge crest.

Setting of posterior teeth depends on the proper anteroposterior setting of anterior teeth.

After the position of the anterior tooth is determined, it serves as a guide for selecting the size of the posterior teeth.

The distance between the distal of the mandibular canine and mesial end of the retromolar pad is measured for the total anteroposterior space that may be covered by the teeth. The occlusocervical length of posterior teeth are determined by the height and fullness of the ridges. The distal extent of the lower teeth is determined by the incline of the lower residual ridge. In addition to this, the buccolingual width of the posterior teeth are less then the width of natural teeth to reduce biting pressure and increase tongue space.

According to Heartwell, the mandibular posterior teeth should be placed before the maxillary posterior teeth for the following reasons:

- There are more anatomic landmarks to locate guide lines in the mandibular arch.
- The lingual surfaces of the mandibular posterior teeth are not placed more in a medial direction than is the medial surface of lingual flange of the denture base.
- The mandibular canines are the turning points of the arch.
- The retromolar pad is used to determine vertical height of the mandibular molars. The posterior occlusal plane is placed at half the vertical height of the retromolar pad when cusp teeth are set on a plane.

According to Winkler, the arrangement of posterior teeth should position them in relation to their three possible dimensions so that they are as close as practical to their original natural positions.

This placement makes it easier for the patient to:

1. Adapt to the dentures.
2. Permit the tongue and cheeks to function effectively during speech, mastication and deglutition.
3. Esthetically more acceptable.

The placement of upper posterior teeth first would make necessary many adjustments and alterations when the lower teeth are arranged in harmony with the oral environment.

The advantages of placing lower posteriors first are:

1. The lower ridge offers reliable landmarks for setting teeth.
2. The lower denture is more difficult to stabilize, has less support, and there are more limitations to placement of lower posteriors.

The criteria used as a guide for setting the lower posterior teeth are:

Anteriorly. The position and height of the right and left first premolar is determined by the lower anterior teeth. The lower canine and first premolar in order to be in proper anatomic and physiologic position should be at or very near the level of the commissure of the mouth at rest and should support the corner of the mouth and modiolus.

Posteriorly. The last posterior teeth should be over foundation tissue that is firm and does not slope steeply upward. This is just anterior to the apex of retromolar pad.

Buccally. The teeth should have passive contact with buccal mucosa and should not displace it. The buccinator then will provide a tooth tissue contact that will seal off the buccal pouch area against impaction of food.

All areas of the posterior teeth that are buccal to the ridge crest should be kept out of occlusal contact for centric and working mandibular positions. This lingualizes the occlusion and prevents lever activity that would tip the denture base.

Lingually. The lower posterior teeth should not interfere with function of the tongue. The lingual cusps of the natural molars are in approximately vertical alignment with mylohyoid ridge. This is a reliable guide to placement of artificial teeth.

Occlusal Plane. The anterior height of occlusal plane is determined by the lower anterior teeth and commissure of the mouth. The posterior height of occlusal plane is at the level of the center of retromolar pad.

With these guides it is possible to:
1. Set lower teeth at a height comparable to the natural teeth.
2. Provide a physiologically and functionally acceptable anteroposterior inclination of the occlusal plane that is nearly parallel to the lower mean foundation plane.
3. Create an occlusal plane parallel to ala-tragus line.

The parotid papilla according to Foley and Latta is on an average 3.3 mm above the occlusal plane and is considered as a guide for height of occlusal plane. If the occlusal plane is too high, upper and lower teeth can bite the papilla during function. If it is too low, the tongue can overlap the lower teeth and cause tongue biting.

At the time of try-in the tongue is a guide for evaluating the height of the occlusal plane. At rest after swallowing with its tip gently touching the lingual surfaces of lower anterior teeth, the tongue assumes a position with its lateral border at the level of lingual contour of lower natural posterior teeth. The dorsal surface of the tongue is nearly level with occlusal surfaces of the posterior teeth.

The tongue should be normal and tacit for it to be used as a reliable guide for evaluating occlusal height of artificial posterior teeth.

In patients who have not worn a denture for a long time or in patients whose arch form of denture is wider than the natural teeth, the tongue will be hypertrophied. In such patients, a new denture will compress the tongue and make it look as if the tongue is high in relation to occlusal plane.

Compensating Curve

The primary function of this curve is to provide balancing occlusal contacts for protrusive and lateral mandibular positions.

Without this curve the entire occlusal plane would have to be tilted at an angle.

1. Elevating the occlusal plane at the distal end would alter the parallel relation between occlusal plane, ala tragus line and mean foundation plane of lower ridge.
2. Altering occlusal plane to an increased anteroposterior angle would favor stability of lower dentures with forces acting on dentures in a downward and backward direction. But these forces would act on the upper dentures in a forward direction causing dislodgement of the dentures. This can damage rugae area and cause increased resorption.

The compensating curve starts with the first molar by raising it at the distal end continuing this with a further raise of second molar (Fig. 20.4).

The radius of curve necessary to achieve balance is the result of the guiding influence of the angle of the incisal guidance and angle of condylar path.

It is functionally advantageous to keep the curve as modest as possible by setting a shallow incisal angle.

Lateral Plane of the Teeth

The lower natural teeth are inclined sightly to the lingual, creating a transverse curve of the occlusal surfaces from side to side. This is known as Monson's curve which is 8 inches in diameter in normal dentition.

This gives prominence for the lower buccal cusps and brings them into heavy contact with upper teeth in lateral working position. The lingual concept of occlusion necessitates a change in the transverse plane of occlusal surfaces of teeth.

Setting Mandibular Posterior Teeth. The key to an ideal anatomically related set-up of upper and lower posterior teeth is the proper relationship between upper and lower canines. In a Class I relation, mesial incline of the upper canine opposes the distal incline of lower canines. This can be accomplished by selecting a compatible width for the lower anteriors to oppose upper

selected anteriors. If the lower anteriors are too wide, the lower canine as related to upper canine is distal to the ideal canine relationship. This will result in spacing between upper first premolar and canine. This can be corrected by selecting and setting smaller lower anterior teeth, grinding distal of lower canine and by narrowing first premolar by grinding.

If the lower anteriors are too narrow, then canine relation will be mesial to normal relation. This will result in maxillary first premolar occluding on mandibular second premolar. This can be corrected by:

1. Selecting and setting wider lower anterior teeth.
2. Grinding distal of upper canine.
3. Narrowing upper first premolar if esthetics permits.
4. Moving lower posteriors distally.

Preparation of Anteroposterior Guides

1. The occlusal rims are removed to evaluate inter-ridge space and arch form.

A mark is placed on distal shoulder of the lower cast as a projection of a line running from the incisal tip of mandibular canine to apex of retromolar pad. This mark is evaluated with the arch form. Then teeth are set.

Establishing Compensating Curve

The compensating curve starts with the first molar. The mesial cusps of the first molar are placed on a curve established by the anteriors and bicuspids. The distal cusps are raised 0.5 mm above this plane. The buccal and lingual cusps are set at the same height to make the transverse plane horizontal. The central fossae are aligned in the center of canine retromolar pad-reference line.

The second molar continues the cuspal elevation of the compensating curve, which is judged by extending the curve created by first molar. The buccal and lingual cusps are horizontal and central fossae are in a line with reference line.

The marginal ridge of adjacent teeth should be at the same height to allow easy transition from one tooth to the other.

Non-anatomic Posterior Set-up

The disadvantage of anatomic teeth is that presence of cusps provides horizontal thrusts. Many resorbed ridges may not be able to stand these potentially destructive forces.

Non-anatomic teeth were designed to favor these types of ridges by minimizing the horizontal component of force during mastication and during parafunctional movements.

Indications

- Flat ridges.
- Knife edge ridges.
- Large inter-ridge space.
- Milling type of chewing pattern with broad excursions.
- Where debilitation has reduced the patient's coordination needed to handle cusped type of occlusion.

Disadvantages

- Flat teeth occlude in two dimensions but the mandible moves in a 3-D arcuate path.
- The loss of the vertical component in flat teeth alters the protrusive and bilateral balance that is possible with cuspid teeth.

The traditional amount of anterior vertical overlap must be eliminated or modified to avoid anterior interferences in lateral and protrusive excursions. The basic anteroposterior guides and anatomic landmarks for monoplane teeth are the same as for cuspid teeth.

Mandibular Set-up

Antero Posteriorly. The position and height of the lower first premolar is governed by the height of the lower canine. The distal of the second molar should be at the height of center of retromolar pad.

Buccolingually. Center of the tooth should be in a straight line from tip of the canine to apex of the retromolar pad. The lower occlusal table should not be buccal or lingual to the mylohyoid ridge.

Maxillary Set-up

The lingual portion of the upper teeth should be in contact with the center area of the lower teeth. This is a modified type of lingual contact occlusion.

Atypical Arrangement of Posterior Teeth

For a Class II relation, the lower ridge will be small and markedly inside the upper ridge. The anterior teeth exhibit a pronounced horizontal overlap when they are arranged properly for esthetics.

The vertical overlap should be kept as small as possible in order to keep incisal guidance as shallow as possible. The lower canine is more distal in its relationship to upper canine than in Class I relation.

In a Class III relationship, the mandible is large with a broad arch form that is outside of the upper ridge. The upper anteriors are placed as forward as esthetics will allow and to set the lower anteriors as far lingual on the ridge as possible without interfering with the tongue. Correct canine relationship can be obtained.

The lower ridge in the molar and premolar region is located buccal to the upper ridge.

This requires placement of teeth in "crossbite occlusion". In this the upper posterior teeth are so placed that the buccal cusp of the upper is in the central fossa of the lower. The crossbite occlusion can be made with anatomic or non-anatomic teeth.

Combination (anatomic and non-anatomic)

The penetrating efficiency of cusp teeth and the favorable control of occlusal forces by non-cusp teeth can be utilized by use of anatomic teeth for upper posteriors and non-anatomic teeth for lower posteriors.

Selection of Teeth. The upper posteriors are steep, cusped 30° tooth and are not modified by grinding. The lower posterior flat teeth should have an occlusal surface design that does not allow the upper lingual cusps to tip in deep sluiceways. This would lock the occlusion and would result in excessive horizontal forces that would traumatize the foundation tissue.

Indications

- It is intended to improve masticatory efficiency
- It can be used with various ridge relationships.

COMPENSATING CURVES

Compensating curves are the artificial curves introduced into dentures in order to facilitate the production of balanced articulation. The term articulation is used in the sense of designating contacts of teeth in motion. The compensating curves are the artifical counterparts of anteroposterior and the lateral curves found in the natural dentition.

Anteroposterior Curve

This curve follows an imaginary line touching the buccal cusps of all lower teeth from the lower canine backwards and approximates to the arc of a circle. A continuation of this curve backwards in the natural dentition (curve of Spee) will nearly always pass through the head of the condyle.

If the posterior teeth are set to an anteroposterior curve rather than in a horizontal plane, then as the mandible moves forwards and the condyles travel downward all the teeth can remain in contact. The posterior teeth will lose contact if they have been set to conform to a horizontal plane.

Lateral Curves

In the natural dentition there are two lateral curves.

Curve of Monson. The curve of occlusion in which each cusp and incisal edge conforms to a segment of the surface of a sphere 8 inches in diameter with its center in the region of the glabella. This curve involves the molar teeth. The curve of Monson has its concavity facing upwards and increases in steepness from before backwards, the occlusal surfaces of the upper molars facing outwards and downwards.

Curve of Wilson

The curvature of the maxillary teeth are convex and that of the mandibular teeth concave

Anterior Teeth

Frontal View (after setting)
- Parallel to interpupillary line
- Incisal edge of maxillary incisors 1-2 mm below maxillary lip at rest.
- No bulging present under nostrils.
- Philtrum should be restored, if possible.
- Full vermillion border of lip should be seen,
- Smile line should follow line of lower lip in smiling.

Sagittal View
- Upper lip should be everted and not fallen in
- Total support of upper lip is from two-third of incisal labial surface of anteriors.

Horizontal View
- Central incisors should be 8-10 mm anterior to midpoints of incisive papilla
- Canines are on a line drawn perpendicular to the mid palatine raphe through the center of the incisive papilla.

Posterior Teeth

Frontal View
- Maxillary posteriors should be placed buccally enough so as to avoid too large a dark buccal corridor upon smiling, but not to eliminate it.
- The occlusogingival length of maxillary first premolar tooth should be long enough so

that the denture base material is not obvious on smiling.
- The occlusal surface of the mandibular first bicuspid should never be superior to the corner of mouth when mouth is open only sufficiently to receive food.
- Posterior plane of occlusion should not drop down posteriorly or maxillary posterior teeth will show too much during smiling.

Sagittal View
- Posterior plane of occlusion should parallel ala tragus line.
- Posterior plane of occlusion is upto two-third height of retromolar pad.

Horizontal View. Lower buccal cusps or central fossae should be placed over crest of ridge.

ARRANGEMENT OF ARTIFICIAL TEETH

The position of the upper teeth (Maxillary)

Central Incisor. Its long axis is parallel to the vertical axis when viewed from the front, and sloping slightly labially when viewed from the side. The incisal edge is in contact with the horizontal plane (Fig. 20.5).

Lateral Incisor. Its long axis is sloping towards the midline of the mouth when viewed

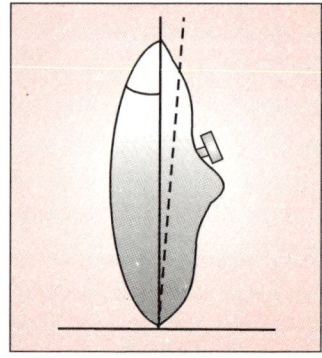

Fig. 20.5. Long axis of the central incisor.

from the front and is inclined labially to a greater degree than the central incisor when viewed from the side. The incisal edge is about 2 mm short of the horizontal plane (Fig. 20.6).

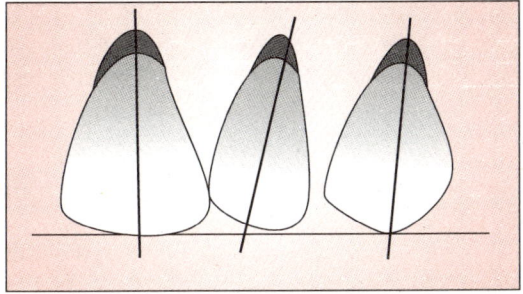

Fig. 20.6. Angulation of maxillary anteriors.

Canine. Its long axis is parallel to the vertical axis when viewed from both front and side. Its cusp is in contact with the horizontal plane.

First Premolar. Its long axis is parallel to the vertical axis when viewed from the front or the side. Its palatal cusp is about 2 mm short of and its buccal cusp is in contact with the horizontal plane.

Second Premolar. Its long axis is parallel with the vertical axis when viewed from the front or the side. Both buccal and palatal cusps are in contact with the horizontal plane (Figs 20.7 and 20.8).

First Molar. Its long axis slopes buccally when viewed from its front and distally when viewed

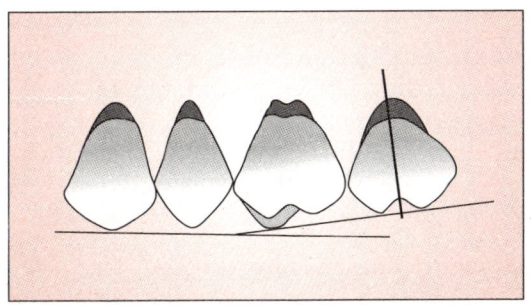

Fig. 20.7. Maxillary posteriors.

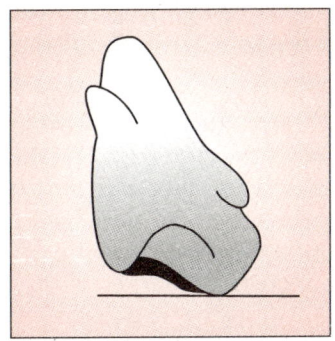

Fig. 20.8. Maxillary first premolar.

from the side. Only its mesiopalatal cusp is in contact with the horizontal plane (Fig. 20.9).

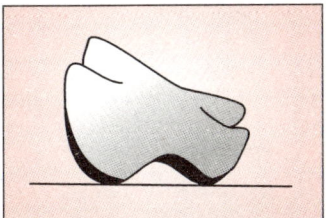

Fig. 20.9. Maxillary first molar.

Second Molar. Its long axis slopes buccally more steeply than the first molar, when viewed from the front, and distally more steeply than the first molar when viewed from the side. All four cusps are short of the horizontal plane but the mesiopalatal cusp is nearest to it (Fig. 20.7).

The position of the lower teeth (mandibular) (Fig. 20.10).

Central Incisor. Its long axis is parallel to the vertical axis, when viewed from the front, and

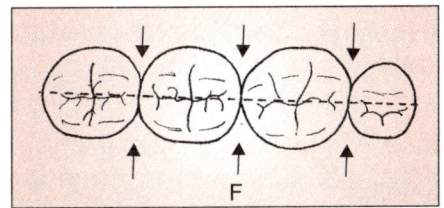

Fig. 20.10. Position of the lower teeth mandibular.

slopes labially, when viewed from the side. The incisal edge is about 2 mm above the horizontal plane.

Lateral Incisor. Its long axis is parallel to the vertical axis when viewed from the front and slopes labially when viewed from the side but not so steeply as the central incisor. The incisal edge is about 2 mm above the horizontal plane (Figs 20.11 and 20.12).

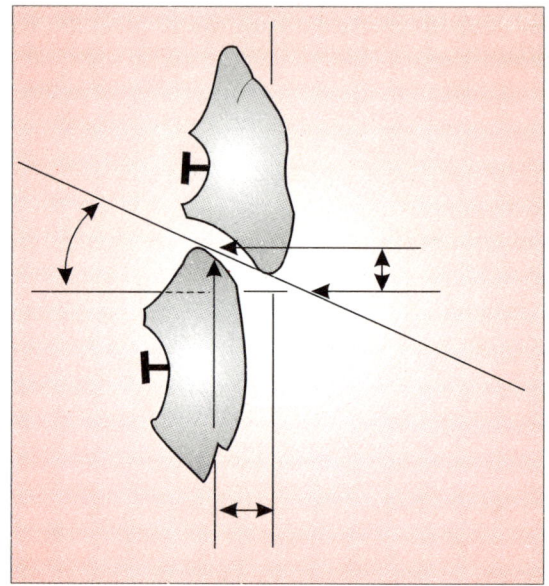

Fig. 20.12. Overjet and Overbite.

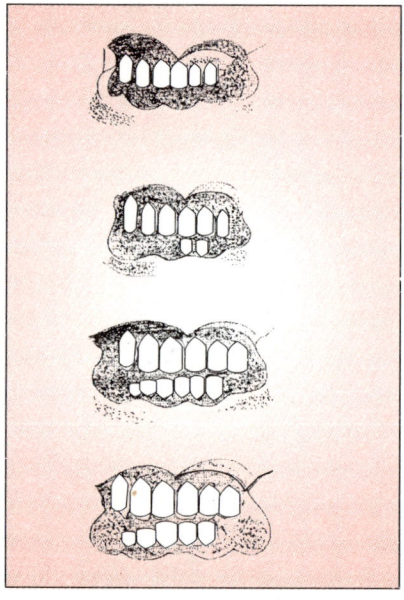

Fig. 20.11. Arrangement of anteriors.

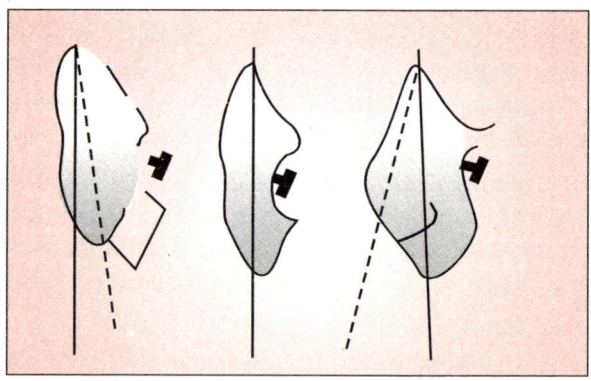

Fig. 20.13. Angulation of lower anteriors.

Canine. Its long axis leans very slightly towards the midline when viewed from the front and very slightly lingually when viewed from the side. Its cusp is slightly more than 2 mm above the horizontal plane (Fig. 20.13).

First Premolar. Its long axis is parallel to the vertical axis when viewed from front and side. Its lingual cusp is below the horizontal plane.

Second Premolar. Its long axis is parallel to the vertical axis when viewed from the front and side. Both cusps are about 2 mm above the horizontal plane.

First Molar. Its long axis leans lingually when viewed from the front and mesially when viewed from the side. All the cusps are at a higher level above the horizontal plane than those of the second premolar, the buccal and distal cusps being higher than the mesial and lingual.

Second Molar. The lingual and mesial inclination of the long axis of the teeth is more pronounced than in the case of the first molar.

All the cusps are at a higher level above the horizontal plane than those of the first molar, the distal and buccal cusps more so than the mesial and lingual.

Further Reading

1. Christensen F T. The compensating curve for complete denture. J Prosth Dent.1960; 10(4): 635-42.

2. Christensen F T. Cusp angulation for complete dentures. J Prosth Dent 1958; 18(6): 910-23.

3. Christensen F T. Balkwill angle for complete dentures. J Prosth Dent .1960 Jan- Feb : Pg: 95-8.

4. Trapozzano V R. Laws of Articulation. J Prosth Dent. 1963; 13(1): 34-48.

5. Weinberg. Tooth position in relation to the denture base foundation. J Prosth Dent. 1958; 18(3): 398-405.

6. Jordan L G. Arrangement of artifical teeth in abnormal jaw relationships. J Prosth Dent. 1974; 32(4): 484-94.

MULTIPLE CHOICE QUESTIONS

1. _____ is a small pear-shaped area of gingival tissue that remains fused to the scar after the loss of the last molar tooth.
   a. Retromolar fossa
   b. Retromolar pad
   c. Retromolar papilla
   d. None of the above

2. The C-P-C line is _____ line
   a. Coronoid-Papilla-Coronoid
   b. Canine-Papilla-Canine
   c. Campers line
   d. Canine-retromolar pad-Canine

3. The labial surface of the natural central incisors lies _____ mm anterior to the center of the incisal papilla
   a. 6-8   b. 8-10
   c. 12-14   d. 4-6

4. Indications for nonanatomic teeth include
   a. Flat ridges
   b. Milling type of chewing pattern
   c. Large interridge space
   d. All the above

5. The curve of Wilson is
   a. A lateral curve
   b. An anteroposterior compensating curve
   c. All are true
   f. a, c are true

21

TRY IN PROCEDURES

INTRODUCTION

By definition a trial denture[1] is the arrangement of teeth in wax, for trial prior to completion of the denture. Three aspects must be considered
1. The functional and esthetic acceptability of the dentures, according to the dentist (dentist's role)
2. The functional and esthetic acceptability of the dentures, according to the patient (patient's role)
3. The competence of the technical delivery (technician's role) (Table 21.1).

THE DENTIST'S ROLE

The first stage is to ensure that the maxillary and mandibular trial dentures are well adapted to the respective master casts and that both bases are stable. The technician is responsible for ensuring the accuracy of fit of bases to casts while the ultimate responsibility for the accuracy of reproduction of the oral tissues rests with the clinician who recorded the definitive impression.

The mandibular trial denture is removed from the articulator and the relationship of the maxillary posterior teeth to the mandibular ridge is assessed. As a general guide to (lower) complete denture stability, the palatal cusps of the maxillary premolar and molar teeth should lie over the mandibular ridge.

When a straight-edged instrument is held over the central fossae of the lower posterior teeth, all the fossae should coincide with the straight edge (this represents the zone occupied by the palatal cusps of the maxillary posterior teeth in retruded contact position). Inspect the intermaxillary space to ensure no unplanned increase or decrease in dimension has occurred

The clinician should also examine the casts to ensure that no laboratory-induced defects have been induced on the denture-bearing areas.

If both dentures are replaced on their respective casts, the clinician may then examine the occlusal relationships of both dentures, to establish that balanced occlusion is present and if required, that balanced articulation has been realized.

With the patient present, and following infection control procedures, the mandibular denture may be inserted in the patient's mouth. Buccinator muscles are ideally restored to their functional width and subsequent insertion of

Table 21.1. Personal responsibilities and factors to be considered in trial insertion of complete denture

Personal responsibilities	Factors to be considered
Dentist's role	1. Ensure that the vital dentures fit the master casts and that the bases are stable 2. Verify the vertical, sagittal and coronal intermaxillary relations 3. Verify the stability of the bases in the mouth 4. Verify the selection of anterior and posterior teeth, their color and that the occlusal planes are correct 5. Verify that speech is lucid 6. Verify that the waxwork is esthetic and functional
Patient's role	1. To record their wishes and expectations 2. Informed consent agreed and that the patient approves of any alteration in form from the previous dentures 3. The patient and any accompanying person, should agree on the acceptability of the trial dentures and that the patient is happy to proceed to completion
Technician's role	4. To have replicated the registration records faithfully 5. To place teeth according to prosthodontic norms 6. To provide stable bases 7. To ensure that balanced occlusion/articulation is provided, according to the prescription by the clinician 8. To have articulated casts appropriately and to have set condylar angles to any prescription given 9. To ensure waxwork is complementary to the age and personality of the patient.

the mandibular denture may stretch the oral commissures.

If the maxillary denture is inserted first, insertion of the mandibular trial denture may dislodge the upper denture, and this may alarm the patient unnecessarily. The verification of stable denture base and, further of a peripheral seal in a lower denture is a source of relief and a confidence builder for patients who have a history of lower denture problems.

The patient may be shown how to use the tongue to control or weigh down the mandibular denture base.

The extension of the mandibular denture base should also be assessed, buccolabially and lingually. The maxillary trial denture is then assessed for stability and for over-underextension.

Four aspects of the denture may be assessed in turn:
- Occlusal relations
- Occlusal planes

- Appearance of teeth and gums (gingival matrix)
- Speech—should not be adversely affected by denture

Incisal Plane. The interpupillary line is an acceptable guideline for this plane, and the clinician and the patient should confirm its acceptability.

Right and Left Occlusal Planes. Fox's occlusal plane guide may be used to confirm these planes (the right may not equal the left). Inappropriately formed planes may result in occlusal errors that may result in pathognomonic symptoms.

Plane of the Mandibular Teeth. Ideally, the resting tongue should overlie the lingual aspects of the lower teeth, and this may be demonstrated to good effect at the trial denture stage to augment (lower) denture stability vide supra. Speech is an important function that in general often receives scant attention from the prosthodontist. Most dentists are aware of the importance of the clarity of sibilant sounds, in particular the test for the 'closest' speaking space, (i.e., ask the patient to say 'Mississippi').

For dentures in balanced occlusion, the following should be checked

- Dentures are in balanced occlusion, and that the incisal guidance post is in contact with the incisal guidance platform.
- Check working, balancing and protrusive occlusions
- Remove the denture from the casts and ensure there are no sharp ridges or acrylic pearls on the 'impression' surface of the denture
- After appropriate infection control place the lower denture in the mouth and assess that no overextensions occur along the periphery of the denture. Gently press on the occlusal surfaces of the lower premolar teeth, and ensure no support problems are evident at this stage.

- Position the upper denture and ensure that no overextensions are present along the periphery. Similarly, ensure no support problems exist at that stage by pressing gently on the occlusal surfaces of the premolar teeth.
- Confirm the occlusal relationships are acceptable as per stages 1 and 2.
- The patient then be re-instructed how to use the tongue to control the lower denture.
- The patient may be instructed to bite on the tip of a cotton wool roll between the first premolar and canine teeth of the upper and lower dentures on a preferred biting side. Instruct the patient to keep a grasp of the roll (unless is painful) and then pull the cotton wool roll away from the patient. Pain indicates either that a support problem exists or that the denture base is unstable (the support problem may be located via pressure relief paste and the denture base relieved appropriately). An acceptable occlusal result is perceived to have been obtained if the cotton wool roll breaks. This will help in training the patient on how to bite.

Further Reading

1. McCord , AA Grant. Trial dentures, insertion of complete denture . Br. Dental J. 2000; 189: 4-8.

MULTIPLE CHOICE QUESTIONS

1. **The technicians responsibilities include all except**
   a. To arrange teeth according to prosthodontic norms
   b. To replicate registration records accurately
   c. Verify that speech is lucid
   d. To ensure waxwork is complimentary to age of the patient

FAQ's

1. **Short notes on Trial insertion of dentures**
2. **Dentist's responsibilities during trial insertion.**

LABORATORY PROCEDURES

DEFINITIONS

Waxing (wax-up). The contouring of a wax pattern or the wax base of a trial denture into the desired form.

Flasking. The act of investing the cast and a wax denture in a flask preparatory to molding the denture base material into the form of the denture.

Processing. The procedure of bringing about the polymerization of appliances, processing of dentures.

WAXING FOR TRY-IN

Preparation of the trial denture for try-in involves contouring the wax on the trial denture to produce a denture base form that reproduces the contours of the original tissues in the dentulous mouth. If carving and contouring are accomplished skilfully, it is much easier to evaluate the appearance and speech of the patient during the try-in appointment.

Waxing the Maxillary Trial Denture (Table 22.1)

Procedure

1. Adapt a softened roll of baseplate wax about 6 mm wide and 5 cm long to the facial surface of one side of the trial denture, and contour with the fingers while the wax is soft
2. Adapt the wax to cover the necks of the teeth and extend it onto the flanges of the trial denture
3. Contour the baseplate wax immediately above the necks of the anterior teeth to produce a gingival bulge, or fullness simulating the attached gingiva
4. Contour the wax above the canine tooth to simulate the canine eminence found in the dentulous mouth. The waxed canine eminence should blend into the peripheral border without producing additional thickness of that border.
5. Develop a slight root prominence over the maxillary central incisors. The prominence should not be as definite as the canine eminence and should fade out before the border is reached.
6. Carve a slight depression, or fossa between the root of the central incisor and the canine eminence. There should be a very slight

Table 22.1. Waxing the trial denture

Problem	Probable cause	Solution
Denture teeth not exposed to cervical finish line	Wax placed above finish line and not carved properly	Use roach carver and trim wax to expose denture tooth
Denture too thick, not contoured to simulate dentulous mouth	Too much wax added during wax-up Failure to carve anatomic contour in wax	Do not overwax Carve anatomic contours in wax-up
	Wax was overflamed	Do not overheat wax when flaming with torch
Denture wax-up unsightly because of discoloration	Wax in waxing tray is old and discolored	Use fresh wax in waxing tray to preserve color
	Incorrect type of alcohol used in torch, causing smoke discoloration	Use proper alcohol in torch

depression and not hollowed out to any extent.

7. Contour the anterior flange of the trial denture to produce a slightly convex effect overall.

8. Wax a gingival bulge immediately above the necks of the posterior teeth. This convexity should resemble the gingival bulge placed in the anterior region, although the gingival bulge area should be almost non-existent in the first premolar area, becoming progressively more prominent in the second premolar and molar region. Vertically the gingival bulge should be approximately 5 to 6 mm wide in the second molar region.

9. Extend the gingival bulge distal to the second molar, and blend it in with the wax, forming the maxillary tuberosity distal to the second molar.

10. Carve a slight depression above the premolar teeth, extending it from the canine eminence posteriorly to the molar process. This depression is the canine fossa and is important if normal facial expression is to be obtained.

11. Carve the area above the posterior gingival bulge to produce a slightly concave surface. This extends from the peripheral roll superiorly to the gingival bulge inferiorly.

12. After adapting and contouring wax on the facial surfaces of the trial denture, seal the baseplate wax around the necks of each tooth with a wax spatula.

13. Use a roach carver, or a No. 7 spatula, to remove excess wax from the facial surfaces of the denture teeth until the finish lines on the necks of the teeth are barely exposed.

14. Use a roach carver, or a No. 7 spatula, held at approximately a 60-degree angle, to carve the gingival margin around the anterior teeth.

15. Carve the gingival margin around the posterior teeth with a roach carver, or No. 7 spatula, held at a 45-degree angle. Follow the finish lines around the necks of the teeth, removing all wax remaining on the teeth above the finish line.

16. Carve the wax to produce a convex gingival papilla. The gingival papilla of the denture should be convex, both occlusogingivally and mesiodistally.

17. Carve the width of the gingival margin around all teeth until it is approximately 0.5 mm in width.

18. Use an alcohol torch to flame the wax surface, taking care to not overheat the wax, thereby obliterating the carved contours.

19. Use a roach carver, a Woodson No. 1 plastic instrument, or small Kingsley scraper, to

remove approximately 0.5 mm of wax, about 1 to 1.5 mm above the necks of the teeth following the contour of the gingival margin. Use care when flaming the gingival roll, otherwise, the wax will be melted and the roll destroyed. Polish this area with a piece of damp nylon stocking.

20. Use the tip of a No. 23 explorer, held perpendicular to the tooth, and carefully follow the gingival margin outline around each tooth, without creating an undercut to remove wax. Any explorer produces a clear separation between the wax and tooth and will result in a more esthetic denture.

21. If desired, the wax denture may be stippled at this time with a modified bristle brush or toothbrush. Stipple the region of the attached gingiva. It is usually more effective if the stippling is confined to the interproximal areas of the teeth.

22. Flame the stippling very lightly, taking care not to melt the wax.

23. Seal the baseplate wax of the palate to the lingual surfaces of the denture teeth.

24. When the wax is cool, use a roach carver, or No. 7 spatula, in a vertical position to remove a sufficient amount of wax in a vertical direction. This will expose the finish line on the lingual surfaces of the teeth.

25. Trim the wax around the necks of the teeth with a No. 7 spatula from a palatal direction at approximately a 20-degree angle below the horizontal.

26. Flame the wax lightly with an alcohol torch and again trim around the necks of the teeth to remove all traces of wax.

27. Polish the wax with a piece of damp nylon stocking until it presents a smooth shiny surface. Check the entire maxillary denture carefully, flame it lightly, and polish any rough areas with a piece of damp nylon stocking. Check the waxed denture carefully for pits. These must be filled with wax using a spatula. The maxillary waxed denture is now ready for try-in.

Waxing the Mandibular Trial Denture

Procedure

1. Flow wax on the lingual surfaces of the lower trial denture and carve the gingival margins to produce a gingival margin angle of approximately 20 degrees below the horizontal.

2. Wax the lingual flanges of the lower denture from the posterior teeth to the peripheral roll to produce an inclined plane that slopes toward the tongue. The contour of the posterior lingual flange should not be convex, but may be slightly concave.

3. Contour and wax the distolingual area of the lingual flange so that it blends into the retromylohyoid space.

4. Wax the peripheral roll to completely fill the peripheral roll outline on the cast. The wax should be contoured to produce a rounded border as will be required in the finished denture.

5. On the labial surface, wax a small gingival bulge just below the gingival margins of the four incisor teeth, similar to that in the maxillary teeth.

6. Develop a canine eminence below each canine tooth.

7. The gingival bulge should be convenient in shape, extreme root prominences should not be present.

8. Contour the area between the gingival bulge and the peripheral roll to produce the concavity. As in the case of the maxillary denture, carve the canine eminences so that they blend with the contour of the peripheral border.

9. Carve the interproximal papilla to completely fill the interproximal space. It should be full bodied and convex mesiodistally and incisogingivally.

10. The free gingival margin, gingival bulge, and interproximal papilla are contoured similar to that of the maxillary trial denture.

11. Contour the space between the posterior gingival bulge and the peripheral border so

that it is slightly concave. Overcarving this area, producing a pronounced concavity, could cause food to be retained on the finished denture.

12. Carve around the individual teeth to produce a slight gingival crevice between the wax and denture teeth.

13. Before the trial dentures are tried in the mouth, check the occlusion on the articulator to be sure that the teeth have not moved during the waxing procedure.

WAXING FOR FLASKING

A plastic palate form can be used to replace the smooth palate of the baseplate (Table 22.2). It will provide anatomic detail for the plate of the maxillary denture and permit better control of palate thickness.

FLASKING THE DENTURE

Procedure

1. Check the seal of the trial denture to the cast, and fill in deficient areas with baseplate wax. Take care to completely fill the peripheral border; however, do not overflow wax into the cast borders.

2. Check the occlusion with tissue paper or plastic tape. Adding wax, cutting out the palate section, and removing and replacing the denture on the cast may produce occlusion errors that should be corrected before flasking the denture (Table 22.3).

3. Select flasks that fit together accurately without rocking. Lubricate the flasks with silicone lubricant to facilitate clean-up after processing.

4. Remove the waxed denture and cast from the articulator, and paint the cast with a separating medium.

5. Place the dentures and casts in the flask to check the height of denture teeth in the flask.

6. Soak the wax dentures on their casts in clear slurry water for a few minutes. The casts will take up slurry water and, as a result, remove less water from the investing stone mix.

7. Proportion artificial stone by weight and mix it with the recommended volume of water. Artificial stone is recommended for flasking because of its superior compressive strength.

8. Place the stone mix in the flask, and settle the wax denture and cast into the mix, center the cast in the flask, keeping the occlusal plane approximately parallel to the base of the flask.

Table 22.2. Adding a plastic palate form		
Problem	*Probable cause*	*Solution*
Palate of finished denture has thick edge at junction of palate form and baseplate	Baseplate not beveled when palate form was adapted	Bevel baseplate to make smooth junction between palate form and baseplate
Midline of palate form, or rugae, not in correct position	Palate form not aligned properly when adapted	Position palate form so that rugae, incisive papilla, midline are located in area of natural counterpart
Palate of finished denture has thick areas not evenly distributed	Air-bubbles trapped under palate form during adaptation	Use care when adapting to minimize air entrapment
		Puncture air-bubbles with sharp instrument; express air

Table 22.3. Flasking the denture

Problem	Probable cause	Solution
Flask halves cannot be separated after removal from boiling water	Undercuts exist in flasking stone or on casts	Examine casts and flasking stone carefully to locate and block out undercuts
Heel broken on mandibular cast on flask separation	Separating medium not painted on stone in lower half of flask. Undercut on cast not blocked out with wax	Paint separating medium on stone in lower half of flask before pouring upper half
Denture has many nodules of acrylic attached when removed from flask	Investing stone not painted on denture during flasking	Check heel area of mandibular denture after half flasked to locate and block out undercuts
	Investing stone not vacuum spatulated	Paint investing stone on teeth wax denture with stiff brush
		Mix investing stone in mechanical spatulator under reduced atmospheric pressure

9. Smooth the stone as necessary, and fill any deficient areas.

10. Allow the stone to complete the initial set, and trim and smooth it with a sharp plaster knife.

11. Remove all stone undercuts that would prevent separation of the flask halves. Undercuts occur commonly in the posterior lingual region of the mandibular dentures. Undercuts should be blocked out with wax before pouring the upper half of the flask to prevent heel breakage on opening of the flask.

12. Place the top half of the flask into position on the lower half to determine that no stone remains on the rim to prevent complete seating.

13. Paint all stone surfaces in the lower half of the flask with a separating medium. Take care not to place the separating medium on the wax denture or teeth. This is particularly true if the denture teeth are plastic, since some separating media can stain resin denture teeth. Soak the lower half of the flask and invested cast in clear slurry water before pouring stone into the top half of the flask.

14. Paint the wax surface with a surface tension reducer and place stone on the occlusal surfaces of the denture teeth and into the interproximal areas with a stiff bristle brush or finger. This procedure reduces voids or bubbles and materially reduces the amount of time required to finish the denture. It can be done while the flask is being held on a vibrator operating at low speed.

15. Pour stone into the flask, allowing time for the stone to flow over the denture and into the lower half of the flask. Take care to avoid air entrapment, which can produce voids. In the absence of a vibrator, the stone may be settled by bouncing the flask on a bench covered with a folded towel. Care must be taken to hold the flask halves firmly together.

16. Fill the flask to within approximately one-fourth inch of the top. Remove the stone with a finger to expose the occlusal surfaces of the teeth in preparation for pouring a stone cap later.

17. Permit the stone to set before pouring the stone cap.

18. After the stone has set, it is sometimes desirable to cut small retentive grooves in

the stone to prevent premature separation of the cap. Carefully paint the stone surface with a separating medium. Do not allow the separating medium to contact the occlusal surfaces or the incisal edges of teeth. This is particularly important when resin teeth are used, because they may become stained.

19. Pour clear slurry water onto the stone surface, and allow it to remain while the stone is being mixed for the stone cap.
20. Pour the slurry water off, and vibrate the stone onto the surface, filling the flask.
21. Place the lid on the filled flask, and tap it gently to be sure that the flask has been completely filled.
22. Allow the stone to set before the wax is eliminated.

Wax Elimination

After the stone has set, the flask is placed in boiling water to soften the wax.

Procedure

1. The flask in a suitable holder is placed in boiling water for approximately 5 minutes.
2. Remove the flask and pry it open with a plaster knife. Be sure to pry on the side opposite to any potential undercuts.
3. Discard the softened wax and plastic denture base, and check that no denture teeth have been dislodged on opening the flask.
4. Place half of the flask in a holder and flow clean boiling water over the surface of the teeth, cast, and stone to eliminate all traces of wax.
5. A brush and soap or detergent solution, can be used to clean the cast and stone, followed by a clean boiling water flush. Place the flask aside to cool.
6. Flush the flask with clean boiling water to remove all traces of detergent water.
7. Place the half flask in an upright position, and allow it to drain and cool.

8. The lower half of the flask is treated in the same manner.

Painting With Tinfoil Substitute

Tinfoil substitute is applied to all stone surfaces of the cast after the flasks have cooled so that they can be handled comfortably.

Procedure (Table 22.4)

1. Pour enough tinfoil substitute into a small container for use on the flasks. Never dip a brush into the main container because it is very easily contaminated and its effectiveness destroyed.
2. Carefully paint the tinfoil substitute on the stone surfaces in the flask. Do not paint tinfoil substitute on the ridge laps of the teeth.
3. Certain tinfoil substitutes are quite thick and can be diluted by adding water. However, take care, to not overdilute, since the effectiveness of the tinfoil substitute may be compromised.
4. After the stone in the flask has been coated with tinfoil substitute, place it aside, and allow it to dry. Be sure that all areas of stone have been painted with tinfoil substitute, or the denture base resin will adhere to the stone, making finishing difficult.

Preparing Ridge Laps. When resin teeth are used in the denture, it is advisable to roughen the ridge laps or make diatorics in these teeth with a bur to provide additional area for bonding between the denture base resin and denture tooth. This is particularly true when highly cross-linked denture base resins are used. 4 or 6 round burs can be used to place indentations in anterior teeth. Grooves or indentations can be placed in resin posterior teeth in order to materially improve the attachment between the denture teeth and denture base resin. After the indentations have been placed be sure to remove all traces of acrylic grinding from the flask.

Table 22.4. Painting the tinfoil substitute

Problem	Probable cause	Solution
Flasking stone sticks tenaciously to cured denture surface	Tinfoil substitute not applied to case or flasking stone	Paint stone and cast with tinfoil substitute
	Tinfoil substitute contaminated with stone	Pour fresh tinfoil substitute in small container for immediate use, do not dip brush in principal storage container
	Tinfoil substitute too diluted as a result of thinning	Do not add too much water to thin tinfoil substitute
	Wax elimination not completed during boil out, rendering tinfoil substitute ineffective	Cleans interior of mold and cast surface thoroughly with boiling water to which detergent has been added; flush with clean boiling water
Resin teeth fail to bond to denture base resin	Tinfoil substitute painted on ridge laps of denture teeth.	Remove any tinfoil substitute that contacts ridge laps of resin teeth.
	Wax residue remains on ridge laps of denture teeth	Cleanse interior of mold, denture teeth, and cast thoroughly with boiling water to which detergent has been added; flush with clean boiling water.

Packing the Denture

Procedure

1. Choose an appropriate shade denture base resin to meet the needs of the patient, and proportion it according to the manufacturer's instructions.
2. Mix the resin in a clean mixing jar with stainless steel spatula. Place it aside until the resin reaches the proper stage for packing. It is important that the mixing jar be airtight to prevent evaporation of the acrylic monomer, which will cause the mix to be grainy. If the lid does not seal well, a sheet of thin plastic can be used to gain a seal.
3. Handle the resin with plastic gloves to prevent contaminating the resin with skin oils and to prevent possible development of contact dermatitis through repeated contacts with the resin.
4. After the resin has reached the dough stage remove it from the jar, form it into a roll, and adapt it to the flask.

5. Place plastic sheets over the resin, place the flask halves in position, and close it slowly in a bench compress to permit the flow of acrylic resin into the minute intricacies of the mold.
6. Open the denture flask and cut away excess resin flash, replace the plastic sheets, and trial pack again
7. Continue trial packing until no more flash is apparent on opening the flask.
8. At this time, when the flask is opened, the resin should exhibit a shiny surface.

Denture Identification

Identification can help reduce losses and could facilitate identification of the patient in the event of a catastrophic accident or illness.

Procedure

1. Type the patient's name and initial on absorbent tissue paper. The name can also be typed on the stainless steel strip material if desired. Cut the name out with scissors.

2. Place the cut-out name strip on the internal surface of the denture and saturate it with acrylic resin monomer.
3. Sift clear acrylic resin polymer over the name strip and wet with monomer.
4. Trial pack the denture again, open the flask, and make certain that the name strip is completely covered with resin. When cured, the embedded name is readily visible and permanently identifies the prosthesis.
5. After the final trial pack, repaint the cast portion of the flask with tinfoil substitute, and allow it to dry. Place a sheet of plastic over the denture base resin to minimize monomer evaporation.
6. Assemble the flask, and close it until metal-to-metal contact between the flask rims is achieved.
7. Place the denture in a compress and bench cure it, before curing it in a curing unit.

Alternate Flasking Procedure

Various silicone molds, or investment coating, materials have been used to flask complete dentures.

Advantages

1. Resultant flexible mold facilitates rapid retrieval of the cured denture from the flask
2. Reduces the finishing time required to remove investing plaster or stone from the denture
3. Serves as a moisture barrier, and does not require application of tinfoil substitute to the mold material.

Procedure

1. Dentures, waxed in the usual manner is flasked in stone.

Curing the Denture

After bench curing the denture for one or more hours, place the denture in water at room temperature and program the curing temperatures according to the manufacturer's recommendations. It is helpful to place a small ball of excess resin around the handle of the compress if the dentures are to be cured overnight in the laboratory. The resin ball is checked the next morning to assure that the power has not been inadvertently turned off during the night, leaving the denture undercured. Cured resin on the handle of the compress, though not infallible is an indicator that the curing unit performed its function.

Deflasking the Denture

After the denture has been cured, it is removed from the curing unit and allowed to bench cool. The denture is then ready for deflasking, finishing, and polishing.

Table 22.5. Packing the denture

Problem	Probable cause	Solution
Cured denture has porosity	Flask underpacked with resin	Fill mold completely before curing; properly packed resin should exhibit flossy surface when flask is first opened
	Thick denture base heated too rapidly	Bench cure followed by long curing cycle
Cured denture has increased processing error	Denture resin packed at late, or rubbery stage	Pack resin during dough stage
	Flask not properly closed prior to curing	Make certain metal-to-metal contact of flask rims is achieved before curing

Denture Base Tinting[1]

Tinted denture base is one that simulates the coloring and shading of natural oral tissues. Several methods have been used to tint denture base resins to achieve a more natural appearance. Usually heat-curing or autopolymerizing resins of various shades or colors are painted on the denture base or are shifted onto the mold during denture construction to obtain a tinted denture.

Procedure. Usually, five stains or tinting resins are adequate to characterize most dentures:

- H, basic color (light pink as in attached gingiva)
- F, light red
- A, medium red, use cautiously
- E, purple, use sparingly in most dentures
- B, brown, used for patients with heavy gingival pigmentation.

1. When waxing the denture, use care in carving appropriate contours on the denture base. Skilful contouring is probably more important for esthetics than tinting. Application of stains is related to carved contours.
2. Flask and boil out the denture, paint it with tinfoil substitute, and allow to try.
3. Modify a glass dropper by heating and drawing to create a smaller orifice and better monomer control. Use heat-curing monomer to wet the resin.
4. Sift H resin over the facial aspect of the flasking stone in the region occupied by the attached gingiva and sature it with monomer. Tint half the denture, then tint the other half.
5. Sift a light coat of F over the H, and extend the F higher on the flange.
6. Sift E sparingly on the area of the attached gingivae/mucosa junction, and saturate it with monomer. Do not overwet the resin, or it may pool in the lower gingival areas.
7. Sift A higher on the flanges to the borders of the denture. Use care, since A is red.
8. After tinting one side of the denture, complete the other side in the same manner. Continually refer to the tinted side for comparison to avoid a pronounced difference in color and distribution of the tinting resin.
9. Place a plastic sheet over the tinted flask, and allow it to set for 15 to 20 minutes before packing the denture base. If the denture is packed too soon, the tinting resin can be squeezed out of the mold, or the distribution modified.
10. Cure the denture, and finish and polish it in the usual manner.

A second method involves the use of brown and purple resins for those with pigmented oral tissues.

Procedure[2]

1. Sift F resin over necks of teeth and saturate with monomer. This should be a very thin layer.
2. Sift a layer of brown resin over the F resin. Take care to correlate the thickness of the layer to obtain desired intensity of the brown tint.
3. Place red fibers above the mucogingival junction on attached mucosal regions and sift A resin over the fibers.
4. Add E resin to the mucosal areas to create a mottled or scattered pattern. A slight amount of yellow can be used as a highlighter over the root eminences. Saturate with monomer.
5. Completed denture simulates color and texture of natural tissue.

Further Reading

1. Kemnitzer D F.. Esthetics and the denture base. J Prosth Dent. 1956; 6(5): 603-15.
2. Johnson H B. Technique for packing and staining complete denture bases. J Prosth Dent. 1956; 16(2): 154-9.

MULTIPLE CHOICE QUESTIONS

1. _____ is the contouring of a wax pattern or the wax base of a trial denture into the desired form.

   a. Waxing   b. Flasking

   c. Processing   d. Staining

FAQ's

1. Denture base tinting
2. Denture identification
3. Methods for identification of dentures
4. Processing of dentures

DENTURE INSERTION

INTRODUCTION

The clinical procedures of this stage mirror those of the trial denture stage, with the exception that the patient takes the replacement dentures home.

When the dentures are placed in the patient's mouth, all the procedures involved in the denture fabrication are subject to review and re-evaluation. The denture is evaluated by

- The dentist who rendered the service.
- The patients who are to use the dentures.
- The friends and relatives of the patient who will be reviewing the result.

Evaluation by the Dentist

Evaluations made by the dentist must be most critical because he knows the potentialities and limitations in the treatment. The dentist must recognize deficiencies, if any in the treatment provided and should institute corrective steps. These evaluations will in the long run help in maintaining the quality of prosthodontic service provided.

Evaluation by the Patient

The patients evaluation of the dentures may be affected by his previous experience with dentures and by comments of friends. Any misinformation or misconcepts about dentures should be corrected.

Evaluation by Friends

The evaluation of dentures by the patients friends may be inaccurate due to a number of reasons.

- The friends do not know how the dentures feel, how they function in mastication.
- They do not know anything about the foundation of the dentures. The denture retention and stability may have been influenced by a poor foundation.
- They may not know anything about the possible lack of coordination of the patient or the ineptness of the patient in following instructions.

The comments of friends may cause the patient to blame the dentist for problems that are beyond the dentist's control. These problems may be overcome by correctly informing the patient. The process is a continuing one and should start at the time the diagnosis is made.

Prior to the placement of dentures, the patient should be instructed to keep his old dentures out for 12-24 hours. This will help heal the distorted tissue and might improve the fit of the denture.

Inaccuracies in the denture may be due to:

1. Errors in judgement made by the dentist.
2. Technical errors developed in the laboratory.
3. Inherent deficiencies of the materials used in the fabrication of dentures.

Before the dentures are inserted, the denture should be inspected to ensure that:

1. The polished surfaces are smooth and devoid of scratches.
2. That no imperfections on the tissue surface remain
3. That the borders are round with no sharp angles in the border areas.

THE INSERTION PROCEDURE

The procedures to be carried out during the insertion appointment should be precise and carried out in an orderly manner.

1. Reviewing of instructions. The first step in the insertion phase is the reviewing of instructions, the patient was given during the diagnostic phase. The instructions given are discussed with the patient and clarification, if needed, are given.
2. Elimination of basal surface errors. The tissue surface of the denture should be evaluated for sharp edges and projections. This may be done using a magnifying glass or gauze. The gauze is run over the tissue surface of the denture. In the areas where projections are present, the gauze will get entangled. These areas are then relieved using a bur.

The dentures are then placed in the patients mouth. In order to evaluate the accuracy of tissue contact, pressure indicating paste is used.

Procedure with Pressure Indicator Paste

This is useful especially in situations where bilateral undercuts in the residual ridge interferes with the initial placement of dentures or when pressure spots are suspected in the final impression.

1. The paste is brushed onto the tissue surface of the denture base in a thin layer so that the brush marks are visible and run in the same direction. In this way, tissue interferences during the placement of dentures or excessive pressure on the residual ridges can be easily interpreted.
2. The painted surface is then sprayed with a silicone liquid or wetted with cold water.
3. The denture is carefully placed in the patient's mouth and pressure is applied by the dentist on the teeth to reveal any pressure spots in the denture base that would displace soft tissue.
4. In areas where tissue interferences are present, marks will be forced on the paste. The denture should be relieved in the areas where marks are present.

The tissue interferences should be corrected before occlusal adjustments are carried out.

When an undercut area is positively established, the denture is relieved by grinding with an acrylic bur. The altered surface is then smoothened with a Burlew wheel revolving at a slow rate.

Evaluation of Borders

The borders and contours of the polished surface are evaluated to determine if: (i) the border extensions and contours are compatible with the available spaces in the vestibules, (ii) borders are properly relieved to accommodate frenum attachment and the reflection of tissues in the hamular notch area, and (iii) the dentures are stable during speech and swallowing.

Procedure

1. Disclosing wax is applied to the borders of the denture in the same manner as green

compound is added during the border molding procedure.

2. The patient is asked to open his mouth as in yawning to protrude the jaw and to move the jaw from right to left.

3. In areas where the denture borders are overextended, the wax will be displaced. The overextended areas are ground and then polished.

4. Disclosing wax is then applied to the remaining borders of the maxillary denture and the patient is instructed to smile, laugh and swallow. This procedure is again repeated for the mandibular denture.

Checking the fullness of the mouth. The facial contour of the denture is evaluated next. If it is found to be excessive, the labial flange of the denture is reduced with a bar. If the correction of the labial flange is put off, it might alarm the patient.

- Checking the degree of tooth and mucosa visibility:
- Checking clearance at the heels of the denture.

The clearance of the dentures in the tuberosity and retromolar pad area of the mouth is evaluated. To evaluate the clearance, disclosing paste is applied on the tuberosity and mandibular movements are carried out. If the paste is perforated, the clearance is considered to be minimal.

- *Checking clearance in the anterior region.* After the dentures are placed in the patient's mouth, anterior clearance should be evaluated. For this an articulating paper is used. When the teeth are in centric relation, the articulating paper should be drawn freely through in the region from canine to canine.
- *Errors in occlusion.* Errors in occlusion may occur due to:
- A change in the state of the TMJ.
- Inaccurate maxillomandibular records by the dentist.
- Errors in the transfer of maxillomandibular relation records to the articulator.
- Ill-fitting temporary record.

- Failure to use a face-bow.
- Incorrect arrangement of posterior teeth.
- Failure to close the flasks completely during processing.
- Use of too much pressure in closing the flasks.
- Warpage of dentures during polishing.

Various errors in the occlusion should be eliminated before the dentures are worn so that the soft tissue interposed between the bone and the denture bases will not be distorted.

Warpage in Dentures During Polishing. Acrylic resins shrink when they change from a moldable to a solid form. They have a high coefficient of thermal expansion and in cooling after polymerization, they shrink, causing dimensional changes. The greatest amount of change occurs when the dentures are removed from the casts. In addition, changes in the denture might occur during polishing and also during use due to absorption of water.

Some of the errors in occlusion can be eliminated by replacing the casts with the processed dentures still on them, in their original mountings in the articulator and by modifying the occlusal surfaces by selective grinding. However errors can also be caused by: (i) inaccurate impressions, (ii) inaccurate jaw relation records, (iii) removal of dentures from the casts, (iv) polishing, and (v) dimensional changes when the acrylic absorbs water.

Therefore it is essential that new interocclusal records of centric and eccentric relations should be made at the time new dentures are first inserted in the patients mouth.

Checking for Occlusal Errors

Procedure. The mandible is guided into centric relation by a thumb placed directly on the anteroposterior part of the chin, with directions to the patient to open and then close until the first feather touch is felt on the back teeth. At the first contact, the patient is instructed to open and then close, stopping the instant tooth contact is felt, and then the patient is instructed to close tight. This procedure will reveal errors in centric relation by touch and slide of the teeth on each other. With this test, occlusal errors can be determined but the amount of occlusal error and the location of deflective contacts cannot be determined. For this, a remounting of the casts is needed.

If articulating paper is used in the mouth to locate interceptive or deflective occlusal contacts, shifting of the denture bases, tissue distortions or eccentric closures by the patient, presence of saliva can prevent the articulating paper from accurately recording occlusal errors. So, a remounting is necessary.

The dentures must be remounted in the articulator using accurate interocclusal records for selective grinding. By remounting the dentures, the errors in occlusion are easily visible, easily located and can be easily corrected.

Advantages of remounting
1. The errors in occlusion can be easily located and corrected.
2. The dentures will be firm on the remount casts in the articulators. If articulating paper is used in the patient's mouth due to various reasons, the errors in occlusion may not be accurately recorded.
3. For remounting of the dentures, the interocclusal records are made in the patient's mouth and then the occlusal errors are corrected without the patient being present. This is a psychological advantage.

Interocclusal Records of Centric Relation

Procedure
1. Two pieces of alu wax are placed over the mandibular posterior teeth. The teeth are dried completely and the wax is pressed firmly onto them to eliminate voids. The alu wax is sealed using a hot spatula.
2. The maxillary denture is placed in the patient's mouth after the occlusal surfaces are lubricated. The alu wax portion is immersed in a water bath at 130°F for 30 seconds. .
3. The mandibular denture is then seated with the index fingers bilaterally positioned on the buccal flanges. The patient is then guided into centric relation position.
4. As contact with the wax approaches, the fingers are raised from the buccal flanges and the patient is instructed to close into the wax until a good index is made.
5. The patient should be prevented from penetrating the wax and making tooth contact.
6. The mandibular denture is carefully removed from the mouth and placed in ice water to chill the wax thoroughly. The wax is then carefully observed. The imprint of the opposing teeth must be crisp and about 1 mm deep. There should not be any penetration of the wax. If the wax is penetrated, it may cause a shifting of the bases or a change in maxillomandibular records.
7. The dentures are reinserted into the patient's mouth and the record is verified. The record is considered acceptable if there is no torquing or tilting of the dentures from initial contact to complete closure.

REMOUNTING OF THE MANDIBULAR DENTURE

1. The maxillary denture is remounted in the articulator by means of the remounted occlusal index.
2. The mandibular denture is positioned on the remount cast and the maxillary denture teeth are carefully positioned in the wax index and secured with a drop of sticky wax in the canine and second molar regions bilaterally.
3. Incisal pin is then adjusted for the thickness of the interocclusal record by dropping the pin.
4. A creamy mix of fast setting plaster is then used to secure the mandibular denture to the lower member of the articulator.

Verification of Centric Relation

Centric relation is verified in order to prevent inappropriate tooth adjustment during selective grinding. If the original record (in alu wax) in the mandibular denture is intact, that record is used. A small amount of molten wax is dripped into the occlusal index. After all the indentations are filled, the wax is smoothened and softened. New centric relation records are then made. After chilling and drying of the records, the dentures are returned to the articulator. With the articulator locked in centric relation, the maxillary teeth should fit precisely into the new record.

If the opposing teeth do not fit exactly into the record, a discrepancy should be suspected. The record should be placed back in the patient's mouth and the centric relation evaluated. If the record still appears correct, it means that the original centric relation registration and mounting were incorrect. In this situation, using the interocclusal record, the mandibular cast should be remounted.

Oral Hygiene with Dentures

Patients should be convinced of the importance of maintaining good oral hygiene for the health of the oral cavity. Plaque, calculus and stains can accumulate on dentures and are considered as the etiologic agents for denture stomatitis, inflammatory papillary hyperplasia, chronic candidiasis, odors and so should be removed.

INSTRUCTIONS FOR THE PATIENT

- Dentures should be rinsed after every meal whenever possible.
- Dentures should be soaked in cleansing solution once a day (for 30 minutes). This helps in the removal of stains and killing of microorganisms. When the dentures are removed from the cleanser, they should be cleaned with a soft brush and thoroughly rinsed. They should be placed over a basin partially filled with water to prevent breakage if they are dropped.
- Patients should be discouraged from using toothpastes as they contain abrasives.
- A denture cleanser can be made by adding 1 teaspoon of Clorox and 2 teaspoons of calgon to 8 ounces of water.
- The mucosal surface of the residual ridge and dorsal surface of tongue should be brushed daily with a soft brush. This prevents accumulation of plaque and debris.
- If the tissues become irritated, the patient should be advised to remove the dentures and to rest the mouth for some while.
- Patients should not attempt to adjust dentures by themselves.
- Dentures should be left out of the mouth at night in order to provide rest to the basal tissues. If rest is not provided, inflammatory papillary hyperplasia or candidiasis may occur.
- Dentures kept out the mouth should be placed in containers of water to prevent drying and possible dimensional change.
- Patients should be advised against the excessive use of adhesives and home reliners. These may alter the relation of the denture to the residual ridge and can alter the vertical and horizontal relation.
- Patients should be instructed to return to the dentist at least once a year for check-up.
- At the denture insertion phase, the patients will be provided with written instructions. The patient should be told to read instructions carefully (Colour Plates 3, 4 and 5 shows pre- and postoperative photos of patients).

DENTURE CLEANSERS

There are a variety of denture cleaners available. These may be classified according to their mode of action, i.e. mechanical and chemical

Requirements of a denture cleanser
A denture cleanser should ideally be:

- Nontoxic and nonirritant
- Be stable in storage with a long shelf-life
- Be bactericidal, fungicidal and viricidal
- Be relatively inexpensive
- Be easy to apply and remove without any residue
- Remove the organic as well as inorganic portion of denture deposits
- Be harmless to all materials used in the fabrication of complete dentures, e.g. PMMA, Co-Cr, etc.

Types of Denture Cleansers

Types

1. Mechanical, e.g. abrasive pastes, and ultrasonic cleansers.
2. Chemical action, e.g. alkaline hypochlorites, acids, effervescent peroxides, disinfectants, enzymes.

Mechanical Action

These include the use of abrasive pastes and brushes and ultrasonic cleansers.

Advantages
- They are easy to use
- Inexpensive.

Disadvantages. Over enthusiastic use of these cleansers can cause damage to denture base material. It cannot be used in patients with impaired manual dexterity.

Chemical Action

Effervescent Peroxides. These are supplied in powder and tablet form and are mixed with water. These are easy to use, have rapid action and are effective. They will also help in denture cleansing by the release of oxygen bubbles which may displace debris. Newer products incorporate enzymes that increase the effectiveness of cleansing.

Alkaline Hypochlorites. Advantages Include:
1. It is effective in the removal of plaque
2. It has inhibitory effects on calculus formation
3. It has superior stain removal properties
4. It has bactericidal and fungicidal properties.

Disadvantages include the bleaching of acrylic resin and corrosion of metal and alteration of taste and odor during use.

Acids. These are supplied as liquids in a plastic container. These are useful for stubborn stains and calcified deposits.

Disinfectants. Disinfectants like chlorhexidine are recommended for use as an adjunct in the treatment of denture-induced stomatitis. They may, however, cause brown staining (due to dietary chromogens).

Enzymes. Enzymes help in cleansing by degradation of enzymes in the plaque matrix.

MULTIPLE CHOICE QUESTIONS

1. **Occlusal correction should be done**
   a. At the time of denture insertion
   b. 24 hours after denture insertion
   c. 48 hours after denture insertion
   d. 1 week after denture insertion

2. **Examples for a denture cleanser that has a chemical action**
   a. Abrasive paste
   b. Ultrasonic cleansers
   c. Alkaline hypochlorite
   d. None of the above.

3. _____ help in denture cleansing by the release of oxygen bubbles that will displace debris
   a. Alkaline hypochlorite
   b. Enzymes
   c. Acids
   d. Effervescent peroxides.

4. _____ are useful for stubborn stains and calcified deposits
   a. Alkaline hypochlorite
   b. Enzymes
   c. Acids
   d. Effervescent peroxides.

FAQ'S

1. **Denture insertion**
2. **Denture cleansers**

24

RELINE AND REBASE PROCEDURES

INTRODUCTION

Maintenance of the adaptation of the denture bases to the mucosa that covers the residual ridges is a critical part of complete denture service. The residual ridges have been described as being plastic in nature, always changing in topography and morphology from many causes. Residual ridges resorb more rapidly in females than in males, and more rapidly in Caucasians than in Negros.

The resorption occurs most rapidly in the first six months following extraction of the teeth and seems to level off at about 12 months only to increase again as the patient reaches age of 65 or above.

The severity of the resorption is not always in proportion to the accuracy of the denture. Resorption frequently results from systemic disease.

Every edentulous patient should be examined on an annual basis to determine the rate of resorption of the residual ridges. The basal seat area should be examined for the presence of abused tissue which may be due to local factors, occlusal disharmony and inaccurate denture bases. The abused tissue should be treated before a reline or rebase is carried out or a new denture fabricated. The most favorable prognosis occurs when the abused soft tissues are allowed to recover to a normal healthy condition before impressions for a rebase or for a new denture are made. If, for any reason the patient cannot remove the denture or will not cooperate, a rebase or new denture may be no more than a temporary expedient. This in turn can cause further soft tissue abuse.

TISSUE RECOVERY ROUTINES

The first step in treating abused tissues is to advise the patient of the treatment plan and to spell out his responsibility in the treatment. The complications and the extensive treatment plan should be explained to the patient, both verbally and in writing, so that he knows what to expect. Treatment plan may include:

1. Surgical removal of hypertrophical tissue, pendulous tissue or fibrous hyperplasia, alterations of the bony support, repositioning of the sulci. Before surgery a tissue

recovery program is instituted a procedure that often reduces the extensiveness of the surgery.

2. The correction of occlusal disharmony by patient remount procedures until tissue recovery occurs.
3. Correction of pressure areas in the tissue surface of the dentures or stabilizing the dentures. This procedure may require a chairside reline.
4. Massage of the soft tissues two or three times a day to stimulate the blood supply and to aid recovery. In addition to this, the patient is instructed to dissolve one half teaspoon of table salt in a half glass of warm water and vigorously swipe the solution against the tissues by inflating and deflating the cheeks. A soft tissue diet is also prescribed.
5. The removal of the dentures from the mouth for atleast 8 out of 24 hours. Patients usually agree to this program, because it can be accomplished during sleeping hours. However, instructing the patient to remove the dentures day and night meets with disapproval in many instances. When a patient properly understands the treatment plan, he usually accepts it readily. When the old dentures are suitable for rebasing procedures and the tissues have returned to an acceptable healthy condition with a program of occlusal correction, tissue rest at night, tissue massage and minor correction of the denture base, rebase procedures are carried out. With this procedure, the dentures may be serviceable for an indefinite period, or the tissues can be maintained in a healthy condition during the construction of new dentures.

TISSUE CONDITIONERS

The most effective method for treating abused basal tissues is for the patient to remove the dentures from the mouth for an extended period of time. Tissue conditioners or temporary soft reliners allow the tissue to return to normal at which time a new denture can be made. For most patients, social and economic considerations preclude this simple but direct approach. The need for rehabilitation of abused tissues without the continuous removal of the patient's dentures has led to the development and acceptance of tissue conditioning materials.

Composition

These substances are soft elastomers that function as short-term reline materials by restoring the fit and stability of a denture base. They are composed of a powdered polymer usually poymethylmethacrylate (PMMA) or one of its copolymers and an aromatic esterethyl alcohol mixture (Braden 1970). These materials when mixed form a gel, the ethyl alcohol having great affinity for the polymer. Optimum properties are obtained when small proportions of alcohol are used and a reasonable gelling rate is obtained that minimizes distortion under masticating conditions. Because of their continuous flow characteristics and viscosity, these materials have to be used within the hard denture base. Denture base should be relieved on the tissue surface. Several compositions are available that exhibit different flow characteristics. The liquid is an aromatic ester (butylphthalate butyglycolate) in ethanol or an alcohol of high molecular weight. Plasticizer is also added to control the flow.

Use of Tissue Conditioners

Tissue conditioners can be used as adjuncts in conditioning (Frisch and associates 1968) and in impression making procedures (Braden), for temporary obturation and protection of surgical areas. They can also find use as a stabilizer of baseplates or of surgical stents to be derived from a specific treatment modality. It also helps to prevent or aid in the treatment of chronic soreness from dentures.

Prerequisites to the use of a Tissue Conditioner

1. Denture should have adequate coverage of the denture-bearing area.
2. A good centric relation.
3. Adequate occlusal vertical dimension.
4. No gross interferences in eccentric jaw positions.

The dentures could have the above mentioned prerequisites incorporated with minimal adjustments.

Preparation of the Denture

Remove from the denture base all undercuts and some of the area immediately on the ridge to a depth of 1 mm or more. Retain the borders or flanges and the hard palatal area in the maxillary denture as vertical stops in seating or placing it on the ridge. If the borders are not well defined, use modeling compound inside the denture and in occlusion, to provide a tripod reference to relate the denture when placing it back in the mouth with the conditioning material in it. Wherever the denture base is short, it should be extended using activated acrylic resin to provide support for the soft material. The important thing to remember is that the dentures should be provided with room for conditioning material that is sufficient to allow the displaced and traumatized tissue to recover to a normal state.

Preparation and Placement of Tissue Conditioner in the Mouth

A three-component system is commonly used:
1. Polymer (Powder) – 1¼ parts of polymer
2. Monomer (liquid)
3. A liquid plasticizer (flow control).

Plasticizer is added to the monomer and mixed prior to mixing it with the polymer. This differs from what the manufacturer recommends. This modification prevents the material from getting rough and hard after 4 to 5 days in use. It makes the material soft, smooth and glossy and it prolongs its durability in use to approximately 4 to 8 weeks.

Technique for using Tissue Conditioners

The powder is added slowly to the liquid in a glass and stirred continuously until the desired amount of polymer is incorporated in the mixture. The material will thicken because of the reaction to form a gel. While the material is still creamy, pour it into the denture. The entire area of the denture base is covered. At the point where the material ceases to flow readily, insert the denture into the patient's mouth. Slowly but firmly carry the denture to place. Use the opposing dentition as a guide to centric relation. Hold the dentures in this position at the desired occlusal vertical dimension for 3 to 7 minutes. Instruct the patient to move his or her lips and cheeks to border mold the material. The excess material that might remain in the mouth is removed. Once the material is set sufficiently, the denture can be removed and the excess material that has come out over the labial and buccal aspects can be removed or trimmed away. This can be done with a sharp knife, scalpel, scissors or an electrically heated spatula. Pressure areas where the pink color of denture base shows through are relieved. Small amounts of the material are added. Where necessary, the denture is returned to the mouth for contouring. The tissue conditioners like the permanent resilient liners can absorb energy elastically and they undergo viscous flow underload. Thus they change their form with the changing contour of the supporting tissue so that good adaptation of the denture to the tissue is maintained. Once an even thickness of 1mm or better of the conditioning material is obtained, cover the sharp edges as well as all the material surfaces with a small amount of the 'flow control' to allow the conditioner to continue to flow and contour itself as the tissues recover. This will also allow the sharp edges to be rounded and become smoother and glossy as the patient functions with the denture.

The denture is returned to the mouth to check for comfort. The patient is instructed for care of the denture. The patient should be asked to return the following day for inspection and correction of pressure areas and this procedure is repeated every 3 to 4 days until the traumatized and irritated tissues have fully recovered. The patient should not eat hard foods in the first 8 hours following the application of the material. This may have a tendency to squeeze the conditioner out of shape destroying what has been previously accomplished.

The tissue conditioner material should not be cleaned by scrubbing with a hard bristle brush since this will have a tendency to tear the material away from the denture base and from itself, and also adversely affect its contour. Soaking in denture cleansers is not recommended since they can adversely affect the physical properties of tissue conditioners and cause premature deterioration. Most of the denture cleansers are mildly acidic. They may be adsorbed by the tissue conditioner and retained even after rinsing with water. This absorbed mild acid may be released later resulting in stomatitis. The denture should be rinsed after every meal and debris removed by brushing with a soft brush. The denture should be soaked in cold water overnight. For disinfection, it should be soaked in alkaline hypochlorite solution for disinfection for 20 minutes.

Demerits

1. The conditioner-lined denture provides immediate relief and comfort. There is a danger that the patient will wear them too long and so cause trauma to the supporting tissue.
2. As the conditioners age they lose their plastic properties, and the elastic characteristics becomes dominant. They harden and roughen within 4 to 8 weeks because of the loss of the plasticizer. The initial mix

is a free flowing liquid which requires 15 to 20 minutes to acquire elastic characteristics. In the end, elastic properties are lost when the alcohol and plasticizer are leached from the resin. This requires close observation of the patient by the dentist.

The different physical stages of tissue conditioner/treatment liner allow the dentist to use them for different objectives (Table 24.1):

Table 24.1. Stages of tissue conditioners

1. Plastic stage (Tissue conditioner)	Tissue conditioner in denture Denture base responds to functional/Parafunctional stresses, and fit is improved (few hours to few days)
2. Elastic stage (Tissue conditioner)	Stress is cushioned. Tissue recovery takes place (1 to 2 weeks)
3. Firm stage (Reline impression)	Surface is similar to polymerized resin surface, except it is vulnerable to deterioration.

RELINING OR REBASING

As the denture foundations change, the impression surface of the denture ceases to fit the tissues properly. The procedure used to correct this is a relining, and dentist achieves this by adding new denture base material to the existing denture base, thereby refitting the denture. Rebasing of dentures is done when the denture needs to be refitted and reoriented as well.

Observed Clinical Changes Include

1. Loss of retention and stability
2. Loss of vertical dimension of occlusion
3. Loss of support for facial tissues
4. Horizontal shift of dentures, incorrect occlusal relationship
5. Reorientation of the occlusal plane.

Preliminary Treatment

Objectives

1. Re-establishment of the vertical dimension of occlusion.
2. Restoration of esthetics by reorientation of the dentures anteroposteriorly.
3. Reorientation of each denture to its foundation.
4. Reorientation of the occlusal plane.
5. Re-establishment of centric relation of the jaws.
6. Correction of the impression surfaces.

In situations where the changes are mild to moderate, tissue conditioners are used. In situations where the changes are more severe, a rebasing may be required. This is carried out by the use of a combination of compound stops, tissue conditioners, occlusal adjustments and autopolymerizing augumentation of the occlusal surfaces.

Indications for Relining or Rebasing[1]

1. Immediate denture at 3 to 6 months after their original fabrication.
2. When the residual alveolar ridges have resorbed and the adaptation of the denture bases to the ridge is poor.

3. When the patient cannot afford the cost of having new dentures fabricated.
4. When the fabrication of new dentures with the accompanying series of appointments can cause physical or mental stress, such as for geriatric or chronically ill patients.

General Considerations

A thorough examination of the patient and of the existing dentures must be accomplished before commencing therapy (Table 24.2). The following should receive special consideration.

1. The occlusal vertical dimension should be satisfactory.
2. Centric occlusion should coincide with centric relation, an error is allowable if it is so slight as to be correctable.
3. The appearance of the denture must be acceptable to the patient and dentist. The size, shape, shade and arrangement of the artificial teeth must be satisfactory.
4. The oral tissue should be in optimum health.
5. The posterior limit of the maxillary denture should be correct.
6. The denture base extensions should be adequate. The denture base extensions ensure distribution of masticatory forces over as large an area as possible.
7. The interocclusal distance is correct.

Table 24.2. Relining techniques

Impression	Advantages	Disadvantages
ZnOE is used; palatal portion with plaster of Paris	1. Opening of the palatal portion will allow better seating of denture and will prevent increase in vertical dimension 2. Premade interocclusal record helps in positioning the denture during impression making 3. Two step impression procedure will prevent movement of maxillarydenture	1. Denture may move up or forward during impression procedure 2. Wax interocclusal record is not accurate
Fluid wax is used; impression is made in two steps	Reduces extreme forward movement of maxillary denture	Wax is susceptible to: 1. Distortion 2. Errors in existing centric occlusion can produce an inaccurate impression

8. Speech is satisfactory with the existing teeth arrangement.
9. There are no existing hard or soft tissue conditions that would preclude the technique.

Contraindications

The dentures should not be relined or rebased when one or more of the following defects exist:
1. When an excessive amount of resorption has taken place.
2. When abused soft tissues are present. The relining is not indicated until the tissues recover and return as closely as possible to normal form.
3. When the patient complains of TMJ problems. Until accurate diagnosis and treatment of the problem has been accomplished, relining or rebasing is contraindicated.
4. If the dentures have poor esthetics or unsatisfactory jaw relationships.
5. When severe osseous undercuts exist (until surgical removal and healing occurs).

Tissue Preparation

With any relining or rebasing technique, the tissues and dentures should be prepared for the necessary procedures as follows:
1. Excessive hypertrophic tissue should be surgically removed. The dentures can be used as a surgical splint.
2. The oral mucosa should be free of areas of irritation.
3. Removal of the dentures from the mouth during sleep is a must for several weeks before treatment commences.
4. The dentures should be left out of the mouth for at least two or three days before making the final impression. Daily massage of the soft tissues is helpful to stimulate their blood supply.

Denture Preparation

1. Pressure areas on the tissue surface of the dentures should be relieved.

2. Minor occlusal disharmony is corrected by selective grinding.
3. Small border inadequacies are corrected.
4. A correct posterior palatal seal area should be established before the final impression.

Principal Pitfalls

The principal pitfalls that must be avoided in any technique to refit a complete denture are as follows:
1. Do not increase the occlusal vertical dimension.
2. Multiple even contacts (maximum inter cuspation) should be present in centric relation.
3. Do not permit the maxillary denture to move forward during impression making.
4. Ensure that centric relation and centric occlusion are identical.
5. Ensure that an accurate posterior palatal seal has been established.
6. An equal thickness of final impression material should be used.

Open Mouth Impression Technique

1. It is a method for relining both maxillary and mandibular dentures at the same appointment.
2. The dentures are essentially used as trays for making the new impressions.
3. The existing centric occlusion is not utilized, and a new centric relation record is accomplished after the impressions are made.

Technique Suggested by Boucher[2]

Centric Relation. Utilizing both dentures as recording bases, the jaw relation is recorded after making the secondary mandibular and maxillary impression

Denture Preparation. A posterior palatal seal is formed in modeling compound on the maxillary denture before any other changes are made on the tissue side of the denture. One millimeter of space is provided inside the denture for the new impression material. The borders are shortened 1mm to allow space for the impression material to form a new border.

Special Suggestion. The lower denture is prepared for the reline impression in exactly the same way as a tray would be prepared for making a new denture. The buccal surfaces of the lingual flanges are ground to minimize the pressure against the mylohyoid ridges and between the tissues of the floor of the mouth and the buccal sides of the lingual flanges. The lingual flange between the premylohyoid eminences is shortened by 1mm. The labial flange between the buccal notches is shortened by 1mm. Two grooves are cut on the buccal sides of the lingual flanges to facilitate removal of the retromylohyoid eminences after the cast is poured. A modeling compound formed over the lower anterior teeth facilitates handling the denture when it is carried to the mouth. Adhesive or masking tape is adapted over the polished surfaces of both dentures and over the teeth.

Closed Mouth Relining Technique (Mandibular Denture)

The hazards in relining a mandibular complete denture are greater than when relining a maxillary complete denture. There are many factors that should be considered during the relining of a mandibular denture. Ridge relations, ridge form, and the characteristics of the mucosa covering the ridges must be considered. There are many factors with which the relined denture must be in harmony.

Technique

Centric Relation. The existing occlusion (inter-cuspation) is used as a means to seat the mandibular denture during the secondary impression. The occlusion is corrected during the establishment of a new occlusal vertical dimension.

Denture Preparation. Not specified.

Special Suggestion. Loss of vertical dimension is corrected by luting softened modeling compound to the occlusal surfaces of the mandibular posterior teeth. The patient is directed to repeatedly pronounce the letter 'm'. The record is chilled, trimmed and slightly heated before returning it to the patients mouth. The procedure is repeated until the occlusal vertical dimension is established to the operator's satisfaction. Then a lower work impression should be made. After pouring the impression and mounting, the lower denture should be removed and cleaned. Any excessive undercuts should be removed. The denture is luted to the maxillary denture in maximum intercuspation. Softened modeling compound is placed inside the mandibular denture and the articulator closed against the lower cast to contact the incisal guide pin. With this procedure, the amount of vertical dimension indicated by the thickness of the compound on the surface of the mandibular teeth is transferred to the base of the mandibular denture. The mandibular denture at this stage is used as tray for making the final impression.

Impression. Modeling compound at the early stage and zinc oxide-eugenol for making the secondary impression are suggested.

Advantages
1. The loss of vertical dimension can be compensated during the relining procedures.
2. The error in centric occlusion can be reduced during the laboratory stages.

Disadvantages
1. This technique is very time consuming from the stand point of clinical and laboratory procedures.
2. The procedure for establishment of occlusal vertical dimension is highly questionable.

Different steps that can be considered as an integral part of a closed mouth reline technique (Table 24.3) are described as follows.

Centric Relation. Existing intercuspation is used to stabilize dentures. Interocclusal

Table 24.3. Closed mouth relining techniques (maxillary denture)

Author	Centric relation	Denture preparation	Special suggestion	Border molding
Shaffer[6]	It is recorded before impression is made using the medium of choice	1. Large undercuts are relieved 2. 1.5-2 mm are relieved from the tissue surface 3. Borders are reduced 1-2 mm (Except PPS)	Large part of middle palatal portion of denture is removed	Low fusing modeling compound is used
Hansen[4]	Existing centric occlusion and intercuspation are used		Large part of palatal portion is removed. A groove is cut outlining the area to be removed. Holes are then drilled at 5-6 mm intervals inside this groove	
Christensen[3]	Same as Hansen's technique		Labial and palatal flange of the denture are perforated. This will help reduce pressure inside the denture	
Jordan[5]	Existing centric relation is used to seat the denture		1. Denture periphery shortened to create a flat border 2. Large opening is created in the palatal portion of the denture 3. Adhesive tape is applied over the labial and buccal surfaces of both dentures 2 mm away from the denture border 4. A deep groove is cut into the buccal and labial surfaces of the denture at the junction of the impression material and filled with molten baseplate wax	

record is made by use of wax or compound and corrected during the re-establishment of a new vertical dimension of occlusion by grinding or use of the autopolymerizing resin.

Denture Preparations. Large undercuts are relieved. Hard resin surfaces are relieved 1.5–2 mm.

• Tissue conditioner removed or relieved.
• Escape holes are drilled (particularly in a

maxillary base), this will also assist in easy removal of the palatal portion during packing and processing. Denture periphery is shortened to create a flat border.

Impression Procedures. Border molding can be achieved with a low fusing compound material. A posterior palatal seal is achieved with low fusing compound. Denture periphery is shortened to create a flat border.

FUNCTIONAL IMPRESSION TECHNIQUE

In this technique, patients usually need a few appointments for adjustments. This technique is based on the use of fluid resins (tissue conditioning) materials as impression material.

Clinical Procedures

1. The patient should be educated concerning the procedure and especially about not wearing the dentures overnight. He should accept his responsibility in the treatment plan.
2. The old denture should be closely examined and errors of occlusion corrected until a satisfactory centric occlusion (maximum intercuspation) is acquired, which should be coincident with centric relation.
3. The basal surface of the denture is reduced to allow room for the tissue conditioning material. The denture borders are reduced to 1-2 mm.
4. This surface is dried before the material is placed into the denture.
5. A minimum thickness of tissue conditioning material is placed over the tissue surface of the denture. The denture is then inserted in the mouth, followed by the usual technique for the use of tissue conditioners. After removal of all the excess material, over extended borders should be reduced and voids on any border of the denture should be corrected by adding additional material with a brush and reinserting the denture into the patient's mouth. The patient is instructed in the care of the resilient lining before being dismissed.
6. When the patient returns to the dentist after 3 to 5 days, the denture should be examined for denuded areas. Mark the denuded areas with an indelible pencil and relieve the pressure areas on the denture before the next application of tissue conditioner. Underextended borders should be corrected with impression compound before the next application of material.
7. The material is reviewed periodically, it is never allowed to remain in a denture for more than a week as the material itself may become a source of irritation. When the tissue has returned to a clinically discernible healthy state, the patient is scheduled for making impressions. At this time, a zinc oxide-eugenol or light bodied polysulfide rubber wash impression can also be used.
8. All of the tissue conditioning material on the tissue surface of the dentures should be replaced with new material. The patient is instructed to wear the dentures for 30 minutes. If there are no pressure areas, this impression could be considered as a master impression for relining the dentures. The manufacturer's instructions should be carefully checked as certain products require a longer time in the mouth when used for making impressions.
9. Laboratory research indicates that these materials begin to harden 30 minutes after mixing and do not have an active effect after three days. The initial reproduction of detail and dimensional accuracy of these materials is excellent. The denture with tissue conditioning material in place should be kept in mouth for 15-45 minutes to assure registration of detail. If kept in the mouth for 60 minutes, the accuracy of detail reproduction may be diminished. A cast must be poured immediately, since the material will undergo some changes in detail even in a humidifier.
10. During one of the appointments, an accurate face-bow transfer of the maxillary denture should be made and kept for future use.

Laboratory Procedure

1. After the final impression is made, a cast must be poured immediately.

2. Mount the maxillary cast on a semiadjustable articulator using the face-bow transfer record. A jig also could be used. Even though this is easier than the use of an articulator, it is less accurate especially when additional occlusal adjustment is required.

Soft lining material: This can be

1. Temporary (Table 24.4) soft materials (tissue conditioners or temporary soft lining materials)
2. Permanent soft lining materials based on silicone rubber or acrylic resin.

Table 24.4. Temporary soft lining materials

Temporary soft material	Constituents	Manufacturer
Viscogel	Polyethyl methacrylate Ethyl alcohol Dibutyl phthalate	Detray division Dentsply Ltd.
Coe comfort	Polymethyl methacrylate Ethyl alcohol Dibutyl phthalate Zinc oxide	Coe Laboratories Ltd.

Further Reading

1. Ostrem C T. Relining complete dentures. J Prosth Dent. 196111(2): 204-12.
2. Boucher. The relining of complete dentures. J Prosth Dent. 1973; 30: 521-26.
3. Christensen F T. Relining techniques for complete dentures. J Prosth Dent. 1971, 26: 373-81.
4. Hensen N.J. Rebasing and relining complete dentures. Dental clinics of North America. 1964; 8: 693-704.
5. Jordan L G. Relining the complete maxillary denture. J Prosth Dent. 1972; 28: 637-41.
6. Shaffer. Relining complete dentures. J Prosth Dent. 1971; 25 : 366-70.

MULTIPLE CHOICE QUESTIONS

1. _____ is the laboratory procedure of replacing the entire denture base on an existing prosthesis.
   a. Reline
   b. Rebase
   c. Repair
   d. None of the above

2. Indications for relining include all except
   a. Unsatisfactory jaw relationship
   b. Immediate dentures 6 months after fabrication
   c. Loss of adaptation of the denture to the tissue
   d. All of the above

3. In christensen's closed month relining technique for the maxillary denture,
   a. Large undercuts are relieved
   b. Labial and palatal flange of the denture are perforated
   c. Large part of palatal portion is removed
   d. All are true
   e. a, b are true

25

MASTICATORY ABILITY

INTRODUCTION

Most patients regard tooth loss as mutilating, and a strong incentive to seek dental care for the preservation of a healthy dentition and socially acceptable appearance. Most Dentists regard the loss of several teeth as posing the hazard of a greater mutilation–the destruction of part of the facial skeleton and the distortion of the morphology and function of the soft tissues.

The edentulous state represents a compromise in the integrity of the masticatory system. The treatment of edentulous patients present a range of biomechanical problems that involve individual tolerances and perceptions.

One of the most desired objectives in complete denture prosthesis is the mastication. When the function of mastication is interfered with or impaired, the digestive organs are necessarily required to do an extra amount of work for which they are unfit. This will eventually result in impaired digestion, systemic disturbances and general ill health that is more or less serious. Many lives may be shortened by years because of the partial or total loss of this most important function. Substitutes for the natural teeth should be made so as to restore, as fully as possible, the function of the natural organs. Ability to masticate and digest food aids in maintaining good health and generally normal body functions, while inability leads to discomfort, ill health, disease and curtailing of the span of life.

The replacement of the lost natural teeth by artificial substitutes is essential to the continuance of a normal life. The essential difference between natural and artificial teeth is that the former are firmly rooted in the bone of the jaws, and as a consequence can incise, tear, and finely grind food of any character because the lower teeth can move across the upper teeth with a powerful shearing action. On the other hand, artificial dentures, merely rest on gums and are held there by weak forces. In addition, they are subjected to powerful displacing forces, so their efficiency as a masticatory apparatus is limited. This efficiency can vary within wide limits depending on the shape and size of the edentulous jaws, the type of soft tissue covering these jaws, the mental attitude of the patient to the dentures, his ability to learn to use them, and the skill of the operator. The main limitations of artificial dentures are that they lack stability, and the masticatory force which can be applied by them is limited by this fact, and also by the pressure which the soft tissue will tolerate.

THE MASTICATORY SYSTEM

The masticatory system can be regarded as a functional unit, the principal components of which include the dentition, the periodontal structures, maxilla and mandible, temporomandibular joints, mandibular musculature; the muscles of the lips, cheeks and tongue; the soft tissues that invest these structures and the innervation supplying all of them.

In addition to mastication, the other functions associated with the masticatory system includes respiration, deglutition, and speech. The system may also engage in occlusal parafunction, which includes such activities as clenching or grinding of the teeth (bruxism), fingernail biting, thumb sucking and pipe smoking. The role of the masticatory system in the perceived esthetics of the individual cannot be disregarded because this factor is often a very important element in patient care.

The mammalian masticatory system is distinguished from those of other vertebrates by the following :

1. A well-developed secondary palate.
2. Separation of masticatory and respiratory pathways.
3. Distinct lips and cheeks that are mobile and prehensile in acquiring of food.
4. A highly evolved tongue that together with the lip and cheek musculature controls the food bolus over the molar teeth during mastication.
5. Salivary glands secrete saliva which not only serves as lubricating agent's but also contain digestive enzymes.

MASTICATION

Mastication[1] consists of a rhythmic separation and apposition of jaws and involves biophysical and biochemical processes including the use of the lips, teeth, cheeks, tongue, palate and all the oral structures to prepare food for swallowing.

In the mastication of food, the movements are (1) "hinge like" used in opening and closing the mouth for introduction of food and to a lesser degree for the crushing of certain types of food, (2) protrusive movements used in the grasping and incision of food, (3) right and left lateral excursion for the reduction of fibrous as well as other types of bulky food. The combination of all these movements appear to be the most effective in the minute trituration of food.

Mandibular Movement in Mastication

1. The basic jaw movement during mastication is rhythmic up and down motion of jaws which involves biophysical and biochemical processes including the use of the lips, teeth, cheeks, tongue and palate (Fig. 25.1).

    From plots of the chewing strokes in the sagittal plane, it can be seen that the opening

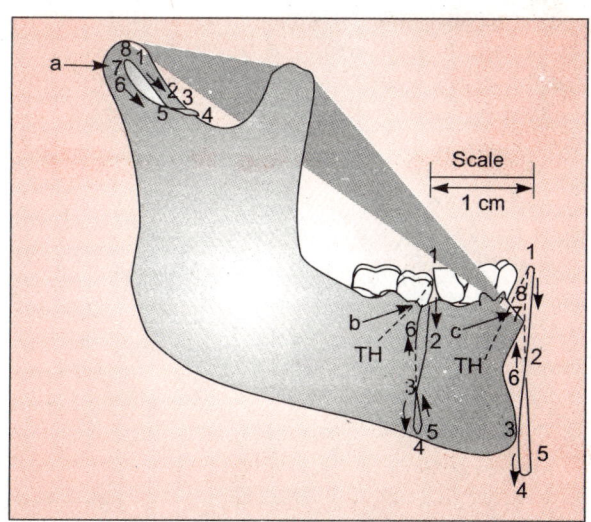

Fig. 25.1. Mandibular movement in mastication.

and closing paths, are all anterior to the terminal hinge position. From these tracings, it is also apparent that there is seldom a pure hinge movement during mastication. Instead, it is a complex movement involving simultaneous hinge, sliding, and rotary motion at the condyles.

Gliding contacts create curved wear patterns on the teeth that are concentric with the condyles. Wear facet patterns are unique to each individual and are changed by extraction of teeth or restorations that alter the occlusion, indicating that the chewing pattern is determined to some extent by the occlusion.

2. The typical adult chewing pattern as represented in the frontal plane is a tear drop shape with the opening phase medial to a more lateral closing phase.

The maximum extent of vertical and lateral movement in normal mastication is about half of the maximum vertical and lateral movements possible.

Figure 25.2 shows the jaw movement patterns of two individuals with different occlusal characteristics. It can also be seen that the closing movements often coincide with the border movements in the vicinity of intercuspal position.

From this it is inferred that there is gliding contact between the teeth as they are guided into the intercuspal position. When the jaws are closed into the intercuspal position, the gliding contacts are greater when lateral movements is larger, which is common when chewing tough resistant foods.

The angle formed between the closing and opening paths (vertex at intercuspal position) is always less or equal to the angle formed by the cuspal inclines.

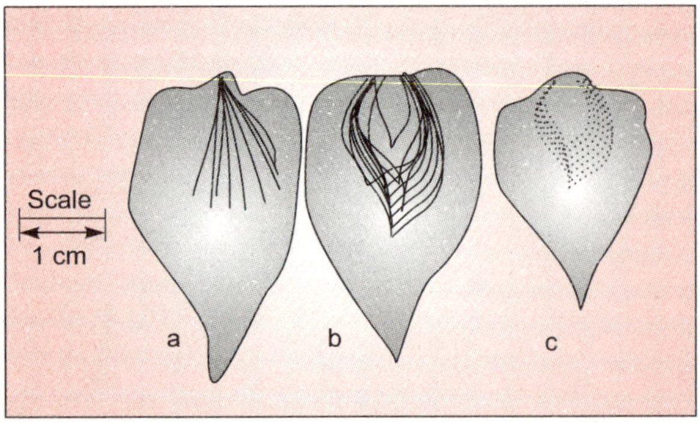

4. Gliding contacts are less frequent and less extensive in the opening phase. Lateral movements with gliding contacts appear to occur in most patients, yet there have been reports that vertical jaw movements are more frequent in Angle Class III prognathic malocclusions and in complete denture wearers.

5. Mastication can be unilateral, bilateral, or bilaterally alternating. The patient will commonly chew on the side with the most teeth. This side is also likely to be the most efficient side to chew on; it is often called the preferred side. Some patients chew on both sides at the same time. This is reported to be common in complete denture wearers.

6. Persons with severely worn occlusion, such as those with a bruxing habit or from a primitive culture with an abrasive diet tend to exhibit wider, lateral chewing movements with longer guide lengths.

Condylar Movements

1. The sagittal view, indicates that the working side condyle moves inferiorly and anteriorly on opening, and then posteriorly and superiorly on closing, with a slight anterior movement on final closure. In the sagittal view, the opening and closing paths of the working side do not coincide.

2. Note the non-working sagittal view of normal chewing movements. The opening and closing paths of the non-working condyle are longer than the movement of the working condyle. The movement patterns nearly coincide on opening and closing.

Scale
1 cm

a   b   c

Fig. 25.2. Jaw movement patterns of two individuals with different occlusal chacteristics.

3. The motion of the mandible during normal chewing in the horizontal plane is shown below:

The distance traced by the working condyle is less. Also, notice that the working side condyle and first molar make a slight anterior movement on final closure. The non-working side condyle, in contrast, does not make an anterior movement on final closure.

The working side anterior and medial movements on final closure are important because they show the likelihood of retrusive range contacts (posterior to intercuspal position) on the working side.

The medial movement represents the Bennett shift occurring when the working side moves from a lateral to a medial position during final closure. It has been shown that there are no terminal hinge contacts in normal mastication.

However, there are retrusive range contacts. Because of this, lateral retruded border registrations for articulator setting have been recommended in restorative dental procedures.

Masticatory Forces

1. Maximum biting forces generally vary from about 20.5 to 104.4 kg, although forces more than 363.7 kg have been reported in some individuals.
2. Maximum biting force appears to be slightly higher in males and is highest when measured in the molar area and lowest when measured at the incisors. Bite force is highest when the teeth are separated by 0-10 mm.
3. Bite force is probably controlled by other factors such as pain thresholds, sensitivity of mucosal and periodontal receptors, emotional status, and area of distribution of force.
4. In complete denture patients, maximum biting forces are much lower than for patients with a full natural dentition. Forces in patients with teeth are 5-6 times greater than in denture wearers. This has been attributed to the fact that denture patients have a much lower area for distributing the forces. It has been shown that anesthesia of the supporting mucosa will increase the maximum biting force recorded in full denture patients, which suggest that the pain is the limiting factor.
5. However, studies on subjects with natural teeth have indicated that anesthesia of the periodontal ligaments of the teeth decrease the maximal biting force. This occurs due to blockage of a positive feedback loop involving the periodontal mechanoreceptors.
6. Chewing speeds range from 49-120 cycles per minute. The usual rate of chewing is 70-80 chews per minute. The speed of the mandible is higher in the opening phase than in the closing phase. The closing speed decreases as the teeth contact the bolus of the food and just before the teeth contact each other. Mandibular movement speeds are generally in the range of 64 to 135 mm per second. There appears to be little change in the chewing rate when teeth are lost or when full dentures are worn. However, if the stability and fit of dentures are not good, the chewing rate can be decreased.

Masticatory Efficiency

1. One of the main functions of mastication is to breakdown food so that it can be swallowed and digested. Masticatory efficiency is a measure of how well, a person can breakdown food.

It is usually measured by sieving a sample of food expectorated by a subject after the person has chewed but not swallowed.
2. Masticatory efficiency (ME) decreases with loss of teeth and is generally lower in complete denture patients. Masticatory efficiency further decreases if the teeth are not replaced.
3. Tough and hard foods are avoided by denture wearers and people with multiple missing teeth. Usually tough foods are avoided by these patients because they are difficult or uncomfortable to chew. However, such avoidance can lead to malnutrition.

4. It is not clear whether there is any difference in chewing efficiency between anatomic and non-anatomic denture tooth forms. However, it is clear that occlusal markings or grooves improve masticatory performance.

Development and Learning of Mastication

1. One theory suggests that mastication develops as an extension and modification of suckling. Like mastication, suckling involves rhythmic up and down jaw movements coordinated with tongue and facial movements and swallowing.

   Proponents of the theory that chewing is an extension of suckling note the cyclic nature of suckling and the coordination of tongue, facial and jaw movements. They suggest that the central pattern generator begins its activity by providing the timing for suckling jaw and tongue movements, and that later, with the eruption of teeth and the appearance of the sensory feedback, mastication develops.

2. Another theory states that mastication is a fundamentally different behavior that develops separately from suckling. Studies have shown that certain electromyographic patterns are linked to specific stages of eruption of teeth. Also, it is noted that infants are able to suckle long after they learn to chew. Adults also maintain the capacity to suckle, suggesting that these two are related but independent behavior.

   Chewing movements in young children with primary dentitions differ from the typical adult pattern. The young children utilize wide lateral gliding movements on opening towards the working side. This pattern changes to a typical adult pattern when the child reaches 10-12 years. The eruption of the adult anterior teeth, which occurs in this time period, has been suggested as a reason for the adoption of the adult chewing pattern.

   In contrast to the relative shallow anterior guidance of the primary teeth, the anterior guidance is usually much steeper in the permanent dentition. It is believed that this steeper anterior guidance reduces the lateral movement component. This is supported by measurements of chewing patterns of adults with anterior-open bite occlusion (and hence lack of anterior occlusal guidance). Patterns in these individuals were found to be very similar to those in children with primary dentitions.

   When the natural teeth are replaced by complete dentures, a number of new factors are brought into play that may have profound influence upon mastication. Among these are loss of periodontal mechanoreceptors, mucosal displaceability, movement of the denture bases, involvement of the tongue and facial musculature in stabilizing the dentures, a decrease in the area of support of chewing forces, and changes in vertical dimension.

Neurological Control of Mastication

1. Early physiologists proposed mastication as control mechanisms based on reflexes. The early reflex theory proposed by Sherrington (1917) was based on the jaw opening reflex. He suggested that the jaw opening reflex coupled with rebound closure would maintain mastication after voluntary closure. Also, it was shown that electrical stimulation of the cortex would initiate chewing. In its simplest forms, a reflex mechanism of mastication would include initiation via cortical influence resulting in jaw opening, stretching of the masticatory muscle spindles, reflex jaw closure, reflex jaw opening, and so on until swallowing.

2. A newer and now more generally accepted theory of the control of mastication suggests that the cyclic pattern of mastication is provided by a central neural program located in the brainstem and which can operate in the absence of afferent information from the oral sites. This was supported by studies in patients who have undergone anesthesia of the gingiva, periodontium, and TMJ.

Anesthesia decreases the ability to control the food bolus, but the cyclical chewing movements are not affected.

3. Although the concept of the brainstem pattern generator is generally accepted, it is also known that the peripheral stimuli have considerable influence on natural chewing. It has been observed that biting on an unexpectedly hard object can interrupt the chewing cycle. Many receptors are implicated in the feedback to the masticatory pattern generator, including periodontal mechanoreceptors, bare pain receptors, TMJ receptors, Golgi tendon organs and muscle spindles.

4. There is evidence for the positive feedback loop that adjusts the chewing pattern and force level depending on the consistency of the food being chewed. As the jaws begin to close on a hard type of food, EMG levels are low. As the teeth contact the food and the crushing phase begins, closing muscle EMG levels rise sharply. As mastication progresses and the food is softened, the high-amplitude EMG activity during the closing phase is reduced.

During normal mastication, there is a great deal of interaction between peripheral inputs, the cerebral cortex, and the brainstem pattern generator to produce the complex behavior of mastication. The pattern generator is thought to be located in the reticular formation of the pons, which is very near the trigeminal sensorimotor complex.

Mastication is a complex neurophysiological activity thought to be dependent on a central pattern generator that programs much of the activity. Chewing is initiated and modified by cortical influence. Peripheral feedback is important in modification and coordination of chewing activity.

Muscle Activity Associated with Mastication

Muscle activity during mastication has been studied by the use of electromyography where the electrodes are mounted on several muscles of mastication, and recordings of these muscles are made simultaneously. EMG measures electrical activity associated with contraction only.

The jaw opening muscles are the mylohyoid, anterior digastric and lateral pterygoid. The lateral pterygoid takes part in jaw closure, lateral movements, and protrusive movements. The two heads of the lateral pterygoid muscle have been shown to act independently, which accounts for the multiple activities of this muscle.

The anterior temporalis on the working side becomes active slightly before the muscles on the non-working side. Because activity is about the same on both sides, it is thought that the anterior temporalis muscle is concerned more with elevating the jaw. The posterior temporalis muscle is thought to be important in lateral movements of the mandible as well as in mandibular closure. The non-working posterior temporalis muscle is involved in the movement of the mandible medially during the closing phase.

The masseter muscle is considered to be primarily involved with force development during mastication. The activity is much higher on the working side, yet the non-working side muscle begins activity earlier and maintains it longer than on the working side.

The medial pterygoid muscles initiate jaw closures. Their activity closely parallels that of the masseter muscle, and outlasts the activity of the anterior temporalis.

The working side lateral pterygoid muscle predominates in the early jaw opening, but later the non-working side muscle dominates, first moving the mandible towards the working side, and then assisting in jaw closure. After initial tooth contact, the working side muscle assists in jaw closure and in bringing the mandible medially towards intercuspal position.

The anterior digastric muscle is active during jaw opening; however, it sometimes appears to be active during the entire masticatory cycle.

The mylohyoid muscle has activity similar to that of the digastric muscle, but also has frequent irregular bursts of activity that may be associated with tongue movement. The tongue muscles are very active and of obvious importance in coordination of the bolus, teeth and jaw muscles.

Types of Mastication

There are basically two types of mastication: carnivorous and herbivorous – with two types of teeth, each functionally and morphologically different and ideally suited to its respective purpose.

Carnivorous mastication with its sharp, penetrating, steep, cuspid teeth is a puncturing type of function. The diet is primarily flesh and it is torn or ripped by sharp incisors and then the bolus is chewed by steep cuspid posterior teeth.

The bolus is not really chewed into small pieces but rather penetrated so that it is sponge-like and can be lubricated by the mucous of the saliva for swallowing and then attacked by digestive juices throughout.

Herbivorous Mastication. It is primarily maceration, grinding and comminuting to small particles. This frees the nutrients locked in the cellulose of the plant food so that digestion can take place. For this type of masticatory function, flat crushing type posterior teeth are needed that incorporate sharp irregular ridges on their surface. The jaw action required with these teeth to function is extensive lateral grinding.

Omnivorous. The human diet is omnivorous and the natural teeth are a compromise between the above two forms.

Functions of Mastication

1. Comminution of food by exerting biting force. This force in dentulous subjects is five to six times greater than in denture wearers.

2. Mastication is necessary for the full appreciation of the flavor of food and is therefore indirectly involved in the excitation of salivary and gastric secretions.

3. Mastication facilitates the digestion of carbohydrates by amylase. Amylase activity, though of minor importance while the food is in the mouth, is nevertheless responsible for the continuation of carbohydrate digestion in the stomach, and this phase can account for as much as 60% of the total carbohydrate digestion.

Clinical Implications of Mastication

1. Chewing efficiency is related to the number of teeth and the number of contacts. Of concern is that patients do not tend to compensate for the lose of occlusal surface by chewing longer. Maintenance of teeth is thus important.

2. Most patients tend to chew bilaterally; however, if patients have missing teeth, they will chew more on the side that has the greater number of teeth.

3. Mandible moves not only vertically during mastication but also anteroposteriorly and laterally. It is this horizontal movement that is most important to restorative efforts. For example, lateral retruded border registrations for articulator settings have been suggested because the working side condyle moves retrusively during mastication.

4. Although forces during chewing average about 22 kg, some individuals bite as high as 360 kg. The implication of these forces for restorative materials and the design of the prostheses is obvious.

5. Forces used by complete denture patients are about five times less than for patients with natural teeth.

6. Finally, regarding the control of masticatory movements, it is believed that mastication is learned early in life, then controlled primarily by a central pattern generator. Although masticatory movement can be

altered by changes in the occlusion, these patterns are relatively automatic and resistant to change, particularly in patients with complete dentures.

It is for this reason it is usually considered wise to make restorations compatible with the functional movement patterns of the patient rather than expect the patterns to adapt to fit the restorations.

FACTORS INFLUENCING MASTICATORY EFFICIENCY[5]

In edentulous patients, masticatory efficiency decreases with the loss of teeth and is generally lower in complete denture patients. The dentulous state represents a compromise in the integrity of the masticatory system.

In the edentulous masticatory system, the factors which influence the masticatory efficiency are:

1. Modifications in the area of support
2. Functional and Parafunctional considerations
3. Changes in morphologic face height
4. Adaptive responses.

Modifications in Areas of Support

Due to the loss of teeth, certain changes occur in areas of support. They are:

Complete Denture Therapy. The patient needing the complete denture therapy is deprived of periodontal support, and the entire mechanism of function and transmission to the supporting tissues is altered.

The Occlusal Forces Exerted on the Natural Teeth. The most prominent feature of the physiologic occlusal forces is their intermittent, rhythmic and dynamic nature.

Abrupt alterations are produced as a result of loss or removal of an opposing or an adjacent tooth; Changes in force acting on the teeth over an extended period of time elicit adjustments in the supporting tissues.

Consequently the application of consistently greater loads during mastication tend to cause an increase in the width of the periodontal ligament.

Stress on Mucosa. In the dentulous state, light loads are placed on the mucosa, but in the edentulous patient with complete dentures, the mucous membrane is forced to serve the same purpose as the periodontal ligaments that provide support for natural teeth.

Selectivity of Food. Prosthetic patients frequently limit the loading of supporting tissues by selecting food that does not require masticatory effort exceeding their tissue tolerance.

Area of Support. The area of mucosa available to receive the load from complete dentures is limited when compared to the corresponding areas of support available for natural dentitions. Watt (1961) has computed the mean denture-bearing area to be 22.96 cm^2 in the edentulous maxilla and 12.25 cm^2 in an edentulous mandible. His estimate of the areas of periodontal membrane of natural teeth is approximately 45 cm^2 in each jaw, more than three and half times the average area of the basal seat of a mandibular complete denture.

Condition of the Mucosa. The mucosa demonstrates little tolerance or adaptability to denture wearing. This tolerance is further reduced by the presence of systemic diseases such as anemia, nutritional deficiencies, hypertension, or diabetes.

Residual Ridge. Alveolar bone supporting natural teeth receives tensile loads through a large area of periodontal ligament. The edentulous ridge receives vertical, diagonal and horizontal loads applied by a denture with a surface area much smaller.

The masticatory efficiency in the edentuous patient is further compromised by the residual ridge resorption. The process of resorption of the mandibular residual ridge makes the flanges of the denture less compatible with functional lip, tongue and cheek movements, leading to less favorable mucosal conditions, this causes deterioration in the masticatory ability. Another problem is the resiliency of the mucosa which causes the inherent instability of the dentures during function.

Functional and Parafunctional Considerations

The masticatory system appears to function best in an environment of continuing functional equilibrium. The prosthesis rests on tissues that will change progressively and irreversibly. The complete denture should be designed so that their occlusal surfaces permit both functional and parafunctional movements of the mandible. This is accomplished by arrangement of teeth to occupy a "neutral zone" in the edentulous mouth.

Parafunctional habits can be harmful to the teeth, such habits in an edentulous patient can cause additional loading on the tissues. Parafunction is a significant prosthetic variable that contributes to ridge reduction.

Stress in denture supporting tissues: During function and parafunction, pressures are applied by the dentures, which will displace the soft tissues. An instantaneous elastic decompression occurs when the pressure is removed. This is followed by a continuing delayed elastic recovery.

Human soft tissues takes as long as 4 hours to recover after moderate loading for 10 minutes. A longer period of time is needed for the recovery of displaced mucosa in elderly people. Therefore leaving the dentures out of mouth during sleeping hours is recommended.

Changes in Morphological Face Height and Temporomandibular Joint

In the facial skeleton, any dimensional changes in morphologic face height or the jaw bones as a result of the loss of teeth are invariably transmitted to the TMJ. Complete dentures should be fabricated to conform to the changes in morphologic face height as a result of the loss of teeth. If this is not kept in mind, masticatory efficiency decreases.

The occlusion of complete dentures should be designed to harmonize with the primitive, unconditioned reflex of the patient's unconscious swallow (i.e. the centric relation). The occlusion in centric relation will be compatible with the forces developed during deglutition to prevent disharmonious contacts that cause decrease in masticatory efficiency.

Adaptive Response

Facility for learning and coordination appears to diminish with age which may affect the masticatory efficiency. Patient motivation will dictate the speed with which adaptation to the denture occurs.

METHODS OF EVALUATING MASTICATORY EFFICIENCY

With the exception of gnathodynamics, the examination of masticatory ability is the oldest procedure used to evaluate the function of the chewing apparatus. Gaudenz devised the first method for determining chewing ability at the beginning of this century. Several others have published their tests.

Masticatory efficiency is basically calculated in terms of the number of chewing strokes required by the subject to achieve the same degree of food pulverization as that obtained by a hypothetical norm. They based this norm on the average values of the masticatory performances at various levels of chewing strokes obtained from a group of dentulous subjects.

Masticatory efficiency can also be assessed by determining the masticatory performance ratio which can be calculated as follows:

$$\frac{\text{Volume of particles passing through a sieve}}{\text{Total volume of food collected from the mouth}} \times 100$$

Review of Methods

Adequacy of masticatory function is difficult to assess. In the absence of any reliable method of measuring masticatory ability, its success generally depends on patient satisfaction and on certain theoretical and arbitrary standards of denture fabrication

Gelman Method (G)

- The chewing ability was determined by requiring the subject to masticate a 5 g portion of hazelnuts for 50 seconds. The pulverized food was expectorated into a glass container and strained through a gauze.
- The food remaining on the gauze was dried over a bath for 40 minutes.
- Sieving was done by shaking the dried mass through a single screen with round openings 2- 4 mm in diameter.
- The weight of the fraction which remained in the strainer was then calculated in percent of the weight of the unchewed portion.
  The coefficient of masticatory efficiency was found by subtracting this percentage from 100.

Dahlberg Method

- The patient was required to chew a piece of flavorless formalin hardened 15% gelatin 10.6 cm^3 in size in 40 masticatory strokes.
- The chewed up gelatin was transferred into an appratus where it was sifted through 10 sieves with openings 1-10 mm in diameter. The holes of each successive screen varied 1 mm in diameter.
- After the sifting was completed, the number of particles was counted on each sieve.
- Special formulas have been used to calculate the total volume of the test portion, its total surface area, etc..

Manly Braley Gravimetric Method

They tested peanuts, carrots, shredded coconuts and raisins as test foods. On the basis of recovery of food after mastication, they concluded peanuts to be the suitable soft food for masticatory performance test.

- 15 g of peanuts were divided into (5)3 g portions, each of which was subjected to 20 masticatory strokes.
- All chewed food was collected into a single container, stirred to break up clumps and washed with 500 cm^3 of water through a 10 mesh screen. The size of the opening of the strainer was 2 mm.
- Both the particles remaining on the screen and the particles passing though the sieve were filtered on separate sheets of filter paper.
- Each fraction was dried in an oven at 100° for 3 hours, transferred into a desicator for 2 hours and weighed.
- Masticatory performance was calculated as the percentage of chewed food which passed through the screen, with the percentage based on the quantity of food that was recovered from the mouth. This test can also be made on a volumetric basis.
- They described masticatory efficiency in terms of the number of extra chewing strokes needed by a deficient person in order to achieve the same pulverization as the standard person.

Kapur and Soman Method

- They replaced the gravimetric sieve analysis by a volumetric method which is time saving and convenient.
- They tested several test foods and found carrots as a reliable test food (because by volumetric method, moisture loss was eliminated.)
- Unlike Manly and Braley they used 95th percentile value of percentage masticatory performance ratio in establishing their efficiency norm.
- They appreciated group differences between dentulous and edentulous subjects and established a separate masticatory efficiency norm for the latter.

Gunne Method[2]

Gunne attempted to determine masticatory efficiency by using gelatin lumps hardened by formalin as a chewed material. After the test pieces were chewed, they were placed in a water soluble dye. The dye diffused into the particles, and eventually the dye concentration in the surrounding solution decreased. The concentration of the dye solution was read from a photometer. A close relation was found between the gelatin particle size and the reduction of the dye solution concentration. Based on this correlation, the breakdown degree of the test material was estimated.

The Graphic Digitizer and Computer

Until now, the degree of particle breakdown has been determined either by using a sieve system or by dyeing chewed particles.

The former method depends on the number of sieves and their mesh size, and the latter method only provides a sum of the breakdown degree and does not show the distribution of the chewed particle size. The graphic digitizer measures the size of the chewed food and analyzes the characteristics of its frequency distribution.

A stereomicroscope is used for making a photograph of the particles. The photographs were magnified. The coordinate values of the diameter of masticated particles were put into a computer with a graphic digitizer and a stylus pen. The real measuring accuracy was within + 0.018 mm.

Masticatory efficiency can be measured by frequency distribution of chewed particle size. This method is convenient, simple and reliable.

Electromyography

This determines changes in bite force and chewing efficiency after denture treatment in edentulous patients. EMG determines the muscle activity after denture treatment which helps indirectly in the estimation of masticatory efficiency.

Low Frequency Sound Transmission

A new system recently has been developed that measures total interocclusal forces during mastication. The system measures low frequency sound transmission through occlusal contacts between the teeth.

This system has the advantage of measuring total interocclusal force in eccentric as well as in intercuspal position. Chewing forces are high in the intercuspal position (about 22.4 kg) and second highest during terminal closure contacts, just before reaching the intercuspal position.

Image Analysis[4]

The occlusal contact area of the complete dentures can be measured using the interactive image analysis system. The results showed that the relation between occlusal contact area and masticatory efficiency was positive significantly, and different regions of occlusal contact area had its corresponding masticatory efficiency.

It is indicated that occlusal contact area is necessary to satisfy the masticatory efficiency needed. If the masticatory load is great, the width of the supporting cusp should be reduced and a definite width of the non-supporting cusp should be preserved for holding the food being masticated.

Masticatory Efficiency Using Artificial Test Food (ATF)[3]

Artificial test food may be preferred to natural foods for the measurement of masticatory performance and efficiency, because the physical properties and shape and size of the particles are more reproducible.

The optosil silicone rubber has been extensively used for studies of masticatory function. ATF offers several additional advantages:

- The food particles can be given distinct shape of a cube.
- The food particles can be given any size.

- It is unaffected by water and saliva.
- The food can be colored so that mixtures containing different sized particles can be composed, each size having its own color.

Further Reading

1. Willam W, Wood A. Review of masticatory muscle function. JJ Prosth Dent. 1987; 57: 22.
2. Slagter et al. Force deformation properties of artificial and natural foods for testing chewing efficiency. JJ Prosth Dent. 1992; 68: 740
3. Shichong Shan. Masticatory efficiency determined with direct measurement of food. J Prosth Dent. 1990; 64: 723.
4. Z.Krysinksi et al. Methods of evaluating masticatory ability. J Prosth Dent. 1981; 46: 568.
5. Klelly E K Factors affecting the masticatory performance of complete denture wearers. J Prosth Dent. 1975; 33(2): 122-31.

MULTIPLE CHOICE QUESTIONS

1. **The maximum biting force varies form**
   a. 10-50 kg
   b. 10-150 kg
   c. 20-104 kg
   d. 100-150 kg

2. **Regarding biting force**
   a. Biting force is maximum in the molar area
   b. Biting force is higher in females
   c. Biting force is highest when teeth are separated by 2 mm
   d. Biting force is higher in complete denture patients.

3. **Biting forces in patients with natural teeth are .... compared to biting forces in complete denture patients.**
   a. 5-6 times lesser
   b. Equal
   c. 5-6 times greater
   d. 8 times greater

4. **The usual rate of chewing is**
   a. 40-50 chews per minute
   b. 14-16 per minute
   c. 70-80 per minute
   d. More than 100

5. **Masticatory efficiency is a measure of**
   a. How well a person can swallow food
   b. How well a person can digest food
   c. How well a person can breakdown food
   d. All the above

6. **The most accepted theory of the control of mastication is**
   a. Mastication develops as an extension and modification of suckling
   b. Mastication is a behaviour that develops separately from suckling
   c. Masticatory control is related to the jaw opening reflex
   d. Cyclic pattern of mastication is regulated by a central neural program.

7. **Gunne determined masticatory efficiency using**
   a. Hazel nuts
   b. Gelatin
   c. Carrots, coconuts
   d. Gelatin hardened with formalin

8. **Graphic digitizer can determine masticatory efficiency within an accuracy of**
   a. Food particles can be given a definite shape
   b. Food particles can be given a definite size.
   c. Food particles are unaffected by water and saliva.
   d. All are true

26

THE GAG REFLEX

INTRODUCTION

Prosthodontists and general dentists frequently come across patients who have extreme oral sensitivity by which they are unable to tolerate a foreign substance in the mouth.

Gagging can be a normal healthy defense mechanism to prevent foreign objects from entering the trachea. However, some patients experience gagging even during the most routine intraoral procedures. Gagging greatly complicates certain prosthodontic procedures, especially maxillary complete denture final impressions.

Gagging or retching is a problem which many dentists have described and analyzed but which has been found extremely difficult to treat. No one cause, has been identified and subjects suffering from the problem have been loosely divided into two groups: (i) the somatogenic—those in whom physical stimulation produces the gagging reflex; and (ii) the psychogenic—those in whom the stimulation appears to be psychic in origin. For the prosthodontist attempting to treat a patient,

the results are the same, the denture cannot be tolerated.

Patients with such sensitivity often complain of nausea, gagging or vomiting during treatment or while wearing dentures. Each of these reactions are part of the same reflex phenomenon and often result from fear. Gagging or retching associated with dental treatment is a normal, healthy reflex and difficult to manage.

GAG REFLEX

The normal gag reflex is an adaptive, vital mechanism for survival, controlled primarily by the parasympathetic division of the autonomic nervous system. Although tactile stimulation of the sensory receptors of the soft palate is the most obvious means by which the reflex may be elicited, gustatory, olfactory, visual and cognitive stimuli may elicit the reflex either as unconditioned or conditioned stimuli.

Gag reflexes that are hyperactive for whatever reason are not uncommon and present a problem for dentists, particularly when it is necessary to make impressions or fit prostheses. The gag reflex is a serious problem because failure to overcome the hyperactive reflex may leave the patient permanently edentulous—an esthetically and nutritionally unsatisfactory outcome.

CAUSES OF GAGGING

Many reasons have been proposed to explain the reaction of gag reflex. Gagging has been found more commonly in men than in women

1. Anatomical Factors. Anatomical abnormalities, and oral and pharyngeal sensitivity predispose a patient to gag when dentures are poorly constructed. A long soft palate and a sudden drop at the junction of the hard and soft palates are associated with the problem.

An atonic and relaxed soft palate elicits gagging by allowing the uvula to contact the tongue and the soft palate to touch the posterior pharyngeal wall.

2. Local Factors Causing Gag Reflex Include. (i) nasal obstruction, (ii) postnasal drip, (iii) catarrah, (iv) sinusitis, (v) nasal polyps, and (vi) congestion of the oral, nasal and pharyngeal mucosa.

3. Sex. Gagging has been found more commonly in men than in women.

4. Medical Conditions believed to contribute to gagging in dentistry include:
- Chronic diseases of the gastrointestinal tract which increase its irritability so that normal subthreshold stimuli elicit the reflex.
- Parasympathetic impulses from severe pain in sites other than the gastrointestinal tract may also cause gagging.
- It has been associated with chronic gastritis, Paterson's dysphagia, carcinoma of the stomach, partial gastrectomy, peptic ulceration, cholecystitis, carcinoma of the pancreas, diaphragmatic or hiatus hernia, and uncontrolled diabetes.

5. Social Causes of Gagging Include: (i) heavy smoking which causes gagging as a result of hypersensitivity, (ii) chronic catarrh, (iii) coughing, and (iv) excessive consumption of alcohol.

6. Fear. Some people who gag with dentures are also unable to tolerate other objects intraorally, with fear acting as a common cause of gagging.

7. Dentures stimulate gagging by moving against the soft tissues or by reducing the tongue space and causing the tongue to be displaced posteriorly into the pharynx.

8. Gagging can also result from a restricted airway. It is difficult for a patient with a very restricted tongue space or a small nasopharynx to tolerate bulky dentures.

MANAGEMENT OF GAGGING

Several treatment approaches (beyond correction of biomechanical factors and reassurance) have appeared in the literature. With a few exceptions, studies have reported little data or small sample sizes. Borkin (1959) described an impression technique using Kerr impression wax over special trays. Techniques designed to divert the patient's attention during unpleasant clinical procedures was used by Krol (1963) and Kovats[4] (1971). Singer (1973) tried to acclimatize his patients to denture wearing by having them keep five glass marbles in the mouth for one week prior to treatment. Re-evaluation of the prognosis took place until impressions could be made, and finally a lower base plate was constructed incorporating a "training bead" on its lingual aspect to maintain the tongue in the correct position during subsequent clinical procedures. This method is not dissimilar to that described by Wilka and Marks (1983).

Jordan (1954) suggested that a matt finish to the denture is more readily accepted. In more than one hundred patients with a retching problem, the freeway space was found to be inadequate by Krol. Kovats considered that great care must be taken to provide an adequate posterior palatal seal by extending the denture to the anterior edge of the soft palate. An inadequate seal will cause the denture to be loose.

A technique for the construction of palateless denture was described by Falmer and Connely (1984) but they noted that it would only be satisfactory if the maxillary ridge is well formed, to minimize horizontal movement.

Hypnosis

Several authors have advocated hypnosis. Relaxation, relaxation and controlled breathing and positive self-statements, and performance of incompatible responses, such as reading aloud, have been used with some success.

Medications[2]

Medications such as sedatives, antihistamines, parasympatholytics and topical anesthetics have been used with some success.

Marble Technique[1]

Singer's "marble technique" is a method by which the gag reflex can be exhausted thereby allowing for gradual exposure to the dental prosthesis or procedure.

The marble technique consists of seven steps which are as follows:

The First Visit. No oral examination of any kind was made at the first office visit. Five round, multicolored, glass marbles, approximately ½ inch in diameter were placed on a tray in front of the patient. The patient was told to put the marbles in his mouth, one at a time, at his leisure, until all five marbles were in his mouth.

Since the fear of swallowing a foreign object can induce the gag reflex, the patient was assured that if he swallowed a marble, it could not harm him. Continual assurance that he would be able to wear dentures was given to the patient at each weekly visit. He was urged to keep the five marbles in his mouth continuously for one week, except when eating and sleeping. Patient's with this problem can be treated with as few as two marbles.

The Second Visit. The patient was again given assurance that he would be able to wear dentures, which further bolstered his own motivation.

The Third Visit. Before the impression making was attempted, the hard palate, the soft palate, the cheeks, the lips, and the tongue were swabbed with 2 percent pentocaine solution in order to produce topical anesthesia.

Preliminary modeling compound impressions were made, refined and completed without a wash. The base plates were not highly polished, but they were sandblasted to give them a dull finish. Highly polished base plates often give a slimy or slippery feeling.

Fourth Vist. The base plate for the lower denture was inserted, and the patient was told to continue to keep three marbles in his mouth in addition to this base plate. A "training bead" (a small bead made of cold-curing acrylic resin) was placed on the lingual aspect of the lower base plate at the normal position of the lower central incisors. The training bead was used to help the patient maintain the proper tongue position. The patient should be reassured that he is making excellent progress.

Fifth Visit. The upper base plate was inserted, It proved to be a little more difficult for the patient to tolerate than the lower one, but he was asked to keep both of them in his mouth continually, except when eating. The use of marbles was discontinued.

The Sixth Visit. The patient will now be able to endure the presence of both base plates. Occlusal rims were used to establish the jaw relations. Try-ins were completed and used to determine esthetic considerations and to verify the occlusion. The patient should continue to wear the upper and lower base plates while the dentures are being processed.

The Seventh Visit. The completed lower denture was inserted first and used in conjunction with the upper base plate. A training bead was placed on the lower denture as a guide to tongue position. The patient should be instructed to keep the tip of the tongue always touching the bead, which would keep the lower denture from lifting. Next the upper denture was inserted.

The "marble technique" is useful in assuring so-called "hopeless" gaggers that it is possible for them to have dentures constructed and then to wear them. The change from the mental rejection to physical acceptance of the dentures can be greatly enhanced by the use of the marble technique.

Reduction of Palatal Coverage of Maxillary Denture

The maxillary denture can be reduced to a U-shaped border situated approximately 10 mm from the dental arch. Denture wearers with the above type of dentures reported that reduction of the palatal coverage influences their sense of taste positively, and gagging tendency disappears.

Modification of the Edentulous Maxillary Custom Tray to Prevent Gagging.[3] The

maxillary custom tray can be modified to prevent gagging as follows:

- Secure a maxillary cast from a preliminary impression in the usual manner.
- Block-out all undercuts on the cast and form a tray with autopolymerizing acrylic resin that is 2-3 mm short of all vestibular extensions. No handle should be placed at this time.
- Place base plate wax on the superior surface of the tray at the posterior segment. The wax should have roughly the same outline as the posterior palatal seal, extending from one tuberosity to the other.
- Attach a disposable saliva ejector to the base plate wax in the midline of the tray. Make sure the tip of the saliva ejector is embedded in the wax. (Border mold the impression in the usual manner. Remove the tray from the mouth after the impression material extruding from the posterior border of the tray has been sucked into the vacuum

chamber that was formed. This modified maxillary custom acrylic resin tray aids in removal of excess impression material.)
- Cover the wax with a thin layer of petroleum jelly.
- Mix a second batch of autopolymerizing tray acrylic resin. Form this material into a thin sheet and place it over the wax and tip of the saliva ejector. The material should extend past the wax and attach to the original tray.
- After the acrylic resin has cured, remove the wax spacer.
- Smooth any roughness on the tray and polish the tray at this time.
- Add a wax occlusion rim to the tray to approximate the position and contour of the teeth in the completed denture.
- Trim the posterior extent of the tray and border mold in the usual manner.
- Mix the impression material and load the tray. As the impression tray is being seated in the mouth, the assistant attaches the low volume evacuation hose to the end of the saliva ejector embedded in the tray.
- Border mold the impression in the usual manner.
- Remove the tray from the mouth after the impression material extruding from the posterior border of the tray has been sucked into the vacuum chamber that was formed.

This modified maxillary custom acrylic resin tray aids in removal of excess impression material as it extrudes from the posterior border of the maxillary custom tray before it can elicit a gag reflex in the patient.

Psychotherapy

Psychotherapy has been recommended for otherwise intractable "chronic or hysterical" gagging.

Analgesics

Analgesics: This causes a rapid, effective elimination of the gagging in denture-wearing patients.

- A cotton swab is used to apply a light coating of oral "antiseptic/analgesic" to the soft palate and rear of the tongue to produce some decrease in sensation.
- Secondly, a tongue depressor was used to repeatedly probe the soft palate and rear of the tongue. When the gag reflex consistently failed to occur, the patient inserted the upper denture. He signals when gagging seems imminent and removed the denture to avoid further associations of proper placement with gagging and vomiting. Four series of timed trials were conducted on the first 2 days of treatment. Fewer trials were conducted on days 3 and 4 because the patient's tolerance of the maxillary denture is likely to increase.

Conditioning Prostheses

A conditioning denture can be used in problematic patients to train the patient to gradually control gagging and adapt to reduced taste sensations.

This conditioning prostheses consists of alveolar palatal prosthesis constructed in acrylic similar to an orthodontic appliance in which ball clasps are included to retain the prosthesis. Such an appliance is worn for 1 week of adaptation, with 1 week of respite between prostheses. This helps the patient in accepting the permanent prostheses to be inserted later.

Controlled Breathing Method

Controlled breathing method advocated by the National Child Trust for use by women in labor is similar to that advocated by Murphy.

- All patients were instructed in controlled rhythmic breathing and told to practice it for one or two weeks before prosthetic treatment has commenced. The breathing was slow, deep and even, and the rhythm maintained by concentrating the mind upon a particular verse or tune with an even tempo. The concentration was particularly important so that if the patient experienced a retching episode, the breathing would become deeper and slower.
- If no satisfactory denture was in existence, a very thin clear acrylic base plate was constructed. Care was taken to provide maximal palatal coverage to just short of the vibrating line, a satisfactory postdam and a very thin posterior border.

Impressions for construction of base plate were taken in two stages: primary impressions using impression compound in stock trays and secondary impressions, usually of plaster, taken in shellac special trays. During impression taking, patient's rhythmic breathing was reinforced. Few problems were encountered at the primary impression stage, and this gave subjects a sense of achievement. At the secondary impression stage, care was taken to ensure that no plaster ran down onto the lower part of the soft palate by waiting until the plaster ceased to 'run' before inserting the impression. At all times the dentist made the subjects concentrate on his or her breathing, and if retching or vomiting occurred, the dentist should maintain a relaxed manner so that the subjects did not get agitated.

- When the base plate was inserted, the breathing technique was explained again and the patient told emphatically that a routine should be adopted whereby a particular time each day was assigned for denture acclimatization.

The length of time the base plate was worn each day should be slowly increased. At first, the base plate was to be kept in for only 5 minutes and under no circumstances removed, even if retching stimulus became very strong. The rhythmic breathing should be maintained for the whole base plate wearing period. Patients had to write down the length of the time the base plate was worn each day so that one particular day's time could be compared with preceding ones. Thus the patient could assess his own progress, and the operator could assess the degree of cooperation.

After the base plate was inserted, the patients were not seen for 2-3 weeks. It took three or four visits before both wearer and dentist were confident enough for treatment to continue and denture construction to begin.

- The models taken from the second impressions were duplicated so that the final denture was constructed on a model identical to that used for the base plate. Thus the base plate could be worn right upto the time the denture was fitted.

Further Reading

1. Singer L. The marble technique. J Prosth Dent. 1973; 29(2): 146-50.

2. Linton et al. Rapid elimination of the hyperactive reflex. J Prosth Dent. 1988; 60(4): 415-17.

3. Gordan N Callison. A modified edentulous maxillary custom tray to help prevent gagging. J Prosth Dent. 1989; 62(1): 48-9.

4. Kovats J J. Clinical evaluation of the gagging patient. J Prosth Dent. 1971; 25(6): 60.

MULTIPLE CHOICE QUESTIONS

1. **Gagging can be caused by**
   a. Long soft palate
   b. Nasal polyps
   c. Partial gastrectomy
   d. All the above

2. **The marble technique for controlling was introduced by**
   a. Kovats
   b. Jordan
   c. Krol
   d. Singer

3. **In the marble technique for gagging, the lower base plate is inserted at the _____ visit**
   a. First
   b. Second
   c. Third
   d. Fourth

4. **The true statement regarding biting force is**
   a. Biting force is highest in the molar area and lowest in incisor area
   b. Bite force is highest when teeth are separated by 1-10 mm
   c. Forces in patients with teeth are 5-6 times lesser than in complete denture patients
   d. All of the above

FAQ's

1. **Definition of masticatory efficiency**
2. **Methods for evaluating masticatory efficiency**

27

IMMEDIATE COMPLETE DENTURES

DEFINITION

An immediate complete denture is a dental prosthesis constructed to replace the lost dentition and associated structures of the maxilla and/or mandible and inserted immediately following the removal of the remaining teeth. It is also defined as a complete denture or removable partial denture fabricated for placement immediately following the removal of natural teeth.

INTRODUCTION

Removable complete or partial dentures fabricated following standard procedures have an undesirable disadvantage in that in the time elapsed between the extraction of the teeth and fabrication of the prosthesis, there is a phase of edentulousness that the patient has to undergo. This time period, not only promotes physiologic changes but also psychologic variations in the patient. This uncalled for experience can be eliminated by fabrication of immediate complete dentures. The immediate complete dentures help in overcoming this deficiency of the conventional complete denture.

REQUIREMENTS

To achieve the maximum degree of success, the immediate denture should satisfy the following requirements:
- Should be compatible with the surrounding environment.
- Should restore the masticatory efficiency within limits.
- Should be in harmony with the functions of speech, respiration and deglutition.
- Should be esthetically acceptable.
- Should preserve the remaining hard and soft tissue support.

The last requirement is the biggest challenge that the dentist and patient have to combat.

The first four can be evaluated by clinical evaluation and analysis.

ADVANTAGES

The advantages of an immediate complete denture include:

1. The denture acts as a bondage or splint to help control bleeding, to protect against trauma from the tongue, food or teeth if present in the opposing arch and aids to keep oral fluids and food particles from entering the sockets.
2. The bondage or splinting action protects not only the wound but also the blood clot there by promoting rapid healing.
3. Patients seem to regain adequate function in speech, deglutition and mastication much sooner than when the lips, tongue and cheeks have gone unsupported for a long time.
4. Many patients are not as reluctant to have diseased teeth removed when they are assured of replacement immediately.
5. For some individuals, it is a financial necessity to continue their businesses with minimal interruption.
6. It is less difficult to make the polished surfaces of the dentures compatible with the structures of the lips, tongue and cheeks when they have not changed their positions (because of lack of support).
7. The natural teeth aid in establishing the VDO and in positioning the artificial replacements.
8. Psychologically there are two outstanding advantages: (i) a patient having an immediate denture rarely fails to be a complete denture user, and (ii) patients do not have to face their families and friends in the edentulous state, therefore their social and business activities can be carried on without embarrassment.

INDICATIONS

1. The edentulous or partially edentulous patient whose remaining natural teeth must be extracted is the prime candidate for immediate denture service.
2. Patients for whom total extractions are required.

CONTRAINDICATIONS

1. Patients with systemic conditions such as cardiac abnormalities, glandular disorders, blood dyscrasias and those with slow healing potential.
2. Patients with limited or poor mental capacity to understand instructions are poor maintenance risks.
3. Patients unwilling to cooperate such as indifferent or unappreciative patients.
4. Emotionally disturbed individuals.
5. Patients with acute periapical or periodontal pathosis
6. Patients who have excessive bone loss.

DISADVANTAGES

1. There is no opportunity to observe the anterior teeth at try-in appointment, Therefore the esthetic result cannot be evaluated until the dentures are inserted.
2. Treatment is more expensive due to: (i) increased office time, (ii) post operative adjustments, and (iii) need to reline or remake the denture following healing.
3. More postoperative care. The surgical site of an immediate denture will change throughout the healing period. This may require more adjustments or the placement of tissue conditioning material to increase retention and stability.
4. Less Retentive. A certain amount of professional guess work is required in contouring the cast after removing the stone teeth. This

can be kept to a minimum, but it does assume that there may be less retention.

5. The immediate denture does not replace the stimulation that was supplied to the bone by the natural teeth.

6. The procedures are precise and time consuming and requires more appointments.

Prior to the start of the treatment, a thorough diagnosis must be completed and treatment plan prepared.

DIAGNOSTIC PROCEDURES

It is advisable to divide the diagnostic procedures into two phases: (1) patient examination, and (ii) consultation interview.

Patient Examination

Patient Examination should include:
- Findings of local and systemic origin
- Roentgenographic study
- Accurately articulated study casts
- Visual and digital appraisal examination
- Appearance of any existing prosthesis and all anatomic entities that influence the procedures incident to the construction of dentures.

Consultation Interview

- Appraisal of patient's mental attitudes and his expectations and needs
- Past dental history
- Existing systemic conditions of which he is aware are determined
- In addition to the information the dentist receives from the patient, the dentist must advice the patient on what to expect from the dentures and must outline the responsibilities of the patient in the use and care of the dentures.

The diagnostic findings are determined by investigating: (i) local oral conditions, (ii) patient's mental attitude, (iii) systemic status, and (iv) past dental history.

Local Oral Conditions

Local factors of particular significance are:
- Condition of the teeth to be extracted
- Position of the teeth
- Presence of foreign bodies
- Presence of bony or tissue undercuts that must be reduced or eliminated
- Exostoses
- Bone loss adjacent to the remaining site
- Muscle coordination.

Patients Mental Attitude

- Philosophical patients are considered ideal.

Systemic Status

Systemic conditions affecting the basal seat include:

1. Neurosis, osteoporosis and xerostomia in patients with poorly controlled diabetes.

2. Poor clotting mechanisms in patients with cardiovascular and cerebrovascular disease.

3. Mucosal disorders such as desquamative stomatitis, developing after menopause.

4. Mucosal disorders, psychogenic symptoms of burning tongue or palate, and carcinophobia in patients undergoing natural menopause.

5. Keratotic lesions, hyperkeratosis and dyskeratosis resulting from vitamin A and B deficiency, hyperestrogenism, hypercholesterolemia and a past history of syphilis.

6. Dermatologic diseases like psoriasis, pemphigoid lesions that ulcerate easily and stand limited pressure and erosive lichen planus.

7. Collagen disorders—arthritis affecting the hand which are so essential in manipulating the denture, sclerodema, lupus erythematosus and disorders requiring steroid therapy.

8. Osteoporosis occurring as a result of bone matrix defects as in malnutrition resulting from colitis, diabetes and hyperthyroidism

9. Defects in the osteoblasts.
10. Ovarian agenesis or atrophy and lack of estrogen and androgen.
11. Poor synthesis of bone matrix in senility and vitamin deficiency of alcoholics.
12. Adult rickets caused by poor absorption of calcium and phosphorous in patients with digestive disorders.
13. Hyperthyroidism
14. Fibrous dysplasia involving the jaws.

Treatment Plan

A Treatment plan is prepared for the patients based upon the diagnostic information that is collected. If immediate dentures are indicated several choices of treatment are possible
1. Remove all the posterior teeth and plan for the immediate replacement of anterior teeth only.
2. Remove all posteriors and plan for immediate replacement of posterior teeth and later replace the anterior teeth by an immediate denture.
3. Remove all the mandibular and maxillary teeth and replace them in the immediate denture.
4. Remove all maxillary teeth and replace them with an immediate complete denture.
5. Remove segments of the dentition and replace them as they are removed by sectional dentures (that are completed and sectioned to replace only the portion of the teeth extracted).

Clinical and Laboratory Procedures

Mouth Preparation

Preparation of the mouth for immediate complete dentures should begin at least six weeks before making the final impression. Procedures to prepare the posterior portion of the residual ridges include the removal of any remaining posterior teeth and residual root tips, correction of interfering exostoses or long under cuts and surgical modification of soft tissue. Although anterior teeth are not removed until immediately before placement of the denture, scaling them at this time will speed the healing of extraction sites.

Impressions

There are two areas that present the greatest challenge to dentists during the fabrication of immediate complete dentures.

The first involves the making of the impression. Since the immediate denture is a hybrid variety which incorporates some of the requisites of a removable partial denture impression and those of a complete denture impression, its management is very critical.

Two basic types of impressions for immediate dentures are:
1. Sectional Impressions
2. Single Impressions
The sectional impressions divides the denture bearing areas into two or more parts for a final impression.

Sectional Impression

Objective. To record the basal seat of the dentures and the adjacent anatomic landmarks.

The irreversible hydrocolloid impression materials have suitable properties to accomplish these objectives.

Preliminary Impression
1. Modify a stock impression tray with wax to provide support for the impression material and stops for the placement of the tray.
2. Outline the hamular notches and the vibrating line in the patient's mouth with an indelible pencil. This indelible line which indicates the posterior extent of the final impression will be transferred to the impression.
3. Place irreversible hydrocolloid into the modified tray and position the tray into the patient's mouth to make the impression.
4. Pour a stone cast.

5. Relieve the lingual surfaces of the remaining dentition, the residual ridges and palatal surface with 20 gauge relief wax.

6. Extend the relief wax about 2 mm anteriorly over the incisal edges of the teeth to provide a ledge in the impression tray for support of the labial vestibular region of the final impression.

7. In case of the maxillary impression, remove the relief wax from the posterior palatal seal area and buccal reflections of the cast and in case of mandibular preliminary casts, the relief wax is removed from buccal shelf areas and the postmylohyoid fossae.

8. Provide stops for repositioning the final impression tray by cutting two windows in the wax ledge opposite to expose the incisal edges of two widely separated anterior teeth.

9. Cover the section of cast (that has not been relieved with wax) with tin foil substitute.

10. Mold an autopolymerizing resin tray over the posterior part.

11. Extend the resin forward to the central incisors to form a handle shaped to fit the fingers.

12. Allow the acrylic resin to harden.

13. Remove the impression tray from the cast.

14. Smooth and polish the impression tray. The trimmed tray should not cover the labial surface of the teeth or the labial vestibule.

Final Impression Technique. The final impression is made in three sections which are reassembled to make the master cast (Fig. 27.1).

The first section which includes all the denture-bearing areas except the labial vestibular region, and the labial surfaces of anterior teeth, is recorded using the individual tray formed by the preliminary cast. The labial surface and the labial vestibules are recorded with a quick setting plaster. This plaster impression is divided into two sections to facilitate its removal from the mouth.

1. Place the individualized tray in the patient's mouth and check for correct adaptation and extension.

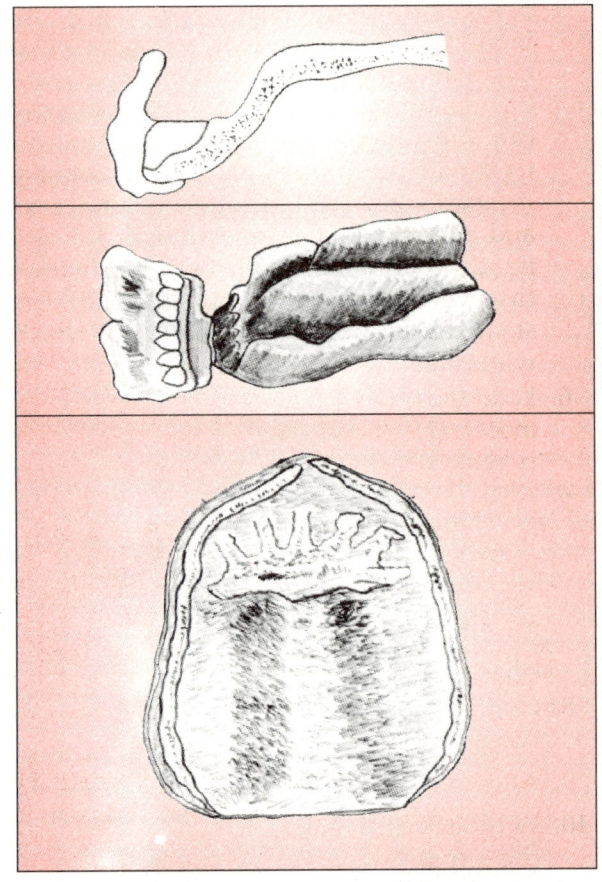

Fig. 27.1. Impression techniques for immediate dentures.

2. Reduce the buccal borders 3-4 mm short of the reflections and perfect them with stock modeling compound. The posterior borders of both upper and lower trays should be checked for correct extensions.

3. Then reduce the height of the perfected border 0.5–1 mm to provide space for the impression material.

4. Drill escape holes for excess impression material through the maxillary tray in areas corresponding to the median palatine raphe and palatal tissue on either side of the palatal raphe. Holes in these areas make it easier to record palatal tissues in the resting state without displacing it. On the mandibular tray, holes are placed over the crest of the ridge.

5. Prior to making the impression, the mobility of the remaining teeth should be evaluated. If the teeth are very mobile and have compromised periodontal attachment, care must be taken to avoid extracting the teeth with the impression. Some preventive measures include blocking out undercuts and interproximal areas with soft wax and lightly coating the teeth with petrolatum. In severe cases, a vacuum formed resin stent can be utilized as protective sheath while making the impression.

6. Load the tray with free flowing impression material such as zinc oxide eugenol or rubber base impression material.

7. Position the maxillary impression tray in the patient's mouth with the incisal stops and the posterior palatal seal area of the tray acting as guides to its proper placement. The incisal stop and the buccal shelves serve as stops in mandibular tray.

8. Gently mold the tissues adjacent to the borders of the impression.

9. Allow the impression material to harden.

10. Without displacing the impression, remove the excess that has flowed around the anterior teeth. A good finish line on the tray will facilitate the removal of the anterior section.

11. Remove the posterior section at this time to check for any discrepancy. If the posterior section is satisfactory the impression is placed correctly back to the mouth.

12. Mix quick setting impression plaster to a medium thick consistency.

13. Moisten the labial mucosa with water and place the plaster impression material in the labial vestibules.

14. Gently manipulate the patient's lips outward and downward (in maxillary impression) and outward and upward (in mandibular impression). The thickness of the labial flange, which occupies the same space as the plaster impression can be determined at this time.

15. When the plaster impression has reached its initial set, make a shallow groove labial to the labial frenum. The grooves should be about half the thickness of the plaster impression.

16. Allow the plaster to harden completely

17. Place a knife in the groove, section the plaster impression and remove the two sections.

18. Remove the posterior section of the impression.

19. Reassemble the three sections to make final impression.

20. Pour a master cast in the final impression.

Variations of the Sectional Technique

1. Variation described by Campagna. The preliminary impression is made in alginate and the final impression in rubber base and alginate.

2. A technique described by Heartwell which differs from Campagna's technique in the design of the custom tray.

Single Impression Technique

Single impression technique can be accomplished by using a stock tray or a custom tray made from the preliminary cast. Disadvantages include:

1. Angulation of the anterior teeth interferes with the correct placement of the tray.

2. This procedure allows little or no border molding.

Freese described a single impression technique in which modeling compound is used to make a preliminary impression in an oversized stock tray. This preliminary impression serves as the final impression tray. The preliminary impression is again border molded by heating the border a little at a time and reinserting the impression in the mouth. Holes are drilled and under cut into the modeling compound to provide for added retention of the final rubber base impression material. A fairly thin layer (3-4 mm) of impression material is added to the tray which is inserted in the mouth and removed after setting. The final casts are poured from this impression.

Appleby and *Kirchoff* described another commonly used single impression technique. A stock tray is trimmed or wax is added to conform to the contours of the mouth. A preliminary alginate impression is made in this tray. A custom acrylic tray is constructed over a preliminary cast poured in this impression. A line extending to within 3-4 mm of the vestibular reflections is drawn to outline the borders of the tray. The acrylic tray is relieved to provide for impression material by adapting shredded wet asbestos to the teeth and then covering the entire cast to the border outline with one layer of base plate wax. The tray is then border molded in sections with low fusing compound. The asbestos and wax are then removed and holes are drilled into the tray to avoid displacement of the tissue by final impression material. Irreversible hydrocolloid impression material is placed in the acrylic tray to make the final impression. Any excess of hydrocolloid is trimmed away before the final cast is poured.

MAXILLOMANDIBULAR RELATION RECORDS

A recording base is fabricated from auto-polymerizing resin and occlusal rim is made from base plate wax.

The maxillo-mandibular relation records for immediate dentures are essentially the same as that of conventional dentures.

Face-bow Transfer

A face-bow transfer is made to orient the maxillary cast on the articulator.

Tentative Centric Occlusion and Centric Relation

Patient's sometimes have enough existing posterior teeth to provide a tentative occlusal dimension. Phonetics is the most reliable way of evaluating an existing vertical dimension. If the patient has no posterior occlusion the tentative occlusal vertical dimension should be determined, as it would be if the patient is totally edentulous.

The centric relation record is made at a slightly increased vertical dimension using a free flowing medium on the occlusal rim (ZnOE impression paste). This contributes to an accurate record and prevents "skids" that might occur as a result of contact between teeth and occlusal rims.

The centric relation record is removed from the mold, trimmed and verified. The mandibular cast is placed using the centric relation record.

Selection and Arrangement of Teeth

Tooth selection for an immediate denture is usually a straight forward procedure. The existing dentition is utilized in selecting a shade and mold that will maintain the patient's natural appearance.

Appropriate posterior teeth are selected. If the immediate denture will oppose natural dentition, an anatomic tooth form is selected. If the immediate denture will oppose a complete denture, either anatomic or non-anatomic teeth can be used. Acrylic denture teeth should be used since it is necessary to: (i) reshape the ridge lap portion of the teeth, (ii) occlusal adjustments are easier, and (iii) acrylic teeth will not cause wear of the opposing natural dentition.

Posterior Try-in

A try-in is scheduled after the posterior teeth are set. The trial base will not be as retentive as it would be for a completely edentulous patient. Denture adhesives may be used sparingly. Centric relation and occlusal vertical dimension are verified. The mandibular cast can be remounted if necessary. The position of the posterior palatal seal is verified and scribed in the maxillary master cast at this time.

Arrangement of Anterior Teeth

The anterior denture teeth are arranged after the posterior try-in appointment. Positioning of the anterior teeth depends on whether the dentist wants to duplicate the patient's natural tooth arrangement. Whereas this is desirable for the majority of the patients, some do present with rather in esthetic arrangement which are usually the result of advanced periodontal diseases and drifting of teeth. Quite clearly in these situations, positioning of prosthetic teeth will be demanded that offers the maximum cosmetic result.

The form, shape and size of the natural teeth are the best guides in the shade and mold selection of anterior teeth. Following this, reference lines for positioning the teeth are made. This is done by drawing a straight line through the middle of the long axis of the tooth from the incisal edge to the border of the impression surface of the working cast on all anterior teeth.

Trimming of the Cast in the Construction of Immediate Dentures

The technique of trimming the cast for an immediate denture should be based on realism. First, the cast must be trimmed in such a way that an immediate denture is to be inserted in order to assure an immediate and favourable adaptation of the denture base to the area from which the teeth are extracted.

Second, it is erroneous to assume that trimming the cast means that it is necessary to reduce the alveolar bony structures to an amount equal to the amount of stone removed from the cast. The procedure was introduced by Frank C Jesbi.

Basically it is a modification of the "rule of thirds" as suggested by Killy who recommends dividing the labial aspects of the ridge into three equal bands of space between the gingival line and at the depth of vestibular space.

The first step is to cut away some parts of the crowns of the teeth that are visible, i.e. the cut is made at a line drawn at the free gingival margin. This amounts to removing the major parts of the crown, but it must be remembered that a portion of the crown still lies beneath the gingiva.

Step two is to trim the cast, so that the sites of the previously removed crowns are recessed approximately 1 mm. With this step the trimming equals the removal of the entire crown of each tooth.

Step three is a flat cut across the facial surface of the ridge, starting the cut at the labial depth of the recess made in Step 2. Stone is removed in a continually diminishing amount from this point to the junction of the gingival and middle third areas of the facial surface of the ridge. The removal of this amount of stone represents the collapse of the labial gingival tissues towards the alveolus.

Step four is another flat cut across the portion of the ridge. This cut begins at the crest of the ridge (labiolingual centers) and extends to the mid points of the cut made in Step 3. This procedure begins the contouring of the labial surface of the ridge.

The fifth step is to trim the part of the cast which is lingual to the teeth. Most of the casts present a reproduction of the continuous roll of gingival tissue that would normally be against the lingual aspects of the teeth and it is the landmark for trimming the cast in this area. This roll of tissue left unsupported after the teeth are extracted will collapse into the alveolus. The roll is completely trimmed away, but care is taken to preserve a part of the cast to represent the incisive papilla in its collapsed position so that the dentures will not place undue pressure on the underlying structures.

The last step is to shape and smooth the surfaces of the cast that have been trimmed in the previous steps. The edge of a knife is used to eliminate acute angles and to carry the contouring into the middle third of the labial aspect of the ridge. The vestibular one-third of the ridge is not trimmed. The contoured areas of the cast are rubbed with fine sandpaper in order to produce a smooth tissue receptive inner surface to the denture.

Positioning of Anterior Teeth

When the dentist decides to position the anterior teeth in their original location, there are two methods that can be used:

1. In the first, alternate teeth are cut away on the cast in the manner explained before. The right central incisor is usually placed first and is secured in wax. Then alternate teeth are removed and replaced until all have been set. By removing only one teeth at a time, the dentist can duplicate in its replacement any delicate irregularities that may exist.
2. In the second method, the trimming is done on one half of the remaining segment and then on the other. The segments of artificial teeth can be set alternatively, or the entire cast may be rendered edentulous and diagnostic cast used as a guide for tooth placement.

Waxing and Flasking

The upper labial border of the denture is filled with wax according to the fullness of the border on the cast. An adequate thickness of the denture border is necessary to protect the patient's tissues if edema follows the removal of teeth and insertion of the denture. The fullness of the denture border is reduced after completion of the denture.

Flasking is performed in the usual way, followed by wax boil out and cleaning.

Processing, Occlusal Correction, Final Preparation of Immediate Denture

The dentures are then processed and resulting changes in occlusion are corrected before removal of the dentures from their casts for finishing. Articulating paper locates any deflective occlusal contacts in centric occlusion, and these are ground away with small mounted stones.

Before any surgery is undertaken, the labial flange of the denture must be thinned to a minimum. However, the border must be well rounded. The prominences on the inner surface, representing the locations of the fresh tooth sockets are trimmed. It is necessary that no early pressure be placed in the regions of the immediate extraction. The anterior portion of the socket is particularly sensitive because the labial plate is so thin and sharp. The inner surface of the denture is reduced whenever socket prominences protrude.

Preparation of the Surgical Template

A transparent surgical template may be used as a guide for shaping the ridge at the time teeth are removed and the denture is inserted. The template will reveal places on the ridge where additional bone must be removed and will minimize the amount of surgery needed.

After the cast has been trimmed an impression of it is made in alginate. Cast is thoroughly soaked in water and the impression material is placed in the same tray in which the original impression was made. The loaded tray is forced into position on the cast in such a way that no air is trapped in the impression material. When the material has set, the impression is removed and plaster is poured into it to form a cast. A clear resin template can thus be made by vacuum formed technique.

Surgical Preparation/Mouth Preparation for Immediate Denture

The technique to be de   ibed causes little or no edema and negligible discomfort and enhances healing. This technique has been used on 179 patients by *William B Linnenberg.*

Preliminary Surgical Procedures

The maxillary and mandibular posterior teeth are extracted 14-24 days before the impressions for immediate dentures are made. This period of time allows for initial healing of posterior ridges.

Premedication

Half an hour before the surgical operation for immediate dentures, the patient is given 1 mg of dexamethasone orally. Dexamethasone is a synthetic analog of prednisolone and is used primarily for its antiinflammatory effects. The low dosage and short period of administration prevent the development of untoward effects of corticosteroids in oral surgery. However a complete patient history must be taken routinely so that the use of corticosteroids may be avoided in patients with active or latent tuberculosis, active peptic ulcer, herpes simplex, congestive heart failure, azotemia and hemorrhagic diathesis.

Careful observation of the patient and the administration of appropriate antibiotics avoid masking infection with the administration of dexamethasone.

Postoperative Instructions

Certain instructions are given to the patient upon completion of surgery

1. Not to remove the dentures for 24 hours and to return at the end of 24 hours.
2. To apply an ice pack on the anterior part of the face for 15 minutes.
3. To take suitable analgesics for postoperative pain.
4. To eat a soft diet and drink large quantities of liquid.
5. To rest if possible.
6. To use no mouthwashes for the first 24 hours.
7. To take dexamethasone as directed.

Postoperative Care

The main reasons that the immediate denture service appeals to the patients are the psychological demands of the patient's social world and masticatory ability. The patient should be cared for on a constant and continuing basis, and the masticatory apparatus must receive continuing maintenance, in order to satisfy these reasons.

The effectiveness of the immediate denture service can be continued after the edema is gone, the pain is minimal, and the patient is pleased with the cosmetic appearance. The initial success can be completely nullified unless, postoperative care is continued through the out healing period.

The term healing period has many different connotations. It can be interpreted to mean that even after the healing is complete from the histologic and physiologic view point, there remains a period of time when supporting tissues will continue to change rapidly for a period of 5 years.

During at least the first six months of this healing period, the dentist should expect to see rather dramatic changes in the shape and in dimensions of the residual alveolar support. To neglect the effects of these changes is to condemn the patients to discomfort and restricted masticatory efficiency.

The prevalent use of tissue conditioners can maintain an accurate denture to tissue contact. The patient's level of comfort can be increased. By increasing the accuracy of fit of the impression physiological values are maintained. Also the established biomechanical dimensions such as correct centric and vertical relations, correct occlusal relationships and balanced interocclusal pressure may be maintained.

CHANGES IN POSITION OF IMMEDIATE DENTURE

In an effort to determine some of the reasons for altered dimensional change Waltz attempted to record the amount of the distal drift of immediate denture. The observations made on the basis of these recordings were as follows.

There appears to be 2-5 times more distal drift of maxillary immediate dentures when teeth were removed for periodontal reasons rather than because of caries.

Anesthesia

Local anesthesia for the area of the maxillary anterior teeth is obtained by bilateral maxillary nerve blocks. This form of anesthesia reduces the edema in the surgical site, the time and pain of injection and the amount of anesthesia solution to be used. The maxillary teeth, alveolar bone and overlying structures, hard palate, upper lip, cheek and side of nose are anesthetized by the injection.

Maxillary nerve blocks. This focus of anesthesia reduces the edema in the surgical site, the time and pain of injection and the amount of anesthetic solution to be used. The maxillary teeth, alveolar bone, hard palate, upper lip, cheek and side of nose are anesthetized by this injection.

Bilateral inferior alveolar, gingival and buccinator nerve blocks are administered for the mandibular anterior region.

SURGICAL PROCEDURE FOR IMMEDIATE DENTURES

After testing of the gingival tissue for adequate local anesthesia, a maxillary labial mucoperiosteal flap is prepared.

The incision for the flap is made several millimeters distal to the last maxillary tooth on the right and left sides and parallel to the mucolabial fold on the crest of the ridge. The interdental papillae are incised. The flap is raised with a periosteal elevator only to the height of bone to be removed.

Once the teeth have been extracted and the flap repositioned, a surgical template made of clear acrylic resin is placed in the mouth. The template fits the posterior part of the ridge and is used to test for impingement of tissues in the anterior part of mouth. Blanched areas that are revealed through the guide indicate pressure spots. These are reduced with a rongeur forceps and smoothened with a file.

A slight periosteal flap is raised palatally to expose the palatal bone of the sockets. Then the surgical guide is reseated. If there are no indications of impingement, the excess soft tissue of the flap is removed with a tissue scissors. The flap is sutured firmly. Gelfoam is placed in each socket to facilitate the formation of a blood dot.

A topical anesthetic jelly is placed in that part of the denture which will be in contact with the teeth sockets before the denture is permanently seated.

MULTIPLE CHOICE QUESTIONS

1. **The advantages of immediate complete dentures include all except**
   a. The immediate denture will serve as a splint to control bleeding.
   b. Anterior teeth can be evaluated at the try in stage
   c. Vertical dimension is maintained mastication
   d. All the above are correct.

2. **In the sectional technique for immediate complete dentures suggested by Campagna, final impression is made using**
   a. Impression compound
   b. Impression plaster and zinc oxide eugenol
   c. Rubber base and alginate
   d. Impression plaster and rubber base.

28

THE DUPLICATE DENTURES

INTRODUCTION

A spare or backup denture is a definite advantage for the patient whose original denture requires repair or modification.

METHODS

There are three methods of duplicating dentures with pour-type autopolymerizing resin. The methods differ principally in the type of flask and the investing medium used. They are: (i) the modified-denture flask method (Brewer and Morrow, 1975), (ii) the pour-resin flask method (Box and Carpenter, 1974), and (iii) the cup-flask method (Wanger, 1970; Singer, 1975).

Modified-denture Flask Method

This method requires the use of a modified denture flask and alginate irreversible hydrocolloid to flask the denture to be duplicated.

Procedure

1. Modify the denture flask by removing a rectangular section from the upper part. This opening will allow access for the sprues.
2. If the denture to be duplicated has thin areas, add wax to the exterior surface of the denture to thicken these areas before flasking.
3. Roll utility wax to form a sprue approximately 75 mm long and 15 mm in diameter.
4. Attach the sprues to the lingual surface of the heels of mandibular dentures and to the palatal surface of the tuberosity region of maxillary dentures.
5. Paint the round plate from the lower part of the flask with an adhesive, and insert it from the exterior surface, rather than from the interior. This insertion prevents distortion of the alginate mold by inadvertent displacement of the plate while handling the flask.
6. Apply the same adhesive to the interior surface of the flask to facilitate retention of the alginate.
7. Mix eight scoops of regular setting alginate with the recommended volume of water for the first pour. Cooling the water will allow additional working time.

8. Mix the alginate with a mechanical spatulator under reduced atmospheric pressure to minimize air inclusions in the material. Hand spatulate thoroughly if a power mixer is unavailable.

9. After mixing, place alginate into the interior of the denture with a finger or a brush, taking care to avoid the entrapment of air and resultant voids. Fill the denture completely.

10. Place the reminder of the alginate mix in the lower part of the flask

11. Settle the filled denture into the mix, as during a routine flasking procedure. The wax sprues can support into the alginate. The alginate should extend approximately 3 mm onto the exterior surface of the denture.

12. After the alginate has set, trim away any excess that flows over the edges of the flask.

13. Place the upper part of the flask in position and adapt the wax sprues to seal the rectangular opening

14. Mix six scoops of alginate with three times the recommended volume of water to make a pourable consistency.

15. Pour the alginate into the flask slowly. Use a finger or brush to wipe alginate onto the teeth of the denture to minimize voids. The second pour will not stick to the first one.

16. Completely fill the flask, and place the top in position. Allow the alginate to set approximately 15 minutes or longer if using cold water.

17. After the alginate has set, open the flask, and remove the denture and sprues.

18. Place the lower part of the flask, i.e. the cast side, in a humidor or under a wet towel.

19. Dry the tooth indentations in the alginate carefully. Use a gentle stream of air or a strip of cleansing tissue to remove water from the tooth imprints.

20. Add autopolymerizing tooth-colored resin of the proper shade to the tooth indentations by the sprinkle-on or paint-on method.

21. Carefully add the tooth-colored resin in increments and fill the indentations to the cervical line. Exercise care to improve materially the resultant duplicate denture. It is possible to add incisal, body, and gingival shading, but it requires considerable skill to achieve good results.

22. Allow the tooth shade autopolymerizing resin to set for a few minutes before assembling the flask.

23. Carefully dry the alginate in the lower flask, then assemble the flask halves, and clamp or secure them with rubber bands.

24. Mix a pour-type resin according to the manufacturer's recommendations, and pour it into one sprue hole

25. Rock the flask gently while pouring to minimize the entrapment of air.

26. Fill one sprue until the resin fills the other sprue, thereby indicating that the mold is full.

27. Attach modeling clay to the filed flask, place it sprues upward in warm water in a pressure container, and cure the denture at 20 psi for 30 minutes.

28. Remove the cured denture, and examine it for nodules and voids.

29. Cut off the sprues, and finish and polish the denture.

Pour-resin Flask Method

It is possible to make satisfactory duplicate dentures by using autopolymerizing pour-type resin, a special flask for these resins, and reversible hydrocolloid.

Procedure

1. Mount the denture to be duplicated on the lower plate of a pour-resin flask, using heat-stable clay. Adapt the clay to form a base approximately 6 mm thick, and develop a land area around the denture border 4 to 5 m wide and perpendicular to the denture flanges.

2. Assemble the pour-resin flask, and fill it with reversible hydrocolloid.
3. Cool the filled flask in water.
4. After the reversible hydrocolloid has gelled, dismantle the flask, and remove the denture and clay.
5. Cleanse the denture, and reposition it in the mold.
6. Switch the bottom plate of the flask to pour the tissue side of the denture.
7. Fill the flask with the hydrocolloid, and cool it in the same manner as before.
8. After the hydrocolloid has gelled, remove it from the cooling bath, and place it in water at 115° F (46° C) for 5 minutes prior to removing the denture.
9. Open the mold, and use a gentle stream of air to facilitate separation of the hydrocolloid pours.
10. Dry the tooth indentations in the mold with a gentle stream of air, or use a thin slip of absorbent tissue to blot the moisture.
11. Place the cast portion of the hydrocolloid mold in a humidor or cover it with a damp towel to minimize dehydration.
12. Paint tooth shade-autopolymerizing resin into the tooth indentations with a brush, and exercise care to avoid the entrapment of air.
13. Fill the tooth indentations with the resin carefully, and pay special attention to maintain the gingival outline. Do not remove the resin teeth from the mold.
14. Using a cork borer, cut sprue holes through the hydrocolloid resin.
15. Assemble the mold, mix and pour the resin into one sprue only, and gently rock the flask to minimize the entrapment of air within the mold.
16. Place the mold with the sprue holes upright in a pressure container of water at 120° F (45.5°C), and cure at 20 psi for 30 minutes.
17. Remove the cured duplicate, and trim it and polish it.

Cup-flask Method

Procedure

1. Slowly pull 16 inch (40 cm) lengths of dental floss through liquefied orthodontic tray wax. This soft wax will enable the floss to adhere to the denture flanges readily.
2. Tie the floss into a loop, and adapt it to the denture flanges 2 to 3 mm from the borders and across the posterior border of the maxillary denture.
3. Use two loops for the mandibular denture. Adapt one loop to the lingual flange approximately 4 mm from the border, and adapt the other loop to the buccal flanges of the denture.
4. Make soft utility wax or chaulking compound sprues approximately 75 mm long and 12 mm thick, and adapt them to the maxillary and mandibular dentures as described previously. An optional vent sprue that extends from the center of the maxillary denture is useful, but it is unnecessary if care is exercised when pouring.
5. For the maxillary denture press the remainder of the loop into the inner and outer surfaces of one sprue.
6. Press the floss loop from the lingual flange of the lower into the inner surfaces of the wax sprue and the floss from the buccal surfaces into the outer surface of the wax sprue.
7. Attach the wax sprue between two ¼ (6 mm) wood dowel rods approximately 6 inches (15.2) long to suspend the denture in a 12-ounce certain cup without contacting the bottom of the cup.
8. Place a modeling clay wedge in the cup opposite the handle to facilitate removal of the mold after pouring
9. Suspend the sprued denture in the cup.
10. Fill the mold with a pourable mix of alginate or reversible hydrocolloid. Alginate mixed with approximately three times the recommended volume of water

makes a pourable mix. A mix of six scoops of alginate and three times the recommended amount of water will fill the 12-ounce cup approximately. A smoother bubble-free mix results from mixing in a mechanical spatulator under reduced atmospheric pressure. An 800 g mixing bowl is recommended. An optional pouring technique involves filling the cup first, then settling the denture into the mix, though there is greater risk of touching the cup with the denture.

11. Allow the irreversible hydrocolloid to set on the bench. Place the reversible hydrocolloid in cool water until gelation occurs.
12. Remove the dowel rods from the mold and the clay wedge from the hydrocolloid.
13. Remove the mold containing the upper denture from the cup. A gentle stream of air directed at the keyway will aid in removal.
14. Pull the dental floss across the posterior border and around the flanges of the upper denture.
15. Open the mold and retrieve the denture.

16. Dry the tooth indentations with a stream of air and with absorbent tissue.
17. Plant autopolymerizing resin of the proper shade into the tooth indentations as described previously.
18. Assemble the mold in the cup in the original position. Mix pour-type resin, and pour it into one sprue as described earlier.
19. Cure the duplicate denture in warm water in a pressure container for 30 minutes at 20 psi.
20. Retrieve the denture, and examine it for voids or nodules.
21. Polish the duplicate denture.

The mandibular denture is handled in much the same way, the main difference is in the placement of the waxed dental floss loops.

1. Cross the inner (lingual flange) dental floss loop, and pull it through the alginate or the reversible hydrocolloid before removing the mold from the cup.
2. Remove the mold from the cup, and pull the floss around the labial and buccal flanges.

Complete the mandibular denture in the manner described for the maxillary denture.

MULTIPLE CHOICE QUESTIONS

1. **The modified denture flask method was introduced by**
   a. Appleby and kirchoff
   b. Box and carpenter
   c. Wanger
   d. Brewer and Morrow

29

THE SINGLE COMPLETE DENTURE

INTRODUCTION

Malposed, tipped[1], or supraerupted teeth in the lower arch make it difficult to achieve a harmonious balanced occlusion. As a result, unfavorable occlusal relationships exist that tend to displace the maxillary denture, causing soreness, mucosal changes, and ultimately ridge resorption. The fixed positions of the mandibular anterior teeth make the esthetic and phonetic placement of the maxillary teeth difficult without introducing anterior interferences in eccentric functional movements. Perhaps the greatest error is to make no attempt to modify the occlusal arrangement of the natural teeth. Failure to diagnose and properly modify the mandibular teeth to achieve occlusal harmony with the denture will result in forces that may exceed the physiologic tolerance of the maxillary residual ridge tissues.

DIAGNOSIS AND TREATMENT PLANNING

Prior to any occlusal modifications of the natural teeth, it is imperative that upper and lower casts be mounted on an articulator. In most situations, it is possible to first make the final maxillary impression and mount the cast on the articulator using a face-bow. This would eliminate the need for mounting an upper cast twice (once for diagnostic purposes and once for treatment) Next, the lower diagnostic cast is mounted using a provisional centric interocclusal record made at an acceptable vertical dimension. Eccentric records are made and the condylar elements of the articulator are set. Whatever adjustments that may be necessary could be properly planned for at this time.

Several techniques have been described in the literature whereby the necessary tooth modifications are determined prior to denture construction. The first method was originally described by Swenson. The maxillary and mandibular casts are mounted on the articulator, using a provisional centric relation record at an acceptable vertical dimension. A maxillary base is made, and denture teeth are set. If the lower natural teeth interfere with the placement of the denture teeth, they are adjusted on the cast and the area is marked with a pencil. The natural teeth are then modified using the marked diagnostic cast as a guide. After the occlusal modifications have been completed, a new diagnostic cast of the lower arch is made and mounted on the articulator. If more adjustment is deemed necessary, the procedure is repeated. Once the occlusal modification appears to be sufficient, the denture teeth are reset and prepared for the try-in. This procedure is time consuming if several impressions and mountings must be made.

A second method, described by Yurkstas involves the use of a metal U-shaped occlusal template that is slightly convex on the lower surface. When placed on the occlusal surfaces of the remaining teeth, the cusps to be adjusted are identified. The stone cast is modified to a more acceptable occlusal relationship and the areas reduced are identified by marking with a pencil. The cast is then used as a guide for modifying the natural teeth.

A third technique for predetermining the amount of the occlusal adjustment of the natural teeth was described by Bruce. The lower diagnostic cast is mounted as in the previous two procedures. The necessary modifications are made on the stone cast occlusal surfaces. A clear acrylic resin template is fabricated over the modified stone cast. The inner surface of the template is coated with pressure indicating paste and placed over the patient's natural teeth. Interferences are readily noted through the template and are removed by reshaping the occlusal anatomy. The process is repeated until the template seats properly.

Boucher et al explained another technique that involves making the natural teeth fit to the established plane and inclines of the maxillary porcelain teeth. The casts are mounted on a programmed articulator as with the other techniques. The maxillary artificial teeth are arranged to obtain the best possible occlusal balancing contacts. If the natural teeth prevent this balancing, the interferences are removed by movement of the maxillary porcelain teeth over the mandibular stone teeth. After the denture has been processed a comparison of the natural teeth and the altered stone cast is made and the areas to be reshaped are noted. The natural teeth are ground at the areas marked on the stone cast. The occlusion is refined using an arch-shaped layer of softened baseplate wax over the lower teeth, and guiding the patient to close in centric relation. Prematurities are identified and removed by grinding the natural teeth. The procedure is repeated for right and left lateral excursions until a harmonious balanced occlusion is established.

COMMON OCCLUSAL DISHARMONIES

A common pattern of tooth loss involves the completely edentulous maxillary area opposing a mandibular complement of natural teeth with missing first molars or second premolars, or both. In these situations the remaining molars are often severely inclined mesially and their distal halves supraerupted. This results in the maxillary denture being easily dislodged during functional movements. Thus the distal portion of the occlusal surface requires severe reduction (often 3 mm or more), while the mesial portion may often be left untouched. When all the molars are missing a removable partial denture is indicated. If all teeth remain from first molar to first molar, then a removable partial denture is usually not indicated. The replacement of missing posterior teeth will enhance the retention and stability of the maxillary complete denture, and help to distribute the functional forces more evenly on the residual maxillary ridge.

METHODS USED TO ACHIEVE A HARMONIOUS BALANCED OCCLUSION

Many techniques[1] have been described explaining ways to achieve a balanced occlusion for a complete maxillary denture opposing natural teeth. They basically fall into two categories: (i) those that dynamically equilibrate the occlusion by the use of a functionally generated path, and (ii) those that statistically equilibrate the occlusion using an articulator programmed to simulate the patient's jaw movement.

The functionally generated chew-in techniques do seem to provide the most accurate method of recording the occlusal patterns. However, they are contraindicated unless the necessary record base stability can be provided by the residual tissues. Also, the patient must have the neuromuscular control to perform the desired jaw movements and the mental competence to effectively cooperate (with the procedure).

Functional Chew-in Techniques

Stansbury described the first functional chew-in technique (1928) for an upper complete denture opposing lower natural teeth. He suggested using a compound maxillary rim trimmed buccally and lingually so that the occlusion is free in lateral excursions. Carding wax is then added to the compound rim, and the patient is instructed to perform eccentric chewing movements. The carding wax is slowly molded to the functional movements, while the compound in the central fossa acts as a guide to preserve the vertical dimension. The generated occlusion rim is now removed from the mouth, and stone is vibrated into the wax paths of the cusps. The upper cast is fastened to the articulator. The stone cusp path record is secured to the lower member of the articulator with plaster. We now have the upper cast mounted on the articulator and two lower casts (one is a duplicate of the lower teeth and the other is a replica of the generated path). The denture teeth are first set to the lower cast of the patient's teeth. After the esthetics have been approved at the try-in, the lower cast is removed and the lower chew-in cast record is

then secured to the articulator. All interfering spots are carefully ground until the incisal guide pin prevents further closure. Thus, in centric and in eccentric movements, maximum bilateral balanced occlusion will be established.

Vig described a similar technique in which he recommended the use of a fin of resin placed into the central grooves of the lower posterior teeth, instead of using compound (as mentioned by Stansbury). The resin fin maintains the vertical dimension and also helps to diagnostically locate the interfering lower cusps. In eccentric movements, the lower cusp tips are ground until equal contact occurs between the teeth and resin. The fin is then built up using a soft wax, and a functional path is recorded. The procedures that follow closely resemble the technique described by Stansbury.

Sharry mentions a simple technique of using a maxillary rim of softened wax. Lateral and protrusive chewing movements are made so that the wax is abraded, generating the functional paths of the lower cusps. This is continued until the correct vertical dimension has been established.

Rudd suggested a technique quite similar to Stansbury's. A compound maxillary rim is formed in much the same way. A thickness of recording matrix made up of three sheets of medium-hard pink baseplate wax and two sheets of red counter wax is added to the buccal and lingual surfaces of the compound rim. He also suggested using two maxillary bases: one for recording the generated path, and the other for setting the teeth. The advantage of this is to reduce the number of appointments necessary for the construction of the upper denture.

Articulator Equilibration Techniques

If the denture bases lack stability or if the patient is physically unable to form a chew-in record, the articulator equilibration method is preferred. This technique is the most common method used.

First, the upper cast is mounted on an articulator using a face-bow with an orbitale pointer. The lower cast is related to the upper by a centric interocclusal record at an acceptable vertical dimension. The buccolingual position of the lower teeth and their relation to the upper arch is studied. A decision whether to articulate the central fossa of the denture teeth to the lower buccal cusps or to the lower lingual cusps must be made. If the denture teeth appear to be placed too far to the buccal cusps, they are reset to oppose the lower lingual cusps. If the denture teeth appear to be placed too far lingually when articulated with the lower lingual cusps, they are reset to oppose the lower buccal cusps. Occasionally, because of tipped and inclined natural teeth, the buccal cusps may be used on some and the lingual cusps on others. Once the holding cusps have been selected the inclines of the remaining cusps are reduced (when the lower buccal cusps are selected for the holding cusps the lingual cusps are reduced. When the lower lingual cusps are selected for the holding cusps, the buccal cusps are reduced). This allows for a cusp-to-fossa relationship between the upper and the lower teeth, simplifying the posterior tooth set-up and facilitating the task of balancing the occlusion.

If any of the natural teeth are supererupted or tipped, they are modified by selective grinding or by restoring with a crown or onlay until an acceptable occlusal plane is established.

As previously mentioned, the central fossae of the upper posterior teeth are set to articulate with the selected holding cusps of the lower natural teeth. Therefore, in centric occlusion the only areas of contact on the denture should be in the central fossae. At the time of the wax try-in eccentric records are made and the condylar inclinations are set on the articulator. The upper posterior teeth are arranged to be as close to being balanced as is possible at this time. After the denture has been processed, it is again related to the mounted lower cast with a new centric interocclusal record. The condylar inclinations previously determined are reset on the articulator. Once the centric holding stops are re-established by selective grinding, eccentric balance is achieved. This is accomplished by selectively grinding the interfering buccal and lingual cuspal inclines of the upper teeth.

It must be emphasized that once the centric contacts have been obtained, they are not to be touched. To avoid the accidental removal of these contacts, it is advisable to use two colors of articulating paper: one color to mark the centric contacts and another color to mark the eccentric contacts. The eccentric contacts are selectively ground until a relatively continuous area of contact is noted on the buccal and lingual cuspal inclines of the upper teeth. If any lower cusps make contact (other than the selected holding cusps), then these interferences are removed by grinding the cast and then the natural teeth. The lower holding cusps should be left unaltered at this time.

The end result is a harmonious balanced occlusion that allows freedom in lateral excursions while maintaining maximum bilateral contacts in functional and parafunctional activities. Perfectly balanced occlusion in all eccentric positions may not be possible in many cases when working with natural teeth in one arch.

OCCLUSAL MATERIALS FOR THE SINGLE DENTURE

The materials available for occlusal posterior tooth forms are porcelain, acrylic resin, gold, acrylic resin with amalgam stops, and IPN (interpenetrating polymer network) resin.

Porcelain Teeth

Porcelain teeth wear very slowly and therefore the occlusal vertical dimension is maintained. However, they are predisposed to fracture and chipping when opposed by natural teeth and are more difficult to equilibrate, since their surfaces do not mark well with articulating paper. They cause rapid wear of opposing natural teeth.

Acrylic Resin Teeth

Acrylic resin teeth cause no wear of the opposing natural teeth and they are the easiest to equilibrate, so they are considered the teeth of choice. The major disadvantage of resin teeth is their wear, which results in loss of vertical dimension. However, wear of the occlusal surfaces is better than resorption of the alveolar ridge.

Gold Occlusals

Although gold occlusals are considered the best material to oppose natural teeth, their expense and the time involved in their fabrication make them impractical for most patients.

Acrylic Resin with Amalgam Stops

The amalgam inserts appear to reduce the occlusal wear, and the technique is simple and much less time consuming and expensive than with the gold occlusals. After the acrylic teeth have been balanced occlusal preparations are made in the acrylic teeth, extending to include as much of the articulating paper tracing as is possible. Amalgam is condensed into the preparations and the articulator is gently closed, going side to side and back and forth until the incisal guide pin is again flush with the guide pin. Thus the centric holding area as well as some of the excursions are recorded in amalgam by the articulator that has been programmed to closely simulate the patient's jaw movements.

IPN Resin

A new tooth material was developed to minimize the disadvantages of acrylic resin and porcelain teeth and enhance certain qualities in each. The material consists of an unfilled, highly cross-linked, interpenetrating polymer network.

DISADVANTAGES OF SINGLE COMPLETE DENTURES

1. The edentulous residual ridge is subjected to more stress from its occlusal counterpart than is an edentulous arch acting opposite a homologous edentulous arch.
2. The residual ridge of a single denture will resorb faster and more extensively than will maxillary and mandibular fully edentulous ridges covered by complete dentures.
3. Patients usually expect more from the denture because the majority of single denture wearers are younger than the average fully edentulous patients, and experience with complete dentures is limited or non-existent.
4. Occlusal harmony is difficult to achieve, because an artificial denture is supported by a soft tissue foundation, acting as one unit, with its occlusal elements occluding natural individual teeth (each of which possess its own proprioceptive mechanism). Occlusal arrangement and coordination is difficult and involves modifications of the buccolingual and mesiodistal positioning of the denture teeth or of the occlusal surfaces of the natural teeth (which usually require grinding).
5. Full occlusal contacts at centric relation and balanced occlusion for a single denture facing natural teeth must be limited to the posterior teeth alone. The anterior artificial teeth are arranged to have 1 mm or more of overjet to avoid contacting in centric relation to minimize the possibilities of dislodgement of the denture when protrusive movements are performed. Theoretically this is imperative in single maxillary denture construction. However, the occluding anterior natural teeth cannot in most cases be reduced extensively at the incisal edges or displaced to provide for an adequate overjet. Labial positioning of the anterior artificial teeth in a maxillary single

denture may create an esthetic problem of protruding teeth. Lingual positioning of the anterior artificial teeth in the single mandibular denture to create an overjet can infringe into the lingual space and cause an unstable prosthesis and a speech problem for the patient.

6. Abrasion of the occlusal surfaces of the natural teeth opposing the single denture porcelain teeth will occur in a relatively short time and may lead to extreme attrition and pulp exposure. Gold surfaces will also wear when occluding with the porcelain complete denture teeth, and the designed occlusal scheme becomes unsettled. Acrylic resin teeth are an acceptable solution, because although natural teeth will abrade the occlusal surfaces of the resin teeth in a relatively short time, in some patients the underlying residual ridge will be preserved.
   a. The artifical teeth may be placed buccal to the crest of the residual ridge near the position of the natural teeth extractions to restore a Class I occlusal relationship.
   b. The tip of the buccal cusps of the artificial teeth may be reduced to direct the occlusal contact of the balancing side on the lingual cusps, which are placed on the same vertical level with the crest of the residual ridge, minimizing dislodging forces on the maxillary denture.

A crossbite-type occlusion may be selected so the artifical teeth are placed on top of the residual ridge. Mechanically, this selection will provide a satisfactory solution, because at lateral movements a buccal-to-buccal and a lingual-to-lingual cusp relation at the balancing side and a buccal–to lingual-natural cusp relation at the working side will convey a stabilizing force for the denture on the top of the ridge. Then the posterior edentulous mandible occludes against a dentulous maxilla.

The artificial mandibular teeth are placed buccal to the crest of the mandibular ridge so the denture teeth are seated in the vertical plane on the buccal flange of cortical bone. In the case of a single denture the resorption seems to be slower and the pathologic changes of epulis enlargement of the tuberosities and flabby tissue are less severe than are the findings described in the combination syndrome.

Further Reading

1. Pietrokovski et al. the single denture. Queintessence international. 1989; 20(11).

MULTIPLE CHOICE QUESTIONS

1. _____ are considered as the best material to oppose natural teeth.
   a. Porcelain
   b. Acrylic resin
   c. IPN resin
   d. Gold occlusals

2. Examples for articulation equilibration techniques are
   a. Stansbury's technique
   b. Sharrys
   c. Rudd's
   d. None of the above

3. The techniques that statistically equilibrate the occlusion using an articulator programmed to simulate the patients jaw movement are
   _____
   a. Functional chew in techniques
   b. Sharrys
   c. Rudd
   d. None of the above

4. **Yurkstas method for correcting occlusal disharmony in single complete dentures involve.**

   a. Modification of natural teeth using a marked diagnostic cast as a guide.

   b. Using porcelain denture teeth and reducing prematurities on natural teeth.

   c. Using a clear acrylic resin template fabricated from the modified cast.

   d. Using a U-shaped metal template to modify the natural teeth.

30

GERIATRIC CONSIDERATIONS IN PROSTHETIC DENTISTRY

DEFINITIONS

Geriatrics. The branch of medicine or dentistry that treats the problems peculiar to the aging patient, including the clinical problems of senescence and senility.

Gerodontics. The treatment of dental problems of aging persons or of problems peculiar to advanced age.

Gerodontology. The study of the dentition and dental problems in aged or aging persons.

People who are above the age of 65 years are termed as geriatric persons.

Geriatric dentistry is part of the health team that is responsible for intervening in and slowing the orofacial aging process or procedures.

Aging. The aging process may be defined as the sum of all morphologic and functional alterations that occur in an organism, leading to functional impairment (which decreases the ability to survive stress). Aging of a human organism is manifested at all levels of the organizational hierarchy, from the macromolecular to that of the population. None of the many changes seen at the macromolecular level is dramatic by itself, but by joining forces these ultimately cause (with time) the exponentially increasing mortality rate seen at the population level. While death is the unequivocal end result of the aging process, an important consequence for healthcare delivery is the increased incidence of impairment, disability and handicap in the aging population.

The origin of this complex aging phenomenon is at the biological levels of the organizational hierarchy. Therefore, it is essential for the development and provision of adequate healthcare and social services to understand these fundamental and causative processes.

The Biology of Aging. Superimposed on the basic biologic changes that occur with age is an increasing vulnerability to disease. The end point of the physiologic decrements that encompass aging is death. Disease may be viewed as the immediate cause of death in the elderly, but ultimately the biologic age changes that make disease more probable determine dying.

FACTORS INFLUENCING AGING

Genetic Factors

The principal evidence that aging as expressed by life span is genetically determined derives from the following kinds of observations.

Mutations. Several mutations reduce the life span.

Species Specific Life Spans. Each species is characterized by its own pattern of aging and maximum life span. The longevity in humans is about 20 years.

Hybrid Vigor. The effect of genetic constitution on longevity is perhaps best exemplified by those experiments in which hybrid vigor has been demonstrated.

Sex. In humans and most animals studied, the male has a shorter life span than the female.

Parental Age. Persons whose parents live to an older age have a greater life expectancy than persons whose parents die young.

Twin Studies. The main difference in life span for monozygotic Twins has been found to be consistently less than that for dizygotic twins.

Premature Aging Syndrome. Single gene changes result in premature senescence in humans.

Cells in Culture. A direct relationship exists between species longevity and replicative capacity of cells derived from the species.

Environmental Factors

Four categories of environmental factors influence the rate of aging in humans:
1. Physical and chemical components of the environment have been implicated as causing differential rates of aging (some investigators claim that even radiation affects aging).
2. Biologic factors such as nutrition is a probable cause for differential aging in humans.
3. Pathogens and parasites have been implicated as influencing the rate of human development and aging, particularly in low income groups and in tropical countries.
4. Socioeconomic factors, such as bad housing, poor working condition, the stress of life are commonly believed to accelerate the aging process.

BIOLOGIC THEORIES OF AGING

Many theories of aging presume that a single mechanism is responsible for all the characteristic changes seen with aging.

Genetic Theories

Error Theories

The error theories of aging propose that senescence is related to the progressive accumulation of metabolic errors in macromolecules. In aging DNA, RNA and protein synthesis are now considered to be interconnected.

Somatic Mutations. The basic assumption of the somatic mutation hypothesis is that just as spontaneous mutations occur in germ line cells, so also they occur on somatic cells.

Redundancies. Medvedev suggested that aging is attributable to the loss of unique, non-repeated genetic information from the genome.

Genetically Programmed Senescence. This theory likens the aging process to the processes involved in the development of the organism. Aging is considered an extension of development. It is the most comprehensive of the genetic theories and is a deterministic theory.

Disposable Soma Theory

It is concerned with the ramifications of evolutionary or adaptive influences on the organism as they become manifested in senescenc. It presents an attempt at a unifying theory for aging.

Non-genetic Theories

Immunologic Theories

With aging, the immune system tends to be less able to distinguish normal molecules from abnormal ones, and so abnormal cells may proliferate and autoimmune reactions take place.

Free Radical Theory

Free radicals are ubiquitous, short lived, highly reactive chemicals produced during normal metabolic reactions. This theory postulates that free radicals combine with essential molecules, causing damage to the DNA or other cellular structures.

Crosslinking Theory

Aging has been postulated to be caused by molecules becoming irreversibly linked as a result of strong crosslinking of substances with a profound effect on the physiologic function.

Metabolic Rate or Wear and Tear Theory

It has been proposed that increased metabolic rate which presumably would result in greater wear and tear on the organism results in shorter life spans.

PHYSIOLOGY OF AGING

Physiological deterioration occurs with increasing adult age although much of the deterioration may be secondary to the increase in prevalence and severity of disease processes. With advancing age, some are the consequence of aging.

However this age-related physiological deterioration during normal aging does reduce physiological capacity and the ability to meet challenges. Since physiological deterioration is progressive, it could well be a major factor contributing to the death of the extremely old.

MANIFESTATIONS OF AGING[1]

Central Nervous System

- A modest impairment of learning and memory is observed.
- Slowing of central processing and sympathetic hyperactivity takes place with increasing age.
- Decrease in the brain size and weight after the age of 60 and widespread loss of neurons with advancing age.
- In the motor systems, there is a deterioration of the functioning of the extrapyramidal system and a deterioration of cerebellar function. Muscular strength diminishes, movement time in and reaction time increases with age.

Sensory Systems

There is age-related loss of vibratory perceptions in the lower extremities:

- Loss of touch and a loss in the sense of taste and smell. The deficits in taste and smell probably contribute to the elderly making inappropriate food choices.
- Hearing loss affects 25% of people above 65 years

- Deterioration of vision with cataracts, glaucoma, and macular degeneration being the major problems.

Sleep. Shortening of sleep time at night, increased multiple brief awakenings, and a shift to an early time of going to sleep and awakening each day.

Neuromuscular System

- Loss of muscle mass.
- Secondary to this is a loss of muscle strength and muscle performance.

Cardiovascular Systems

- Decrease in intrinsic heart rate.
- Mean maximum heart rate during exercise also decreases considerably with age.
- Cardiac output in the reclining position decreases with age.
- Decrease in peripheral resistance with age.
- Heart becomes stiffer and contraction of cardiac muscle is prolonged with increasing age.
- Decrease in thickness and luminal size of the aorta and a loss of distensibility of its walls.
- Mean arterial blood pressure increases with age but not in all people.
- During dynamic exercise, the maximum cardiac output and oxygen consumption declines with advancing age.

Respiratory System

- Residual volume increases with age.
- No change in total lung capacity (TLC).
- Expiratory reserve volume decreases with age.
- Marked changes in airflow occur with age.

Kidney and Body Fluids

- Progressive deterioration of kidney structure and function with advancing age.
- Change in composition of body fluids with age.

- Loss of weight of kidney and loss of glomeruli with increasing age.
- Progressive decline in renal blood flow and glomerular filtration.

Gastrointestinal System

- Disordered constructions and spontaneous gastroesophageal reflex occurs.
- Gastric emptying is slower.
- A higher fat intake, young people absorb more fat than older people.
- Very slight impairment of protein digestion
- Reduction in calcium absorption with increasing age.
- Gastric glands decrease secretion with age that is less volume and concentration of HCl intrinsic factors and pepsin.

Endocrines

- Secretion of thyrotrophin by the adeno-hypophysis is blunted in humans.
- Greater release of antidiuretic hormone (ADH) by neurohypophysis.
- Slight decrease in plasma thyroxine (T4) concentration in advanced age.
- Rate of secretion of cortisol does decrease with age, but there is a proportional decrease in the metabolic rate of disposal of cortisol.
- Decreased rate of secretion of aldosterone and there is decreased plasma concentration of aldosterone.
- Elderly subjects have a diminished medullary response to stresses such as insulin hypoglycemia and vasomotor conditioning.
- Glucose intolerance occurs with advancing age due to a decreased sensitivity of the target tissues to the action of insulin.

Reproduction

- Sexual interest, drive and vigor decline in men with increasing age.
- Plasma concentration of luteinizing hormone (LH) and follicle-stimulating hormone (FSH) increase in men with age.

- In females there is a marked decline in the plasma estrogen concentrations after menopause.

Miscellaneous

- Loss of lean body mass from the age of 30 with the rate being greater in men.
- Body fat increases with age.
- Decrease in basal metabolic rate (BMR).
- Reduced ability to maintain body temperature appropriately in advanced age.

The immune system appears to play a role in the pathogenesis of a number of dental diseases such as periodontal disease and oral lesions observed in systemic lupus erythematosus (SLE). Neither has the precise role of the immune system and detailed chronological sequence of the pathogenesis of these diseases known, nor has a primary causative event been unambiguously identified.

It is unclear whether the immune system plays a primary or secondary role in the pathogenesis of the disease. Changes occurring in the immune system with age might predispose to an increase in periodontal disease.

ORAL ASPECTS OF AGING

Oral Mucosa and Skin Changes

With age, the oral mucosa may become increasingly thin, smooth and dry have a Latin like appearance with loss of elasticity and stippling and become more susceptible to injury.

The clinical picture of the oral mucosa is one of atrophy. The epithelial layers are less in number and mucosa and submucosa show a decrease in thickness. This actual thinning of the tissues, coupled with its depleted repair potential renders the denture-bearing mucosa of the basal seat friable and easily traumatized. Edentulous areas of the elderly are frequently thin and tightly stretched and it blanches easily. Rate of wound healing is decreased.

An atrophied denture-bearing mucosa is frequently encountered in females during menopause. Tissues need extra care, i.e. frequent application of soft liners, as well as counseling in tissue handling and cleaning.

Skin Changes

With aging, skin undergoes progressive clinical changes. The skin of old individuals is wrinkled, dry and shows areas of patchy pigmentation. The epidermis of the face and dorsal surface of the hands has been reported to be generally thicker with few layers of cells in old persons than in the young. As the skin ages, its surface loses its fine pattern and the skin loses its elasticity. The concomitant atrophy occurring in the structures beneath the skin leads to even more noticeable changes in the face. The muscles, fat and connective tissue all diminish in bulk. As the elasticity of the skin is decreased, the lines in the base of the creases become more permanent.

The skin changes cannot be compensated for by the prosthesis as they can severely compromise the esthetic opportunities of the denture service. The skin changes should be brought to the patient's attention before denture treatment is started.

Gingiva

With age, the gingiva shows a loss of stippling, edematous appearance and the keratinized layer is thin or absent. Tissue is friable and easily injured.

Lips

Angular cheilosis is very common and is probably related to vitamin B deficiency than to aging. Cheilosis and purse string mouth may also result in dehydration.

Changes in Teeth[4]

Microscopic changes include alterations in form due to wear and in color due to secondary dentin formation, pigmentation and altered light reflection patterns.

The surface enamel exhibits certain acquired properties such as the increase in fluoride content, which are slowly built up with age. The number of enamel cracks or acquired lamellae also increase with age.

The cementum increases in thickness with age. Gingival recession leads to the exposure of cementum to the oral environment. Age changes in dentin constitute two independent processes: secondary dentin formation and obturation of dentinal tubules.

The main pulp changes include a change from a cell rich/fiber poor to a cell poor/fiber rich connective tissue. The blood supply is reduced with age and the frequency of pulp stones increase.

Salivary Changes

Reduced salivary flow has been reported during aging. The xerostomia seen in the aged can be due to medication for gastric complaints, depression or insomnia. Regardless of the cause, this can lead to a diminished facility for mastication, digestive upsets and poor retention of dentures. The dryness of the mucosa renders it more susceptible to frictional irritation from denture movement and may interfere with the patient's ability to wear dentures.

Some patients may produce excessive saliva on the insertion of dentures. This is usually a transient effect and can be controlled by the explanation of the cause to the patient, reassurance and antisialogogue administration if necessary.

More recent studies on salivary gland function during aging have involved individual glands of healthy people. Reports show that there is no reduction in the salivary output from the parotid gland in different aged persons. However, the submandibular salivary flow output has been found to be reduced in older individuals. As submandibular flow accounts for 45% of the whole saliva, this may provide an explanation for earlier reports of diminished salivary output in older persons.

The diminished function of the glands also result in a change in the saliva itself which shows a decrease in ptyalin content, an increase in mucin content and becomes very viscous and dry. This change in character of saliva contributes to plaque formation and creates a favorable environment for the growth of cariogenic bacteria.

Treatment of Xerostomia

There is no specific treatment as such if the xerostomia results from loss of glandular function. Increased intake of water can be helpful. Coating of the tissue surface with lubricating jelly silicone, fluid or commercial semisolid denture adhesive can temporarily increase denture retention and decrease irritation of underlying soft tissues. Pilocarpine hydrochloride or nitrate 5 mg before meals and sucking on a sour candy can also help. If xerostomia is due to a nutritional deficiency, a therapeutic dose of nicotinamide 250-400 mg thrice daily for a period of 2 weeks can be used.

Since saliva is critically important in the maintenance of oral health, any general disturbance in salivary gland function, whether due to age related changes or pathology would result in severe morbidity. Clinicians must take care not to actually ascribe complaints by older patients, which are suggestive of salivary gland disorders, to aging, but rather to include age as one possibility in a differential diagnosis.

Changes in Bone Tissues[2]

The osseous structure consists of compact or cortical bone and the spongiosa or the trabecular or cancellous bone. Skeletal involution takes place by cortical thinning of the bone and increase in porosity. Resorption is an inevitable accompaniment for denture wearers.

As the maxillary residual ridges are reduced, the maxilla becomes smaller in all dimensions and the denture-bearing surface decreases. The mandibular arch remains stable or static or appears to become wider posteriorly. This discrepancy in relative jaw sizes can pose several technical problems in the placement of artificial teeth as failure to place the artificial teeth in the position of the natural teeth can jeopardize denture support and stability. The attempt to restore the original arch contour can also be limited by the effects of aging.

Muscle changes coupled with residual ridge resorption bring about spatial alteration in the position of the mandible relative to that of the maxilla. These changes must be recognized to make an accurate measurement of the interarch and interocclusal distances in order to attain a proper vertical relation and in turn comfort to the patient.

Tongue and Taste Changes[3]

Tongue shows clinical changes with the loss of filiform papilla and disturbance of the sensory elements resulting in the deterioration in the sense of taste. The tongue frequently becomes smooth and glossy or red and inflamed in appearance. Sensations of soreness, burning or abnormal taste can be encountered on the lingual mucosa which is common in the elderly as well as in postmenopausal women. A common nodular varicose enlargement of the superficial veins on the undersurface of the tongue is frequently seen.

With age, the number of tastebuds decrease. The foliate papillae may appear red and in case of persistent soreness, excision of these papillae is advised. Vitamin B therapy is successful in treating a burning tongue.

The tongue size does not vary with age, but tooth loss can lead to a wider tongue by virtue of an overdevelopment of some parts of the tongue's intrinsic musculature. Constant and habitual attempts to keep a loose maxillary denture in place can cause these changes.

Gingival tissue changes may be accompanied by alterations in the sense of taste. Tastebud atrophy leads to loss of appetite. Older persons frequently blame their dentures for a changed sense of taste and burning sensation of the tongue. Reassurance and diet counseling are necessary to overcome these symptoms.

Cardiopulmonary Disorders

Several cardiac problems have implications for dental practice. Vascular heart disease is perhaps the most common of these. It is generally recommended that every person with a significant heart murmur (regardless of etiology) should receive prophylactic antibiotics prior to the dental procedure. Another common cardiac problem among the elderly people is the existence of cardiac arrhythmias. Sometimes these patients are treated with anticoagulants and they may need a modification in their anticoagulant therapy prior to any operative dental procedure. Occasionally, elderly persons may suffer syncopial episodes from a hypersensitive carotid sinus reflex syndrome. A common disorder the dentist will encounter in the elderly population is ischemic heart disease (IHD). Angina is the term which describes chest pain produced by ischemic heart disease. Anginal pain in the jaw can easily be confused with a local disorder of the mouth or throat rather than being interpreted as a cardiac symptom. Hypertension is another frequent disease experienced by the elderly. Persons with severe hypertension should not undergo medical or dental treatment till hypertension is controlled. Therapy of hypertension, particularly clonidine and other centrally acting agents can induce oral symptoms, (most prominently dry mouth).

Patients who have a chronic cough due to chronic bronchitis/emphysema may create difficulty for dentists by constant interruption for coughing. Chronic lung disease frequently causes asthophen, an inability to lie flat. For those patients, it will be necessary to perform dental work in the sitting position.

Nervous System Disorders

Cerebral vascular disease (or strokes as they are commonly termed) whether on the right side or left side, hemianopsia prevents the patient from seeing one half of the visual field. Patients with hemianopsia should be treated from the functional side of their visual field. Some stroke patients are also anticoagulated for their condition. Dentists should be watchful of such cases.

Tardive diskinesia is a spasmodic movement disorder which primarily involves the lingual, facial and muscles and may be sufficiently severe to interfere with eating and cooperation during dental care. These spasms can be moderated by the administration of relaxing drugs. Tardive dyskinesia may be associated with abnormal teeth wear, eating dysfunction and temporomandibular joint dysfunction.

Dentists should be alert to hearing impairment and loss of vision which are commonly seen in sensory disorders in the elderly.

Rheumatologic Disorders

Among the elderly patients perhaps the most important disease dentists need to be aware of is temporal arthritis. This disorder which can be easily confused for TMJ disease may progress to blindness unless treated aggressively. Symptoms are vague or localized pain on one side of the temporal region.

The most common rheumatologic disorder among elderly women is the decrease in bone mass called osteoporosis. The process is accelerated at menopause in women and eventually leads to fractures of the radius and ulna, femoral head and vertebral bodies of the spine. Some individuals have considerable difficulty in lying flat and/or sitting in dental chairs, take extra time for proper positioning and need extra pillows.

Some individuals with severe osteoarthritis as well as some who have fractured femoral necks will have prosthetic joints in place. These patients should receive antibiotic chemoprophylaxis to prevent infection of these prostheses.

GEROPSYCHIATRIC DISORDERS AND ITS RELATION TO DENTISTRY[5]

Dental conditions most often associated with emotional crisis or prolonged situational stress are those resulting from improper oral hygiene and sustained muscular tension (bruxism, atypical facial pains). Burning mouth and/or tongue is associated particularly with intense grief and will persist until the patient has reached the emotional crisis.

Affective Disorders

The depressed patients are usually cooperative in the dental chair but may seem hard to reach or appear to forget clear instructions. Depressed patients fatigue easily and require several short appointments.

The dental practitioner is in an excellent position to detect the side effects of antidepressant medication. The side effects like burning mouth, falling due to postural dizziness excitement, simulating mania, tachycardia, overactivity, rapid speech and confusion all occur and interrupt dental treatment. In case of oral surgical or restorative work, the antidepressant therapy has to be discontinued for a time. The lithium dosage has to be temporarily lowered and blood levels monitored during cases of prolonged dental treatment.

Anxiety Disorders

Anxiety disorders are characterized by apprehensiveness, worry, agitation, somatic symptoms like tachycardia, dizziness, weakness, visual and gastrointestinal disturbances, fatigue and headache and sometimes insomnia and may contain depressive elements.

Treatment includes the use of benzo-diazepines and tricyclic antidepressants. Benzodiazepines cause oversedation, apathy, and confusional states in the elderly.

AGING AND NUTRITION

Nutrition is one of the factors under human control which can influence the health of the aging. A good general diet is essential to the health of the elderly and to the supporting tissues of the teeth.

Dietary problems can be due to:

1. Low income and lack of knowledge on how to spend the money available for food to the best advantage
2. Physical handicaps, disability and a lack of mobility which makes shopping and food preparation difficult.
3. Poor facilities for food preparation
4. Poor dentitions, especially dentures, which may cause the wearer to reject some essential foods that are difficult to chew, without the inclusion of a suitable substitute.
5. Existing food habits which may result in the choice of a poor diet.
6. Depression, boredom, anxiety and lone-liness which give little or no incentive for the preparation of the nourishing meals.
7. Studies of the elderly have shown that they are susceptible to subclinical, if not frank clinical malnutrition.

The geriatric patient must be prevented from changing his/her diet to softer food which require little or no chewing and are easy to swallow. This can result in a loss of proteins. A reduction of foods in the diet limits the deposition of cholesterol in the arterial walls. Low fiber intake in the elderly can cause constipation, colon cancer and diabetes. Insufficient vitamin intake may give rise to atrophy of the oral mucosa.

The geriatric patients must include the proper amounts of proteins, fats, carbohydrates, sufficient minerals and an adequate quantity of water. Adequate nutrition is vital in the health of the aging oral tissues, which in turn influences the progress of any prosthetic treatment. Oral and dental disease in the elderly, like angular stomatitis, denture stomatitis, glossitis and bone resorption can be related to insufficient dietary habits.

DRUGS AND AGING PHARMACODYNAMICS

There are no significant pharmacodynamic difference between the younger and older subjects. The frequency of adverse drug reactions is greater in the elderly. But older persons take more medications and this must be taken into consideration.

DRUGS IN DENTAL PRACTICE

Antibiotics

The elimination of water soluble antibiotics namely penicillins, cephalosporins, amino-glycosides, tetracyclines will be affected by an age-dependent decrease in renal function. No general prediction can be made with regard to age and changes in kinetics for lipid soluble antibiotics, erythromycin and chloramphenicol.

Penicillins

Excretion of these compounds is much reduced in the elderly. Normal doses of all penicillins can be safely prescribed to all patients regardless of age. But high does should be reduced in the elderly.

Erythromycin

Normal doses can be prescribed, irrespective of age.

Metronidazole and Tinidazole

Lower doses of metronidazole should be prescribed for the elderly. The excretion of tinidazole is unchanged even in renal failure.

So, normal doses of tinidazole can be prescribed.

Sulfamethizole

Sulfamethizole is normally used for a short period of time and the toxicity is low. Both young and old patients can be treated with upto 4 g daily of this drug.

Analgesics

Usual amount of paracetamol, i.e. 3 g daily can be prescribed as it is completely and rapid absorbed after oral administration and eliminated by hepatic metabolism.

Acetyl Salicylic Acid (Aspirin)

Clinically, normal dosages upto 3 g m (daily) can be prescribed in older patients. But they should be monitored for chronic salicylate toxicity which causes mental confusion and hyperventilation, which can be mistaken for a result of age itself or a disease.

Dextropropoxiphene

Normal dosages can be prescribed to the elderly.

Opioid Analgesics (Morphine, Pentazocine)

Initial dosages of opioid analgesics should be reduced in the elderly patients as compared to young subjects.

Benzodiazepines

Moderation of dosage of benzodiazepines to the elderly should be exercised when it is considered how easily elderly patients develop mental confusion and loss of memory.

Local Anesthetics

Clearance of lidocaine is reduced in elderly males. Concentration greater than 0.5% should not be administered.

Non-steroidal Antiinflammatory Drugs (NSAIDs) (Phenylbutazone, Azapropazone)

There are a few small alterations in the kinetics of NSAID which take place with advancing age. It is prudent to administer smaller doses to the elderly, or they are more prone to adverse reactions like gastrointestinal hemorrhages and edema than younger patients.

Anticoagulants (Warfarin)

Anticoagulant treatment of the elderly is difficult. The dosage should be low (3 mg daily), and the patients monitored carefully for drug interactions.

ORAL AND DENTAL DISEASES CAUSED BY DRUGS

A number of drugs such as salicylates, potassium, corticosteroids, pancreatic enzymes, tetracycline, clindamycin and phenylbutazone can cause ulcerations of the oral mucosa. These drugs should be swallowed immediately. Oral herpes may be seen in immunosuppressive treatment. *Candida* infections can occur due to corticosteroids and antibiotics. Decreased salivary secretion with increased frequency of caries is seen with therapy of drugs with anticholinergic effect like antihistamines, cyclic antidepressants, neuroleptics and some opioids.

SENSORY CHANGES AND ITS IMPLICATIONS FOR DENTAL PRACTICE[5]

As we get older we cannot see, hear, touch, taste or smell as we did when we were young. The rate of decline varies among the five senses and among individuals. Compensatory mechanisms are more difficult if the decline in any one system is severe or if all the sensory channels deteriorate concurrently.

The changes in visual function include the decline in accommodation or the ability to focus from near to far. Another major change of visual function is the difficulty with adaptation from light to dark. The changes in auditory function due to old age include.

Presbycresis. Progressive bilateral loss of the ability to hear high frequency tones.

Tinnitus. A high pitched ringing that is particularly acute at night or in quiet surroundings.

The dental team must be sensitized to the difficulties experienced by the aged person who must constantly compensate for poor visual and auditory function. The practical suggestions to ensure more accurate reception of the communication by the aged patients are:

1. Use of bold large print to write down a message. This is an effective way to assist the older patient's vision.
2. Use contrasting colors when preparing written messages in blue letters against a pale yellow background or a black print can be used.
3. When speaking with aged patients, one can aid the patient's use of compensatory mechanisms by facing the patient directly and maintaining eye contact. It will permit older persons with hearing loss to read lips and also in orienting the individual with poor visual function.
4. Standing closer to older patients than with younger patients may also aid their reception of information through auditory and visual channels.
5. The pattern and volume of speech has to be considered. It will aid the older person's comprehension if the dentist speaks more slowly and clearly. Raising one's voice slightly may be helpful.
6. Finally it would be helpful to speak with aged patients in a quiet, unhurried manner. Avoid any physical barrier such as a desk between the patient and the dentist.

7. In listening to the aged patients, the dental team must be sensitive to the individual's concerns with pain, time involved, transportation to the dental office and sometimes, the inadequate home care which has resulted in the extensive decay or periodontal destruction. It is upto the dental team to ask questions and emphasize with the patient's social and psychological situation.

By responding to the patient's concerns, the dentist can go a long way in establishing rapport with the older patient, thus making it more likely that the patient will return for preventive visits and practise the suggestions made by the dental team about home care.

ASSESSMENT OF THE OLDER ADULT

The delivery of quality-based oral health care to the older adult patient requires the effective utilization of assessment and evaluation skills by the dental team.

The patient should be encouraged to talk freely, not only about his/her chief complaint but other possible symptoms too. If possible, the assessment should be performed in a consultation room or private office where the patient is seated comfortably, and the furnishings are warm and less threatening than the dental operatory. The dentist himself should take the history and he/she should be an active listener, exhibiting responses when appropriate.

Steps in the Assessment Process

Assessment of the patient should begin the moment the patient enters the office. The first impression of the patient's physical appearance, nutritional status, gait, posture, attitude and behavior should be noted by the practitioner.

Patient's Identification Data

This has to include name, date, age, birth date, address, telephone numbers, third party information, and the name, address, telephone number of a relative, not living with the patient for emergency purpose.

The name, address and telephone numbers of the patient's other healthcare providers should be noted. If the patient has been referred by another practitioner, his/her address and telephone number should be obtained so as to forward the consultation results.

Medical History and Physical Examination

This includes a patient questionnaire and patient interview.

Patient Questionnaire

Essential patient medical data should be obtained as listed:
1. Under the present care of a physician
2. Previous hospitalization
3. Current medicines (including non-prescription)
4. Allergy history
5. Heart disease, heart murmur, high blood pressure or rheumatic fever history
6. Diabetes
7. Tuberculosis or other lung diseases
8. Hepatitis or other liver diseases
9. Bleeding problems or other blood disorders
10. Kidney disease
11. Sexually Transmitted Diseases (STD)
12. Pregnancy.

Patient Interview and Summary

Medical Review. The information obtained from the questionnaire should be transferred and summarized. Specific symptoms noted in the history may initiate a more detailed review of various organ systems. The type of prophylaxis required for the patient as such should be noted. Non-dental signs and symptoms of nutritional deficiency may also be highlighted.

Vital Signs

- Blood pressure should be recorded
- Measure pulse rate and rhythm (a rate under 60 or one over 110 should be investigated)
- Respiration rate (if above 20 per minute, check)
- Temperature reading (96.8°f to 98.6°f are within normal limits).

Important clinical signs associated with organ systems.

Organ Systems

Clinical Signs

CNS. Fainting, convulsions, headache, dizziness, tremors, paralysis, anesthesia.

CVS. Exertion causing chest pain, palpitations, ankle swelling, dyspnea and orthopnea.

Pulmonary. Cough, sputum, wheezing, infections.

GI and hepatic. Appetite level, nausea, vomiting, dysphagia, heart burn (pyrosis), indigestion, pain, jaundice, food intolerance.

Renal. Dysuria, nocturia, polyuria, hematuria, frequency, infections.

Hematopoietic. Bruising, bleeding, anemia, radiation or toxic agent exposure.

Mobility

The mobility status of the patient, i.e. ambulatory, wheelchair, assisted and others should be assessed.

Drug History

A pre-examination request for the patient to bring the containers of all current medication contributes significantly to the correct drug and dose charting. An attempt should be made to determine the patient's compliance with the prescribed medication regimen.

Updates

Before each appointment, the dentist should enquire regarding any recent medical change.

Dental History

Chief Complaint. The major reasons for the dental visit should be thoroughly investigated.

Extraoral Examination

Extraoral examination should include:
- Skeletal form and symmetry
- Neck (evidence of thyroid enlargement)
- Skin (cyanosis, pallor, flushing, character)
- Hair (texture, amount, and color)
- Eyes, conjunctivitis and scleras (for jaundice, pallor or exophthalmos)
- Head and fingers (tremors, finger clubbing and hair bed cyanosis)
- Ankles (swelling, dermatitis)
- Chest (breathing rate, wheezing, expirations)
- Abdomen (ascites)
- Ears (MPDS, referred mandibular molar pain)
- Lymph nodes (enlargement, tenderness, mobility)
- Salivary glands (enlargements, symptomatic)
- Paranasal sinuses
- TMJ
- Breath (halitosis, local causes and systemic causes).

Intraoral and Perioral Soft Tissue Examination

Oral soft tissue
- Lips and corners of the mouth
- Buccal mucosa and mucobuccal fold
- Dorsal and ventral surface of the tongue
- Salivary flow (dry mouth)
- Hard and soft palate
- Oropharynx.

Alveolar ridge and periodontium
- Changes in alveolar bone
- Presence of periodontal disease
- Mobility of teeth.

Caries, restorations and teeth structure loss
- Type of caries and extent
- Existing restorations
- Types of loss of teeth structure namely abrasion, erosion or teeth fracture.

Occlusion
- Occlusion examination should include a clinical as well as a laboratory component
- Midline deviations should be checked far.

Diagnostic aids
- Radiographic evaluation
- Assessment of pulp
- Laboratory testing, Microbiologic testing, blood tests, urine analysis, contact allergy testing, oral exfoliative cytology and oral biopsy.

Prosthesis. Evaluation of existing prosthesis. Patient should be queried regarding satisfaction with denture esthetics, chewing function, history of prosthesis use and associated discomfort if any, as well as an interest in receiving prosthodontic treatment.

TREATMENT PLANNING FOR THE OLDER ADULT

The knowledge base required to manage the oral problems of the elderly patients does not depend on the development of new technical skills but rather on the following.
1. An understanding of aging
2. An understanding of pathologic aging
3. The recognition of oral implications of systemic disease
4. A knowledge of drug-induced dental disease
5. Interpersonal skills
6. Special communication techniques with older persons who have secondary deficits
7. Decision making skills.

Based on the assumption that since persons become increasingly compromised because of various medical, social and psychologic problems, a modified system of dividing the care provided (into four broad categories) is listed:

Class I–Comprehensive treatment.

Class II–Intermediate care (maintenance of dentition and prevention of disease).

Class III–Emergency care (alleviation of pain and infection)

Class IV–No treatment.

One of the difficulties encountered in treatment planning is that dental treatment options are continuously evolving, and new information and techniques are becoming available to the clinicians.

Even after diagnosis, there is a question as to what treatment should be rendered and what modifying factors should be assessed before a rational treatment plan is developed. For this some patient related factors are assessed.

Patient Attitude. To what degree does the patient desire dental treatment, and will he/she give informed consent to institute treatment?

Quality of Life. How much is the patient affected either physically or emotionally by the dental problem and how/will his life respond to the different levels of treatment?

Limitations of Treatment. How much of the existing medical, psychologic or social problems limit the patient's ability to benefit from the treatment?

Iatrogenic Potential. How much possibility is there of creating iatrogenic problems, either a medical emergency, a drug reaction or a dental problem associated with the treatment plan?

Prognosis. What are the consequences of not treating the dental problem and how long should the treatment continue?

Dentist's Limitations. Does the dentist have the equipment, the skill, or the experience to provide the appropriate therapy at the appropriate site?

Staged Treatment Plan

When all the requisite information has been gathered including medical consultations, a staged dental treatment plan can be evolved.

Stage I: Emergency Care

1. Life-threatening emergency–immediate referral to a hospital for care
2. Referral to hospital for stressful elective care
3. Oral emergency–alleviation of pain and infection
   a. Perform biopsy of the lesion.
   b. Extract high risk teeth.
   c. Perform pulpectomy of symptomatic teeth
   d. Debride periodontal tissue and follow up with chemotherapy
   e. Control caries with temporary dressing or stainless steel crowns for symptomatic teeth
   f. Repair damaged denture or reline with a tissue conditioner.

At this point the dentist should evaluate the long-term needs of the patient and undertake the following:
1. Consider the potential life span of the patient
2. Undertake special investigations, such as blood tests
3. Consult with specialists
4. Evaluate on mounted study casts
5. Evaluate need for stress reduction.

Stage II: Maintenance and Monitoring Care

1. Management of chronic infections
2. Required preprosthetic surgery
3. Root canal therapy
4. Roat planning and curettage
5. Patient education to improve oral health (such as changes in dietary habits, plaque control and use of topical fluorides
6. Restoration of carious lesion
7. Reline, rebase or remake dentures or construct new dentures as required.

Stage III: Rehabilitative Phase

1. Orthognathic surgery or implants
2. Surgical endodontics

3. Surgical periodontics
4. Esthetic dentistry
5. Reconstruction of the occlusal plane and restoration of vertical dimension with fixed and removable prosthesis.

If the practitioner carefully stages his provision of dental care, the patient can receive the requisite treatment in increments that are appropriate to the resolution of the immediate problem. Once a critical dental problem is stabilized, the dentist can provide comprehensive dental care.

PROSTHETIC CONSIDERATIONS IN GERIATRIC DENTITION

Diagnosis and Treatment Planning

A careful history and clinical examination of the elderly patient are necessary in attempting to clarify the patient's demands and needs for prosthetic treatment. It is also important to consider systemic and local factors as well as the patient's previous experience with dentures before deciding treatment and establishing prognosis

Systemic Factors

1. *Nutrition*
2. *Debilitating disease.* Systemic diseases such as gastrointestinal disorders, diabetes mellitus or arteriosclerosis may enhance the signs and symptoms of debility. As a consequence, patients will often totally neglect oral and prosthetic care. Under these circumstance's prosthetic treatment should be postponed until the patients general health is restored. For chronically ill and febrile patients, professional oral hygiene care is necessary.
3. *Neurophysiological changes.* Adaptation to prosthetic treatment in aged patients is achieved very slowly. The patient's existing dentures can be used as a template for the design of new dentures and this makes adaptation to the new dentures more easy.
4. *Psychic changes.* Mentally ill patients try to deceive the dentist in order to attract attention. With such patients it is important to collaborate with the patient's physician in order to select an appropriate time for the prosthetic treatment.

Local Factors

There is a wide variety of local and systemic conditions which affect the masticatory system and the oral mucosa of the elderly denture patient. During clinical examination of the elderly denture patient, the following factors and conditions should be considered:
• Function of the TMJ
• Size and tone of musculature
• Quantity and quality of saliva
• Tissue tone
• Health of the oral mucosa.
• Dental and periodontal health
• Oral and denture hygiene
• Size and shape of the alveolar ridge
• Inter ridge space and inter ridge relation
• Occlusal conditions
• Fit and extension of existing denture.

GUIDELINES FOR REHABILITATION WITH COMPLETE OVERLAY DENTURE

It is a complete (or partial) denture prosthesis which is constructed over existing teeth or root structures.

Today, with the stress on preventive measures in prosthodontics, this type of treatment is a realistic alternative to conventional complete dentures in most patients with some teeth remaining. Advantages of overdenture treatment in elderly patients are:
• The natural roots provide support, stabilization of dentures during occlusion and

mastication and reduce trauma of the denture supporting oral mucosa.

- The roots and the periodontal ligament membrane will aid in minimizing future loss of the alveolar bone. The existence of periodontal membrane preserves the proprioceptive response.
- The roots can be provided with devices for added retention of the denture.
- If the periodontal ligament is significantly reduced a complete overlay denture is more favorable than an RPD. With an overdenture, the reduction in the crown/root ratio has a favorable effect on tooth mobility and on the stability of the tooth in the jaw.

There are no serious advantages of treatment with an overlay denture in elderly patients. The need for endodontic treatment and subsequent care will cause added expense. Occasionally an overlay denture may be bulky due to the presence of bony undercuts adjacent to the overlay teeth. This may result in improper fullness of the lips.

In geriatric dentistry, treatment with over dentures is particularly relevant in the following situations:

1. In patients with clinical signs of muscular hyperfunction of the masticatory apparatus, e.g. severe attrition, bruxism.
2. In patients where there are no overt signs of a decreased vertical dimension of occlusion but where an increased vertical dimension is indicated to create sufficient space for a denture.
3. In patients where severe difficulties of using conventional complete dentures can be anticipated, e.g. pronounced gagging reflex.

To prevent problems in treatment with overlay dentures, it is important to carry out a proper examination and treatment planning with regard to selection of abutment teeth.

1. The abutment teeth should have at least 3-5 mm of periodontal support and at least 2-3 mm of attached gingiva.
2. Proper endodontic treatment of abutment teeth should be possible.

3. Canines and second molar teeth are both ideally located and numerous enough to provide optional dental support for the denture.
   a. The abutments should have a height of 2-3 mm with a dome-shaped contour. If this is not possible, coping should be cemented.
   b. When a significant improvement of retention is desired and the abutment teeth have sufficient root length, the cast coping can be fitted with a precision attachment. But because of the added cost and the risk of technical failures, this procedure should be reserved for patients with a favorable dental prognosis.

Immediate Complete Denture

Conventional immediate complete denture is a dental prosthesis to replace the lost teeth and associated structures immediately after the last tooth is removed.

In elderly patients, this treatment is indicated if no teeth can be retained. This treatment procedure is advantageous compared with treatment with a conventional complete denture, the latter starting 2-3 months after extraction when healing of the edentulous ridge is completed. Thus after treatment with immediate dentures, adaptation to the dentures will be more easy, the patient will suffer less from the psychologic distress of becoming edentulous, and the denture will act as a bandage to control bleeding and to protect against injury from food and direct mechanical injury.

In otherwise fit elderly patients, there is no definite contraindication for treatment with maxillary immediate complete denture's. However treatment with immediate mandibular dentures may give complications such as pain and progressive resorption of the alveolar ridge.

In elderly patients it is often advisable to plan a sequential approach to the treatment to achieve uncomplicated adaptation to the dentures. Such treatment procedures may include stepwise extraction of teeth with adjustment of existing partial dentures.

The clinical treatment plan includes:

1. Removal of posterior teeth 3-4 weeks prior to denture construction, leaving behind 1-2 occlusal contacts to maintain the vertical dimension of occlusion
2. Primary impression
3. Functional secondary impression
4. Recording of jaw relations
5. Arrangement of posterior teeth and try-in
6. Arrangement of anterior teeth
7. Alteration of cast to compensate for soft tissue changes
8. After extraction and adjustment of the alveolar ridge, the denture is inserted, the occlusion corrected and the patient is asked to return the following day.

Postoperative care includes instruction in oral hygiene and regular review of occlusion and fit of the dentures. Soft tissue changes are usually completed 3-6 months after extraction. At that time a permanent denture is constructed or the immediate denture is relined or rebased.

Complete Denture Wearers

In elderly patients, treatment with complete dentures most frequently involves replacement of existing complete dentures. These patients may require prosthetic treatment because the existing dentures have broken, because of excessive wear of teeth or for esthetic reasons. For these patients, the treatment procedures must be done with much delicacy as it will be difficult for most elderly patients to adapt to significant changes of existing dentures.

In well-adapted denture wearers with relatively well-fitting dentures, i.e. an acceptable vertical dimension of occlusion and relatively stable occlusal relationship but poor adaptation between the denture base and the conderlying mucosa, relining and rebasing is the treatment of choice.

In well-adapted elderly denture wearers with severe tissue deterioration or poorly fitting existing dentures, i.e. significant decrease of vertical height and unstable occlusal conditions, it is realistic to consider restoring the inadequate esthetics and occlusal conditions. In this situation, a temporary relining of the dentures are done and the patient is asked to wear the dentures for 1-2 weeks. If denture function and esthetics are acceptable, the altered dentures could be rebased. If the esthetics are poor, new dentures should be constructed.

In elderly patients who have no existing denture or who do not accept the diagnostic dentures, prognosis for prosthetic treatment is questionable. It may be advantageous to use an impression technique for the mandibular jaw which records the supporting mucosa as well as the shape of the polished denture surfaces and which also allows determination of the horizontal and vertical dimensions of occlusion in the same treatment period. Here an occlusal rim is used as an individual tray after having been adjusted to the correct vertical dimension of occlusion. A functional impression is then made using a closed mouth technique.

In elderly patients who had a number of recent unsuccessful prosthetic treatments, prosthetic treatment should not be considered if there is an underlying psychiatric disease, if there are no major faults of the existing dentures, or if the patient does not accept the diagnostically altered dentures. Regular recall of denture wearers should take place for the following reasons:

1. In order to control development of microbial plaque on tooth surfaces and on dentures
2. In order to control development of functional disorders of the masticatory system resulting from changes in occlusal relationship
3. In order to prevent mechanical injury to periodontal and denture supporting tissues.

Plaque Control

Plaque control is planned by proper motivation and instruction of the patients and secured by employing an individual recall system for the professional care of the oral hygiene.

In elderly patients one should be reluctant to introduce new brushing techniques as the patients may have difficulty in conforming to these.

Chemical agents can be used for oral hygiene maintenance in patients who cannot be motivated or who are physically unable to maintain sufficient oral and dental hygiene. Thus daily mouth rinsing with chlorhexidine solutions, applications of chlorhexidine gel are effective means in chemical plaque control. Hypochlorite denture cleansers can be used but may cause bleaching, tarnish and have a bad taste.

ORAL IMPLANTS IN THE AGED

An implant can be defined as an alloplastic device placed in the body for a specific functional purpose. The purpose of an oral implant is to create a stable retention of a prosthetic appliance.

In the aged patients, morphological prerequisites for retention of dentures are limited. New dentures with a low retention capacity demand complicated functional patterns which the patient has limited ability to learn. This warrants the use of implant dentures. Further, old age, anxiety provides an additional burden. In such clinical situations, the development of soundly documented implantology provide and offer real prognosis in the rehabilitation of geriatric dental patients.

The implant treatment in the aged must be performed by a specially trained team including a prosthodontist, oral surgeon, radiologist, physician and auxillaries.

Surgical and Medical Aspects

Preoperative measures for improving the prognosis of implant therapy should be undertaken, the nutritional status should be improved, anticoagulation therapy stopped and antibiotics administered for the prevention of infections.

Surgical procedure can be done under local anesthesia, Nervous patients should be sedated with an appropriate preparation, for example, a benzodiazepine.

Surgery must be performed as quickly and as atraumatically as possible to reduce strain on the aged patient and tissues in question. Aseptic surgical procedures should be followed to prevent postoperative complications. When the osseous implant sites are being prepared, heat due to friction has to be reduced to a minimum by continuous irrigation with sterile saline and by minimizing drill speed.

It is also important to give the patient or his next of kin careful and detailed instructions to be followed during the postoperative period.

If all the above said principles are followed, implant surgery seems to be successful.

Indications

Indications for treatment with implants in the aged are:
1. Insufficient retention of prosthetic devices due to:
   - Extensive resorption of alveolar bone
   - Hypersensitive and highly vulnerable mucosal conditions
   - Defects of the jaw after trauma or tumor resection
   - Disturbed innervation of the oral and perioral muscles following trauma or cerebrovascular disease.
2. Functional disturbances preventing the patient from wearing prosthetic devices due to:
   - Age-related adaptation difficulties to dentures
   - Severe nausea and vomiting reflexes.
3. Psychosocial inability to accept a prosthetic device in spite of adequate morphological and functional prerequisites.

Contraindications

These are:

1. Oral rehabilitation with conventional prosthetic devices which have already been accepted
2. Insufficient residual bone volume and quality
3. Lack of motivation for sufficient oral hygiene measures
4. Lack of motivation for sufficient oral hygiene measures
5. General medical conditions, e.g. diabetes and severe osteoporosis
6. Alcoholic and/or narcotic misuse
7. Special oral conditions as seen after radiation therapy
8. Certain psychological conditions and other mental conditions that might indicate negative psychological outcome
9. Inability to perform meticulous postoperative care and long-standing maintenance programs.

Implant Procedures

There are at different well-documented implant designs which have been shown to be successful in the aged patients. Osseointegrated titanium implants are especially suitable for edentulous cases.

Implants[6]

After a careful preoperative analysis regarding the patient's general, physical and psychological health including an evaluation of the oral condition, from a prosthodontic, surgical and radiographic point of view, the treatment is performed in three stages:

Stage I: Titanium threaded implants are installed. An undisturbed and relatively long period (5-6 months) of healing and osseointegration of the implants is necessary in the treatment of the aged.

Stage II: After the healing period the abutment connection is surgically achieved.

Stage III: About 2 weeks later, the prosthetic procedures should be finished.

Implants AD Modum Schulte

These implants are made of aluminum oxide and produced in different sizes.

The implants are inserted according to the surgical principles to achieve ossointegration.

During healing the implant is not protected by covering mucosa. After a healing period of about 3 months, treatment is completed by application of a prosthetic reconstruction of the implant.

The frequency of successful cases is about the same as for titanium implants and covers a period of 8 years. Both systems have their special advantages and indications.

Implant therapy is a promising alternative method of treatment of aged patient, but the geriatric aspects of this therapy have not yet been sufficiently tested. It is extremely important to make a careful preoperative evaluation of the general and local conditions with respect to both the surgical and prosthetic therapy.

Only longitudinally well-documented implant methods should be used, and any approach other than a team approach in implant management is poorly grounded.

Further Reading

1. Jamieson C H. Geriatric and the denture patient. J Prosth Dent. 1958; 8(1):8.

2. Lamie G A. Aging changes and the complete lower denture. J Prosth Dent. 1956; 6 (4): 450-65.

3. Ramsey W O. Nutritional problems of the aged. J Prosth Dent. 1983; 19(1): 16-9.

4. Nedelman et al. The significance of age changes in human alveolar mucosa and bone. J Prosth Dent. 1978; 39: 495.

5. Hygeal I M. Geriatrics and dental service. J Prosth Dent. 1951; (1): 295.

6. Massler M. Geriatric dentistry; the problem. J Prosth Dent. 1978; 40: 234.

MULTIPLE CHOICE QUESTIONS

1. _____ theory is concerned with the ramifications of evolutionary influences on the organism as they become manifested in senescence.
   a. Genetically programmed sensecence
   b. Disposable soma theory
   c. Redundancies
   d. Somatic mutations

2. **Free radical theory states that**
   a. Increased metabolic rate results in reduced life span.
   b. Free radicals combine with essential molecules causing damage to DNA and other cellular structures.
   c. Molecules become irreversibly linked as a result of cross linking substances.
   d. None of the above.

3. **Stage I of a staged treatment plan is**
   a. Rehabilitative
   b. Monitoring
   c. Repair of denture
   d. Root canal therapy

31

BIOMECHANICS OF MANDIBULAR MOVEMENT

INTRODUCTION

Mandibular movements are complicated in nature and vary greatly among persons and in each person. Many different mandibular movements occur during mastication, speech, swallowing, respiration and facial expression. The dentist is the scientist who must understand the factors that regulate the motion of the jaws. These include: (i) contacts of opposing teeth, (ii) the anatomy and physiology of TMJ, (iii) the axis around which mandible rotates, (iv) the action of muscles and ligaments, and (v) the neuromuscular integration of all these factors. The dentist is also a health clinician, who understands the mandibular movements and is able to relate these movements with their useful clinical applications for the satisfactory treatment of the patients, especially those who are edentulous.

SIGNIFICANCE OF UNDERSTANDING MANDIBULAR MOVEMENTS

A knowledge of mandibular movements is essential to developing tooth forms for dental restorations, understanding occlusion, arranging artificial teeth, treating TMJ disturbance's, preserving periodontal health and the designing, selection and adjustment of articulators.

When dental operations replace more than single restorations, restorative procedures can be developed more accurately, conveniently and quickly on the articulator than in the patient's mouth. The articulator then must closely simulate jaw movement with the range of contacts between opposing teeth, so the occlusion planned on the instrument will function well in the patient's mouth. Difference can be expected between the manner in which opposing tooth surfaces contact on a simple non-adjustable articulator and the manner in which they contact in the patient's mouth. The decision whether most adjustments of occlusion in eccentric jaw relations for finished restorations should be made on the articulator or patient's mouth will determine the selection of an appropriate articulator for restorative procedures.

METHODS OF STUDYING MANDIBULAR MOVEMENTS

Mandibular and particularly condylar activity has been studied for many years by a variety of methods, ranging from direct clinical observations to sophisticated electronic instrumentation. In 1899 Luce photographed the reflection of sun light from beads placed opposite the condyle. Walker in 1896, used a facial clinometer to measure the condylar movements.

Bennett in 1908 traced the pathway of light positioned opposite the condyle.

Hildebrand recorded condylar movements by roentgenofluoroscopy in 1931. Studies have been conducted using mechanical and cinematographic techniques. Several of these techniques have been coupled with computer analysis to provide valuable information relative to the manner of the mandibular movements. Motion pictures of markers attached to the teeth and others positioned adjacent to the condyles have been made in single planes and with a prism beam splitter. Three-dimensional motion picture photography has depicted movement of markers attached to the teeth and to a pin inserted directly in the condyle. Light emitting diodes, computer-monitored radionuclide tracking and optical pantography have been used to study mandibular movements. In addition, electronic instruments (including gnathic replicator, a dynamic duplicator an ultrasonic probe, and other sensing devices have been computerized and programmed to cause casts of the patient to move in the same manner as the patient's mandible.

The studies have included the effects of tooth contact on condylar movements, the movement of working and balancing condyles during linear mandibular excursions and the presence or absence of opposing tooth contacts during masticatory mandibular movement from the vertical relation at rest to vertical relation at occlusion. Studies of mandibular movement have revealed important information regarding factors that regulate jaw movement which then have clinical implications on all aspects of occlusion.

FACTORS REGULATING JAW MOTION

When opposing teeth are in contact, the mandibular movement is controlled by the neuromuscular system as limited by the movement of the two condyles and the guiding influences of the contacting teeth. When the opposing teeth are not in contact and mandibular movements occur, the direction of movement is controlled by the mandibular musculature as limited by the condylar movement alone. The condyles and teeth modify only the mandibular movement initiated by the neuromuscular system.

Any mandibular movement is the result of the interaction of a number of biologic factors. These include contacts of opposing teeth, the anatomy and physiology of TMJ, the rotational arcs of mandible, and the action of the controlling and moving muscles as directed by the associated neurophysiologic activities.

Influence of Opposing Tooth Contacts

An important aspect of many jaw movements include the contact of opposing teeth. The manner in which the teeth occlude is related not only to the occlusal surfaces of the teeth themselves but also to the muscles, TMJ and neurophysiologic components including the patients mental well-being.

When patients wearing complete denture's bring their teeth together in centric or eccentric positions within the functional range of mandibular movements, the occlusal surface of the teeth should meet evenly on both sides. In this manner neither is mandible deflected from its normal path of closure nor are the dentures displaced from the residual ridge.

When mandibular movements are made with opposing teeth in contact, the inclined planes of the teeth should pass over one another smoothly and not disrupt the influence of the condylar guidance posteriorly and incisal guidance anteriorly. Condylar movement is limited not solely by anatomy of TMJ but also by contacts of opposing teeth. Variations in condylar movement have been observed concomitantly as deflective occlusal contacts or steep incisal guidance from opposing canines (change the pathway of mandibular movement). So the inclined planes of the artificial teeth must be placed so that they will be in harmony with the other factors that regulate jaw motion. A failure to develop this kind of occlusion can disrupt the stability of complete dentures and cause denture bases to move on the soft tissues of the residual ridges.

Influence of Temporomandibular Joints

Each temporomandibular joint is divided into a superior and inferior compartment by the articular disk in effect making two joints within each temporomandibular articulation. The basic type of mandibular movement in the two compartments is different. In the upper compartment, it is translation and in the lower compartment, rotation. This difference is related to the anatomic attachments of the articular disks to the lateral surface of the condyle and to the lateral pterygoid muscle.

All mandibular movements are either rotation or translation. A rotational movement is one in which all the points in a body describe, concentric circle around a common axis. A translatory movement is one in which all points in a body are moving at the same velocity and in the same direction. Rotational movements of the mandible take place in the lower compartment between the superior surface of the condyle and inferior surface of the articular disk. Translatory or gliding movements take place in the upper compartment between the superior surface of the articular disk and the inferior surface of the glenoid fossa. The condyle can translate anteroposteriorly for ¾ inch (18 mm).

AXES OF MANDIBULAR ROTATION

Rotational movement of the mandible are made around 3 axes (transverse, vertical and sagittal) that move constantly during normal jaw functions.

During opening and closing, the mandible moves in a sagittal plane around a transverse axis that passes near or through both the condyles. The transverse axis can be located when opening and closing the mandible in its most posterior position. In a lateral excursion the mandible rotates around a vertical axis passing through or near the condyle on the working side as the condyle on the balancing side moves forward and medially. Since it is physiologically impossible to make a lateral mandibular movement with no translation of the condyle on the working side, the vertical axis is moving and tilting along with the mandible.

During a lateral mandibular movement, the condyle on the balancing side that is moving forward and medially also move downward because of the slope of the articular eminence. This downward movement of the condyle on the balancing side causes the mandible to rotate around a sagittal axis passing through or near the condyle on the working side. As the condyle on the working side rotates around the vertical axis and translates, the sagittal axis moves in a corresponding manner.

Another important mandibular translatory movement, the direct lateral side shift that occurs simultaneously with a lateral excursion was first described by Dr Norman Bennett and is known as Bennett shift. The primary cause of Bennett movement is the contraction of the external pterygoid muscle. Its origin is located medial to its insertion as well as anteriorly and thus it appears inevitable that some side shift takes places when the muscle contracts.

When the mandible shifts to the side its movement can be described in two segments: (i) immediate side shift, (ii) progressive side shift.

During immediate side shift the major direction of movement is mediolateral, although some anterior direction is evident. As progressive side shift begins and continues the major direction of movement is anterior although some mediolateral direction continues.

The location of the axis of rotation, the establishment of horizontal and lateral condylar guidance and the provision for direct lateral shift of the mandible must be closely approximated on the articulator if they are to be simulated.

MUSCLE INVOLVEMENT IN JAW MOTION[2,3]

The muscles responsible for mandibular motion generally show increased activity during any jaw movement. This increase in activity may be associated with movement of the mandible and fixation in a given position.

The temporalis muscles have broad fan-shaped origins in the skull. The fibers that form the posterior part of each muscle run mostly horizontally than those in the anterior and middle parts. When the posterior fibers contract they tend to move the mandible posteriorly into centric relation.

The lateral pterygoids move the mandible forward if acting jointly or to the opposite side if acting individually. During conscious effort, required in mandibular terminal hinge opening movement, the lateral pterygoid remains relatively inactive. During uncontrolled opening movements the lateral pterygoids are responsible for forward movement of the condyles and mandible. They are also responsible for the lateral and protrusive movements necessary for making an eccentric interocclusal record or pantographic tracing.

The superior belly of each lateral pterygoid acts to fix or stabilize the disk during elevation of the mandible.

NEUROMUSCULAR REGULATION OF MANDIBULAR MOTION

The muscles that move, hold or stabilize the mandible do so because they receive impulses from CNS. The impulses that regulate mandibular motion may arise at the conscious levels and result in voluntary mandibular activity. They also may arise from subconscious levels as a result of the stimulation of oral and muscle receptors. The impulses initiated at the subconscious level can produce movements or modify voluntary movement.

Certain receptors in mucous membrane of the oral cavity and other receptors located principally in the periodontal ligaments, mandibular muscles and mandibular ligaments provide information as to the location of the mandible in space and are called pro-prioceptors. The impulses generated by these oral receptors travel to the sensory nuclei of the trigeminal nerve, or in the case of proprioceptors to the mesencephalic nucleus. From there they are transmitted: (i) by the way of the thalamus to the sensorimotor cortex to produce a voluntary change in the position of mandible, (ii) by way of a reflex arc to the motor nuclei of the trigeminal nerve and directly back to the mandibular muscles to cause an involuntary movement of the mandible, or (iii) by a combination of these two under the influence of subcortical areas such as hypothalamus, basal ganglia or reticular formation. Involuntary movements of the mandible away from a source of pain during the making of jaw relation records or a modification of the physiologic rest position of the mandible because of denture soreness are examples of this activity.

The loss of receptors in periodontal ligament when teeth are removed eliminates this source of control in positioning the mandible for edentulous patients. Such loss of control is an important biological factor that must be compensated by construction of complete dentures that have centric occlusion in harmony with centric relation.

Mastication was formerly believed to be the result of interaction between jaw closing and jaw opening reflexes as influenced by sensory input and conscious control. Recent evidence indicates that mastication is a programmed event residing in a chewing center located within the brain stem.

THE BORDER MOVEMENTS

Definition. Any extreme compass of mandibular movement limited by bone ligaments or soft tissue.

The border movements are most often executed on command and rarely as habitual exercises. The total border movement path has been called the envelope of movement which is a three-dimensional space inside which all the movements of mandible take place.

Pantography

The best way to study lateral border movement is by pantography. The pantograph is an apparatus consisting of two face-bows one fixed to maxilla and other to the mandible. One holds the writing devices and other the recording table. Six writings or records are made at three planes on each side of the head. One is anterior for an arrow point tracing (Fig. 31.1). One is near the condyle to trace the horizontal movement path of a point near the condyle and the last is usually fixed to the second to record the vertical movement path of a point near the condyle.

There are presently three appliances available: one designed by Stuart one by Granger, and third by Guichet.

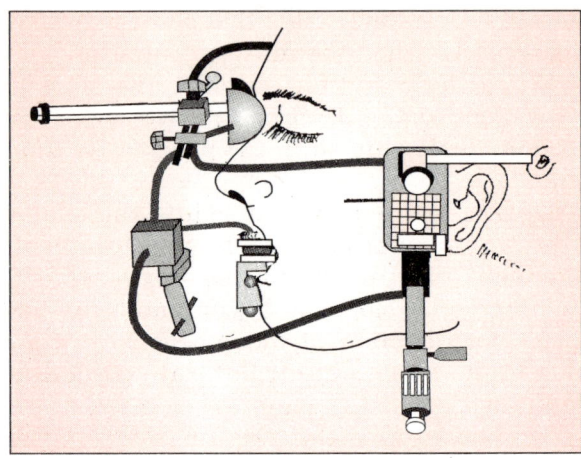

Fig. 31.1. Pantograph on patient.

Clinical Understanding of Mandibular Movement

Parallelogram of Forces. Parallelogram of forces are executed by the muscles of mastication. The parallelogram of forces can be studied only in relation to the entire skull. The direction of these forces has much to do with the seating or unseating of dentures. The occlusal vertical dimension affects this direction of forces, a fact that makes the positioning of the mandible after the loss of teeth so important.

Envelope of Motion in the Sagittal Plane

In an explanation of the clinical implications of mandibular movements, it is helpful to define the limits of possible motion and certain mandibular reference positions.

Figure 31.2 shows envelope of motion in sagittal plane.

The tracing starts at 'P', which represents the most protruded position of the mandible with teeth in contact. As the mandible is moved posteriorly while tooth contact is maintained, a dip in the top line of the tracing occurs as the incisal edges of the upper and lower anterior teeth pass across one another. CO (centric occlusion) is reached when the

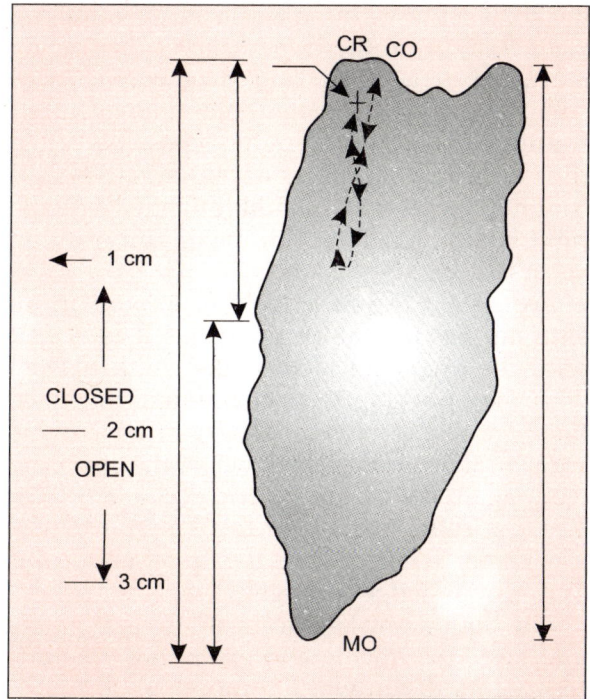

Fig. 31.2. Envelop E of motion in the sagittal plane.

CR-MHO represents the posterior terminal hinge movement. This movement is used clinically to locate the transverse hinge axis (Fig. 31.3).

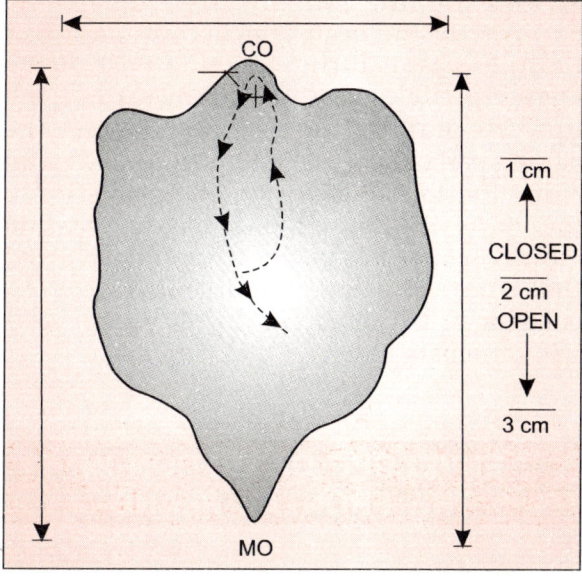

Fig. 31.3. Envelop E of motion in the frontal plane.

opposing posterior teeth are manually intercuspated. When the mandible is further retruded the most posterior relation of the mandible to the maxilla is depicted by CR (centric relation). Centric relation and mandibular position where centric occlusion occurs are two reference positions that are of extreme importance in constructing dental restorations. Single restorations are generally constructed to be in harmony with centric occlusion. Multiple restoration and complete dentures are so constructed that their occlusion will be in harmony with centric relation.

As the teeth separate, the mandible moves to its most retruded position, CR, and the patient can continue to open in this retruded position, with no apparent condylar translation to approximately MHO (maximum hinge opening) position. Any opening beyond MHO will force the condyle to move forward and downward from their most posterior position.

At approximately MHO, the patient can no longer retain the mandible in the most retruded position, and as further opening occurs, the mandible begins to move forward with translation of condyles in a forward direction. At MO (maximum opening), the jaws are separated as far possible and the condyles are in or near their most anterior position relative to the mandible. The most forward line of the tracing running from. MO to P represents the pathway of mandible as it is moved from its most open position upward to its most protruded position until the teeth contact at P which was the starting point for tracing the envelope of motion.

Intraborder Movement

The dotted line beginning with the teeth in centric occlusion (CO) at and extending downward and then upward anterior to the path of the posterior terminal hinge movement line (CR–MHO) is a tracing of the masticatory cycle viewed in the sagittal plane and superimposed on the envelope of motion. The arrows pointing downward indicate the pathway of the bead attached to the lower central incisor during opening part of the chewing cycle, and the arrows pointing upward indicate the pathway during the closing part of the cycle. For most persons with natural teeth, the pathway occurs anterior to the line representing terminal hinge movement. However if restorations are so constructed that centric occlusion and centric relation coincide at CR, many of the chewing cycles will terminate at CR.

ENVELOPE OF MOTION IN THE FRONTAL PLANE

The envelope of motion as seen in the frontal plane roughly resembles a shield. The tracing in the diagram begins with the teeth in centric occlusion (CO). As the mandible is moved to the right with the opposing teeth maintaining contact, a dip in the upper line of the tracing is created as the upper and lower canines pass edge to edge. The mandibular movement is continued as far to the right as possible. Then the opening movement is started and continued with the mandible in the extreme right lateral position until maximum opening occurs (MO) (Fig. 31.3).

From MO the mandible is moved in an extreme left lateral excursion as it is closed until the opposing teeth make contact. Then with the opposing teeth maintaining contact, the mandible is moved back from the extreme left lateral position back to where the opposing teeth again contact in centric occlusion (CO). The dip in the left side of the superior border movement is made when the upper and lower canines pass edge to edge.

The dotted line beginning at approximately middle of the tracing and extending upwards represents the upward component of masticatory cycles as the subject chews a bolus of food on the left side. The masticatory cycle moves to the right when the subject opens from centric occlusion as indicated by downward dotted line.

Further Reading

1. Lundeen JC, Gibbs. An evaluation of the mandibular border movements; their character and significance. J Prosth Dent. 1978; 40:442-52.
2. Guichet NF. Biologic laws governing functions of muscles that move the mandible. J Prosth Dent. 1977; 37: 648-56, 1977.
3. Raymond Cohen. More on Bennett movement. J Prosth Dent. 1959; 9(5): 778-94.
4. Yaeger J A. Mandibular path in the grinding phase of mastication. J Prosth Dent. 1978; 39: 569.
5. Mahan et al. Superior and inferior bellies of lateral pterygoid muscle EMG activity at basic jaw positions. J Prosth Dent. 1983; 50: 710.
6. Masserman T et al: Investigation of functional mandibular movements. Dental clinics of North America. 1969; 13: 629.

MULTIPLE CHOICE QUESTIONS

1. _____ used a facial clinometer to measure condylar movements

   a. Luce   b. Walker
   c. Hildebrand   d. Bennett

2. _____ photographed the reflection of sunlight from beads placed opposite the condyle

   a. Luce   b. Wildebrand
   c. Walker   d. Bennett

3. _____ movement is one in which all points in a body are moving at the same velocity and in the same direction.
   a. Rotational
   b. Translatory
   c. None of the above

4. _____ muscles help to retrude the mandible
   a. Anterior fibres of temporalis
   b. Posterior fibres of temporalis
   c. Middle fibres of temporalis
   d. Masseter

5. A pantograph is
   a. The most accurate method to study border movement.
   b. Apparatus consists of 4 face bows, 2 fixed to the maxilla and 2 to the mandible.
   c. 6 records are made at three planes on each side of the head.
   d. All are true

6. The factors that influence the movement of the jaws include all except
   a. Periodontal ligament
   b. Opposing cusps
   c. Neuromuscular control
   d. Temporomandibular joint

7. The direct lateral side shift that occurs with a lateral excursion was first described by
   a. Luce
   b. Wildebrand
   c. Walker
   d. Bennett

8. Any extreme compass of mandibular movement limited by bone ligaments or soft tissue is referred to as
   a. Border movements
   b. Envelope of motion
   c. Bennett shift
   d. None of the above

FAQ's

1. Factors influencing mandibular movement
2. Envelope of motion in the sagittal plane

32

DENTAL IMPLANTS FOR THE EDENTULOUS PATIENT

research findings provide a better understanding of the biologic principles that govern the development of the dynamic interface between living tissues and an artificial substitute.

INTRODUCTION

The phase of prosthodontics concerning the replacement of missing teeth and/or associated structures by restorations that are attached to dental implants is known as implant prosthodontics.

In the early days, extracted teeth, animal teeth, teeth made of wood, rubber, gutta percha, were used for replacing missing teeth. The scientific foundation for implant dentistry was established only in the 1960's with the work of Branemark and colleagues[1,2,3] using the titanium chamber. He coined the term osseointegration. Later various designs and criteria were also proposed. Currently endosteal implants are an accepted treatment modality for oral and craniofacial reconstruction, serving as transmucosal structures to support single teeth, fixed partial dentures, complete arch reconstructions, complete dentures or to reconstruct maxillofacial defects. Implant technology is evolving continually as new

BRIEF HISTORY OF DENTAL IMPLANTOLOGY

Since the age of prehistoric man, humanity has suffered from dental pathology and decay. Treatment for these afflictions can be traced historically to the Babylonian era. These afflictions frequently result in the loss of teeth. The quest for the replacement of missing teeth has intrigued man through the ages. Implant materials used by early practitioners included gold, lead, ivory, iridoplatinum, porcelain, silver, wood and others.

Intraosseous implantation[5] of animal teeth and artificial teeth carved of ivory were performed in court women of ancient Egyptian dynasties. The Mayans inlaid precious stones while the South American incas tribes practised reimplantation and implantation of teeth. Therefore the dental implant history can be traced to Africa (the Egyptians) the Americans (the Mayans and Incas) and to the Middle-East. The medieval period (1000-1799) were primarily concerned with the transplantation of teeth. Pioneers like Ambroise Pare, used this procedure. Endosseous oral implantology was given an impetus in the 18th century when Maggilio in 1809 inserted a gold implant into a freshly extracted tooth socket. Later teeth made of porcelain, gutta percha, rubber and gold were implanted.

In the 20th century, two innovative clinicians, **NE Payne** and **EJ Greenfield** proposed various procedures. Payne presented his capsule implantation technique in 1901 at the third international dental congress. Greenfield, who considered implant dentistry as the missing link of dentistry, manufactured an artificial root of 20 gauge iridoplatinum wire soldered with 24 carat gold. Other designs introduced during this period included making of designs using porcelain, and design by Venable who inserted rubber pins into artificially prepared sockets.

The 1930's saw the introduction of various designs by Venable, Strock, Dahl, Gershkoff and Goldberg. This period is regarded as the beginning of the modern era. Venable developed vitallium alloy which was used for manufacturing implants. This alloy was used by Strock and Alvin for developing a screw type implant. **Dahl, Goldberg** and **Gershkoff** helped in popularizing the subperiosteal implant. The evolution of industrial implant designs were accelerated in the 1940's. In 1947, Formiggini developed a single helix wire spiral implant made of stainless steel or tantalum. Linkow developed the vent plant implant and followed it with the development of the Linkow bladevent implant in 1967. He also played a pivotal role in the formation of the American academy of implant dentistry.

In Sweden, PI Branemark[14,15] introduced the concept of osseointegration following the culmination of a series of studies that began in 1952. This was followed by the tubingen-aluminum ceramic implant by Schulte and Heimke in 1976, the aluminum oxide implant by Sandhous in 1969, single crystal aluminum oxide endosteal implants in Japan in 1983. The ITI implant (developed by the international term of oral implantology) in 1974 (also known as the Swiss hollow basket implant) and the IMZ implant in 1989. The IMZ (intramobile zylinder) implant developed by Kirsch and Ackermann had a special stress breaking mechanism called the *intramobile element* (IME)[9] made of polyoxymethylene. Designs at use presently include the external hex type, internal connection, threaded and non-threaded cylindric or "pressfit" types.

DIAGNOSIS AND TREATMENT PLANNING[11,12]

Over the years, several diverse methods, of prosthodontic treatment of edentulous patients have evolved. The search for a substituted attachment mechanism has led to the osseointegration method which significantly improved the clinical ability to treat edentulous patients.

In these patients, a proper diagnosis and treatment plan is essential (Fig. 32.1).

1. Diagnosis
Patients examination by the prosthodontist, History, examination, radiographic evaluation
2. Patient examination by the oral surgeon
Treatment
1. Fixture operation
   Healing period
   Three months minimum for the mandible
   Six months minimum for the maxilla.
   Prosthodontic maintenance.
2. Abutment operation
   1 week later: Change of surgical pack
   preliminary impressions.
   Weekly change of pack for 3-4 weeks
   prosthodontic maintenance.
3. Routine prosthodontic clinical/laboratory protocol.
4. Patient's recall and maintenance program.

Case history

1. Patient data
   Name: Age:
   Address: Sex:
   Cosmetic index:
   Personality:

2. Chief complaint:
   History of present illness:
3. Posture and walking pattern:
   Neuromuscular coordination:
Voice:
Breath:
Vital signs:
Heart rate: Breathing rate:
Blood pressure: Pulse rate:
Systemic examination:
History of any illness:
History of medication:
Examination of systems:
CVS: GI Tract:
Urinary: Brain:
Others:
External Examination:
Face form: Face profile:
Examination of the lips:
Fullness: Visibility:
Contour:
TMJ examination:
Salivary gland:
Mandibular movements:
Examination of lymph nodes:
Intraoral examination:

Evaluation of the height, width and contour of the ridges.

Fig. 32.1. Proposed flowchart outlining the sequence.

The presence of concavities, depressions on the labial or lingual expects of the ridge are noted. In situations, where fibrous tissue is present, accurate assessment of bone width is difficult (e.g. in the palate). Clinical procedures like simple palpation or ridge mapping may be done. Palpation is simple but prone to error.

Procedure for Ridge Mapping

1. The area under investigation is given local anesthesia.
2. The thickness of the soft tissue is measured by puncturing it to the bone using either a graduated periodontal probe or specially designed calipers.
3. The information is transferred to the cast sectioned through the ridge area.

4. This method gives an indication of bone profile but is still prone to error.

Radiographic Evaluation

Angulation of the Ridge. Proclined ridge forms will tend to lead to proclined placement of the implants. This can affect esthetics and loading.

Relationship of the Jaws. Large horizontal discrepancies between the jaws (Class III) may not be suitable for placing implants.

Distance between the Maxillary and Mandibular Ridges. There should be adequate space for the placement of restorative components.

Evaluation of Soft Tissue Thickness. An adequate soft tissue thickness should be present for good esthetics. Keratinized tissue is also preferable.

Evaluation of the Length of Edentulous Span. This will provide an indication of the number of implants that can be placed. This should be correlated with the radiographic evaluation.

Study Casts and Diagnostic Set-ups

1. Study casts that are articulated allow detailed measurement of the various factors observed clinically
2. The proposed replacement teeth can also be positioned on these casts. The diagnostic setup will therefore determine the number and the position of teeth to be replaced
3. The occlusal relationship of these teeth to the opposing dentition can also be determined
4. It can be used to construct a stent or guide for radiographic imaging and for surgical placement of implants
5. A diagnostic set-up can be done on study casts. These will help in determining the esthetic placement of teeth and potential functional speech disturbances.

Traditional Treatment Plan

1. Examination—clinical and initial radiographic
2. Diagnostic set-up, provisional restorations and specialized radiograph, if required
3. Discussion of treatment options and decision on final restoration
4. Completion of necessary dental treatment extractions, restorative treatment, periodontal treatment, etc.
5. Construction of provisional or transitional restorations if required
6. Construction of a surgical stent or guide
7. Surgical placement of implants
8. Allowing adequate time for osseointegration
9. Prosthodontic phase.

Use of the Biomodel in Treatment Planning

Recent developments in computer software and derived hardware products have expanded the possibilities of visualizing residual structures. Computer-guided implant dentistry can optimize transfer from the preoperative plan to actual surgery and facilitate the clinical outcome via collaboration between the prosthodontist and the dental lab technician. Along with clinical evaluation, radiological assessment will determine whether augmentation procedures are needed to re-establish adequate bone mass for implant anchorage and adequate contour to fulfill the esthetic expectations of the treatment objectives. So, a 3-D format can be used to fabricate a life-sized replica or biomodel of the edentulous jaw.

Advantages

1. For planning bone graft treatments—the location and volume of bone required can be predetermined.
2. Can be duplicated, mounted on the articulator and can be used to generate proposed occlusal schemes to plan the situation with respect to implant installation sites and provisional or transitional interim appliances.

3. Can be used to develop an accurate surgical template after a simulated operating procedure.
4. Can be used to develop the provisional restoration used in single stage surgery and immediate loading protocols.

Biomodels are solid plastic replicas of anatomical structures. They were originally produced by stereolithography.

Radiographic Evaluation

Bone Quality. Bone quality is on a four-point scale:

Type 1—mainly cortical

Type 2—is a dense cortex and cancellous type

Type 3—thinner cortex and less dense cancellous type

Type 4—a very thin cortex and sparse bone trabeculae in the medullary space.

Bone Quantity

1. Based on the classification of ridge resorption by Zarb and Lekholm (1985). The ridge resorption has been classified from A to E. A is the ridge shortly after tooth extraction, and E is the ridge that is grossly atrophic.

Advantages

1. It allows the clinician to make an initial assessment of the bone levels available for implant treatment
2. In combination with clinical examination, they may provide enough information to plan treatment
3. They provide information regarding bone quality, especially the thickness of the cortices and density of cancellous bone
4. Provide an assessment of osseointegration and of long-term maintenance.

Disadvantages

1. They are two-dimensional images and do not provide any indication of bone width
2. Patient may be exposed to radiation.

Screening Radiographs

Uses

1. Gives an indication of the overall status of teeth and supporting bone
2. Those sites, where it is possible to place implants with a straight forward protocol
3. Those sites where other surgical procedures such as grafting may be required
4. Those sites which are contraindicated for placing implants
5. Anatomical anomalies or pathological lesions.

Orthopantomographs (OPG)

Orthopantomograph radiographs provide an image of both upper and lower jaws. They provide an indication of the bone height, position of structures such as the inferior alveolar nerve, the size and position of the maxillary antrum and presence or absence of pathological conditions.

Advantages

1. Provide an ideal view for initial treatment planning
2. Radiation dose is approximately 0.007 to 0.014 msv
3. Provide more information about associated anatomical structures.

Disadvantages

Include magnification all images (about 1.3%) and distortion in the anteroposterior dimension. Information provided by the OPG can be supplemented by occlusal views or lateral cephalograms (distortion 50-70% horizontally and 10-32% vertically).

Computerized Digital Radiovisiography[14]

Advantages

1. Detectors are solid state, so the doses can be greatly reduced
2. Manipulation of the digitally derived image may provide information regarding bone density.

Computerized Tomography (CT scan)

The CT scan uses radiograph to produce sectional images as in conventional tomography (OPG). The radiation is detected by highly sensitive crystals or gas detectors which is then converted to digital data. This is then stored and manipulated by computer software to produce a gray-scale image. The software then allows multiplane sections to be reconstituted. The images can be produced as:

- Standard radiographic negative images on large sheets
- Positive images on photographic paper
- Images for viewing on a computer monitor.

Disadvantages

1. Heavy metals will produce a scatter-like interference pattern in all general sections rendering a CT scan unreadable. So, metal containing radiographic stents should not be used
2. Magnification produced may vary
3. Images of implants may be produced and placed within the CT scan. So, the relationship of the implant to adjacent teeth and anatomic features can be evaluated (Simplant, a computer-based image software program).

Scan ORA[14]

Scan ORA is a new generation of tomographic devices which can generate high quality sectional images. The scanora produces a tomographic image directly onto film. It uses complex broad beam spiral tomography and is able to scan multiple planes.

Factors that Determine an Accurate Image

Patient Positioning. Even though the scans are computer controlled with automatic execution, good patient positioning is essential. The patient's head is carefully aligned within the device, and this position is recorded with skin markers and light beams.

Advantages

1. The scan area magnification is × 13 for routine DPTs and × 1.7 for all sectional images
2. Tomographic sections are 2-4 mm in thickness.
3. The scan sections are thicker and fewer, so the overall patient dose is less than for a CT scan
4. The amount of detailed information obtained is sufficient for all but the most complex cases.
5. To facilitate planning using imaging at different magnifications, transparent overlays depicting implants of various lengths and diameters at the corresponding magnification can be superimposed directly on the radiograph. These provide a simple method of assessing implant sites and implant placement at different angulations.

Medical History. The medical history is one of the most important and revealing aspects of patient evaluation. The questionnaire should have references to the following:

1. History of rheumatic or congenital heart disease, rheumatic fever, angina, myocardial infarction or arrhythmias
2. History of diseases of the kidney, urinary tract, gastrointestinal tract, respiratory system, endocrine system and nervous system
3. History of abnormal bleeding tendencies, e.g. prolonged bleeding
4. History of allergy such as sensitivity to certain drugs or dental material
5. History of abusing drugs, alcohol or chemical substances
6. History of psychological problems
7. History of treatment by a physician. The present illness and history should be determined.

Dental History

History of extraction. The reason for extraction, date of last extraction should be determined

Intraoral examination should include. A thorough oral examination should include evaluation of the soft tissue, oral hygiene and periodontal health. The remaining teeth should be evaluated for caries, relative positions, mobility plaque index, and presence of calculus. Edentulous areas should be evaluated for undercuts, pathology and size and shape of the residual bone. Parafunctional habits such as bruxism should be evaluated. These can have detrimental long-term effects.

In patients with severe bone resorption, the position of the mental foramina and neurovascular bundles should be noted.

Fabrication of Radiographic Splint

There are two methods for the fabrication of a resin splint.

One method involves the duplication of the patients present prosthesis (such as a complete denture). This can be used as a radiographic and surgical splint.

Procedure

1. Silicone putty material is mixed according to the manufacturer's instructions and placed into the tissue surface of the denture. Enough material is added to denture. Enough material is added to obtain a land area around the denture.
2. After the material has set, the denture is removed and notches are cut. One notch is placed in the anterior region and one in the posterior region. The notches serve to orient the halves of the putty mold for duplication.
3. The denture is repositioned into the set material and a separating liquid is applied to the denture surface and the exposed area of the impression material.
4. A similar amount of putty is mixed and pressed onto the denture surface and into the orientation notches to form the top half. After the material sets, the denture is removed. The orientation notches help in repositioning the two halves of the mold.

5. Holes are then cut to gain access into the duplicate denture area. The two halves are luted together or held together with rubber bands and self-cure acrylic resin is poured into the mold to obtain a duplicate denture.

A second method for obtaining a radiograph stent involves fabrication of a resin denture from study casts.

A resin splint is fabricated using the diagnostic set-up on the study cast. Two procedures can be used: (i) the first procedure involves the investing of the diagnostic set-up in denture flasks and processing using a clear resin (as in complete denture fabrication). The second procedure involves the use of a silicone putty mold (as described for the first procedure).

Procedure

1. The diagnostic cast is duplicated and the diagnostic set-up is luted to the cast to create a smooth transition to the land areas
2. The exposed stone areas are lubricated and the cast is boxed with boxing wax. The opposing half is poured using dental stone
3. The two casts are placed in a bowl filled with warm water for five minutes and then separated
4. The record base is pried off the cast
5. Residual wax is then rinsed off using a brush with detergent or wax solvent. The teeth are also removed from the cast
6. After the casts have had residual wax removed, the two stone molds fit well together
7. An access hole is drilled into the joined casts. The hole creates access to flowing material. The casts are separated, lubricated and allowed to dry
8. The casts are then sealed together using wax or rubber bands. The only area not sealed is the access hole
9. Clear self-cure acrylic resin is mixed and poured into the access hole
10. After the acrylic resin has set, the two halves can be separated or the top half is chiseled off the duplicate cast. The clear surgical guide splint is removed from the cast. The splint is finished and used as a radiograph measuring device or during the surgical appointment.

Uses of a Resin Splint

1. As a radiograph measuring device
2. As a surgical guide splint.

This will help in determining the location and direction for fixture installation and is used during the second surgical procedure to identify positions of buried fixtures.

Resin Splint with Ball Bearings

This is used to determine the amount of distortion. After the splint is fabricated, holes are drilled into the splint at desired locations and small metallic balls are luted over the holes. This splint is then inserted into the patient's mouth before the orthopantomograph is obtained. The diameter of each metal ball is measured and compared with the diameter of the balls measured directly from the orthopantomonograph. These two measurements create a ratio equivalent to the distortion factor of the orthopantomograph. The height of bone in the desired area is determined on the radiograph and then multiplied by the distortion factor previously determined and calculated to get the actual bone height (Colour Plate 3).

SITE CLASSIFICATION FOR IMPLANTS

Class A Site

1. The site has 10 mm or greater vertical bone present, and 6 mm or greater of horizontal bone available
2. The implant does not penetrate into the sinus or nasal fossa, impinge on the inferior alveolar nerve, or perforate the inferior border of the mandible
3. *Bone quality.* Both cortical and marrow vascular bone is present, overall bone density is good, and bone has viability and strength

4. The Angle's orthodontic classification of malocclusion is limited to Class I occlusion. The angulation of the implant is near to ideal (90 ± 5 degrees to the plane of occlusion)
5. Sufficient access of jaw-opening and inter-arch vertical clearance is available to provide for both surgical and prosthetic preparation
6. No proximal jaw or tooth pathosis is present
7. The general health and compliance (competence to follow oral hygiene instructions) of the patient is good.

Class B Site

1. The site has 7 to 10 mm of vertical bone and at least 4 mm of horizontal bone available
2. The implant may penetrate slightly (1 to 2 mm) into the sinus or nasal fossa or extend beyond the inferior border (1 to 2 mm) as long as the respiratory epithelium or periosteum is not perforated
3. Bone quality is satisfactory
4. Malocclusions are limited to Class I and modest degrees Class II and III as long as a maximum of 15 degree angulation of the implant is not exceeded
5. Sufficient interocclusal clearance and vertical mouth opening is available
6. No associated jaw pathosis is present
7. The general health and compliance of the patient is good.

Class C Site

1. The site has less than 7 mm of vertical bone or less than 4 mm of horizontal bone, especially where grafting procedures might be used (the implant should at minimum be 50% in native bone).
2. There is a total lack of cortical stop with a greater than 2 mm penetration into the sinus or nasal fossa, a greater than 2 mm penetration through the inferior border of the mandible has occurred, or minor nerve transposition surgery is desired.
3. Bone quality or density is poor (e.g. highly dense avascular bone or regions of large marrow spaces)

4. Extremes of malocclusion (Class II or III) require long cantilevers
5. Interarch space and mouth opening are limited
6. Associated jaw disease such as chronic periodontitis is present
7. The patient may have medical conditions such as diabetes or there may be limited patient compliance.

Class D Site

1. There is absent alveolar process or severe basal bone loss requiring bone graft reconstruction, e.g. discontinuity defects or sites with only a few millimeters of bone available in horizontal or vertical dimensions. Class D sites have less than 50% of the implant in non-graft bone.
2. Near total aerification of the maxillae requires sinus lift and graft procedures. In posterior mandibular sites, extensive nerve repositioning would be required.
3. Bone density and quality is poor—bone is lacking in marrow- vascular component, or there is osteoporosis, reactive bone, or proximal periendodontic scar lesions.
4. Extreme orthodontic malocclusion would require orthognathic surgery before placement.
5. Inadequate interocclusal space or jaw opening would require dentoalveolar or temporomandibular joint (TMJ) surgery before the placement of implants
6. Lesions are present near the site of placement, the patient is receiving postradiation therapy, or there are alveolar cleft sites.
7. The patient is in poor medical condition and/or may be non-compliant.

A single-site approach to the osseointegrated implant receptor location limits the treatment planning focus to the region being restored. Site classification need not supersede the total jaw classification, but gives a more detailed field in dealing with the relatively small endosseous implant. Each site can be catalogued to aid in preoperative treatment planning. The intraoperative findings and postoperative implant status in bone is better defined for each implant at each site. Individual implant prognosis is thus better estimated according to specific receptor site morphology.

IMPLANT MATERIALS AND DESIGN

Implant Materials

Materials used in the fabrication of dental implants can be categorized:
1. From a chemical point of view:
   - Metals
   - Ceramics
   - Polymers
2. Based on the type of biologic response they elicit when implanted, and the long-term interaction that develops with the host tissue. Three types of biodynamic activities have been reported.
   - Biotolerant. Materials are those that are not necessarily rejected when implanted into living tissue but are surrounded by a fibrous layer in the form of a capsule
   - Bioinert materials. Allow close apposition of bone on their surface, leading to contact osteogenesis
   - Bioactive materials. Allow formation of new bone on their surface, but ion exchange with host tissue leads to the formation of a chemical bond along the interface.

Osteoconductive. The bioinert and bioactive materials are osteoconductive. They act as scaffolds allowing bone ingrowth on their surfaces.

Osteoinductive. Capacity refers to the ability of materials to induce bone formation, e.g. recombinant human bone morphogenetic protein (rh BMP-2).

Biocompatible. All three types (Biotolerant, Bioactive and bioinert) are biocompatible and result in a predictable host response in specific application.

Biomimetics. These are tissue engineered materials designed to mimic specific biologic processes and help optimize the healing/ regenerative response of the host microenvironment. These can be any combination of the chemical and biodynamic activity categories, depending on the therapeutic strategy and type of host tissue.

Ceramics. Hydroxyapatite, tricalcium phosphate and bioglass are some of the commonly used bioactive ceramics. Ceramics can make up an entire implant or may be added in the form of a coating onto a metallic core.

Metals. Earlier metals like cobalt, chromium, stainless steel and gold were used, but these produced adverse tissue reactions. Endosseous parts of dental implants are now made with titanium and its alloys. Prosthetic components, including abutment screws, abutments, cylinders, prosthetic screws and other attachments are still made from gold alloys, stainless steel and cobalt chromium.

Titanium interacts[18,23] with oral fluids through its oxide layer which forms the basis for its exceptional biocompatibility. When exposed to air, titanium forms an oxide layer immediately, that reaches a thickness of 2-10 nm by one second and provides corrosion resistance. Titanium is considered as an ideal implant material because of its high passivity, controlled thickness, rapid formation, ability to repair itself instantaneously if damaged, resistance to chemical attack, catalytic activity for a number of chemical reactions, and a modulus of elasticity compatible with that of bone. The stoichiometric composition of titanium allows its classification into four grades that vary in oxygen and iron content. Traces of nitrogen,[26] hydrogen and iron help in improving the mechanical, and physiochemical

Chemical composition			
Biodynamic activity	*Metals*	*Ceramics*	*Polymers*
Biotolerant	Gold Co-Cr alloys Stainless steel Zirconium Niobium Tantalum		Polyethylene Polyamide PMMA PTFE Polyurethane
Bioinert	CPTitanium Ti-6 Al 4V	Aluminum oxide Zirconium oxide	
Bioactive		Hydroxyapatite Tricalcium phosphate Tetracalcium phosphate Calcium pyrophosphate Flurapatite Brushite Carbon, vitrus pyrolytic Carbon silicon Bioglass	

Titanium and its alloys[2,16]	
	There are actually five grades of titanium that may used for dental implants. Grade 1 through 4 are medically pure titanium and grade 5 is a titanium alloy (Ti6A14V). The higher the number, the stronger the metal but the more impurities are found. Type 1 titanium is too soft for dental implants and Type 2 might also be too soft. Type 3 seems to approach the ideal in terms of strength and level of impurities.
Advantages	The stronger the metal, the less problems with breakage and stripping. Grade 5 is the strongest.
Recommendations	Grade 3 titanium or above seems to be acceptable for endosseous dental implants.

properties and also improve stability. Low flexural strength and various degrees of dissolution of an all ceramic implant have made its use restricted to a coating on metallic implants. Coatings can be dense or porous, depending upon the chemical composition of the parent material and the coating method that is employed. Surface-coatings can be incorporated by plasma sprayed technique or by surface induced mineralization.

Polymers. Polymers like ultra high molecular weight polyurethane, polyamide fibers, polymethyl methacrylate resin, polytetrafluoroethylene, and polyurethane have been used. Inferior mechanical properties, lack of adhesion to living tissues, and adverse immunologic reactions have resulted in the elimination of this material. Polymeric materials are nowadays used as stress absorbing components incorporated into the superstructures supported by implants.

Basic Implant Design

1. Threaded
2. Non-threaded (cylinders).

Specific Micro-surface Design

1. Plain
2. Machined
3. Acid etch
4. Sand-blasted
5. Titanium plasma spray
6. Hydroxyapatite (HA) plasma spray
7. Porous sintered surfaces.

IMPLANT CLASSIFICATION

Implants have been classified in different ways; (i) implant/abutment interface, (ii) the body shape, and (iii) implant-to-bone surface

The Implant-abutment Interface

The implant/abutment interface connection is generally described as an internal or external connection. The feature that distinguishes between the two is the presence or absence of a geometric feature that extends above the coronal surface of the implant. An external connection may extend 1-2 mm above the coronal area of the implant and an internal connection may extend approximately 5.5 mm into the body of the implant.

The connection may be a slip fit joint, where a slight space exists between the mating parts and the connection is passive or as a friction fit joint where no space exists between the mating components and the parts are literally forced together. The mating surfaces can also be categorized as being a butt joint which consists of two right angle flat surfaces contacting or a bevel joint, where the surfaces are angled either internally or externally.

The joined surfaces may also incorporate a rotational resistance and indexing feature, the geometry of which may be octagonal, hexagonal, cone screw, cone hex, cylinder hex, spline, cam tube, cam and pinslot.

The Body Shape or Geometry. The body geometry of the endosteal implant is cylindrical

in shape. Three basic types were initially available.

1. A threaded screw (e.g. ad modum Branemark).
2. A press fit cylinder (ad modum IMZ)
3. Hollow basket cylinder. (ITI–Straumann)

1. Threaded screws can be categorized as:
   - Straight
   - Tapered
   - Conical/tapered
   - Ovoid
   - Expanding (based on body geometry). The thread pitch, pattern depth, thickness, thread face angle and thread helix angle are varying geometric parameters that determine the functional thread surface and affect the biomechanical load distribution of the implant. Thread thickness and thread face angle determine the shape of the thread, which can be V-shape, square or a reverse buttress thread.

     Various manufacturers have introduced double-threaded and triple-threaded implants which are faster to thread into the osteotomy site, generate less heat upon placement, provide increased initial stability and require more torque for placement.
2. Non-threaded cylindric or press fit implants can be categorized as: (i) straight walled, (ii) tapered, (iii) conical, (iv) trapezoidal, and (v) trapezoidal step (based on body geometry).
3. Hollow basket cylinder. The implant body can also be distinguished by the presence of a flared or straight neck.

Cervical Geometry Patterns

1. Standard cervical collar with tapered neck.
2. No collar.
3. Straight collar with no neck constriction.
4. Bevel cervical collars.
5. Reverse bevel with no cervical collar.
6. Tapered cervical collars with and without threads.

Surface Topography

The quality of the implant surface can influence the wound healing at the implantation site and so affect osseointegration. Surface topography can produce orientation and guide locomotion of specific cell types and can influence cell shape and cell function. The surface of implants can be smooth (as in machined CP titanium) or rough (as in plasma sprayed titanium).

A Rough Surface May be Produced by

Plasma Sprayed Titanium. It is one of the most common methods for surface modification. Plasma spraying is used for the application of both titanium or hydroxyapatite on metallic cores with a coating thickness of 10-40 micrometer for titanium and 70 micrometer for hydroxyapatite. It is welded to a thickness of 0.3-0.4 mm.

The external hex[2]	
Description	The external hex is the original prosthetic connection for the dental implants designed by Dr Branemark. Actually the hex itself was only on the implant to enable the operator to screw the implant into the bone. It subsequently became important as a prosthetic connection as various forms of prosthetic restoration evolved.
Prosthetic advantages	Most common type of prosthetic attachment. Has the most options available. While there are some variations in the actual size of the external hex from manufacturer to manufacturer, this has proven to be a liable and useful prosthetic attachment for all kinds of restorations.
Prosthetic disadvantages	Poor techniques will allow for loosening of this attachment and premature wear of the hex.
Economics	The ubiquity of this attachment interface makes it the most economical in the market although there are variations that are somewhat more expensive.

The internal hex	
Description	The internal hex was designed as a more stable and retentive alternative to the external hex. This attachment provides a recessed portion in the top of the implant.
Prosthetic advantages	It is very stable and retentive.
Prosthetic disadvantage	Possible fracture of the head of the implant.

Two stage procedure[2]	
Description	In a two-stage procedure, the implant is surgically placed and covered over with the gum tissue. Three of four months later, the gum tissue is opened and a second piece is screwed into the implant to allow the soft tissue to heal around the site. The teeth can then be made or attached.
Advantages	The implant remains protected throughout healing and there are some people who believe this might be advantageous.
Disadvantages	Require a second surgery. Additional time is necessary for healing from the second-stage surgery.

Single stage procedure[2]	
Description	A one-stage technique refers to the placement of a dental implant with one surgical procedure. When the implant is inserted, it is not covered up with the soft tissues. It is allowed to protrude through the gingiva. This technique implies that the implant is not loaded in any way.
Advantages	There is no need for an additional surgery and the gingiva tissue is completely matured when the implant is ready to load.
Disadvantages	Possible accidental loading of the implant (Colour Plates 6, 7).

Sintered titanium	
Description	Sintering titanium alloy powders to a machined titanium surface using a high temperature and controlled atmospheric pressure produces a uniform porous surface that greatly increases surface area.
Advantages	The surface is said to induce rapid bone in growth and more complete osseointegration.

Hydroxyapatite coated titanium	
Description	HA is sprayed onto the surface of a machined implant to produce a rougher surface configuration.
Advantages	The HA increases the surfaces and it also provides an accelerated biointegration. There is a definite advantage to using HA on dental implants because it is osteoconductive and promotes rapid and more complete osseointegration.
Disadvantages	HA is soluble in oral fluids and if the HA is exposed, it will cause implant failure with accelerated bone loss.
Recommendations	Acceptable with proper technique to prevent exposure of the HA.

Thickness depends on particle size, speed and time of impact, temperature and distance from the nozzle tip to the implant surface area.

Blasting with Particles of Various Diameters. The implant surface is bombarded with particles of aluminum oxide (Al_2O_3) or titanium oxide (TiO_2) and by abrasion. A rough surface is produced with pits and depressions. Roughness depends on particle size, time of blasting, pressure, and distance from the source of particles to the implant surface.

Chemical Etching. The metallic implant is immersed in an acidic solution, which erodes its surface creating pits of specific dimensions and shape. Factors determining the roughness include the concentration of the acidic solution, time and temperature. Implants that have been etched with a mixture of hydrochloric acid and sulfuric acid have been introduced.

Sandblasted and Acid Etched. Surfaces that have been sandblasted with 500 micrometer particles followed by etching with hydrochloric acid-sulfuric acid.

Combination of Two or More Different Surfaces on the Same Implant Body. The rationale is to achieve better soft tissue response, stability and attachment in cortical bone with a machined or etched coronal implant surface and better mechanical locking in medullary bone with a roughened TPS surface in the apical and middle portions of the implant.

Porous Sintered Surfaces. These are produced when spherical powders of metallic or ceramic material become a coherent mass with the metallic core of the implant body. Pore surfaces are characterized by pore size, pore shape, pore volume and pore depth. Advantages include:

- ability to use shorter endosseous implants because of a three-fold increase in surface area.
- may be impregnated with growth factors and act as delivery vehicles because of increased surface volume.

Abutments. Can be categorized as:
- One and two piece flat top
- One and two piece conical shouldered
- UCLA type plastic castable
- UCLA machined/plastic cast to cylinders
- UCLA gold sleeve castable
- One piece fixed post
- Two piece fixed shoulder
- Prolonged fixed
- Telescopic malleable post
- Ceramic
- Single tooth direct connection
- One and two piece overdenture abutments.

IMPLANT RESTORATIONS FOR EDENTULOUS PATIENTS

Osseointegrated implant[8] treatment was originally designed for the edentulous patient to support a fixed detachable prosthesis. Now, alternative designs have evolved. Preoperative evaluation of the structure and quality of the edentulous ridge, intermaxillary relationship, esthetics, phonetics, hygiene and cost considerations can influence the selection of the design.

Various Implant-supported Prosthesis: These include the following
- The fixed ceramomet al prosthesis
- The fixed detachable prosthesis
- Overdenture
- The fixed removable prosthesis.

The Fixed Ceramometal Prosthesis

This prosthesis is similar in design to the conventional fixed prosthesis used to restore partially edentulous arches. The ceramometal prosthesis can be cemented to transmucosal abutments or secured with gold alloy screws. Beumer has recommended a minimum of six implants to be placed in an antero-posterior span of 20 mm with sufficient bone in the second premolar position to house a 10 mm implant

Advantages

- Optimal esthetics
- Phonetics is good
- Oral hygiene can be easily maintained.

Variables Influencing the Treatment Planning[8]
- *Considerable labial bone resorption.* The prosthetic teeth may appear very long with large spaces apparent interproximally.
- *High lip line.* Esthetics may be affected along with speech.
- *Bone density.* Less dense maxillary bone may require more implants.
- *Intermaxillary relationship.* Can affect the design and use of the fixed ceramometal design.
- Ungrafted patients with advanced bone loss are not candidates for this prosthesis.

Disadvantages

- Cost may be prohibitive.
- Loss of a pivotal implant can compromise the entire prosthesis.
- Long span frameworks are prone to casting errors.
- Porcelain fracture is challenging and difficult to repair.
- Short crowns on cementable abutments can pose retention problems.

Cement Retained and Screw Retained Implant Prosthesis

Advantages

- Easy retrievability.
- Provide a passive, stable environment because they are cemented on well-adapted machined abutments with discrepancies in fit of the castings of the abutments being negated by the grouting action of the cement.
- Non-passive framework can be seated and adjusted by routine chairside clinical procedure and indicating materials.
- Sectioning and soldering is not required routinely.
- Absence of screw holes provides a design that enhances the physical strength of porcelain and acrylic resin, resulting in less fracture.
- Occlusion is devoid of screw holes and so the occlusion can be developed as required.
- Provide easy access to the posterior of the mouth.
- Reduced costs.
- Reduced complexity of components.
- Reduced complexity of lab procedures.
- Reduced chair side time.
- Superior esthetics.

Disadvantages

Retention depends upon factors like taper, parallelism, surface area and height. For example, if the height of the abutment is less, retention may be compromised.

Screw-retained Prosthesis

Advantages

- In areas of limited inter ridge space, a screw is more effective than a cement-retained prosthesis.
- Retention may be better than for a cement retained prosthesis.

Disadvantages

- Screw loosening is a major disadvantage.
- Sectioning and soldering are routinely required.
- Presence of screw holes can compromise the strength of porcelain and acrylic resin.
- The occlusal surface may have screw holes that can affect the occlusion.
- Increased cost.
- Complexity of components and lab procedures.
- Poor esthetics.

Fixed Detachable Prosthesis

The fixed detachable implant prosthesis consists of denture teeth connected to a metal framework with acrylic resin.

Advantages

- In moderate to advanced ridge resorption, this prosthesis can replace hard and soft tissue.
- Can be used in poor quality load-bearing soft tissue.
- Retention is better.

Disadvantages

Phonetics may be affected.

Interabutment spaces and bar placement can result in breaks in the palatal contour and speech disturbance.

Hygiene may be compromised.

High lip line can create esthetic complications.

In patients with severe bone resorption, the lack of facial scaffolding and cheek biting can present esthetic and functional problems.

Fractured acrylic resin matrix, loose gold alloy screws and occlusal wear are common complications.

Overdenture Prosthesis

This prosthesis is used in patients with advanced ridge resorption. This requires four to six implants in the anterior region connected with a bar superstructure.

Advantages

- Can provide facial support.
- Access will be provided for oral hygiene maintenance.
- Load capacity of the implants may be increased.

Indications

- Patients with high muscle attachment
- Sensitive mucosa
- Knife-edged ridges
- Sharp mylohyoid projections
- Superficial placement of mental nerve.

Implant and Tissue-supported Overdenture. When overdenture prostheses are supported by both implants and the mucosa, fewer implants may be needed.

Indications

- In medically debilitated patients, who cannot tolerate long surgical procedures (fewer implants need to be placed).
- Economic considerations.
  The advantages include greater stability.

Fixed Removable Prosthesis

It was first reported in 1982. The spark erosion prosthesis is a combination of two technologies. First a meso-bar is waxed, cast and precision milled with a two degree taper on both sides, which provides the frictional retention for a metal superstructure. The primary bar is constructed to allow the principles of a rotational path prosthesis to be used in stabilizing the superstructure. Retention is provided by three frictional pins in the anterior segment of the primary bar and also by two swivel latch attachments.

Electrical discharge machinery is used to achieve close tolerances of fit between the meso-bar and superstructure.

Indications

- Extensive ridge resorption.
- Ridge prosthesis is required but phonetics, hygiene and esthetic demands preclude the use of a fixed detachable prosthesis.
- The superstructure can be removed to facilitate hygiene procedures.
- In unfavorable ridge relations, where better retention is needed.

Disadvantages

- Cost
- Technique-sensitive lab fabrication
- Patient dexterity to remove swivel latches.

SURGICAL PROCEDURES IN IMPLANT DENTISTRY

Corrective or reconstructive surgical procedures in implant dentistry may be needed for functional and/or esthetic purposes. These may involve the hard and soft tissue. Sufficient bone (hard tissue) must be present to allow placement of an implant of suitable dimensions. The soft tissue around the implant should be capable of maintaining functional integrity and should withstand oral hygiene procedures.

Alveolar Bone Deficiencies. The bone height, width, quality should be assessed prior to implant placement. In situations where an adequate amount of bone is absent, it may be difficult to place an implant. Implant placement at alternative sites such as zygomatic process and pterygoid plates may present surgical and prosthodontic problems.

Deficiencies in bone may be restricted to small, well-defined defects involving one or more sites or may be much more generalized involving an entire jaw. Different techniques and materials are used to augment bone into these areas.

Autogenous Bone Grafts

These remain the gold standard by which all other materials are judged.

Advantages

- Readily available from adjacent or remote sites.
- Sterile.
- Biocompatible/non-immunogenic.
- Osteoinductive/conductive.
- Easy to manipulate.

Sources

Intraoral sites such as the retromolar pad and symphysis region. These are harvested using trephines, surgical bone traps attached to the suction apparatus.

Advantages

- Environment in which the surgeon works, will be familiar.
- Graft is of the same developmental origin.
- The disadvantage is that large blocks of bone cannot be obtained. So, these can be used only for small defects.

Extraoral Sites

For example, the iliac crest. Optimization of grafting is achieved by ensuring that there is close apposition between the graft and host bed and that the graft is stable. Stability can be achieved by using guided bone regeneration (GBR) membrane (the most widely used is Gore-tex, an expanded polytetra-fluoroe-thylene—PTFE).

Ideal Properties of GBR Membranes

- Should be biocompatible.
- Should be totally occlusive (non-permeable) to prevent passage of cells during the healing period.
- Physical properties which allow the space under the membrane to be maintained. This is achieved by using titanium reinforced membranes.
- Should enhance wound stability and protection of the initial clot and delicate granulation tissue. The membrane can be stabilized by using screws or pins.

Uses of Guided Bone Regeneration

- In its simplest form, GBR membrane can be used to promote bone fill of a defect before implant treatment.
- Can be used to regenerate bone in dehiscences and fenestrations around implants at the time of placement.

Technique

It is one of the most common techniques used for the treatment of localized ridge deficiencies. This technique employs barrier membranes which allow the creation of a confined defect into which the bone progenitor cells may migrate, allowing bone to form in the void. A membrane is positioned in the wound in such a way that it separates the overlying gingival connective tissue from the implant, creating a space.

Alloplastic Graft Materials

For example, the hydroxyapatite, tricalcium phosphate and bioactive glass.

Advantages

- Easy to use
- Provide an osteoconductive framework for bone.

Disadvantages

- These are not osteoinductive and do not contribute to osseointegration.
- Efficacy when used alone as grafting materials has not been proven clinically.

Allografts

e.g. DFDB's, freeze dried bone.

Advantages

- Used as a scaffold for bone repair.
- Are resorbable.

Disadvantages

- Small fragments remain.
- Sterility may be difficult to achieve.

Xenografts (graft materials derived from other animal species)

Bio-Oss is bovine bone in which the organic component is completely removed to leave the mineralized bone architecture. Corals and nacra (the calcium carbonate shell of molluscs) have also been used with promising results.

Bone Promoting Molecules

Identification and production of bone morphogenetic proteins are a recent advancement in implantology. They have been used for bone regeneration in the maxillary antrum. They are also present in the natural form in demineralized freeze dried bone.

Management of localized deficiencies in the alveolar ridge. Implant placement in thin ridges may result in incomplete bone coverage of the implant surface. These may be managed using grafts or by guided bone regeneration.

Management of large deficiencies of the alveolar ridge. Large deficiencies of the alveolar ridge may arise as a result of tooth loss and trauma, developmental anomalies, and pathological conditions. These deficiencies may be managed by:

Onlay grafting. Onlay grafts can be used to augment bone in the vertical and lateral dimension. Grafts may be harnessed from the symphysis and retromolar pad areas. Larger grafts are harvested from the iliac crest.

Procedure

- Grafts are harvested from the donor site.
- The recipient bed is perforated with a small bur to allow a blood clot to form.
- The donor graft is secured to the recipient bed using miniscrews, plates or wires.
- Remaining voids are packed with cancellous bone chips to maximize the healing potential.

Modified technique. A modified technique was introduced by Breine and Branemark in 1980. They described onlay composite bone grafts for reconstruction of the severely atrophic edentulous arch. These grafts were secured to the recipient bed using endosseous titanium implants.

Procedure

- An iliac crest graft is taken in one piece. It is of the same dimension as the proposed area.
- The graft is secured to the residual ridge using five or six implants.

Requirements for onlay grafting with implants (Collins)
- Presurgical/prosthetic work-up to determine the desired definitive prosthesis. This will allow.
- Fabrication of a surgical splint.
- Identification of the area of augmentation.
- Direction for the surgeon to provide an adequate site for precise implant placement.
- Flap closure without tension. The flap should drape the graft loosely, with an approximated margin prior to suturing the wound edges.
- Provisional restoration without pressure. Pressure on grafts or transmucosal loading of implants within grafts causes shrinkage of the grafts and may lead to loosening of the implants.
- Reasonable expectations by the patients.
- Minimum 1.5 mm thickness of bone graft covering the implant. If thickness is less, the exposure of the implant surface can occur.
- Anatomic replacement. Should replace alveolar bone and adnexal basal bone.

- Intimate interfacial mortising. The graft and host bed interface should be adjusted for complete contact without dead space.
- Rigid fixation. Without rigid fixation, resorption or infection can occur.
- Solid graft anchorage in native bone.

Bone Grafting Concepts

- *Gentle bone harvesting (Albrektsson)*. All three graft healing mechanisms, bone induction, bone conduction and transfer osteogenesis can occur in the same grafted site depending on the status and the type of graft and the ability of the recipient site to provide nutrition, cellular viability and rapid revascularization. Bone harvesting should be done reducing heat production.
- Graft should be transported to the recipient site as soon as possible or should be stored in a cool, moist environment if there is a delay.
- At the recipient site, the following factors which influence bone healing should be considered.
  1. Proper incision and flap design to avoid extensive surgical undermining.
  2. Conservative use of cautery.
  3. Conservative periosteal reflection in mandibular discontinuity because the residual mandibular blood supply is primarily from the periosteum.
  4. Avoiding overheating of residual bone.
  5. Use of an aseptic technique.
  6. Rigid skeletal fixation of bone grafts.
  7. Watertight, tension-free, everted closure.
  8. Meticulous hemostasis, elimination of dead space.

Maxillary Sinus Grafting

The sinus lift or sinus elevation is similar to a Caldwel-Luc procedure combined with grafting of the floor of the maxillary sinus. Boyne in 1960 described the first use of bone grafting to the maxillary sinus to increase depth and bulk of osseous tissue for prosthetic reasons. Three anatomic locations are used for performing the maxillary sinus floor graft.

- The classic Caldwel-Luc opening located just anterior to the zygomatic buttress and above the apices of molar and premolar teeth.
- The midmaxillary entrance, between the crest of the alveolar ridge and zygomatic buttress.
- A low position along the anterior surface of the maxilla, (at the level of the existing alveolar ridge).

Procedure

- Local anesthesia is given.
- A window is cut in the lateral antral wall using surgical burs. The integrity of the sinus membrane is maintained.
- Window is then fractured to create a discrete cavity on the superior aspect of the residual alveolus.
- Graft material is then inserted which keeps the elevated bone in its elevated position.

Indications. In situation where initial implant stability is difficult to achieve, e.g. maxillary ridge with less than 5 mm bone.

Inlay Graft Combined with Maxillary Osteotomies

Class III skeletal relationship with gross resorption of the maxilla can be managed with an inlay graft combined with a Le fort Type I osteotomy.

Newer Developments

Zygomatic Implants

Prosthetic rehabilitation of an extremely atrophic maxilla may involve the use of large autologous graft combined with nasal floor augmentation. Frequently the patient's systemic condition or attitude may preclude use of these procedures. In these patients, zygomatic implants have been used. These implants are designed to engage the zygoma, and enter the oral cavity in the premolar/molar region to provide stabilization for a fixed prosthesis.

These are placed in patients under general anesthesia. They are available in lengths of 30, 35, 40-45, and 50 mm. An osseointegration time of 6 months is allowed before the implants are loaded. The ideal prosthetic restoration supported by zygomatic implants is a fixed, palateless, unit with crossarch stabilization.

Recombinant Human Bone Morphogenetic Protein 2 (rh BMP-2)

It is an osteoinductive protein that when administered locally results in new bone formation at the site of implantation.

Implants for Orthodontic Anchorage

The concept was first introduced in 1945 and involves the use of osseointegrated implants as anchorage.

SURGICAL PROCEDURES IN PLACEMENT OF DENTAL IMPLANTS

Since this chapter deals with implants for edentulous patients, the following part represents graphically the armamentarium and surgical procedure involved in implant placement (Colour Plate 8 shows pre- and postoperative views of a patient).

Armamentarium

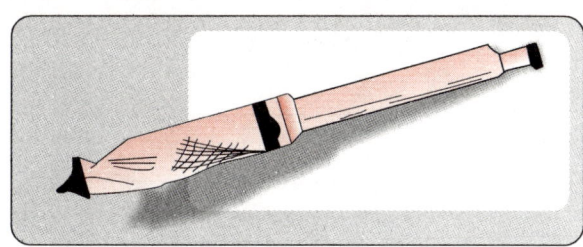

Twist drill

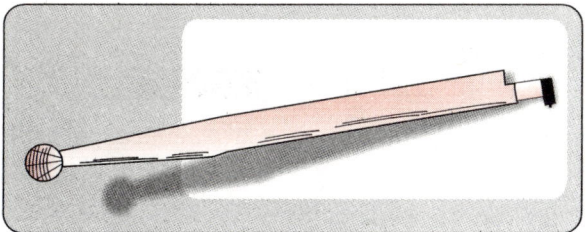

Round bur

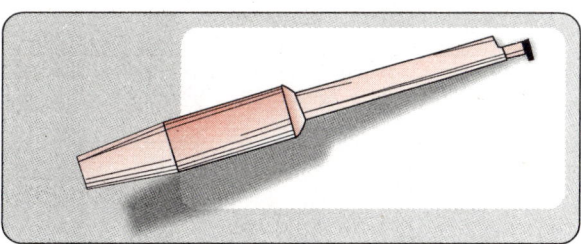

Drill extension

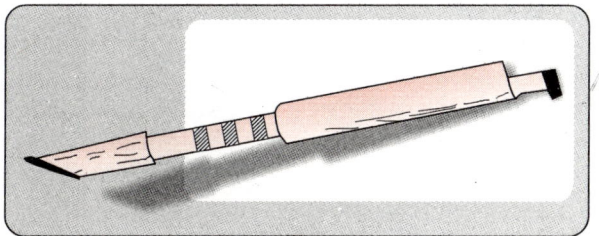

Pointed starter drill

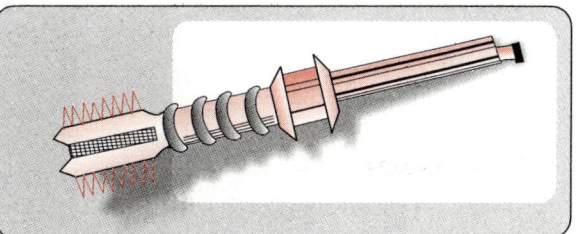

Tap drill

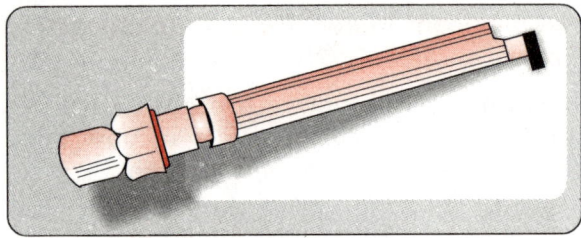

Crestal bone drill

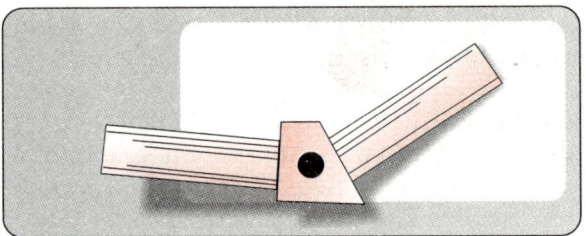

Paralleling pin (angled)

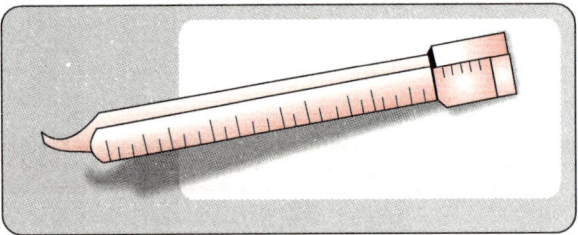

Depth probe

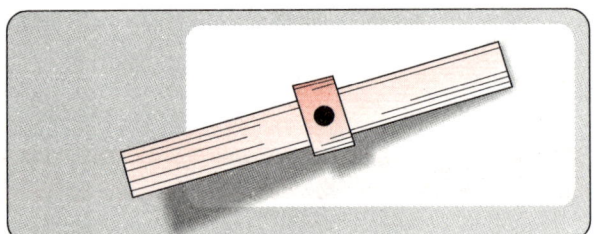

Paralleling pin (straight)

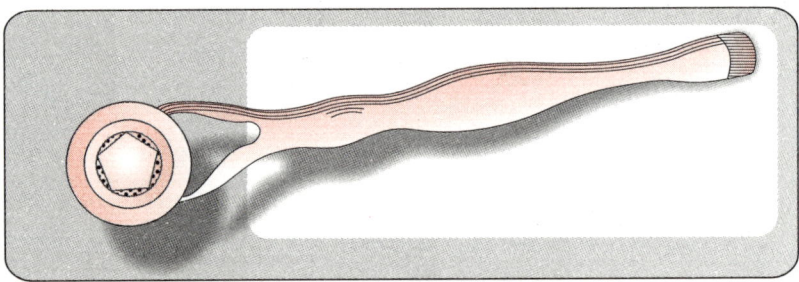

Rachet

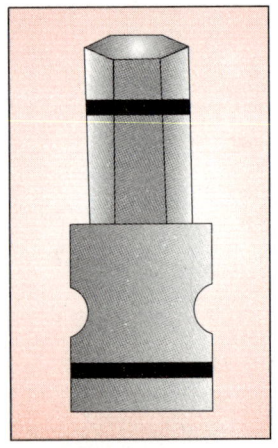

Ratchet adapter

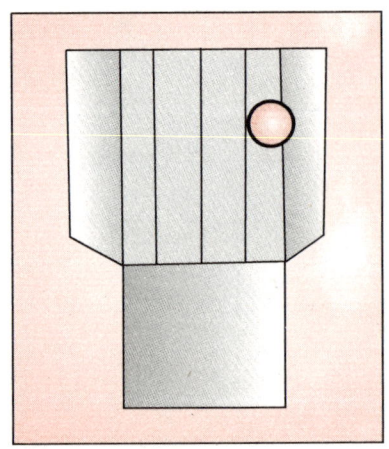

Hand wrench

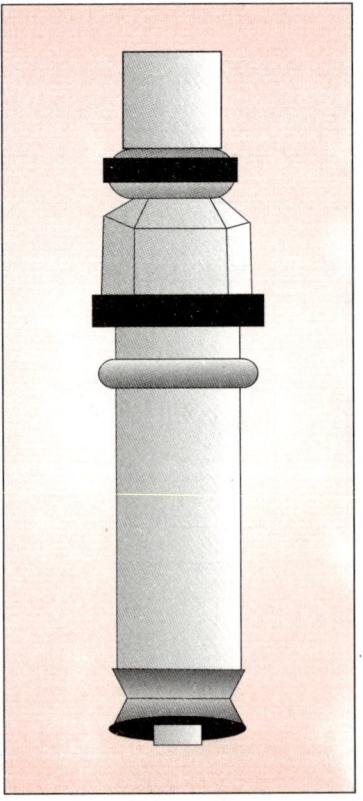

Insertion tool

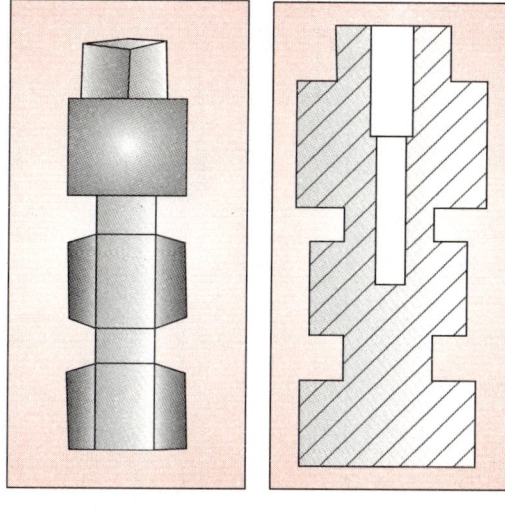

Implant analog

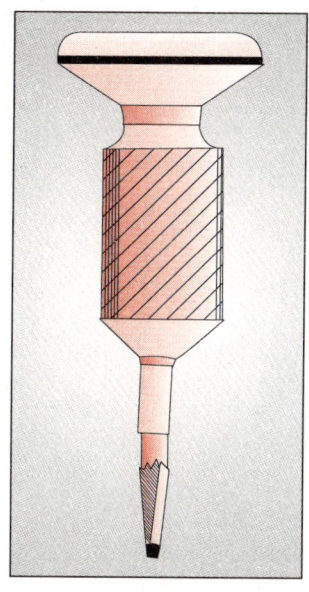

Hex driver

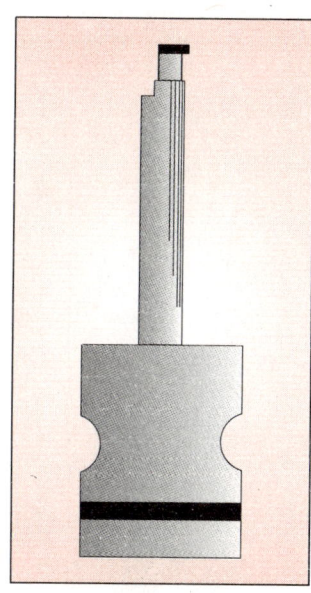

Handpiece adapter

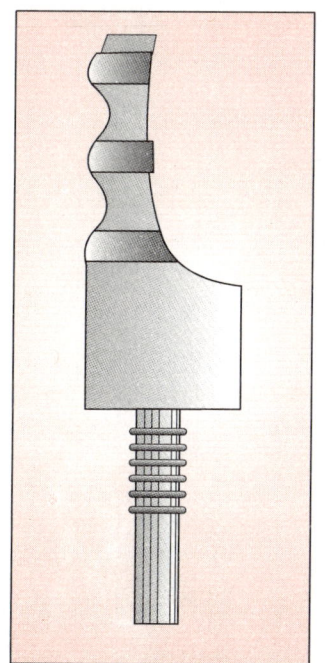

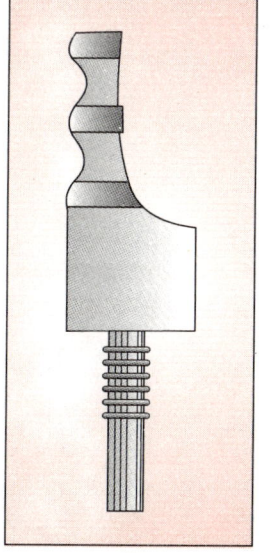

Indirect transfer coping (non-flexed)

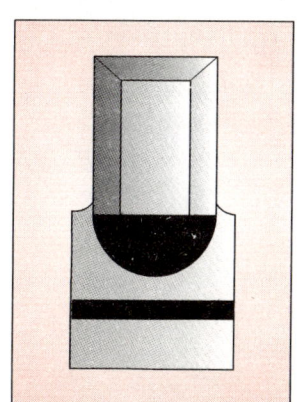

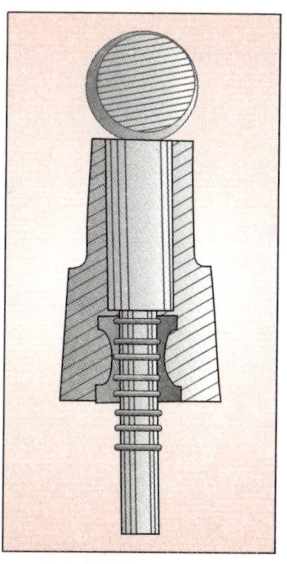

Direct transfer coping (ball top)

An implant System

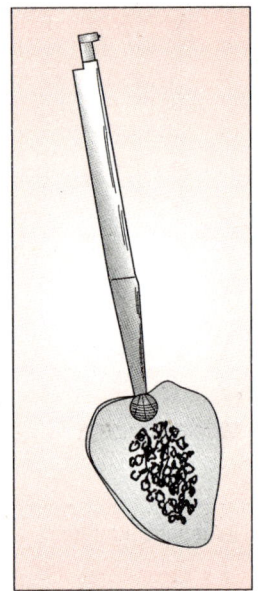

Round bur

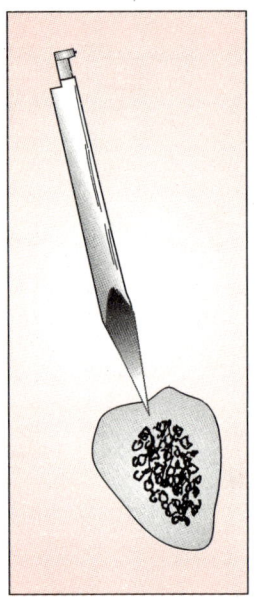

Pointed starter drill

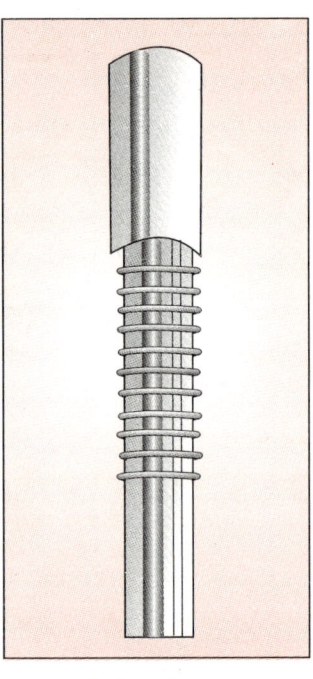

Abutment screw

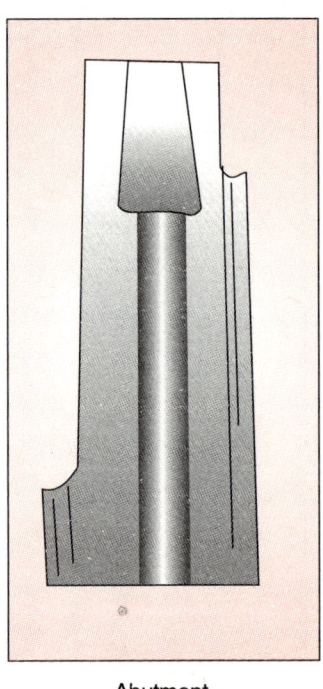

Abutment

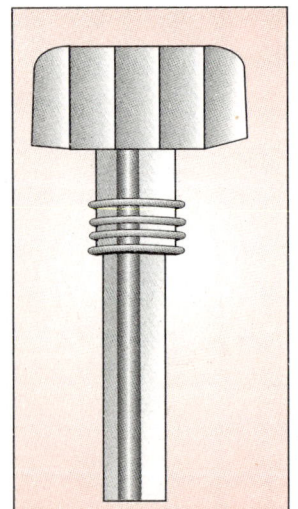

Cover screw

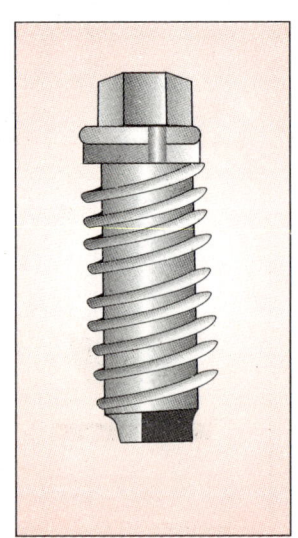

Implant

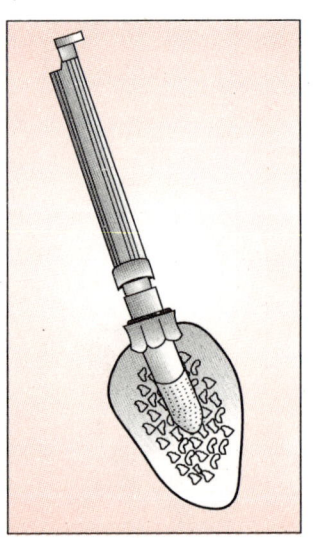

Crestal bone drill

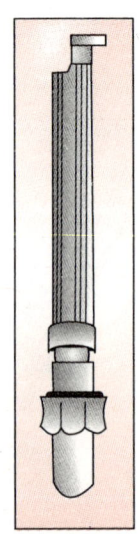

Crestal bone drill – design

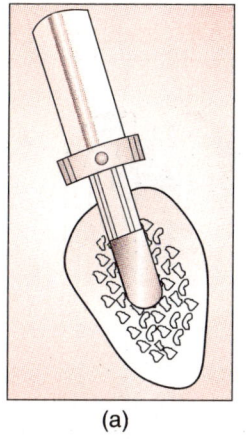

(a)

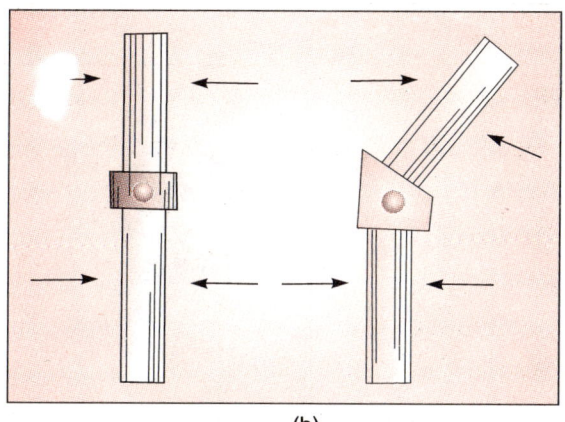

(b)

Force direction indicator

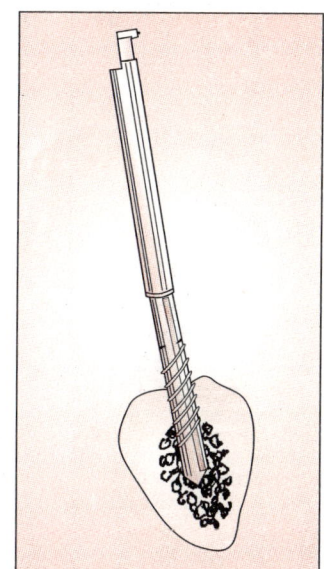

Twist drill

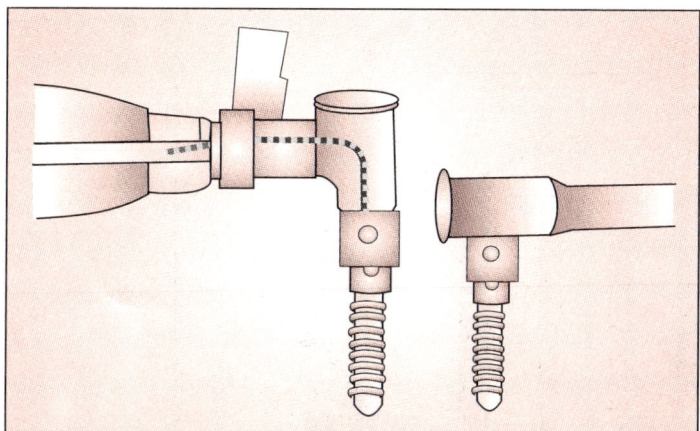

Implant placement using various means

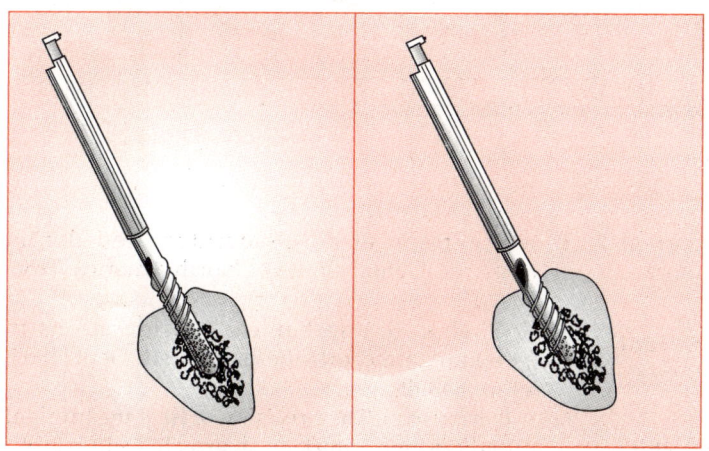

Drills of increasing diameter

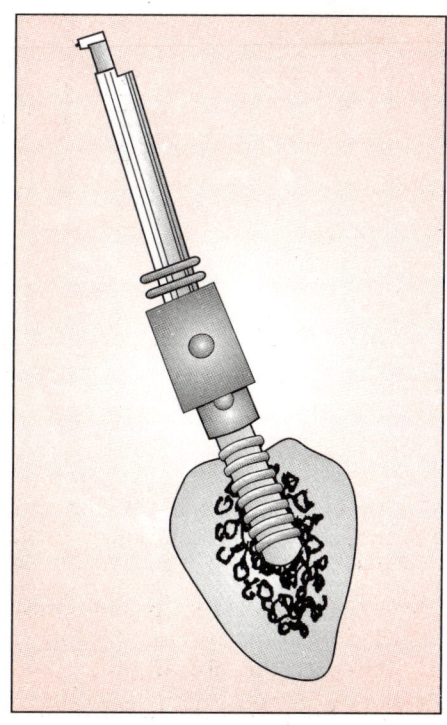

Surgical tap

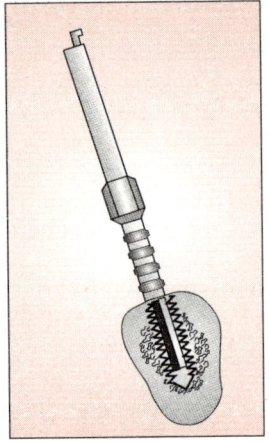

Surgical tap

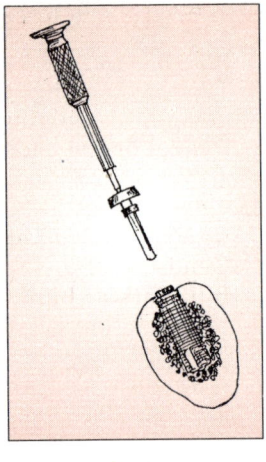

Placement of the cover
screw

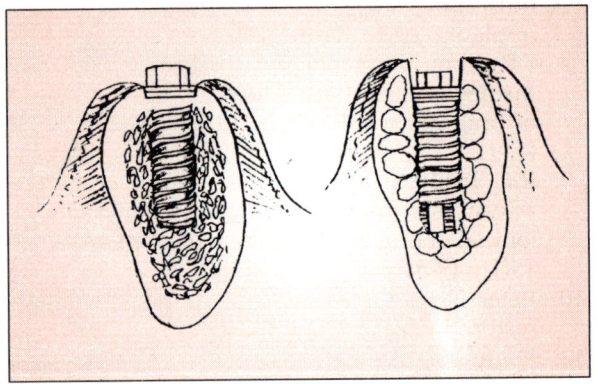

Implant placement level

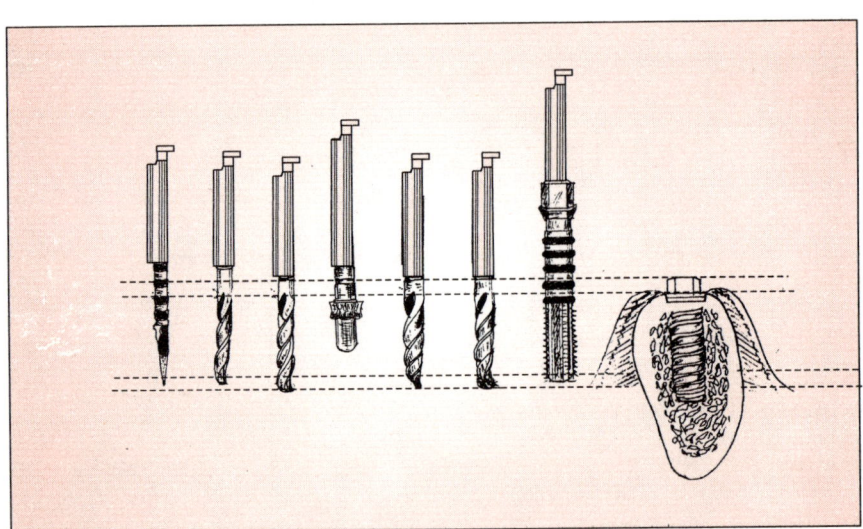

Drilling sequence for placement of implants

Further Reading

1. Albrektsson. T et al. Osseointegration, current state of the art. Dental clinics of North America. 1989; 1(4):33.

2. A prosthodontic based implant patient classification system. http://www.dental-implants.com/clsfcart.htm.

3. C.D. Kopp. Branemark osseointegration. Dental clinics of North America. 1989; 33(4).

4. Albrektsson et al. Osseointegrated dental implants. Dental clinics of North America. 1986; 30(1).

5. R. Skalak. Biomechanical considerations in osseointegrated prosthesis. J Prosth Dent. 1983; 49(6): 843-48.

6. K.B. May et al. The precision of fit at the implant prosthodontic interface. J Prosth Dent. 1997; 77: 497-502.

7. Brunski et al. Biomaterials and biomechanics of oral and maxillofacial implants. The international journal of oral and maxillofacial implants. 2000; 1(15):15-41

8. P.P. Binon. Implants and components entering the new millennium. The international Journal of oral and maxillofacial implants. 2000;11(1): 76-91.

9. R.G. Triplett et al. Oral and maxillofacial surgery advances in implant dentistry. The international journal of oral and maxillofacial implants. 2000; 15(1): 47-54.

10. Peter Floyd. Treatment planning for implant restoration's. Br. Dental J. 1999; 187(6) : 297.

12. Diagnosis and treatment planning. British Dental Journal. Vol. 187, 1999.

13. P.J. McMillan. Variables that influence the relationship between osseointegration and bone. International Journal of oral and maxillofacial implants 200, Vol.15, pg. 651-661.

14. P. Floyd. Radiographic techniques. British Dental Journal. Vol. 187, 1999.

15. Lars Linder et al. Electron microscopic analysis of the bone titanium interface. Acta Orthop Scand. 54: Pg. 45-52, 1983.

16. Gregory Parr. Titanium. The mystery metal of implant dentistry. Journal of Prosthetic Dentistry. 1985, Vol.54, No.3.

17. T. Albrektsson et al. Bone metal interface in osseointegration. Journal of Prosthetic Dentistry. 1987; Vol.57, No.5.

18. Alberktsson et al. Osseointegrated titanium implants. Acta Orthop. Scand 52, 155-170, 1981.

19. Tayler et al. Implant prosthodontics current perspective and future directions. International Journal of oral and maxillofacial implants. Vol. 1:15, No.1, 2000.

20. Goodacre et al. Clinical complications of osseointegrated implants. Journal of Prosthetic Dentistry. 1999, Vol. 81, Pg. 537-52.

21. B.B. Balkin. Implant dentistry- A historical overview. Journal of Dental Education. Vol. 52, No.12, 1988.

22. T. Nomura et al. Current evaluation of Dental implants; A review of literature Journal of long term effects of medical implants. 8(3-4). Pg. 175-192.

23. Russel R, Wang. Titanium for prosthodontic application's. A review of literature. Quintessence International Vol.27, No. 61, 1996.

24. M. Jarcho. Biomaterial aspects of calcium phosphates. Dental clinics of North America. Vol. 30, No.1, 1986.

25. Esposito M et al. Biological factors contributing to failures. Eur.J. Oral Sci. 1998, 106, Pg. 527-551.

26. H.A. Hansson et al. Structural aspects of the interface between tissue and titanium implants. Journal of Prosthetics Dentistry. 1983, Vol: 50, No.1.

MULTIPLE CHOICE QUESTIONS

1. **The bladevent implant was introduced by**
   a. Dahl
   b. Schulte and Heimke
   c. Linkow
   d. Goldberg

2. **The implant that has a special stress breaking mechanism is the**
   a. ITI implant
   b. IMZ implant
   c. Aluminium oxide implant
   d. None of the above

3. **Type II bone quality is**
   a. Mainly cortical
   b. A dense cortex and cancellous space
   c. A very thin cortex
   d. None of the above

4. **_____ are tissue engineered materials designed to mimic specific biologic processes and help optimise the healing response.**
   a. Bioinert
   b. Bioactive
   c. Biomimetic
   d. Bioactive

5. **Polymers used for dental implants are considered as**
   a. Bioinert
   b. Biotolerant
   c. Biomimetic
   d. Bioactive

6. **Grade _____ Titanium is considered acceptable for dental implants**
   a. 1
   b. 2
   c. 3
   d. 4

7. **Plasma spraying is done on titanium implants to a thickness of _____ mm.**
   a. 1-2
   b. 3-4
   c. 0.1-0.2
   d. 0.3-0.4

8. **Advantages of cement retained prosthesis are**
   a. Easy retrievability
   b. Occlusion can be developed adequately
   c. Provides access to the posterior of the mouth
   d. All of the above

9. **Zygomatic implants**
   a. Engage the zygoma
   b. Are used in severe atrophy of maxilla
   c. Available in lengths of 30-50 mm
   d. All are true

33

INTERIM DENTURES

ADVANTAGES OF INTERIM DENTURES

- They should be compulsory for patients with severe periodontal disease. When these dentures are used with proper exodontic treatment, there is a minimum of trauma, and the resultant ridge is almost unbelievably good after healing. Most patients have some malocclusion and probable changes in the temporo mandibular joints when they arrive at the stage where complete dentures are necessary. Those who have been without posterior teeth for a long time have changes in the muscles, tongue enlargement, and abnormal chewing and swallowing habits. The placement of interim dentures allow the dentist, by progressive occlusal adjustment and lining by tissue conditioners—to help the basal seat tissues, muscles and joints to reach a more nearly normal and healthy condition. If desired, the occlusal vertical dimension can be altered by grinding or adding acrylic resin to the occlusal surfaces of the teeth.

- For patients who have posterior stops in their own dentition prior to extraction, the placement of the interim dentures preserves the health of the joints, muscles, and oral physiology, instead of forcing the patient to become accustomed to the edentulous state with its abnormalities in diet, speech, and appearance.

- Interim dentures can be worn during the fabrication of new dentures and can act as spare dentures should an accident befall the new dentures at any time. They make excellent temporary substitutes and can be worn to maintain the oral tissues during rebasing or repairing of the second dentures.

- The cost of the interim denture in terms of time and services is not excessive; in fact, it can be compared with the cost of refitting immediate dentures which usually is necessary during the first year. With no substitutes, a patient faced with the loss of his dentures for a week, or even a weekend, becomes almost panic-stricken.

- One of the most important advantages is the preservation of the maximum amount of ridge bulk with the minimum of trauma and swelling. The dentist should attempt the most delicate and gentle extraction of the teeth. No flaps should be turned and no sutures should be used under ideal conditions. No deliberate trimming of bone should be undertaken. The gingival and interseptal tissue should be retained because this tissue provides good cushioning for the denture. Interim dentures should not be made for patients whose ridges are extremely bulky, where numerous and heavy undercuts exist, or where the bone is very dense and the problem is not one of periodontal disease. There is too much difficulty in doing non-traumatic surgery for these patients and the consequent swelling may be too great. On the other hand, when the teeth can be removed very gently, there is almost never any significant swelling or pain.

TECHNIQUE

An alginate (irreversible hydrocolloid) impression is made of the jaws and the remaining teeth and the excess moisture is blown off the impression. A light pink or white wax is heated in a small ladle and poured into the impressions of the teeth up to their gingival margins. As soon as the wax has hardened, the remainder of the cast is poured in stone.

The cast is separated from the impression very carefully after 20 minutes, and a second cast is immediately made in stone. This will provide two casts, one with wax and one with stone teeth, both made from the same impression. The second (the stone cast) serves two purposes: (i) it is used to form a baseplate for making jaw relation records, and (ii) it will serve as a reference cast for the second set of dentures.

A centric jaw relation record is made on wax occlusion rims with minimum pressure. The casts and the interocclusal wax record are now mounted on a plane line articulator. Artificial teeth and clasps (if needed) are placed. The waxing is completed, using a double thickness of wax at the border and thinning it out near the necks of the teeth. The gingival margins are sharply carved on the labial, buccal, palatal, and lingual surfaces so that the tooth color resin can be more easily delineated from the pink resin when the denture is packed. The pattern for the palate of the denture is formed of one thickness of wax. The wax dentures are flasked with a stone matrix over the wax. This is then dewaxed. The prosthetic teeth that may have been added are now removed from the flask. All the teeth will be made with tooth-colored acrylic resin which will be packed in the molds provided by the wax teeth and any prosthetic teeth that may have been used temporarily.

A liquid tin-foil substitute is applied to the stone mold so that it provides a good sheen on the surface of the stone.

Packing the Tooth Colors

The flasks should not be allowed to dry out, before packing the acrylic resins. The investment takes up the monomer and makes the stone stick to the cured resin. Therefore, as soon as the flask is separated and a sheen is produced by the tin-foil substitute, the tooth color resins are sprinkled into the molds for the teeth and wet with monomer. It is usually best to use a light incisal color of acrylic resin and a neutral body shade. This color is not too light for the mouths that have been badly stained, and it is not too dark for the mouths where the teeth were fairly light. It gives the dentist an opportunity to make improvements in the second set of dentures. If the interim dentures look too attractive, the patient may not be anxious to have the second set made at the proper time after healing. The tooth-colored resin is allowed to begin its jelling process.

With a small sharp knife, the bulges on the cast remaining from the teeth should be removed just down to the gingival margins, but a convex contour must be retained where the teeth are to be removed. Overtrimming of the cast should be avoided as this denture should have a very passive fit. The posterior part of the cast should be scraped from hamular notch to hamular notch to form the posterior palatal seal and to allow for the dimensional change in the cured acrylic resin.

Packing the Resin

The pink denture base resin is packed when it is still fairly soft. If it is too soft, it may stick to the stone; if it is too hard, it may displace some of the tooth-colored resin in the tooth molds. As an added precaution, the upward facing surfaces (the cervical ends) of the tooth-colored resin are flamed to form a slight crust on the resin. This is done just before the pink resin is packed. With the proper amount of resin in the mold, the flasks are placed in the press and cured for nine hours at 165°F and allowed to cool to room temperature.

The cured dentures are removed from the flasks and polished. Any undercuts on the tissue side are removed so that the dentures may go to place without binding. The borders are shortened to avoid any overextension. Adequate relief is provided in any region of impingement, such as on the labial and buccal frenula. The margins are made very thin but well rounded so that the possibility of cutting tissues is minimized.

THE SURGERY

Many patients prefer to have the operation done in the hospital under general anesthesia. This works extremely well because it offers the maximum of convenience and serenity for the patient. The patient's activity is curtailed by rest so that complications are minimized. There is usually no swelling and, immediately after release from the hospital, the patient can carry on all activities, very well. A soft but nutritious diet should be followed for a few days until the blood clots are well established.

Esthetically, no attempt is made to change the positions of the teeth. This makes the transition to dentures as little noticeable as possible. Over a period of time, gradual modifications of tooth positions can be made. The patient must be seen at frequent intervals during the healing period in order to adjust the occlusion as required, to place conditioning linings in the denture as soon as the sockets close, and to keep the patient functioning as well as possible.

Interim dentures are worn for a minimum of 12 weeks, but they can be used for as long as four or five months. By this time, however, they become quite clumsy from the linings, and sufficient alteration has occurred so the patient is quite anxious to have the second dentures constructed. Usually, when the second set of dentures is started, the mouth is in an ideal condition. The tissue covering the residual ridges has healed and is maintained in good contour and firmness by the treatment liners. The patient's vertical dimension and muscle function have been maintained, along with proper lip support and other appearance factors.

Construction of the Second Dentures

The posterior teeth are not changed very much from their positions in the interim dentures.

The second set of dentures should have minimum modifications and yet improve the appearance of the teeth and the patient.

34

COMPLICATIONS AND FAILURE OF IMPLANTS

Introduction
Complications in general
Failure in implants (Abdel Salam el Askary)
Failures in general

INTRODUCTION

Failure of implants have been related to biologic, microbiologic, biomechanical, biomaterial implant surface treatment and characteristics. Implant failure is defined as the total failure of the implant to fulfill its purpose (functional, esthetic or phonetic) because of mechanical or biologic reasons.

Classification

1. Swedish Team (Branemark et al)

a. Loss of bone anchorage
- Mucoperiosteal perforation
- Surgical trauma

b. Gingival problems
- Proliferative gingivitis
- Fistula formation

c. Mechanical complications
- Fixture fracture
- Fracture of prosthesis gold screws, abutment screws

2. UCLA Team (Beumer Moy)

a. Complication in Stage 1 surgery
- Mental nerve damage
- Penetration into sinus, nasal cavity
- Excess countersink
- Thread exposure
- Eccentric drills, taps
- Stripping of threads
- Jaw fractures
- Echymosis
- Wound dehiscence
- Facial abscess
- Suture abscess
- Loose cover screw

b. Complications in Stage II surgery
- Poor retention
- Incorrect placement (more than one cannot be used)
- Damaged hex nut on top of fixture
- Loose abutment
- Fractured abutment screw
- Early loading of prosthesis
- Poor airflow pattern with high water tight dressing
- Aspiration of instruments
- Thread exposure
- Fixture fracture
- Excess bone resorption

- Plaque or calculus formation
- Periodontal problems
- Poor selection of abutment height

c. Prosthetic complications
- Insufficient space for fully bone anchored prosthesis
- Abutment penetrating through unattached mucosa
- Jaw fracture
- Acrylic/porcelain fracture

3. Prosthodontic Complications (by Thomas D. Taylor)

- Loss of osseointegration
- Lack of presurgical planning
- Complication of bridge design
- Malalignment
- Component fracture
- Occlusal wear
- Soft tissue complications
- TMJ and muscle pain

4. Hubertus Spiekermann

a. Surgical, Intraoperative
Haemorrhage
Nerve injury
Sinus perforation
Jaw fracture
Osseous dehiscence
Osseous perforation
Damage to adjacent teeth
Lack of initial stability

Postoperative
- Mucosal perforation
- Surgical emphysema
- Implant mobility

Late postoperative
- Implant pathology
- Implant fracture
- Chronic pain
- Chronic sinusitis
- Secondary nerve damage
- Mucosal irritation

Prosthetic Complications

Unfavourable implant location
Loosening and fracture
Framework fracture
Esthetic complications
Functional complications
Implant loss

COMPLICATIONS IN GENERAL

Haemorrhage. Proper planning prevents haemorrhage. Presurgical investigation is mandatory. Copious artery or venous haemorrhage indicates vascular injury.

In the maxilla damage to the greater palatine vessels may result in excessive bleeding. The mandibular canal may deviate from its normal course and location occasionally. If instruments during the preparation for the implant placement contact the nerve the patient will experience pain even under anesthesia.

The best way to avoid lingual nerve damage is to place a broad elevator between the lingual cortical plate of the mandible and mucoperiosteal flap.

Opening into Sinuses. The posterior maxilla is the most challenging area to restore with implants. A perforation into a sinus may be detected by asking the patient to hold the nose and blow. This will locate the area of perforation. Appropriate radiographs should be taken and shorter implants should be used.

Jaw Fracture. This is relatively rare. Nevertheless this danger exists especially when multiple implants are placed and when the bone is mechanically weakened. Treatment is reduction and stabilization with splints.

When placing endosseous implants in the severely resorbed mandible several precautions must be taken to avoid fractures. The inferior border of the mandible should be engaged without perforation. The shortest possible implants should be used and spaced so that there is atleast 3 mm of space between the implants and 2 mm between buccal and lingual cortical plates. When inserting implants, increased tightening must be avoided.

Dehiscence and Perforation

As much bone as possible should be preserved. Bony dehiscence exceeding 3 mm will affect long-term success. Perforation is due to lack of proper axis for placement of implant. It can be treated by shorter implants and by GBR techniques.

Damage to Adjacent Teeth

Damage to adjacent teeth occurs commonly with single tooth implants due to lack of proper axis of placement. The damaged tooth should be endodontically treated. Proper radiographic evaluation with stents in place should be done. The distance of at least 1 mm should be maintained between implants and the periodontal ligament of adjacent tooth.

Lack of Initial Stability

If initial stability is not achieved, the implant should be removed, bone grafting procedures or implants of wider diameter, longer length should be selected after proper assessment.

Periimplant Pathology

Periimplant pathology is because of poor oral hygiene, lack of use of healing caps, presence of dead spaces under the superstructure and lack of attached mucosa. These problems are more with implant over dentures. The keratinised mucosa should be preserved as much as possible. Inflammatory and infected tissues should be removed. Implant components should be disinfected by chlorhexidine solution.

Implant Fracture

Implant fracture can occur due to inadequately aligned bridges or by use of less number of implants than necessary.

Sinusitis and Pain

Localised dull feeling of pressure along with diffuse headache and radiopacity of maxillary sinuses. Treatment consists of antibiotic regimen and removal of implant.

Esthetic Complications[22]

Esthetic complications are seen mainly in the maxilla, mostly due to labial inclination of implants or subsequent gingival recession. Faulty implant inclination can be compensated by angulated abutments. Gingival recession often occurs if the facial plate of bone is lost or if it is extremely thin. It may also result from improper oral hygiene as well as from high frenal attachments in case of inadequate attached gingiva. Treatment consists of surgical placement of free gingival grafts and flaps.

Functional Complications

Functional complications are usually rare and occur after placement of implant super-structure. Phonetic problems occur when there is a large space between the mucosa and the base of the prosthesis. This can be solved by the use of shorter posts or placement of gingival epithesis.

FAILURE IN IMPLANTS
(ABDEL SALAM EL ASKARY)

Classification

1. According to Etiology

- Host factors-history
- Medical status
- Habits
- Parafunctional habits
- Oral status
- Irradiation therapy

Surgical Placement
- Off axis placement
- Lack of initial stabilization

- Impaired healing and infection
- Overheating the bone and excess pressure
- Minimal space between implants
- Implants in immature bone
- Implants in pathologic sites
- Contamination of implant

Implant Selection
- Improper implant types
- Length of implant
- Width of implant
- Number of implants
- Improper implant design
- Restorative problems

2. According to Timing of Failure

- Stage I surgery
- Stage II surgery
- After restoration

3. Origin of Infection

Peri implantitis (infective process, bacterial) Retrograde perimplantitis (traumatic occlusion) excess pressure, premature loading

4. Condition of Failure

- Clinical
- Radiographic

5. Responsible Personnel (prosthodontist, surgeon, technician, hygienist)

6. Failure Mode

- Lack of osseointegration
- Unacceptable esthetics
- Functional problems
- Psychological problems

7. Supporting Tissue Type

- Soft tissue problems
- Bone loss

FAILURES IN GENERAL

Medical Status

Bone disorders are contraindications for implant treatment. Uncontrolled diabetes mellitus impairs healing. The liability of infection is probably caused by thinning and fragility of the blood vessel.

Habits

Long-term smoking predisposes to poor quality of healing. Parafunctional habits such as bruxism and clenching create mechanical and biologic problems related to prosthetic components, materials and osseointegration.

Oral and Periodontal Status

Plaque is main factor for implant failure. Spontaneous loss of permucosal seal leads to increased accumulation of spirochaetes that release proteolytic enzymes dissolving fibrin, trypsin like enzymes disrupting cell adhesion and metabolic end products that are cytotoxic to gingival tissues. Periodic recall at 3 months interval is necessary. Tissue debridement should be performed by means of plastic curettes and plastic tips.

Transmission of periodontopathogenic organisms from periodontal sites to implant sites is possible. Therefore the need for a clinical protocol, including the elimination of periodontal disease in prospective implant patients is mandatory.

Radiation therapy: Irradiation for the treatment of oral cancer does not seem to reduce the survival rate of implants as compared with those placed in the non-irradiated site. If necessary hyperbaric oxygen treatment has to be done.

Off Axis Placement[25]

Improper implant placement can result in a framework design that compromises esthetics and proper distribution of the forces onto the implants. During implant placement problems may occur due to alveolar resorption. The solution for this is to do grafting procedures at that site. Prerestoring the implant site by grafting to avoid offset loading is recommended. Endosseous root from implants distribute occlusal load ideally in an axial direction, but if the occlusal load is in a lateral direction, damaging stresses are generated.

Based on finite element analysis increased stress concentration have been observed for implants not placed perpendicularly in relation to applied forces.

Healing and Infection

Improper flap design would lead to an early infection at implant site. Other systemic conditions also play a role in healing. Hunt stated that good surgical procedure, flap design, blood supply, visibility, access and the primary closure are the factors that should be regarded in implant placement. Overheating of bone, and excessive pressure should be avoided.

Temperature control during osteotomy preparation is needed when osseous drilling is done. Bone cell death occurs at a temperature of 47°C and higher when drilling is performed for 1 minute. Excessive pressures on the implant will lead to bone loss and cell necrosis. Death of bone cells, causes formation of a connective tissue interface between the implant and viable bone thus leading to loss of integration.

Speed recommended that be no more than 2,000 rpm with a graded series of drill sizes is to be used.

Placement

A space of 4 to 7 mm between neighbouring implants is required to allow for sufficient biologic space.

Implantation at Specific Sites

One of the main causes of implant failure is the immediate loading of the implant supported prosthesis. The problem with placing implants in grafted bone is that if the implant is loaded before the surrounding bone matures from woven into lamellar bone, then the failure incidence is much higher because of the nature of woven bone. Woven bone is the first and fastest to form around the implant interface. It is partly mineralized and demonstrates an unorganized structure unable to withstand full scale stresses. Lamellar bone is ideal for implant prosthesis support.

Implants can also fail if they are placed in infected socket or existing pathologic lesion.

During the initial stage of osseointegration the implant is particularly vulnerable to infection from an adjacent endodontic lesion. The implant may have the ability to withstand any bacterial challenge during the first stage of osseointegration. An endodontic lesion can travel through marrow spaces and contaminate the adjacent implant fixture.

Placement into a socket with a chronic lesion does not necessarily result in failure if certain precautions are taken. Removal of the causative agent with debridement, use of antibiotics, eliminates the chances of bacterial contamination and subsequent failure.

Contamination

Contamination of the head of an implant may alter the surface chemistry. Autoclaving a contaminated implant will bake the bacteria onto the implant surface, so that when the implant is placed in the body it becomes almost impossible for phagocytic cells to clear. This prevents close adaptation with bone. The implant should be cleaned by a radio frequency glow discharge unit or plasma cleaner.

Implant Selection

Qualitative and quantitative consideration of bone must be evaluated before placing the implant. Type I and Type II situations could use titanium without HA coating. HA coated implants are preferred in Type III and Type IV bone. HA coated implants have 66.3% of their surface in contact with bone whereas grit blasted Ti implants have only 50.2% their surface in contact with bone.

On comparison between screw and cylindrical non-coated Ti implants, it was found that the screw design had increased surface contact with the same overall implant length, whereas HA implant had a higher percentage of bone along a length than the Ti implant.

The titanium screw type implant is recommended in the anterior mandible when depth exceeds 12 mm, and the cortical layer was thick and dense. The HA-coated screw is recommended in the anterior maxilla and the posterior mandible where the depth exceeds 10 mm and when the cortical layer was thinner. HA-coated cylinder is recommended in the posterior maxilla when the cortical layer is very thin with (Type 4 or D4) bone.

The unusual length of the implant is indicated by the amount of available bone height. The success rate is proportional to implant length and quantity and quality of available bone. The rate of failure can be expected to rise proportionately as the depth of bone diminishes to less than 10 mm. Placement of a short implant where bone permits longer implant would result in higher stress concentration leading to subsequent failure of the implant.

Crown implant body ratio. This affects the appearance of the final prosthesis along with the amount of moment of force on the implant and the crestal surrounding bone. Greater the crown implant ratio, greater will be the amount of force, with any lateral force.

Maximum implant length must be used for the greatest stability of the overlying prosthesis. It has been recommended that 1 mm of bone surrounding the fixture labially and lingually is mandatory for the long term success. Diameter of the implant should be properly selected in the preoperative phase, according to available bone width, esthetic requirement, stress analysis, neighbouring natural teeth and the arch space available. It is advisable to use a large diameter implant that improves the ability of fixed restoration to withstand forces. Maximum osseous surface area and bone density are requirements for long-term resistance and occlusal overload.

Hollow implants affect the success rate negatively more than the solid cylinders because of the dead space that is susceptible to infection.

Problems in Restoration

Excessive cantilevering, is a major problem while restoring the completely edentulous arch. It places offset loads to implant abutments and results in greater tensile and shear forces on cement or screw fixation. Problems encountered are fracture of prosthesis, loss of osseointegration and bone fracture. They can be in mesial or distal orientation opposed by natural teeth. Fixed bridge or a complete denture with occlusal forces acting on the cantilever implant become a fulcrum and is subjected to axial, rotational and torsional forces. Implants are also used as pier abutments.

The breakdown of supporting tissues is extremely rapid because the dental implant will take most the loads as a result of differences in mean axial displacement. Treatment consists of the use of a non-rigid connector between pontics.

Achieving a passive fit during prosthesis insertion is considered to be one of the keys for the success of dental implants. A passive fit reduces long-term stresses on the superstructure, implant components and bone adjacent to the implants. Absence of passive fit is manifested by pain, discomfort, loosening or fracture of the implant.

Dimensional changes in a ceramometal restoration during firing cycles, improper impression techniques, improper spaces and improper metal for casting are responsible for misfit. There is a direct correlation between implant abutment, rotational misfit and screw joint failure, probably because of the micromovement between implant components. So, it is recommended that the fit of dental implant components be checked before the impression is made by clinical and radiographic examination that could lead to such complications.

Proper Prosthetic Design

The ideal implant treatment plan is based on the patient's needs, desires and financial commitment. Broad knowledge, proper patient selection, better psychological understanding, proper presurgical prosthetic planning and a very good biomechanical background are the main components for achieving a good prosthetic design.

Premature Loading

One of the main reasons for fracture is premature loading. Branemark stated that strict protocol required a stress-free healing period of 3 to 6 months for osseointegration to occur. Micromovements of more than 100 micrometer should be avoided.

Threaded implants can be placed immediately to support a provisional fixed prosthesis in edentulous arches during the 4-6 month healing period in both arches. A delayed loading protocol remains the treatment of choice, immediate loading for multiple implants splinted across the arch may prove to be a conditional successful therapy.

Timing of Failure

Failure during Stage I is less likely. Causes may include placing the implants in an infected socket, pathological lesion, immature bone, previously irradiated bone, lack of biocompatibility, surgical trauma and lack of primary stability.

It can fail in Stage II surgery during healing, abutment placement or before prostheses placement.

According to Condition of Failure

Mellert proposed a classification of failure. This involves ailing, falling, and failed implants. Ailing implants are those showing radiographic bone loss without any inflammatory signs or mobility, failing ones are those characterized by progressive bone loss, signs of inflammation and no mobility. These are reversible situations when the etiologic factor is controlled. Failed ones are those with progressive bone loss with clinical mobility and that are not functioning as intended. They are encapsulated by fibrous capsule and radiographic evidence shows radioluency around them.

Surviving is a term applied to implants that are still in function but have not been tested against success criteria. It is an intermediate position between successful and failing implants.

Personnel Responsible

Dental surgeon is responsible for patient selection and is also responsible for placement of fixture, prosthodontic plan, evaluation of available bone, patient's health history, and surgical complication that arises during any phase of treatment.

Prosthodontist is responsible for planning, loading biomechanics, selection of proper abutments, occlusion and prosthetic complications.

Periodontist is responsible for proper oral hygiene care, evaluation of soft and hard tissues, maintenance care.

Hygienist is responsible for recording and monitoring implant status (bleeding and pocket index) and oral hygiene, lab technician contributes to longterm success of dental implant therapy both esthetically and functionally.

Patient is responsible for keeping the implants surviving by following oral hygiene instructions, reporting any discomfort pain, odour or taste.

Failure Mode

Esthetics. An implant with successful osseointegration and biointegration can still be a failure if the facial prosthesis does not provide optimal required esthetics. Esthetics outcome is affected by implant placement, soft tissue management, bone grafting considerations and prosthetic considerations.

Functional. Proper function of implants is dependent on two main types of factors: anchorage-related factors compromise osseointegration and marginal bone height. Prosthetic related factors result mainly from improper prosthetic design. Improper occlusal scheme will result in improper load distribution, improperly restored vertical dimension will cause temporomandibular joint disorders and inability to chew and speak.

Supporting Tissue Type

Absence of keratinised soft tissue and implant failure are related. Marginal periabutment tissues should constitute a functional barrier between the oral environment and lost bone by thermal and mechanical trauma.

Bone loss. Bone loss occurs during the healing period and after abutment connection. Bone loss in the mandible is higher during healing period and in maxilla it is after abutment connection. The difference is due to higher vascularity of maxilla which allows faster remodelling during the healing period and the compact nature of mandible which withstands applied torsional forces much better.

Factors contributing are trauma, improper stress distribution, occlusal trauma, ridge resorption, gingivitis.

Prognostic Factors for Success with Implants

- Implants featuring an external hex connection with abutment are prone to screw loosening.

- Material-commercially pure titanium is better than blasted, etched surfaces because of electrochemical events at the tissue implant interface, another consequence is release of metallic species into tissue fluids. These may interfere with the differentiation of osteoblasts or osteoclasts.
- Interfacial zone containing non-collagenous bone native to prosthesis such as bone sialoprotein (BSP). The absence or relative paucity of serum proteins such as albumin indicates osteoclastic action at the interface.
- Physiochemical method, surface energy, surface charge, surface apposition are physical, chemical characteristics that have been altered with the aim of optimising the implant interface. Increased surface energy has not been shown to increase bone implant interfacial strengths.

Morphogenic

- Porous coatings were developed with the rationale that because of mechanical interactions, bone ingrowth would increase formation and stability. Research revealed that relatively a small portion of the available bone volume is filled with bone. Surfaces with grooves can induce contact guidances where the direction of cell movement is affected by the morphology of the substrate. The highest bone interface was formed with sandblasted large gritted, acid attack with (HCL/HNO_3) and HA flame spraying.
- *Biochemical.* Understanding the biology and biochemistry of cellular function and differentiation.

Ideally design goals should create an implant interface so that anticipated loading does not damage the implant or surrounding tissue when the implant is loaded. Bone implant interface can be damaged if stress strain are not controlled.

MULTIPLE CHOICE QUESTIONS

1. Speed recommended for drilling should be no more than _____
   a. 2,000 rpm   b. 4,000 rpm
   c. 10,000 rpm   d. 500 rpm

2. A space of _____ mm is required between neighbouring implants
   a. 2-3   b. 4-7
   c. 10 mm   d. 1-2 mm

35

SEQUELAE TO COMPLETE DENTURE USE

Introduction
Direct sequelae, Indirect sequelae

INTRODUCTION

The response of human skin to everyday wear and tear is to become keratinised and tough. The oral mucosa does not behave in a similar manner. If the tolerance of the mucosa is low and exceeded, injury and inflammation will result and the denture cannot be worn. If the tolerance of the tissue is high, a fibrous response may be elicited (flabby, hyperplastic tissue). The wearing of complete dentures can result in direct and indirect sequelae.

Direct sequelae these include: (i) burning mouth syndrome, (ii) denture stomatitis, (iii) soft tissue hyperplasia, (iv) mucosal reactions, (v) gagging, and (vi) residual ridge resorption.

Indirect Sequelae these include:(i) disturbances in speech, (ii) poor chewing ability, (iii) atrophy of masticatory muscles, and (iv) nutritional disturbances.

Mucosal Reaction

Mucosal reaction may result from:
1. Mechanical irritation of the dentures
2. Accumulation of microbial plaque on the dentures
3. Toxic reaction to the constituents of the denture material.

Denture Stomatitis

This is also referred to as denture sore mouth, denture induced stomatitis. It is defined as the chronic inflammation of the denture bearing mucosa. It is seen in 50% of complete denture wearers.

Classification (by Newton)

Type I   A localized simple inflammation or pin-point hyperemia

Type II   An erythematous or generalised type presenting a more diffuse erythema involving part of the denture-bearing mucosa

Type III A granular type involving most of the denture bearing area, e.g. Inflammatory papillary hyperplasia.

Aetiology

- Trauma from ill-fitting denture
- Nocturnal denture wear
- Allergic response to denture material
- Infection with *Candida albicans*
- Poor oral hygiene.

It may be asymptomatic and is seen more in the maxilla than mandible.

Infection with *Candida albicans*

Strains of *Candida* are frequently involved in denture stomatitis. *Candida*-associated denture stomatitis is associated with-cheilitis. The diagnosis for *Candida* associated denture stomatitis is confirmed by the finding of mycelia or pseudohyphae in a direct smear or by isolation of *Candida* species in high numbers. The factors predisposing to this condition include systemic factors like old age and diabetes mellitus, and local factors like the presence of dentures in the mouth and xerostomia.

Management

Improving oral and denture hygiene
1. Tissue rest. This can be obtained by: (i) removal of dentures, and (ii) use of tissue conditioners
2. Occlusal adjustment
3. Technical improvement of existing denture.

Use of Antifungal Therapy

The presence of the condition is first confirmed by a palatal smear. Once confirmed, the condition is managed by antifungal drugs like nystatin. The denture may be kept in a chelating agent or a mixture of chlorhexidine and enzymes.

Surgical Excision

1. Electrosurgery
2. Cryosurgery

Preventive Measures

1. Patients should avoid wearing dentures day and night
2. Reduce denture trauma (by regular recall appointments)
3. Dentures should be kept clean

4. Proper oral hygiene should be maintained.

The patient should be instructed to remove the dentures (after meal) and to scrub it vigorously with soap before reinserting it. The mucosa in contact with the denture should be kept clean and massaged with a soft brush.

Soft Tissue Hyperplasia

Soft tissue hyperplasia is a chronic sequelae to the wearing of complete dentures. This may be seen in tissue around the borders of the denture.

Etiology

1. Changes in the alveolar socket after extraction
2. Trauma from denture wearing
3. Gradual residual ridge reduction
4. Habits and duration of wear
5. Change in soft tissue profile and TMJ function
6. Changes in relative proportion of the jaws
7. Excessive force on limited segments of the arch because of the lack of balancing contacts in lateral excursions. The treatment consists of surgical excision in severe cases.

Epulis Fissuratum

Epulis fissuratum is hyperplasia (in the form of fibrous growth) occurring around the borders of dentures. It is frequently seen at the junction of free and attached mucosa.

Etiology

Epulis fissuratum results from chronic irritation from ill-fitting dentures or over extended borders. As the residual ridges resorb, even the most well-fitting denture may develop over-extension.

Treatment

1. Tissue rest
   - Keep the denture out
   - Reduction of the offending flange
   - Massage of the damaged site.

2. Surgical excision

After surgical excision, the old dentures is relined and worn. Adequate epithelialization is obtained in 6-8 weeks.

Angular Cheilitis (perleche)

Angular cheilitis may be seen with denture stomatitis.

It can also occur due to: (i) reduced vertical dimension, and (ii) riboflavin and thiamin deficiency.

The management includes fabrication of new dentures and antifungal therapy.

Traumatic Ulcers

Traumatic ulcers develop frequently within 1-2 days after placement of new dentures. The ulcers are small, painful, covered by a grey necrotic membrane and surrounded by an inflammatory halo.

Etiology

- Overextended dentures border
- Unbalanced occlusion
  The sore spot may heal in a few days.

Burning Mouth Syndrome

Burning mouth syndrome is characterised by a burning sensation in one or more oral structures in contact with dentures.

Symptoms

1. Symptoms have a gradual onset.
2. Pain is present, this may increase as the day progresses.
3. Dry mouth and altered taste sensation.
4. Aggravating factors include tension, fatigue, hot foods.
5. Pain is reduced by sleep, distraction, eating.

Etiology

Causes may be:
1. *Local*
   - Mechanical irritation
   - Allergy
   - Infection.
2. *Systemic*
   - Diabetes
   - Iron deficiency anemia
   - Vitamin deficiency.
3. *Psychogenic*
   - Depression
   - Anxiety
   - Psychosocial stressors.

Management

1. Refer to physician for systemic analysis
2. High protein diet
3. Vitamin supplement
4. Avoiding of local irritants.

36

TOOTH SUPPORTED COMPLETE DENTURES

Definition
Synonyms
Types

DEFINITION

A removable complete denture that covers and rests on the one or more remaining natural teeth, the roots of natural teeth and/or dental implants, a prosthesis that covers and is partially supported by natural teeth, natural tooth roots and/or dental implants.

SYNONYMS

Overlay dentures, overlay prosthesis, super-imposed prosthesis.

Preventive prosthodontics emphasises the importance of any procedure that can delay or eliminate future prosthodontic problems. The over denture is a logical treatment alternative in preventive prosthodontics. It has been found that the remaining natural teeth provide directional sensitivity, tackle sensitivity to load, dimensional discrimination in addition to support.

Advantages

1. It is an equally effective or superior method of treatment. It is specially effective in patients with congenital defects such as oligodontia, microdontia, cleft palate and also in Class III patients.
2. *Simplicity of construction.* The procedures used are similar to that of conventional dentures. The retained roots in addition will help in tooth placement, in maintaining vertical dimension and will provide stability to the record bases during maxillo-mandibular relations.
3. *Ease of maintenance.* Repair, refitting and alterations can be easily accomplished.
4. Stability and retention are better compared to conventional dentures.
5. Esthetically pleasing.
6. Cost is reasonable.
7. The palate can be kept open, when both anterior and posterior teeth are present to support and retain over dentures. The palate can be kept roofless.
8. Maxillomandibular records can be easily recorded. When teeth are retained for an immediate overdenture, the vertical dimension of occlusion can be maintained accurately. The roots will also help in improving the stability of record bases.
9. Occlusion can be properly developed.
10. Excellent patient acceptance. Patient acceptance can be improved.

11. ***Ease of cleaning.*** The denture can be removed and so is easier to clean than a fixed prosthesis. The abutments retaining the denture can also be cleaned.
12. ***Conversion to complete denture.*** When the retained teeth or roots are lost, the over denture can be relined or rebased and converted to a complete denture.
13. ***Reversibility.*** Occasionally, overdentures are placed over a complete natural dentition. The teeth may require minimal adjustment. Later the over denture, if required, can be removed and the patient's teeth are brought back to their original status.
14. ***Less trauma to supporting tissues.*** The use of an overdenture will reduce residual ridge resorption and will reduce soft tissue trauma.
15. ***Stabilisation of existing structures.*** Bone resorption will be minimal under existing roots. As a result of this, vertical dimension and soft tissue support are maintained.
16. Minimal adjustments are required.

Disadvantages

1. It is more expensive than conventional complete dentures. This is because orthodontic treatment may be required followed by copings.
2. It is bulkier and heavier compared to conventional dentures.
3. Some patients may not accept removable prosthesis psychologically.
4. Caries and periodontal disease can develop in the retained teeth/roots.

Indications

1. Presence of few natural teeth.
2. In situations where the anatomy of the denture bearing area is unfavorable, e.g. high palatal vault.
3. In situations where better retention is required.
4. When teeth are of questionable value as conventional abutments because of unfa-vourable crown root ratio, they can be treated endodontically and clinical crown can be reduced.
5. To improve support and stability.
6. To improve function and esthetics.

Contraindications

1. An overdenture is contraindicated when another method promises superior results.
2. In patients who cannot tolerate a removable partial denture psychologically.
3. When oral hygiene and motivation to improve oral hygiene are poor.

Types of Overdentures

Transitional Overdentures (Interim Overdenture). It is made from the existing removable partial denture, the patient's own teeth or both.

Advantages

1. Converting an existing prosthesis into an overdentures is less costly.
2. Patient's previous experience with the prosthesis permits a smooth transition to the new prosthesis.

Disadvantage

1. Border extension, esthetics, occlusion, support, stability are inadequate.
2. Use of autopolymerising resin results in a prosthesis that is weak.

Immediate Overdenture. It is an overdenture fabricated for insertion immediately after the removal of natural teeth. It may be used as an interim prosthesis.

Advantages

1. Increased support and stability.
2. Preserve natural ridges by retention of natural teeth.
3. Are favourably accepted by the patient.
4. Function is not interfered with.

5. Construction technique is simple.
6. When used as an interim prosthesis, it allows the dentist the opportunity to evaluate the response of the abutments and supporting tissues to the overdenture.
7. To observe the effect of oral hygiene measures.

Disadvantages

1. Not as strong as conventional dentures.
2. Remote overdentures.

It is fabricated for insertion at some time remote from the removal of hopeless natural teeth. It is placed over well-healed ridges.

37

CLINICAL PROBLEMS AND SOLUTIONS IN COMPLETE DENTURES

Failures in complete dentures

FAILURES IN COMPLETE DENTURES

Problems may arise subsequent to the insertion of complete dentures. These may be transient (may be disregarded by the patient) or serious enough resulting in the patient being unable to tolerate the denture.

There are four major causes for this.
1. Adverse intraoral anatomic factors, e.g. atrophic mucosa[1]
2. Clinical factors, e.g. poor denture stability
3. Technical factors, e.g. failure to preserve the peripheral roll in a master cast.
4. Patient adaptational factors.

The major problems seen in complete dentures are discomfort associated with the dentures, looseness of dentures, and poor adaptation (Tables 37.1 and 37.2).

Table 37.1. Factors resulting in discomfort associated with dentures

Problem	Cause
Related to the impression surface	
Discrete painful areas	Pearls or sharp ridges of acrylic on the fitting surface. These may be located with a dry finger or dry cotton wool and rounded
Pain on insertion and removal	Denture not relieved in undercut regions. These may be located by disclosing material and reduced (excessive removal should be avoided as it can affect retention)
Areas painful to pressure. mucosa relieved. If	These may result from faulty impressions, warpage of denture, base, residual, pathology, lack of relief for active frena, displaceable (over tori). These are located with disclosing material and severe, a remake may be required
Generalised pain over denture bearing area	These may be due to an under extended denture base or inadequate free way space. These can be managed by extending the denture to optimal denture bearing area. If freeway space is inadequate, a remake will be required
Overextension of the lingual flange (denture lifts on tongue protrusion, painful to swallow)	Over extended, impression. These can be detected using disclosing material and relieved

413

Problem	Related to the impression surface Cause
Lack of relief for frena or muscle attachments	Peripheral over extension, relieve with the aid of disclosing material
Pinching of tissue between denture base and tuberosity	Post dam is too deep, management is similar to above

Related to occlusal surface

Problem	Cause
Pain on eating. (Occlusal imbalance is present but no support problems)	Anterior or posterior prematurity, incisal locking or lack of balanced articulation. The occlusion is adjusted by selective grinding. If the error is severe, a remount with new interocclusal records is needed
Pain lingual to the lower anterior ridge	This may be due to protrusive slide from centric occlusion to centric relation. The deflective inclines of posterior teeth are marked with articulating paper and if the slide exceeds half the cusp width, teeth are reset
Pain or inflammation on the labial aspect of lower ridge	This may be due to a lack of incisal over jet causing incisal locking. This may be managed by reducing the incisal vertical overlap or by resetting the incisors
Pain about the periphery of dentures along with pain in masseter and temporalis muscles	Vertical dimension of occlusion may be more than the patient can tolerate. If the vertical dimension excess is less than 15 mm, the freeway space can be obtained by grinding teeth. If the vertical dimension excess is greater than 1.5 mm, teeth will have to be reset
Cheek biting	The functional width of the sulcus mass not restored. This should be restored
Lip biting	Poor lip support or inadequate anterior horizontal overlap.
Tongue biting	Lack of lingual overjet. This is managed by 1. Removing lower lingual cusps 2. Resetting teeth
Related to polished surfaces. Pain at the posterior aspect of the denture on opening	Distobuccal flange of the denture may be too thick impinging on the coronoid process. Disclosing material is used to identify the area and then relieved

Miscellaneous factors causing discomfort

Problem	Cause
Burning sensation over upper denture supporting tissues	Burning mouth syndrome management 1. Correction of denture faults 2. Multivitamin advice 3. Refer to a consultant
Glossodynia	Vitamin B_{12} or folate deficiency. Refer for medical advice
Tongue thrusting or empty chewing	Neurological or psychological occlusal adjustment or occlusal pivots may be needed
Herpetiform ulcers	Due to herpes simplex or herpes zoster history and distribution of lesions should be considered. Antiviral therapy may be required
Frictional lesions related to dentures, mucosa, may adhere to probing finger, dry mouth	Xerostomia. In conditions where some saliva is present, citrus lozenges may be given. In the absence of saliva, artificial saliva is given
Painful clicking sound in TMJ on opening or closing	TMJ disfunction syndrome. This may be due to: (1) Sudden change in VDO (2) Psychological
Allergy to denture material	This may be due to a higher residual content of monomer. A rebasing using heat cured acrylic or use of polycarbonate resin should be considered

Problem	Cause
Factors causing looseness to dentures	
Lack of peripheral seal	Border under extended in width and depth. Modelling compound is added to the relevant border, moulded, and then replaced by acrylic resin
Inelasticity of cheek tissues	Due to aging or diseases like scleroderma and submucus fibrosis. Denture borders are moulded incrementally so as to slightly underextend denture periphery in width and depth
Air beneath impression surface; denture rocking	Due to deficient impression, damaged cast, warped denture, residual ridge resorption, undercut ridge, excessive relief chamber, managed as required
Xerostomia	Causes: 1. Medication 2. Irradiation of head and neck region 3. Salivary gland disease use artificial saliva or citrus lozenges
Neuromuscular control	Basic shape of the denture may be incorrect. Denture faults should be corrected
Overextended lower denture borders causing slow rise of the lower denture, or inflammation ulceration at sulcal tissue	Thickened flanges. These are managed by slightly underextending the denture flange and by moulding with modelling compound
Deep posterior palatal seal causing pain or ulceration	This can be reduced, denture should be worn sparingly till inflammation clears
Overextension in width	Design error reduce overextension
Denture not in optimal space	1. Molars on lower denture lingual to the ridge 2. Optimum triangular shape of dentures absent 3. Posterior occlusal table too broad, causing tongue trapping 4. Thick lingual flanges causing lifting

Table 37.2. Failure due to poor adaptation to denture

Symptoms	Cause	Treatment
Noise on eating/ speaking may be apparent on first insertion	May be lack of skill with new dentures, excessive OVD, occlusal interference, loose dentures, or poor perception of patient to denture wearing	Reassurance and persistence recommended
Eating difficulties Dentures move over supporting tissues	Unstable dentures	Construct dentures to maximize retention and minimize displacing forces
'Blunt teeth'	Broad posterior occlusal surfaces which replaced narrow teeth on previous denture. Non-anatomical type teeth used where cusped teeth previously used	Routine use of narrow tooth moulds recommended
Jaws close too far	Lack of OVD so that mandibular elevator muscles cannot work efficiently	May increase up to 1.5 mm from occlusal plane by grinding but if more is required, remake denture.
Speech problems	Cause may not be obvious. May be unfamiliarity-check	Check for vertical dimension accuracy, and that vertical incisor overlap not excessive. Palatal

Symptoms	Cause	Treatment
		contour should not allow excessive tongue contact or air leakage assess using disclosing paste over denture palate while sound is made
Gagging	May be loose dentures, thick distal border of upper denture, lingual placement of upper, posterior teeth or low occlusal plane causing contact with dorsal aspect of tongue	Construct denture to maximise retention and minimise displacing forces. Psychological assessment if indicated
Appearance complaints may arise from patient or relatives. Common complaints include, shade of teeth too light or dark; mould too big/small; arrangement too even or irregular or lacking diastema	Patient failed to comment at trial stage, or has subsequently been swayed by family or friends	Accurate assessment of patient's aesthetic requirements
Too much visibility of teeth	Level of occlusal plane[2] unacceptable, teeth placed on upper anterior ridge and no/poor lip support	Accurate prescription to laboratory via optimally adjusted occlusal rim
Creases at corners of mouth	Labial fullness and anterior tooth position may be inaccurate. OVD may be inadequate.	Adjust tooth position as appropriate. If OVD is a problem, re-register jaw relations
Colour of denture base material 'unnatural'	Patient's skin colour not taken into account in determining colour of base material	Remake using suitable base material

Further Reading

1. J.J. Sharry. Denture failures related to occlusion. Dental Clinics of North America. Vol. 16, No.1, 1972.

2. C.H. Heartwell. Complete denture failures. Dental Clinics of North America. Vol: 16, No.1, 1972.

MULTIPLE CHOICE QUESTIONS

1. **Pain while swallowing after insertion of the mandibular denture may be due to**
   a. Overextended buccal flange
   b. Overextended distolingual flange
   c. Overextended distal flange
   d. Under extended distolingual flange

2. **A frequent cause for dislodgement of the mandibular denture is**
   a. Use of non-anatomic teeth
   b. U-shaped residual ridge
   c. Use of the mucocompressive impression technique
   d. Occlusal disharmony

38

PHARMACOTHERAPEUTICS IN PROSTHODONTICS

Sialagogues
Antisialogogues
Analgesics
Antibiotics
Antianxiety agents
Centrally acting muscle relaxants

SIALAGOGUES

Xerostomia may result from disease states (Sjogren's syndrome, rheumatoid arthritis diabetes insipidus, pernicious anemia), from radiation, as a side effect of a wide variety of drugs, or from natural aging. The condition can lead to complications that reduce denture wearing time and cause difficulty in swallowing and speaking, loss of taste, stomatitis, burning tongue, rampant caries, and periodontal disease. Edentulous patient may experience problems with dentures and an increased incidence of intraoral infection with *Candida albicans*.

The obvious treatment rationale for xerostomia is to activate muscarinic cholinergic receptors of the parasympathetic nervous system to increase salivary flow. Pilocarpine, a naturally occurring cholinergic agonist, produces a short-duration (3 hour) increases in salivary flow without accompanying side effects. Use of pilocarpine has been limited to patients with Sjogren's syndrome and rad-

iation. It is not used in patients with drug-induced xerostoma. Pilocarpine commonly causes mild to moderate sweating. It should not be used in patients with uncontrolled asthma. Some relief of antidepressant drug-induced xerostomia has been reported with the use of citric acid. Anethole-trithione and bromhexine are direct-acting cholinergic agonist with a degree of salivary gland selectivity.

Saliva Substitutes

Most contain either carboxymethylcellulose or hydroxyethylcellulose as lubricant and a variety of artificial sweeteners, preservatives, and chloride or fluoride salts.

All commercially available preparations have a limited duration of action, making frequent application necessary. Additionally, short-term relief is obtained for some, but not all patients, and compliance is a major problem.

Milk has many properties that make it a useful saliva substitute.

ANTISIALOGOGUES

Agents used to decrease salivary secretion are cholinergic antagonists and thus block the same receptors that are activated by the cholinergic

417

agonists (sialagogues). Atropine and scopolamine are naturally occurring alkaloids contained in a tincture made from the leaf of Atropa belladonna. Both methantheline and propantheline are synthetic atropine derivatives that have similar pharmacologic characteristics but propantheline is more potent. For the desired reduction in salivary flow, the oral administration of atropine, scopolamine, or methantheline and propantheline should precede the clinical procedure by 1 to 2 hours one-half to 1 hour, or one-half hour, respectively.

Side effect of the antisialogogues are rare in dentistry because salivary glands are quite responsive to the blocking action of the agents, and the desired effect is obtained at low doses. An increased incidence of side effects could be expected in the geriatric patient population, who may already have xerostomia. Anticholinergic drugs are contraindicated in patients with glaucoma, prostatic hypertrophy, severe gastrointestinal atophy and myasthenia gravis. Drugs such as tricyclic antidepressants and antihistamines which have anticholinergic activity can have an additive effect. Centrally acting anticholinergic drugs used to treat Parkinson's disease, would interact with antisialogogues. Also, anticholinergic drugs, used to treat Parkinson's disease antagonize the desired therapeutic effect of blockers such as propranolol.

Atropine is the prototype anticholinergic drug. A reduction in salivary flow may be expected for 4 to 6 hours after oral administration. It differs from scopolamine in that at high doses it causes CNS stimulation, whereas scopolamine causes sedation.

Methantheline and propantheline are pharmacologically identical except propantheline is approximately five times more potent. Neither drug offers any particular advantages over atropine. Side effects and precautions are similar to those for atropine. Nicotinic cholinergic receptors can be blocked by methantheline, which if insufficient, lead to blockade of ganglionic transmission followed by orthostatic hypotension and syncope. Both agents have been used as antisialogogues.

ANALGESICS

Non-steroidal Antiinflammatory Drugs (NSAID)

The NSAIDs have antiinflammatory, analgesic and antipyretic properties. NSAIDs are referred to as peripherally acting because their analgesic and antiinflammatory effects are, to a large extent, produced through a peripheral mechanism. The most popular NSAIDs are aspirin and ibuprofen. Although varying slightly in degree of activity, all the NSAIDs share the same mechanism of action, side effects, contraindications, and enzymes involved in a biosynthetic cascade in which arachidonic acid is converted to eicosanoids, such as prostaglandins, which are involved in pain mechanisms. The prostaglandins thus sensitize nociceptors to neuropeptides such as histamine, bradykinin, substances, and serotonin, which are released in response to painful stimuli. There are two isoforms of cyclooxygenase (COX-1, COX-2), and although all currently available NSAIDs inhibit both forms, the two isoforms differ slightly in their sensitivity to NSAID inhibition. This difference is therapeutically important because COX-2 appears to be more involved in synthesis of prostaglandins at sites of inflammation, whereas COX-1 is more involved at sites where adverse effects of NSAIDs are expressed, such as the gastrointestinal tract.

All the NSAIDs cause gastric irritation, which can become severe enough to cause ulceration, occult blood loss, and occasionally iron-deficiency anemia. Gastrointestinal irritation is caused by a direct irritation effect and NSAID induced reduction of gastrointestinal prostaglandins that normally have a dual action to increase the secretion of a protective mucus from the gastric mucosa and decrease the secretion of gastric acid. Gastric irritation is prominent with aspirin but less of a problem with the propionic acids. For patients with a peptic ulcer, aspirin is contraindicated and the propionic acids should be used cautiously. Gastric irritation may be reduced by taking NSAIDs with meals. NSAIDs prolong bleeding time because inhibition of cyclo-oxygenase results in decreased formation of thromboxane A2 a compound that causes platelet aggregation.

Hypersensitivity to aspirin is not uncommon and usually manifests as rhinitis, urticaria, bronchoconstriction and laryngeal edema. The hypersensitivity can be as severe as an anaphylactoid-like reaction. The reaction occurs more commonly in patients who have other allergies, nasal polyps, and asthma, thus patients with documented cases of asthma should not be given NSAIDs.

Salicylism is a toxic reaction to long-term use of high doses of aspirin. This reaction might occur during the treatment of arthritis or as a result of drug overdose. Classic signs and symptoms of salicylism are tinnitus, confusion, dizziness, delirium, nausea, vomiting, and respiratory irregularities with accompanying disturbances in acid-base balance. Aspirin given to children who have chicken pox or influenza can cause fatal hepatotoxicity and encephalopathy.

NSAIDs cause a number of drug interactions, most of which are from displacement of drugs from protein binding sites. Drug interactions that are of particular significance occur with phenotoin, penicillin, anticoagulants, and oral hypoglycemics. Aspirin is also contraindicated in patients with diabetes because it can cause hypoglycemia. Alcohol sensitizes the gastric mucosa to the deleterious effects of aspirin, and patients should be advised accordingly.

Ibuprofen, for example, appears to have a higher "ceiling effect" than aspirin and causes fewer gastrointestinal side effects. The convenience of once-or twice-a-day dosing with longer-acting and newer NSAIDs such as naproxen, is offset by their higher cost.

Acetaminophen

Acetaminophen, an analgesic and antipyretic with little or no antiinflammatory activity, is not an NSAID. When administered at doses of 650 mg, acetaminophen and aspirin, both produce approximately the same degree of analgesia, but greater doses of acetaminophen (100 mg) have a higher "ceiling effect" than aspirin. It is a valuable alternative analgesic when NSAIDs are contraindicated, such as for patients with allergies, bleeding disorders, or a peptic ulcer. Acetaminophen overdose causes hepatotoxicity from the accumulation of a toxic metabolite. Under normal circumstances the metabolite is detoxified after reacting with glutathione, but in acetaminophen overdose, the excess metabolite depletes hepatic glutathione.

Opioids

Opioid analgesics can be classified according to their profile of activity at opiate receptors. There are four, major classes of opiate receptors: mu (μ), Kappa (k), delta (δ) and sigma (σ), all of which have subtypes. These receptors are responsible for both the therapeutic and side effects of opioids. Opioids-induced analgesia results from agonist action at one or more of these receptors at the level of the brain and spinal cord, whereas side effects result from their activation at both central and peripheral sites.

Morphine and codeine, produce analgesia and euphoria by an agonist action at μ-receptors and side effects of respiratory depression and constipation by an agonists. Opioids, which are agonists act at some receptors and antagonists at others, are called "mixed" agents or partial agonists. Pentazocine, for example causes analgesia by an agonist action at-μ-receptors and dysphoria by an agonist action at μ-receptors. The third class of opioids antagonists act at opioid receptors and are therefore primarily used to treat opioid overdose.

Opioids are effective for all types of pain but are particularly effective for pain that has a strong emotional component, such as cancer pain. Morphine is rarely used in dentistry, because it undergoes significant first-pass metabolism and is therefore usually parenterally administered. Interestingly, first pass metabolism of codeine results in the formation of small amounts of morphine. Codeine is frequently used in dentistry as an analgesic, particularly in combination with aspirin or acetaminophen. Codeine is an excellent antitussive at doses less than those used for analgesia.

Side effects of all opiate analgesics are similar. Respiratory depression is the most important side effect of upload analgesics. These are contraindicated for patients with any condition in which respiration is compromised. Opiate-induced CNS depression is additive with that caused by other CNS depressants. As the response of the CNS to depression of inhibitory mechanisms may be expressed as excitation, opioids should be used with care in patients with epilepsy. Opioid-induced nausea and vomiting, particularly in the ambulatory patient, is caused by direct stimulation of the chemoreceptive trigger zone and opioids–induced hypersensitivity of the vestibular system. Opioids cause the peripheral release of histamine and may precipitate bronchospasm in patients with asthma. Opioids cause spasm of gastrointestinal smooth muscle, which may preclude their use in patients who have preexisting conditions involving this musculature. Spasm of the intestine causes constipation an advantageous side effect for the treatment of diarrhoea; spasm of the sphincter of the bladder causes urinary retention. Opioid-induced hyperglycemia may preclude use in patients with diabetes. Individuals receiving opioids who are not in severe pain frequently experience dysphoria rather than euphoria.

Meperidine is a synthetic opioid that is frequently used alone or in combination with other drugs as a preoperative sedative. In contrast to other opioids, meperidine overdose causes signs of CNS stimulation, including tremor, hyperactive reflexes, and convulsions. Meperidine has anticholinergic activity that results in significantly less pupillary constriction than that occurring with other opioids and that is why it is a drug of choice for abuse by health professionals. Fentanyl is a synthetic meperidine derivative that is approximately 80 times more potent than morphine. It is frequently administered intravenously as a preparative sedative for induction of anesthesia.

Loperamide and diphenoxylate are meperidine derivatives that are used to treat diarrhoea. Neither drug has abuse potential, and loperamide can be purchased over the counter. Petazocine is a mixed opioid that can precipitate withdrawal in a patient who is opioid dependent. Because of its opioid receptor-antagonist properties, pentazocine was thought to be free of abuse potential, but abuse has been reported.

Tramadol has a low affinity for m-receptors and inhibits both serotonin and norepinephrine-uptake. Its therapeutic efficacy is approximately equivalent to that of combinations of codeine with either aspirin or acetaminophen. Combining tramadol (100 to 200 mg) with ibuprofen (400 mg) extends analgesic effects up to 5 to 6 hours for several types of dental pain. Tramadol has been considered to be free of abuse and is not a controlled substance, but abuse potential may be dose dependent.

Steroids

Corticosteroids act within the biochemical cascade of events leading to the formation of prostaglandins, but at one step earlier than that of the NSAIDs. Corticosteroids inhibit phospholipase A2, an enzyme involved in the formation of arachidonic acid. As a result, the formation of both prostaglandins and leukotrienes is inhibited by corticosteroids, which may account for their greater antiinflammatory effect compared with NSAIDs. Suppression of growth factors necessary for inflammation offer additional anti-inflammatory effects. Topical preparations are available for application to ulcerations in the oral cavity, but the potent corticosteroids cause pituitary-adrenal suppression; therefore administration on an alternate-day schedule is recommended. Topical application is less likely to cause pituitary-adrenal suppression unless a large inflamed area is involved and prolonged application with an occlusive dressing is used.

When administered orally, corticosteroids are usually taken in the morning to coincide with normal diurnal rhythms and with food to prevent peptic ulcers. Corticosteroids may cause restlessness, insomnia, euphoria, and changes in mood.

Table 38.1. Drug standard regimen dosing regimen

Amoxicillin	3.0 g orally 1 hr before procedure; then 1.5 gm 6 hr after initial dose.
	Patient allergic to Erythromycin ethylsuccinate amoxicillin/penicillin 800 mg or erythromycin stearate 1.0 gm orally 2 hr before procedure; then half the dose 6 hr after initial dose 6 hr after initial dose.
Clindamycin	300 mg orally 1 hr before procedure and 150 mg 6 hr after initial dose.

ANTIBIOTICS

Systemic Antibiotics

Antimicrobial agents are broadly classified into bacteriostatic or bactericidal agents. Bactericidal agents by inhibiting synthesis of the cell wall or membrane kill bacteria. Therapeutically, antibiotics are used in dentistry either to treat oral infections, most of which are caused by aerobic gram-positive cocci (*Staphylococcus aureus*) and anaerobic microorganisms (*Peptostreptococcus*) or as a prophylaxis to prevent bacterial endocarditis caused by alpha-hemolytic streptococci.

Antibiotics do not "cure" infection but instead assist the host in riding itself of the infecting organism.

Penicillin V is the drug of first choice in dentistry because it is more acid-stable than penicillin G and is therefore more efficiently absorbed orally. Peak plasma levels are reached about 1 hour after oral administration. Penicillin is widely distributed in the body and is secreted rapidly from renal tubules. Probenecid which inhibits renal tubular secretion, is sometimes used to slow penicillin's secretion rate. Penicillin causes few adverse side effects, and claims of allergic reactions to penicillin may be exaggerated. A true allergic reaction usually manifests as an irritating rash. Anaphylactoid reactions only rarely occur, but in suscepetible patients the reaction occurs within 30 seconds of an intramuscular injection. Signs and symptoms of anaphylaxis include oral paresthesia, cold hands and feet, bronchospasm and wheezing circulatory collapse, and unconsciousness.

Erythromycin is acid-sensitive and therefore has an enteric coat or is the form of an insoluble ester. Erythromycin is best given with food because it causes stomach irritation, nausea, and vomiting. Some anaerobes that cause dental infections are resistant to erythromycin, making it somewhat less effective than penicillin. Bacterial organisms rapidly develop resistance to erythromycin. Erythromycin estolate and erythromycin ethylsuccinate can cause a unique allergic reaction clinically expressed as cholestatic hepatitis. These two salts are therefore contraindicated in the presence of liver dysfunction.

Cephalosporins are structurally similar to penicillin, and cross-sensitivity occurs in <10% patients. Cephalosporins can be used in patients who have had mild reactions to penicillin, but they are contraindicated if penicillin has caused anaphylactic shock. The mechanism of action and spectrum of activity of first-generation cephalosporins are similar to those of penicillin. Second generation cephalosporins are somewhat more resistant to enzymatic degradation, and third-generation agents have become widely used because of their extended spectrum of activity and relative safety.

Clindamycin's antibacterial spectrum is similar to those of erythromycin, but it distributes well to bone and is therefore useful for osseous infections. Diarrhoea, a common side effect of clindamycin, may progress to pseudomembranous colitis a potentially fatal condition. Pseudomembranous colitis responds to treatment with vancomycin or oral metronidazole.

Tetracyclines are a poor choice as an alternative to penicillin because they are bacteriostatic rather than bactericidal. Because their absorption is erratic and incomplete, tetracylines are useful for intestinal infections. Milk and other dairy products are contraindicated with the tetracyclines because chelation with divalent metals such as calcium impede absorption. The use of tetracyclines during pregnancy and in children < 8 years of age should be avoided because of permanent staining of deciduous and permanent teeth and retardation of bone growth. Other adverse effects include gastrointestinal upset, hepatotoxicity, nephrotoxicity, and photosensitivity.

Topical antibiotics

Topical use of drugs is more apt to evoke a local tissue response and an allergic reaction than other forms of administration. The topically applied antibiotics are not rapidly absorbed when applied to the mucous membrane of the oral cavity, but small amounts are swallowed and are subject to systemic absorption. Anaphylaxis has been reported after topical application of a bacitracin/ polymyxin B combination preparation to a braded skin of the leg, and it can only be assumed that a similar effect could occur after topical application to abraded mucous membrane. Three topical antibiotics are used in dentistry: polymyxin B (absorption), bacitracin, and neomycin sulfate.

Bacitracin inhibits cell wall synthesis and is most effective against gram-positive cocci. Bacitracin is frequently combined with polymyxin, neomycin, or hydrocortisone, hypersensitivity reaction to bacitracin are infrequent. Polymyxin B is effective in treating gram-negative bacteria. The drug kills cells by distorting bacterial membrane to cause leakage of essential cellular components. Bacterial resistance develops to polymyxin B, and superinfections have occurred after its topical use. Neomycin has a broad spectrum of activity and is bactericidal. Neomycin causes little local reaction when applied topically but is the most toxic of the aminoglycoside antibiotics when systemically administered. Deafness and renal tubular necrosis have resulted from systemic use and after topical application of excessive amounts to abraded skin.

Antifungal Antibiotics

The most common drug used in dentistry to treat fungal infections of the oral cavity is nystatin. Nystatin has a dose-dependent fungistatic or fungicidal effect on several fungi, including *Candida albicans C. albicans* causes oral moniliasis and can also infect prosthetic devices. Tablets are usually held in the mouth for several minutes until they dissolve. Colonised dentures can be treated by soaking then in a solution of nystatin.

Clotrimazole (Mycelex), a fungistatic, is an effective treatment for oral, skin and vaginal infections caused by Candida albicans. A 10 mg troche is dissolved in the mouth five times a day for 14 days. Clotrimazole is not absorbed and causes minimal side effects.

Fluconazole (diflucan) and itraxonazole (Sporanox) are broad-spectrum antifungal agents that are chemically classified as triazoles. Fluconazole is rapidly absorbed into body fluids, including saliva and cerebrospinal fluid, after oral administration. Fluconazole is effective against oropharyngeal Candidiasis at doses of 50 to 100 mg/day; esophageal Candidiasis typically requires 100 to 200 mg/day: Fluconazole causes few side effects, but nausea and vomiting are common at doses of more than 200 mg/day.

Mouth Rinses Containing Local Antiinfective Agents

Mouth rinses that contain local antiinfective agents also have a variety of other ingredients, including flavorings, sweeteners, dye, preservatives, and wetting agents. Most mouth rinses tend to be acidic and many contain ethanol. Ethanol is the major local antiinfective agent in many over-the counter mouth rinsers. Preparations containing phenolic derivatives such as thymol have limited usefulness and objectionable taste. Hydrogen peroxide has no antibacterial activity but any loosen debris by the physical action of oxygen that is released by its decomposition. Cetylpyridinium, a surface-active agent, is a quarternary ammonium derivative that has slight bacteriostatic activity. Cetylpyridinium has a bitter and unpleasant after taste. Povidone-iodine, an iodophore, is a halogen-releasing compound combined with a surface active agent. It is probably the most effective antibacterial agent of any of the ingredients in over the counter preparations. The iodophores do not stain or sting as iodine solutions do, but they have an unpleasant taste. At concentrations of 7.5% to 10%, povidone–iodine is used as a surgical scrub. It is most effective against gram positive organisms, less effective against gram negative organism and fungi and ineffective against spores and viruses, Chlorhexidine digluconate at concentrations of 0.12%, has been approved for the treatment of gingivitis and suppression of the formation of plaque. Chlorhexidine binds to hard and soft tissue and salivary protein and is then slowly released, a desirable characteristics for plaque control. Undesirable effects include a reversible, altered taste perception, staining of teeth, tongue, and margins of anterior restorations that cannot be removed by brushing with toothpaste; and local irritation if applied to abraded tissue. The therapeutic use of chlorhexidine–containing mouth rinses are useful adjuncts that may facilitate healing after insertion of dentures.

Antiseptic and Disinfectants

Antiseptic drugs are applied to body surfaces to prevent infection by killing or inhibiting the growth of pathogenic bacteria. Disinfectants are substances that are intended to kill pathogenic bacteria when applied to non-living materials. Neither agent absolutely guarantees sterility. The antimicrobial action of antiseptics disinfectants is a result of protein denaturation; enzymes may thus be destroyed, or the cell membrane may be disrupted. The effectiveness of these agents depends highly on their concentration (which is immediately altered by wet instruments or dilution by saliva), time of exposure, and degree of contamination which can be decreased by preplanning.

The halogens (chlorine and iodine) are used as antiseptics and disinfectants. Common bleach (5% sodium hypochlorite) is one of the most practical disinfectants for general use. Sodium hypochlorite finds greatest use as a disinfectant for surgical instruments but is corrosive on prolonged contact. Sodium hypochlorite has been used to debride the root canal during endodontic therapy, but it cannot remain in contact with mucous membrane because it is a strong irritant and causes tissue damage. A 5% sodium hypochlorite solution is virucidal and had sporicidal activity, but it is quickly inactivated by organic material. Chloramine-T is another chlorine containing agent that is less corrosive and causes less tissue irritation than sodium hypochlorite. The iodine compounds are probably the most effective of the antiseptics, being bactericidal, virucidal, fungicidal and sporicidal with extended exposure. Their activity depends on the generation of free iodine. Iodine, unlike chlorine, is not readily inactivated by organic material. When applied to mucous membranes iodine tinctures cause erythematous necrosis, staining, and patient discomfort. Iodophores such as povidone-iodine, are organic iodine compound that provides a sustained release of free iodine on contact with organic material. Iodophores are used as antibacterial surgical scrubs and cause less tissue irritation and staining than inorganic iodine compounds.

Glutaraldehyde, the most commonly used agent from the aldehyde group finds use as a disinfectant for dental instruments, particularly rubber and plastics, that cannot withstand heat sterilization. It is bactericidal exposure of more than 12 hours may be necessary to kill spores. Glutaraldehyde is also virucidal and fungicidal. Alkalinity increases biocidal activity, and preparation are available with an activator that increases pH to 8. Glutaraldehyde although less irritating than formaldehyde, would not be used on skin or mucous membrane.

Hexachlorophene is the most important of the phenol derivatives. It is a weak antiseptic, effective only against gram-positive organisms. It has no virucidal or sporicidal activity. At one time, hexachlorophene was widely used in hospitals to routinely wash newborns. The practice was terminated after several deaths occurred, and the product was removed from all over the counter preparations.

Ethanol and isopropyl alcohol are probably the most widely used disinfectants. Their primary use are as skin antiseptics and solvents. Both are bactericidal but have little effect on spores, viruses or fungi. The alcohol, which when applied to areas of tissues damage, precipitates proteins and may form a protective layer under which bacteria can multiply.

Soaps are anionic surface-acting agents that have weak bactericidal action against gram-positive bacteria. Their most important properties are emulsification of fats and oils and physical removal of bacteria. Soaps neutralize cationic surface-active agents such as benzalkonium chloride, and the two preparations should not be combined. Benzalkonium chloride, a cationic surface-active agent has weak bactericidal activity against gram-positive organisms and is ineffective against spores, viruses and gram-negative organisms. The cationic surface active agents are commonly and inappropriately referred to as "cold sterilizing" solutions. They can be inactivated in the presence of hard water, and once prepared have a shelf-life of only about 2 weeks.

ANTIANXIETY AGENTS

Antianxiety agents are perhaps most appropriately used in clinical dentistry for those patients who become unusually apprehensive to the stress of a pending operative procedure. All benzodiazepines appear to act by facilitating the binding of the major inhibitory transmitter of the brain, γ-aminobutyric acid (GABA), to GABA receptors. Both $GABA_A$ and $GABA_B$ receptors have been identified in the CNS. CNS is mediated by the $GABA_A$ receptors. Under physiologic conditions, GABA, by a direct agonist action at $GABA_A$ receptors, cause opening of chloride channels and a subsequent influx of chloride ions into the neuron. Physically this action results in hyperpolarization (inhibition) of the neuron and decreased synaptic activity. Benzodiazepine receptors are a component of the GABA receptors complex, and subtypes are found throughout the CNS. Under the influence of benzodiazepines, GABA binding to its receptors is facilitated causing chloride channels to open much more frequently.

All benzodiazepines cause a dose-dependent depression of the CNS. As a result, any benzodiazepine leads to coma and (rarely) death. The therapeutic index of the benzodiazepine that is promoted as an antianxiety agent can in higher doses, be used as a hypnotic. Overdose with benzodiazepines leads to coma and (rarely) death. Barbiturates may be considered obsolete and, in fact, have been taken off the market in several countries. Nonetheless, three barbiturates, amobarbital and secobarbital, used as primary for the treatment of insomnia, and methohexital, used intravenously as a general anesthetic, are accepted as sedatives and hypnotics. Midazolam (versed), an intravenously administered, ultra short-acting benzodiazepine, is superior to methohexial for most short operative procedures in dentistry. In fact, intravenously administered midazolam or diazepam is adequate for most procedure that can be performed in <40 minutes administered benzodiazepines for conscious sedation.

Flumazenil (Mazicon) is a benzodiazepine antagonist available for the treatment of benzodiazepine overdose and should be available as an emergency drug if benzodiazepines, especially midazolam, are used clinically. Benzodiazepines are absorbed well after oral administration. The majority are metabolized to active and long-acting metabolites of diazepam The half-life of diazepam consists of two phases. 1) a phase of approximately 2 to 3 hours that results form rapid distribution to the brain and a subsequent rapid and 2) a second phase of approximately 20 to 60 hours caused by a combination of slow release from storage sites and subsequent metabolism to active metabolites. This second, or so called elimination phase, accounts for the well-known "hangover" on the day after the initial benzodiazepines dose. Patient should be made aware of the prolonged half-life of benzodiazepines because the potential for drug interaction lasts for many hours after the initial dose. Diazepam and its metabolites, as well as most other benzodiazepines, are conjugated with glucuronic acid and excreted, but oxazepam and lorazepam are simply conjugated and excreted. Oxazepam and lorazepam are therefore more suitable for geriatric patients or others who may have compromised liver function.

Adverse effects of benzodiazepines are minimal. In therapeutic doses, they have little effect on cardiovascular function and respiration. Because they are CNS depressants, they can cause drowsiness and impaired function, and patients should be cautioned. The safety of benzodiazepines when used alone, is remarkable. However, in combination with some CNS depressant drugs, can be lethal. Alcohol causes potentiation of the CNS depressant effect of benzodiazepines rather than an additive effect. Because of the pharmacokinetics of benzodiazepines, this drug interaction may occur long after the initial benzodiazepines dose, and patients should be advised accordingly regarding alcohol intake. Although benzodiazepines abuse is a major concern, the acute and short duration of their use in dentistry minimize the problem of abuse.

Hydroxyzine, an antihistamine, is the only antianxiety agent approved by the Council of Dental Therapeutics. Most antihistamines cause sedation, and this effect likely accounts for a non-selective antianxiety effect. Hydroxyzine finds use in pediatric dentistry and as an alternative for the extremely rare individual who is allergic to the benzodiazepines. Hydroxyzine has anticholinergic properties that may be advantageous in maintaining a dry operative field. Promethazine, an antihistaminic phenothiazine, is commonly added to preanesthetic "cocktails" primarily for its sedative and anticholinergic effects. Antianxiety agents such as buspirone (Buspar), although therapeutically effective for the treatment of anxiety disorders, are of little value in dentistry because it takes 2 to 3 weeks before therapeutic effects are observed.

CENTRALLY ACTING MUSCLE RELAXANTS

Muscle relaxants may act at the level of the CNS or the peripheral nervous system (PNS). Only one peripherally acting agent, dantrolene sodium, has been accepted by the Council on Dental Therapeutics. It acts by interacting with the release of calcium from the sarcoplasmic reticulum, which prevents excitation coupling. Dantrolene is used to treat spasticity characteristic of multiple sclerosis, cerebral palsy and malignant hyperthermia. It has little effect on non-spastic muscle. Dantrolene and the centrally acting agents find limited use in dentistry.

Diazepam is by far the safest and most useful of the centrally acting agents. The dose, duration of action, and pharmacologic characteristics of diazepam are the same whether it is used as a skeletal muscle relaxant or as an antianxiety agent. Diazepam relieves spastic skeletal muscle but has relatively little effect on normal muscle tone. The centrally acting muscle relaxants are sometimes used in treating temporomandibular disorder, but their efficacy is not consistent, predictable, or well established. Centrally acting muscle relaxants can be abused, and dependence occurs. Carisoprodol (Soma) has a high potential abuse rate, and suspicion should be aroused if a patient requests both carisoprodol and an opiate for pain relief. Because of their abuse potential, prolonged administration of centrally acting skeletal muscle relaxants should be tapered off rather than abruptly stopped because withdrawal, not unlike that seen with alcohol and barbiturates, occurs in the patient who is dependent. Baclofen ralgia, especially in combination with carbamazepine.

KEY TO MCQs

Chapter 17

1. (b)	2. (c)	3. (b)	4. (a)
5. (d	6. (b)	7. (d)	8. (a)
9. (d)	10. (b)	11. (c)	

Chapter 18

1. (d)	2. (d)	3. (b)	4. (b)
5. (c)	6. (a)	7. (d)	8. (c)
9. (b)	10. (b)	11. (d)	

Chapter 19

1. (a)	2. (e)	3. (b)	4. (d)
5. (b)	6. (b)	7. (a)	8. (b)

Chapter 20

1. (c)	2. (b)	3. (b)	4. (d)
5. (a)			

Chapter 21

1. (c)

Chapter 22

1. (a)

Chapter 23

1. (a)	2. (c)	3. (d)	4. (c)

Chapter 24

1. (b)	2. (a)	3. (d)

Chapter 25

1. (c)	2. (c)	3. (c)	4. (c)
5. (c)	6. (d)	7. (d)	8. (d)

Chapter 26

1. (d)	2. (d)	3. (d)	4. (b)

Chapter 27

1. (d)	2. (c)

Chapter 28

1. (d)

Chapter 29

1. (d)	2. (d)	3. (d)	4. (d)

Chapter 30

1. (b)	2. (b)	3. (c)

Chapter 31

1. (b)	2. (a)	3. (b)	4. (b)
5. (d)	6. (a)	7. (d)	8. (a)

Chapter 32

1. (c)	2. (b)	3. (b)	4. (c)
5. (b)	6. (c)	7. (d)	8. (d)
9. (d)			

Chapter 34

1. (a)	2. (b)

Chapter 37

1. (b)	2. (d)

INDEX